J. E. Oliver, Jr., D.V.M., M.S., Ph.D.

Professor and Head
Department of Small Animal Medicine
and Professor
Department of Physiology and Pharmacology
College of Veterinary Medicine
University of Georgia
Athens, Georgia

Diplomate, American College of
Veterinary Internal Medicine,
Neurology

B. F. Hoerlein, D.V.M., Ph.D.

Professor and Director Emeritus
Scott-Ritchey Research Program
School of Veterinary Medicine
Auburn University
Auburn, Alabama

Charter Diplomate, American College of
Veterinary Surgery and American College of
Veterinary Internal Medicine, Neurology

I. G. Mayhew, B.V.Sc., Ph.D.

Professor
Departments of Medical Sciences and
Comparative and Experimental Pathology
College of Veterinary Medicine
University of Florida
Gainesville, Florida

Diplomate, American College of
Veterinary Internal Medicine,
Neurology

Veterinary Neurology

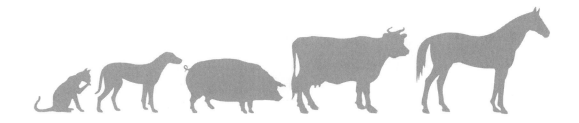

1987
W. B. Saunders Company
PHILADELPHIA / LONDON / TORONTO / MEXICO CITY
RIO DE JANEIRO / SYDNEY / TOKYO / HONG KONG

W. B. Saunders Company: West Washington Square
Philadelphia, PA 19105

Library of Congress Cataloging-in-Publication Data

Veterinary neurology.

1. Veterinary neurology.   II. Oliver, John E. (John Eoff),
   1933–   II. Hoerlein, B. F.   III. Mayhew, Ian G.

SF895.V48 1987   636.089′68   86–15436

ISBN 0–7216–1314–4

Editor: Darlene Pedersen
Designer: Karen O'Keefe
Production Manager: Bill Preston
Manuscript Editor: Terry Russell
Illustration Coordinator: Lisa Lambert
Page Layout Artist: Meg Jolly
Indexer: Elizabeth Gittens

Veterinary Neurology   ISBN 0–7216–1314–4

Last digit is the print number: 9   8   7   6   5   4   3   2   1

*To our wives, for their love, support, and
understanding.*

Contributors

D. L. BARBER, D.V.M., M.S.,
DIPLOMATE, A.C.V.R.
Professor of Veterinary Radiology, Virginia-Maryland Regional College of Veterinary Medicine, Virginia Tech, Blacksburg, Virginia; Coordinator, Radiology, Veterinary Medical Teaching Hospital, Blacksburg, Virginia
Neuroradiography

J. M. BOWEN, D.V.M., Ph.D.
Associate Dean for Research and Graduate Affairs, College of Veterinary Medicine, University of Georgia, Athens, Georgia
Electrophysiologic Diagnosis

K. G. BRAUND, D.V.M., M.S.,
Ph.D., F.R.C.V.S., DIPLOMATE,
A.C.V.I.M.
Professor of Neurology, Department of Small Animal Surgery and Medicine, Auburn University College of Veterinary Medicine, Auburn, Alabama; Director, Neuromuscular Research Unit, Scott-Ritchey Research Program, Auburn University College of Veterinary Medicine, Auburn, Alabama
Degenerative and Developmental Diseases; Inflammatory, Infectious, Immune, Parasitic, and Vascular Diseases; Neoplasia; Diseases of Peripheral Nerves, Cranial Nerves and Muscle.

B. D. BREWER, D.V.M., M.S.,
DIPLOMATE, A.C.V.I.M.
Assistant Professor of Large Animal Medicine and Neurology, Department

of Medical Sciences, University of Florida, Gainesville, Florida
Inflammatory, Infectious, Immune, Parasitic, and Vascular Diseases

D. B. COULTER, D.V.M., Ph.D.
Professor, Department of Physiology and Pharmacology, College of Veterinary Medicine, University of Georgia, Athens, Georgia
Electrophysiologic Diagnosis

J. R. DUNCAN, D.V.M., Ph.D.,
DIPLOMATE, A.C.V.P.
Professor and Head, Department of Pathology, College of Veterinary Medicine, University of Georgia, Athens, Georgia
Laboratory Examinations

C. E. GREENE, D.V.M., M.S.,
DIPLOMATE, A.C.V.I.M.
Professor, Department of Small Animal Medicine, College of Veterinary Medicine, University of Georgia, Athens, Georgia
Principles of Medical Therapy

I. R. GRIFFITHS, B.V.M.S., Ph.D.,
F.R.C.V.S.
Reader in Veterinary Surgery, University of Glasgow, Glasgow, Scotland
Central Nervous System Trauma

B. F. HOERLEIN, D.V.M., Ph.D.,
CHARTER DIPLOMATE, A.C.V.S.,
A.C.V.I.M.
Professor and Director Emeritus, Scott-Ritchey Research Program, School of

Veterinary Medicine, Auburn University, Auburn, Alabama
Intervertebral Disk Disease; Cranial Surgery

C. D. KNECHT, V.M.D., M.S., DIPLOMATE, A.C.V.S., A.C.V.I.M.
Professor and Head, Department of Small Animal Surgery and Medicine, College of Veterinary Medicine, Auburn University, Auburn, Alabama
Principles of Neurosurgery

J. N. KORNEGAY, D.V.M., Ph.D., DIPLOMATE, A.C.V.I.M.
Professor of Neurology, North Carolina State University School of Veterinary Medicine, Raleigh, North Carolina; Veterinary Medical Teaching Hospital, North Carolina State University, Raleigh, North Carolina
Metabolic, Toxic, and Nutritional Diseases

I. G. MAYHEW, B.V.Sc., Ph.D., DIPLOMATE, A.C.V.I.M.
Professor, Departments of Medical Sciences and Comparative and Experimental Pathology, College of Veterinary Medicine, University of Florida, Gainesville, Florida
Neurologic Examination and the Diagnostic Plan; Laboratory Examination; Neuroradiography; Inflammatory, Infectious, Immune, Parasitic, and Vascular Diseases; Metabolic, Toxic, and Nutritional Diseases

L. J. MYERS, II, D.V.M., Ph.D
Assistant Professor, College of Veterinary Medicine, Auburn University, Auburn, Alabama
Electrophysiologic Diagnosis

J. E. OLIVER, JR., D.V.M., M.S., Ph.D., DIPLOMATE, A.C.V.I.M.
Professor and Head, Department of Small Animal Medicine, and Professor, Department of Physiology and Pharmacology, College of Veterinary Medicine, University of Georgia, Athens, Georgia
Neurologic Examination and the Diagnostic Plan; Laboratory Examination; Neuroradiography; Electrophysiologic Diagnosis; Seizure Disorders and Narcolepsy; Disorders of Micturition; Cranial Surgery

R. W. REDDING, D.V.M., M.Sc., Ph.D., DIPLOMATE, A.C.V.I.M.
Professor Emeritus, Scott-Ritchey Research Program, School of Veterinary Medicine, Auburn University, Auburn, Alabama; Small Animal Clinic, Auburn University, Auburn, Alabama
Electrophysiologic Diagnosis

D. SORJONEN, D.V.M., M.S., DIPLOMATE, A.C.V.I.M.
Associate Professor, College of Veterinary Medicine, Auburn University, Auburn, Alabama
Vertebral and Spinal Cord Surgery

S. F. SWAIM, D.V.M., M.S., DIPLOMATE, A.C.V.S.
Professor, Small Animal Surgery, and Director, Scott-Ritchey Laboratories, College of Veterinary Medicine, Auburn University, Auburn, Alabama
Vertebral and Spinal Cord Surgery; Peripheral Nerve Surgery

P. C. WAGNER, D.V.M., M.S., DIPLOMATE, A.C.V.S.
Associate Professor, Department of Large Animal Surgery, College of Veterinary Medicine, Oregon State University, Corvallis, Oregon
Vertebral and Spinal Cord Surgery

Preface

Clinical veterinary neurology is built on the foundation of Hoerlein's Canine Neurology. Our goal was to develop a comprehensive reference and textbook of neurology, including medicine and surgery of all domestic animals. To maintain a book of reasonable size with that goal required reducing duplication, being selective in the coverage of some topics, and eliminating some material included in *Canine Neurology*, such as some information on anatomy and physiology. The organization of the book has been changed to include sections on Diagnosis, Diseases of the Nervous System (following an etiologic classification), and Medical and Surgical Therapy. A major change is the addition of material on all species of domestic animals.

We hope this book serves as a useful reference and text for students, practicing veterinarians, and specialists.

Acknowledgment

It is not customary to recognize one of the authors of a book, but two of us (JEO and IGM) felt it necessary. Frank Hoerlein provided veterinary medicine with the first comprehensive textbook on canine clinical neurology, including neurosurgery. His work raised the standard of clinical neurology throughout the world. This book would not have been possible without the effort that made *Canine Neurology* a standard for three editions. Although it has been completely revised, much of *Canine Neurology* is still here.

To Frank Hoerlein, we say thank you.

Contents

Chapter 1   *BF Hoerlein, DVM, PhD*

Introduction

The nervous system has for centuries been one of the most perplexing systems of the body to understand, and nervous disorders have always been regarded as mysterious and difficult to diagnose. However, throughout history scientists have observed various portions of the nervous system, and these milestones form an appropriate introduction to the various clinical subjects presented in this text.

EARLY HISTORY

The first neurologic record was made by the ancient Egyptians about 3000 years BC when they used the term "brain." Hippocrates, Plato, Aristotle, and others in the fifth and fourth centuries BC wrote accounts of neurologic disorders, such as epilepsy, spinal injuries, and head injuries, as well as descriptions of the brain, its cerebral and cerebellar hemispheres, and its ventricles and membranes.[17]

Despite these observations, the physiologic function of the nervous system was not recognized. The brain was believed to be only a gland that secreted "phlegm" into the pituitary gland and nose. The *heart* was the central organ, and the blood vessels, not the nerves, were the channels by which motion and sensation were transmitted. This belief was even shared to some degree by William Harvey some 2000 years later.[17]

The true role of the nervous system was first suspected by Galen of Rome (130–210 AD). He sectioned the spinal cord of newborn pigs and noted the loss of movement and feeling in the limbs. The brain was believed to be the seat of intelligence and imagination, the principal organ for sensory perception. It was also the source of one of the vital spirits that flowed down the nerves' invisible channels transmitting motion and sensation.[17]

Although the anatomists of the Renaissance—Vesalius, Falloppio, Willis, Sylvius, and Morgagni—laid the foundations for our knowledge of the structure of the nervous system, it was not until the nineteenth century that the mode of transmission of nervous impulses was discovered.[17]

Through the experimental stimulation of exposed tissue of animals and humans by mechanical, thermal, and chemical means, the concepts of sensitivity, irritability, and contractility emerged. Nevertheless, the wasting of tissues distal to nerve disruption could still be explained by the loss of nourishing nerve juices, which were thought to flow from the brain, although microscopic studies (1674) failed to reveal nerve channels through which they were said to pass.[17]

Physical explanations of anatomy were more persuasive than concepts of the body's humors, and the body was viewed as a machine. Nerve threads connecting the brain to the periphery of the body were supposed to be the bases of movement and sensation. However, the discovery of electricity provided a new solution to the mystery of nerve conduction. Galvani (1737–1798) applied this discovery to neurophysiology by using the humble nerve-muscle preparation of the frog to demonstrate that nerve conduction was electric in nature. Just a century ago it was shown that the nerve impulse results from a self-propagating depolarization of nerve membrane.[17]

The synapse was unknown until Sherrington's work in 1897. The peculiar histology of motor end plates and the delays in conduction that occurred there raised the possibility of some form of nonelectric transmission. The roles of adrenalin and acetylcholine in the sympathetic and parasympathetic synapses were discovered by the physiologists Elliott, Loewi, and Dale. The ancient neurohumoral theory thus eventually proved to contain some small truth.[17]

The sequential knowledge of the physiologic

1

functions of the spinal cord was made possible by such investigators as Flechsig and Gowers, Schwann and Purkinje, Marchi, Golgi, Ramón y Cajal, Waller, Brown Séquard, Magendie, and Bell. Magendie and Bell showed that the spinal roots possessed different functions—the anterior root was a motor nerve, and the posterior root was sensory. The neurohistologists Golgi, Marchi, Weigert, and Ramón y Cajal, using silver and gold impregnations, aniline dyes, and osmic acid techniques, portrayed the extraordinary complexity of nervous tissue. The development throughout the last century of knowledge of spinal tracts, sensory and motor conduction, and reflex activity of the spinal cord by scientists such as Babinski and Sherrington laid the groundwork for modern neurophysiology and neurologic diagnosis.[17]

Although cranial trephination was performed by the ancients, the birth of modern neurosurgery began with Sir William Macewen in 1879. This surgery was based on anatomic, physiologic, and clinical observation because the techniques of radiology and lumbar spinal fluid puncture were unknown before 1891 and 1895, respectively. The ancients studied and named many of the now well-known parts of the brain, such as the vein of Galen and the dura and pia mater (the "hard" and "devoted" protecting "mother" membranes). Later, the ventricles were thought to be concerned in the processes of neurologic respiration and excretion, which were essential to Galen's doctrine of the three spirits. The casts and drawings of the ventricles by Leonardo da Vinci (about 1500) were centuries ahead of practical usefulness to medicine. Sylvius, Monro, Magendie, Luschka, and Willis are remembered in the names of the ventricles.[17]

As development of the concepts of the 12 cranial nerves progressed, William Harvey in the seventeenth century was asking whether the substance of the brain or the ventricle had the chief role in mental functions. By 1840, the cells in various parts of the nervous system had been recognized and described. Myelinated and unmyelinated fibers had been demonstrated. By the end of the nineteenth century, Virchow, Waldeyer, Forel, and Ramón y Cajal had prepared splendid atlases of the gross and microscopic anatomy of the brain, showing that the nervous system was not a simple network of tissue but a highly complex system.[17]

Persons prominent in the development of modern human neurology (and their studies) include Charcot (cerebral localization and spinal joint disease), Erb and Westphal (peripheral nerve and tendon reflexes), Friedreich (hereditary ataxia), Head (dermatome), Huntington (chorea), Jackson (seizures), Landry (sensory nerve function), Oppenheim (tabes, syphilis, polio), Parkinson (palsy), Sicard (contrast radiography), Spiller (neurovascular occlusion), and Wernicke (encepalopathy).[6]

The title of father of modern neurosurgery is usually given to Harvey Cushing. A few other prominent neurosurgeons include Dandy (ventriculography), Elsberg (vertebral surgery), and Horsley (decompressive procedures for inoperable brain tumors). Many other neurologists and surgeons have made momentous contributions to the modern clinical practice, but space does not allow extensive review. Historians will find Haymaker and Schiller's text *The Founders of Neurology* most fascinating.[6]

HISTORY OF VETERINARY NEUROLOGY

Veterinary neurology is a younger profession. Notable progress in neuropathology was made in Europe in the latter 1800s and early 1900s. Such names as Dexler, Scherer, Frauchiger, Hofmann, Fankhauser, Lugenbuhl, Aruch, Joest, and Cohr are among those of the early contributors to the knowledge of neuropathologic lesions. Many of these persons correlated the clinical signs with the lesions, thus furthering the cause of clinical neurology. Unfortunately, most of these works were printed only in German.[5] However, American veterinarians translated some of these works into English, notably the translation in 1920 by Mohler and Eichhorn of Hutyra and Marek's *Special Pathology and Therapeutics of the Disease of Domestic Animals*[8]; discussions of diseases of the nervous system were excellent, comprehensive, well illustrated, and remarkably accurate.[8]

Some of the later works that proved to be helpful to English-speaking clinicians are Schnelle's text *Radiology in Canine Practice*[16] and McGrath's *Neurological Examination of the Dog*.[11] The latter work gave the practicing veterinarian a firm system of neurologic examination and a correlation of clinical signs with pathologic lesions. Innes and Saunder's *Comparative Neuropathology*[9] is a comprehensive treatise valuable to pathologists and clinicians alike. One must not overlook the early work of Dukes[4] in neurophysiology (1933) as a basis for clinical understanding.

From the 1960s to the present time, there have been innumerable contributions to veterinary neurology, some of which have been published in monograms and texts. These include Palmer,[13] Hoerlein,[7] Pettit,[13] deLahunta,[3] Chrisman,[1] and Oliver and Lorenz[12] in clinical neurology, and Klemm,[10] and Redding and Knecht[15] in electroencephalography. Many veterinarians have contributed or are currently contributing a tremendous volume of knowledge to the science and art of clinical neurology. The author has of necessity limited this historic discussion and is not able to acknowledge all who have been productive in this area.

INCIDENCE OF NEUROLOGIC DISEASE

According to the Veterinary Medical Data Retrieval Program (VMDP)* (through 1981) the incidence of nervous disease in common domestic animals is 2.1% (4364 cases out of 204,492). The largest recorded species in this retrieval is the dog at a total population of 122,897, with 3138 neurologic cases seen, for an incidence at 2.6%. The cat, with a population of 37,292, had only a 1.1% incidence of neurologic disease (Table 1–1). Infectious (18.9%) and traumatic (27.8%) disorders were much more frequently noted than genetic (5.1%) and neoplastic (6.7%) neurologic diseases (Table 1–2). The cat at 38.8%, the dog at 29.2%, and the horse at 24% had surprisingly high incidences of traumatic neurologic disease.

The incidence of small animal neurologic diseases for 1 year (1982–1983) at the Auburn University (AU) Small Animal Teaching Hospital paralleled the VMDP data (Table 1–3). Per-

*American Association of Veterinary Medical Data Program Participants, Inc. New York College of Veterinary Medicine, Cornell University, Ithaca, NY.

centages of trauma cases in the dog were 32.6% at AU and 29.2% in VMDP; infectious cases at AU, 12.9% and VMDP, 16.2% (Tables 1–2 and 1–3).

Considering the multitude of pathological diagnoses possible in domestic animals seen at university teaching hospitals, those attributable to nervous system constitute a considerable number. Thus neurology represents an important discipline in veterinary clinical practice.

EXPANDING AREAS OF CLINICAL VETERINARY NEUROLOGY

A short discussion of the expanding areas of knowledge in clinical veterinary neurology is appropriate for this introduction to the balance of the text. The neurologic examination in recent years has been aided substantially by newer techniques and special diagnostic aids.

The ocular fundic changes in infectious, metabolic, and toxic diseases are better documented. Neuroelectric diagnostic testing in institutional and group practices now includes electroencephalography, electromyography, cortical and spinal evoked potential testing, electroretinography, electroencephalographic audiometry, brain stem auditory evoked response, cystometrograms, and nerve conduction velocity studies. The laboratory testing of cerebrospinal fluid for exfoliative cytology and chemical composition and electrophoretic studies of immune responses are becoming much more common.

The use of routine radiography is being enhanced by special radioactive imaging or scanning techniques, tomography, normal and contrast computerized axial tomography (CAT scan), and nuclear magnetic resonance imaging (NMR). Although some of the equipment re-

Table 1–1. TOPOGRAPHIC INCIDENCE OF NEUROLOGIC DISEASE IN DOMESTIC ANIMALS

	Population	Nervous Diseases		CNS Disorders		Peripheral Nerve Disorders	
		Number	Percentage	Number	Percentage	Number	Percentage
Bovine	12,769	317	2.5	266	2.1	51	0.4
Equine	26,949	325	1.3	281	1.1	44	0.2
Porcine	1111	33	2.9	30	2.7	3	0.2
Ovine	1105	50	4.5	49	4.4	1	0.1
Caprine	1055	38	3.6	37	3.5	1	0.1
Other large animal	102	10	9.8	10	9.8	0	0
Canine	122,897	3138	2.6	2584	2.1	554	0.5
Feline	37,292	418	1.1	336	0.9	82	0.2
Other small animal	2212	35	1.6	34	1.5	1	0.1
TOTAL	204,492	4,364	2.1	3,627	1.8	737	0.3

Data furnished by the American Association of Veterinary Medical Data Program Participants, Inc. New York College of Veterinary Medicine, Cornell University, Ithaca, NY. Veterinary Medical Data Retrieval Program (VMDP), 1981.

Table 1–2. ETIOLOGIC INCIDENCE IN NEUROLOGIC DISEASE IN DOMESTIC ANIMALS

	Population	Infectious		Traumatic		Genetic		Neoplastic	
		Number	Percentage	Number	Percentage	Number	Percentage	Number	Percentage
Bovine	317	132	41.6	36	11.4	13	4.1	7	2.2
Equine	325	60	18.5	71	24.0	19	5.8	20	6.1
Porcine	33	13	39.4	4	12.1	6	18.2	—	—
Ovine	50	15	30.0	5	10.0	3	6.0	—	—
Caprine	38	19	50.0	7	18.4	1	2.6	1	2.6
Other large animal	10	5	5.0	4	40.0	1	10.0	—	—
Canine	3138	509	16.2	918	29.2	156	4.9	230	7.3
Feline	418	56	13.4	162	38.8	23	5.5	32	7.6
Other small animal	35	14	40.0	8	22.8	1	2.8	1	2.9
TOTAL	4364	823	18.9	1215	27.8	223	5.1	291	6.7

Data furnished by the American Association of Veterinary Medical Data Program Participants, Inc. New York College of Veterinary Medicine, Cornell University, Ithaca, NY. Veterinary Medical Data Retrieval Program (VMDP), 1981.

Table 1–3. INCIDENCE OF NEUROLOGIC DISEASES IN SMALL ANIMALS

	Popu-lation	Nervous System		Central Nervous System		Peripheral Nervous System		Infectious		Traumatic		Genetic		Neoplastic	
		Number	Percentage	Number	Percentage	Number	Percentage	Number	Percentage	Number	Percentage	Number	Percentage	Number	Percentage
Canine	7325	193	2.6	154	2.1	39	0.5	25	12.9	63	32.6	4	2.0	13	6.7
Feline	1450	25	1.7	24	1.6	1	0.1	2	8.0	7	28.0	—	—	1	4.0
Other small animal	207	11	5.3	11	5.3	—	—	1	9.0	10	90.9	—	—	—	—
TOTAL	8982	229	2.5	189	2.1	40	0.4	28	12.2	80	34.9	4	1.7	14	6.1

Retrieval of data from Small Animal Surgery and Medicine, Auburn University, 1982–1983, and Auburn University Computer Services.

quired is costly and requires expensive maintenance, a few teaching institutions have access to this equipment. In larger cities, veterinarians could explore the possibility of using medical center facilities for their patients. The results of such examinations have proven helpful in localizing brain lesions for more successful surgical relief.

The use of thermography and echography will no doubt become routine in many veterinary clinics. The use of the laser beam and microsurgical equipment certainly offer bright prospects for future methodology. All of these techniques involve expensive equipment, but practicing veterinarians must promote the value of comparative medicine to their counterparts in human medicine. They must take advantage of the possible use of human medical center facilities for their patients for comparative clinical investigations. Many of these techniques are available at veterinary referral institutions as well.

In a recent listing, 35 of 281 animal models for human disease[1] are of primary neurologic importance. More of the future veterinary medical research support will come from the study of these animal models of human disorders. Diseases such as globoid cell leukodystrophy, neuronal glycoproteinoses (Lafora's disease), neuronal gangliosidosis (Tay-Sachs disease), ceroid lipofuscinosis, demyelinating diseases, spinal dysraphism, and idiopathic polyradiculoneuritis (Landry-Guillain-Barré syndrome) are examples. Veterinarians can make a tremendous contribution to comparative medicine by studying these models.[1]

Great advances have been made in studying the pathogenesis of central nervous system trauma. The role of neurotransmitters and the action of endorphin in acute spinal trauma have been clarified. More effective medical and surgical therapy has evolved. Even more exciting are the advances in nerve transplantation and grafting, and central nervous system neuronal regeneration as a result of advanced microsurgical techniques. The methods to inhibit re-

jection of transplanted tissues and organs are improving at an unbelievable speed. The emerging science of genetic engineering will involve future advances in neurology, as well as other disciplines. Replacement of enzyme systems offers the hope for treatment of inherited diseases such as the storage diseases.

REFERENCES

1. Capen CC, Hackel DB, Jones TC, and Migaki G: A twelfth fascicle for handbook: Animal Modes for Human Disease. Washington, DC, Registry of Comparative Pathology, Armed Forces Institute of Pathology, 1983.
2. Chrisman CL: Problems in Small Animal Neurology. Philadelphia, Lea & Febiger, 1982.
3. deLahunta A: Veterinary Neuroanatomy and Clinical Neurology. Philadelphia, WB Saunders Co, 1977, 1983.
4. Dukes HH: The Physiology of Domestic Animals. Ithaca, NY, Comstock Publishers, 1933.
5. Fankhauser R and Luginbuhl H: Pathologische Anatomie Des Zentralen Und Peripehren Nervensystems Der Haustiere. Berlin, Verlag Paul Parey, 1968.
6. Haymaker W, and Schiller F: The Founders of Neurology, 2nd ed. Springfield, IL, Charles C Thomas, 1970.
7. Hoerlein BF: Canine Neurology. Philadelphia, WB Saunders Co, 1965, 1971, 1978.
8. Hutyra F, and Marek J: Special Pathology and Therapeutics of the Diseases of Domestic Animals, 2nd English translation of 4th German Edition by Mohler, JR and Eichorn A. Chicago, Alexander Eger, 1920.
9. Innes JRM and Saunders LZ: Comparative Neurology. New York, Academic Press, 1962.
10. Klemm WR: Animal Electroencephalography. New York, Academic Press, 1969.
11. McGrath JT: Neurologic Examination of the Dog. Philadelphia, Lea & Febiger, 1956, 1960.
12. Oliver JE Jr and Lorenz MD: Handbook of Veterinary Neurological Diagnosis. Philadelphia, WB Saunders Co, 1983.
13. Palmer AC: Introduction to Animal Neurology. Philadelphia, FA Davis Co, 1965, 1976.
14. Pettit GD: Intervertebral Disc Protrusion in the Dog. New York, Appleton-Century-Crofts, 1966.
15. Redding RW and Knecht CD: Atlas of Electroencephalography in the Dog and Cat. New York, Praeger Scientific Publishers, 1984.
16. Schnelle CB: Radiology in Canine Practice. Evanston, IL, The North American Veterinarian, Inc. 1950.
17. Spillane JD: An Atlas of Clinical Neurology, 2nd ed. New York, Oxford University Press, 1975.

I Diagnosis

Chapter 2

JE Oliver, DVM, MS, PhD
IG Mayhew, BVSc, PhD

Neurologic Examination and the Diagnostic Plan

The objectives of this chapter are to outline a systematic approach to neurologic diagnosis, describe each step in sufficient detail so that it can be performed by the veterinarian, and explain how to integrate the results into a diagnostic plan. To make a diagnosis (Table 2–1) it is necessary to determine whether a lesion is present in the nervous system, and, if so, to ascertain its location. Results of the physical and neurologic examinations enable localization of the lesion. The cause of the problem must then be identified. Signalment and history provide most of the information needed to determine the type of disease process. The extent of damage to the nervous system, based on the neurologic examination, and the cause of the problem indicate the prognosis and need for treatment.[17]

FUNCTIONAL ORGANIZATION OF THE NERVOUS SYSTEM

Appreciating some fundamentals of structure and function of the nervous system is necessary for lesion localization. The more understanding of neuroanatomy and neurophysiology the ex-

aminer has, the more precise and accurate the diagnosis can be. However, a minimal level of knowledge is adequate for solving most clinical problems. These fundamentals are reviewed here.[15] More details are included in the description of each test in the neurologic examination. For comprehensive coverage one of the references should be consulted.[4, 7]

Lower Motor Neuron and Segmental Signs

The lower motor neuron (LMN) is an efferent neuron connecting the central nervous system (CNS) to an effector muscle or gland. Any

Table 2–1. OUTLINE OF NEUROLOGICAL DIAGNOSIS

Collect minimum data base
Identify problems
Identify one or more problems related to nervous system
Localize level of lesion
Estimate extent of lesion within that level
Determine cause or pathology
Determine prognosis with and without therapy

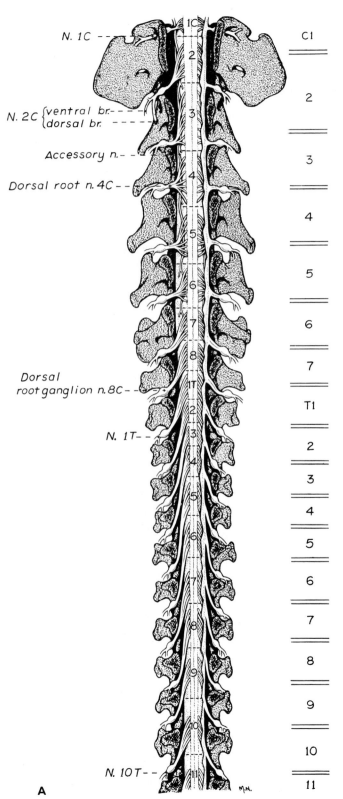

N. 1C

N. 2C { ventral br.
       { dorsal br.

Accessory n.

Dorsal root n. 4C

Dorsal
root ganglion n. 8C

N. 1T

N. 10T

A

C1

2

3

4

5

6

7

T1

2

3

4

5

6

7

8

9

10

11

Figure 2–1. A, Dorsal roots of spinal nerves and spinal cord segments, cervical 1 to thoracic 11, dorsal aspect. The dura mater has been removed except on the extreme right side. The figures on the right represent levels of the vertebral bodies.

Illustration continued on opposite page

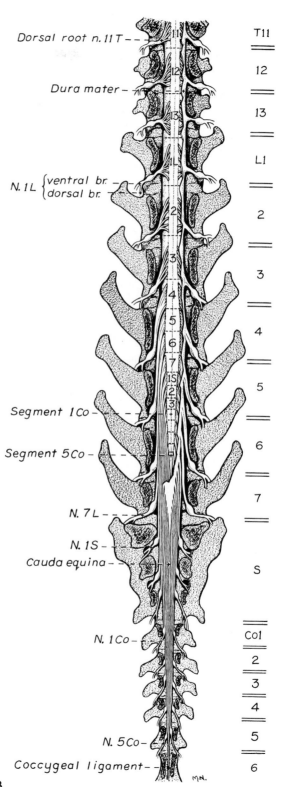

Figure 2–1. *Continued* B, Dorsal roots of the spinal nerves and spinal cord segments, thoracic 11 to caudal 5, dorsal aspect. The dura mater has been removed except on the extreme right side. The figures on the right represent levels of the vertebral bodies. (From Fletcher TF and Kitchell RA: Anatomical studies on the spinal cord segments of the dog. Am J Vet Res 27:1759, 1966.)

activity of the nervous system must ultimately be expressed through an LMN to be recognized as a movement or secretion. The cell bodies of the LMN are located in all spinal segments in the intermediate and ventral horns of the gray matter and in the nuclei of the cranial nerves (III, IV, V, VI, VII, IX, X, XI, and XII) in the brain stem. The axons extending from these cells join the peripheral spinal and cranial nerves.

Sensory neurons are located in the ganglia of the dorsal roots along the spinal cord and in the ganglia of some of the cranial nerves, with the exception of the special sensory pathways (olfaction, vision, hearing, balance).

The nervous system is arranged in a segmental fashion. A spinal cord segment is demarcated by a pair of spinal nerves, each spinal nerve having a dorsal (sensory) and a ventral (motor) root (Fig. 2–1). The brain has less uniform segmentation, but anatomically and functionally distinct segments can be identified (Fig. 2–2). The muscle or group of muscles innervated by one spinal nerve is called a myotome. Myotomes are arranged segmentally in the paravertebral muscles but are more irregular in the

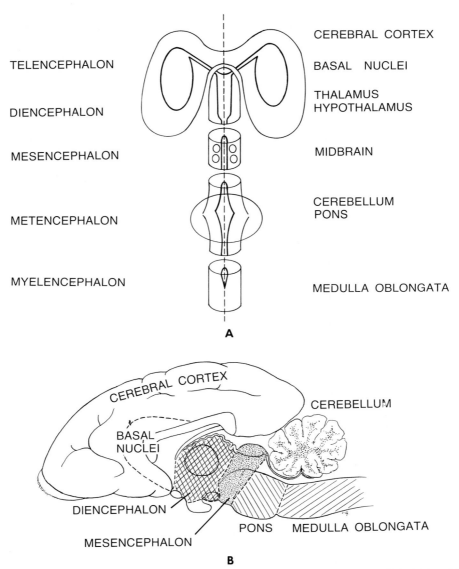

Figure 2–2. Subdivisions of the brain. (*A* modified from Elliott HC: Textbook of Neuroanatomy. Philadelphia, J. B. Lippincott Co, 1963.)

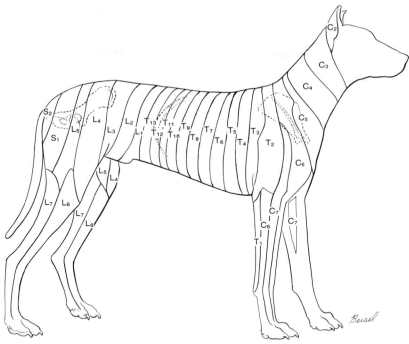

Figure 2–3. Dermatomes of the dog. This illustration represents results of several studies. Dermatomes vary among individuals, and overlapping innervation of approximately three segments is present in most areas. The distribution to the thoracic limb is tentative.

limbs. Comparison of clinically affected groups of muscles with tables of distribution of spinal nerves can be used to localize a lesion of a spinal nerve, ventral root, or cord segment.

The area of skin innervated by one spinal nerve is called a dermatome. Dermatomes are also arranged in a regular, segmental fashion, except on the limbs, where there is some variation (Fig. 2–3). Alterations in sensation of a dermatome can be used to localize a lesion of a spinal nerve, dorsal root, or cord segment.

Lesions of the LMN, whether of the cell body or the axon, produce a characteristic group of clinical signs. LMN signs include (1) paralysis of the muscles innervated, (2) areflexia, (3) early and severe muscle atrophy (neurogenic), (4) flaccidity of muscle, loss of tone, and loss of resistance to passive manipulation, (5) electromyographic (EMG) changes after 5 to 7 days (fibrillation potentials and positive sharp waves [see Chapter 5]), and (6) contracture and fibrosis of the muscles after several weeks (Table 2–2).

Table 2–2. SUMMARY OF LMN AND UMN SIGNS

	Lower Motor Neuron–Segmental Signs	Upper Motor Neuron–Long Tract Signs
Motor function	Paralysis—loss of muscle power, flaccidity	Paresis to paralysis—loss of voluntary movements
Reflexes	Hyporeflexia to areflexia	Normal to hyperreflexia (especially myotatic reflexes)
Muscle atrophy	Early and severe—neurogenic; contracture after several weeks	Late and mild—disuse
Muscle tone	Decreased	Normal to increased
Electromyographic (EMG) changes	Abnormal potentials (fibrillation, positive sharp waves) after 5–7 days	No changes
Associated sensory signs	Anesthesia of innervated area (dermatome), paresthesia or hyperesthesia of adjacent areas	Decreased proprioception, decreased perception of superficial and deep pain

From Oliver JE Jr and Lorenz MD: Handbook of Veterinary Neurologic Diagnosis. Philadelphia, WB Saunders Co, 1983.

LMN signs are easily recognized on the neurologic examination. Paralysis, loss of tone, and loss of reflexes are present immediately after the neuron is damaged. LMN signs are especially significant in localizing a lesion. The differentiation of a lesion of the cell body or nerve root (spinal cord or brain stem) and of the axon (peripheral spinal or cranial nerve) is based on the distribution of signs.

Lesions of the sensory neurons also produce characteristic clinical signs. Segmental sensory signs include (1) anesthesia (complete lesion), (2) hypesthesia, or decreased sensation (partial lesion), (3) hyperesthesia, or increased sensation or pain (irritative lesion), or (4) loss of reflexes. Increased or decreased sensation of a dermatome can be mapped by pinching the skin. With practice, lesions of sensory roots can be accurately localized to within three spinal cord segments.

Upper Motor Neuron (UMN) and Long Tract Signs

The collective term upper motor neuron (UMN) is applied to the motor systems originating in the brain that control the lower motor neurons. The UMN systems are responsible for initiation and continuation of normal movements and for maintenance of tone in extensor muscles used to support the body against gravity. The cell bodies are located in the cerebral cortex, the basal nuclei, and the brain stem. The classic pathways include the corticospinal and corticorubrospinal tracts, which are primarily responsible for initiation of voluntary motor activity, and the reticulospinal and vestibulospinal tracts, which are primarily responsible for muscle tone and posture.

The classic concepts of pyramidal (corticospinal) and extrapyramidal motor systems are not useful when considering function in animals. Spinal stepping centers are located in the brachial and lumbosacral enlargements (C6–T2 and L4–S2, respectively). These centers generate rhythmic stepping movements of the limbs. They are controlled by brain stem locomotor centers (midbrain and pons), which coordinate the gait.[22, 23] The distinction between *voluntary initiation* of movements, which is generally thought to be a function of the cerebral cortex, and the relatively normal walking movements of decorticate animals is not easy. It is clear that decorticate animals have poor postural reactions. An animal with a relatively normal gait and severe postural reaction deficits usually has a lesion rostral to the midbrain.

Sensory pathways of clinical significance include those responsible for proprioception (position sense) and pain. Sensory neurons from the body are located in the dorsal root ganglia and synapse in the spinal cord gray matter. Proprioceptive pathways are found in the dorsal and lateral portions of the spinal cord. Relays are present in the spinal cord, medulla oblongata, and thalamus before projecting to the cerebellum and cerebral cortex. Pathways for transmission of superficial pain (discrete pain, pin prick, skin pain) are primarily located in the lateral portion of the spinal cord, with a relay in the thalamus. The pathway ultimately extends to the cerebral cortex for conscious recognition of pain. The pathway for deep pain (which includes severe or crushing pain and joint, bone, or visceral pain) is a bilateral, multisynaptic system that projects to the reticular formation, thalamus, and cerebral cortex.

Lesions of the UMN, whether at the origin of the pathway in the brain or of some portion of the tract in the brain or spinal cord, produce a characteristic group of clinical signs. Signs of UMN deficits include (1) poor performance of postural reactions, (2) normal or hyperactive spinal reflexes, (3) increased tone in extensor muscles (spasticity), and (4) abnormal reflexes, eg, crossed extensor reflex or extensor toe response (Table 2–2). UMN signs are present caudal to the level of the lesion.

UMN signs are more common than LMN signs in neurologic diseases. They are not as useful in localizing a lesion as LMN signs, but it is possible to identify the region of the CNS responsible for a lesion on the basis of UMN signs.

Signs of sensory long tract lesions are valuable for establishing prognosis of CNS disorders, as well as localization. Conscious proprioceptive deficits are usually the first signs observed with compressive lesions of the spinal cord. Abnormal positioning of the feet and ataxia may be present before there is any significant loss of voluntary motor activity. Superficial pain (conscious perception of pin prick) is often lost at about the same time as voluntary motor activity. Deep pain (strong pinch of bone or joint) is the last clinically useful sign to be lost when the spinal cord is compressed. Sensory deficits are present caudal to the level of the lesion.

OVERVIEW OF NEUROLOGIC EXAMINATION

Traditionally, the neurologic examination has been described as a series of tests that are done after a history has been taken and a physical examination performed.[2-4, 12, 13, 17] In some instances, this may actually be the way the clinician works. More often, the neurologic examination is done as a part of the physical examination. The sequence of the tests is not important, although a logical sequence may assist in interpretation. It is important that all results are recorded so that important tests are not overlooked. Depending on the species of animal, the preferences of the veterinarian, and other individual circumstances, the sequence may vary. The signalment and history are usually obtained first.

A brief description of an examination will be presented to illustrate one method. Detailed descriptions of the various tests will follow. An outline of a complete neurologic examination is presented in Table 2–3.[17]

The first steps in the physical and neurologic examinations include *observation* of *mental status, posture,* and *movement.* Observation of movement is of utmost importance in evaluation of large animals.

Palpation is a routine part of any physical examination. Special attention is devoted to symmetry of muscles, contour of the skull and vertebral column, and wear on the toes.

Assessment of *postural reactions* is not a part of the routine physical examination. Proprioceptive positioning can be tested while palpating the limbs by knuckling each foot in turn. Hopping must be tested separately. If results of these tests are normal (screening examinations, Table 2–3), the other postural reactions are not usually evaluated. Postural reactions are sensitive indicators of the presence of neurologic disease. If they are normal, the animal's problem is frequently not attributable to defects of the nervous system.

Evaluation of *spinal reflexes* also requires special tests, although the flexion reflex is often performed when the examiner touches the foot. If the animal withdraws the limb in response to touch, it is not necessary to crush the digit with a hemostat. The quadriceps and extensor carpi radialis reflexes are tested if there is evidence of paresis.

Most of the *cranial nerves* can be assessed during the routine physical examination. The face is observed for symmetry (CN V, trigeminal nerve, and (CN VII, facial nerve) and the head for normal posture (CN VIII, vestibular nerve). The eyes are observed for symmetric position of the globes (CN III, IV, and VI; oculomotor, trochlear, and abducent nerves, respectively) and size and symmetry of the pupils (CN III,

Table 2–3. NEUROLOGIC EXAMINATION

I. Observation*
Mental status
Posture
Movement
II. Palpation*
Integument
Muscles
Skeleton
III. Postural Reactions
Proprioceptive positioning*
Wheelbarrowing
Hopping*
Extensor postural thrust
Hemistanding and hemiwalking
Placing (tactile)
Placing (visual)
Tonic neck
IV. Spinal Reflexes
Myotatic
Pelvic limb
Quadriceps femoris muscle*
Cranial tibial muscle
Gastrocnemius muscle
Thoracic limb
Extensor carpi radialis muscle
Triceps brachii muscle
Biceps brachii muscle
Flexor*
Extensor thrust
Perineal*
Crossed extensor
Extensor toe
V. Cranial Nerves
Olfactory
Optic*
Oculomotor*
Trochlear
Trigeminal*
Abducent*
Facial*
Vestibulocochlear*
Glossopharyngeal*
Vagus*
Accessory
Hypoglossal*
VI. Sensation
Touch
Hyperesthesia*
Superficial pain*
Deep pain†

*Included in a screening examination.
†If superficial pain is absent.
From Oliver JE Jr and Lorenz MD: Handbook of Veterinary Neurologic Diagnosis. Philadelphia, WB Saunders Co, 1983.

and sympathetic nerve). The head is moved from side to side, producing normal vestibular nystagmus (CN III, IV, VI, and VIII). Shining a light in each eye allows evaluation of pupillary light reflexes (CN II, optic nerve, and CN III). A menacing gesture is made at each eye, producing a blink (CN II and VII). The medial and lateral canthus of each eye is touched, producing a blink (CN V, trigeminal nerve, and CN VII). The mouth is opened, noting jaw tone (CN V); a gag reflex is induced (CN IX, glossopharyneal nerve, and CN X, vagus nerve), and the nose is touched, which will usually induce a lick (CN V, sensory, and CN XII, hypoglossal nerve). In large animals the examiner should look for food at the nares and stimulate swallowing by palpating the larynx.

Every cranial nerve except CN I, olfactory nerve, and CN XI, accessory nerve, can be tested with minimal additions to a routine physical examination of the head. The olfactory nerve is rarely tested. Atrophy of the brachiocephalic or trapezius muscles innervated by the accessory nerve could be noted during palpation.

The examination of *sensations* is partially completed during palpation as areas of hyperesthesia are noted. Behavioral responses to stimulation of the limbs to assess the flexor reflex also were observed. More detailed evaluation is necessary if abnormalities are found.

These components of the neurologic examination can be integrated into the routine physical examination regardless of the sequence the examiner prefers. Minimal additional time is required. Abnormal findings indicate the need for a more thorough assessment.

SIGNALMENT

Species, breed, age, sex, and use of the patient are important considerations in the diagnosis. There are diseases specific to certain species and breeds (see Appendix II). Many are more common in certain age groups. A few diseases have a predilection for one sex.

HISTORY

The history of the animal's problem may provide more information than the various examinations. General concepts related to taking a history may be found in the references.[2-4, 11, 17, 18] Basic information can be obtained on a questionnaire filled out by the owner.[17]

After some general information is obtained about past medical problems, questions should center around the primary complaint. The examiner should inquire about the nature of the problem, whether it is specific and localized, or multifaceted, and its location. These ques-

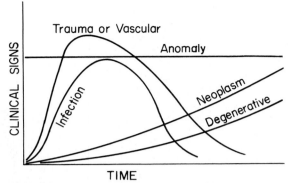

Figure 2–4. Sign-time graph of neurologic diseases. Progression of metabolic, nutritional, and toxic diseases is variable, depending on the cause. (From Oliver JE Jr and Lorenz MD: Handbook of Veterinary Neurologic Diagnosis. Philadelphia, WB Saunders Co, 1983.)

tions will elicit information related to the localization of the lesion, which will be verified by the neurologic examination.

Chronologic data are valuable for determining the cause of the problem and, in some cases, the ultimate prognosis. The onset and course of the problem are used to mentally construct a sign-time graph (Fig. 2–4), which often indicates the general category of disease responsible for the problem. For example, vascular lesions and trauma are almost always acute in onset and nonprogressive, whereas degenerative and neoplastic diseases are more likely to have a gradual onset and be progressive.

Information regarding signalment and history, along with data related to the animal's environment, should limit the number of categories of disease to be considered. The neurologic examination provides the information to localize the lesion and determine the severity of the problem. Integration of these findings into a diagnostic plan should be accomplished (see The Diagnostic Plan below).

NEUROLOGIC EXAMINATION

This section will review each of the tests, including the method of performance, the anatomy and physiology, and the assessment. Responses may be different in young animals. Most reflexes and postural reactions resemble those in the adult by the age of 3 to 4 weeks in the dog and foal. Examples of forms for recording results of neurologic examinations of large animals are presented in Tables 2–4A and B.

Observation

The animal's mental status, posture, and movement are observed carefully while taking the history. Additional observation, especially of gait, may be necessary.

Mental Status

Method. The levels of consciousness, behavior, and contact with the environment are observed. Normal variations for species, breed, and age must be considered. The history is an important source of information related to behavior.

Anatomy and Physiology. The reticular activating system in the rostral brain stem receives projections from most sensory pathways.[4] It projects diffusely to the cerebral cortex through relays in the diencephalon, maintaining a level of activation that characterizes consciousness (Fig. 2–5). Loss of this projection results in a loss of consciousness. Disruption can occur in the brain stem or by diffuse, severe damage to the cerebral cortex.

Assessment. The level of consciousness is recorded as *alert, depressed, stuporous,* or *comatose*. Abnormal behavior includes expressions of *fear, aggression, withdrawal,* or *disorientation*.[16] Other signs related to abnormal behavior include yawning, head pressing, compulsive walking, circling, and "stargazing."

Depression characterizes an animal that is awake but relatively unresponsive to the environment. It may be seen in animals that are ill from any cause.

Stupor describes an animal that sleeps except when aroused by strong stimuli. Painful stimuli may be necessary to arouse stuporous animals. Stupor is seen with partial disconnection of the reticular activating system from the cerebral cortex.

Coma is a state of deep unconsciousness. The animal cannot be aroused even with noxious stimuli. Reflexes are usually intact. Coma indicates complete disconnection of the reticular formation and cerebral cortex, usually from a severe brain stem lesion.

Behavioral disorders may be functional or related to primary brain disease. They are rarely localizing because lesions in many areas will produce similar behavioral abnormalities. The limbic system, including the hypothalamus, hippocampus, amygdala, other subcortical structures, and portions of the cerebral cortex, is associated with complex behavior.[3, 7]

Posture

Method. Abnormal posture, such as a head tilt, may be the primary complaint. Subtle alterations in posture may be seen as the animal moves about.

Anatomy and Physiology. Normal posture is maintained through sensory inputs to the central nervous system from various kinds of receptors in the limbs and body, vision, and the vestibular system. Vestibular receptors are important for sensing alterations of the animal's head in relation to gravity and for the detection of motion. Sensory information is processed through the brain stem, cerebellum, and cerebral cortex. Finally, the integrated output to the muscles of the neck, trunk, and limbs through the motor pathways maintains normal posture. The cerebellum and vestibular system are especially important in maintaining normal posture.

Vestibular influences are present in the newborn animal. Puppies and kittens can maintain a sternal position to nurse. Large animals are normally ambulatory shortly after birth.

Assessment. Posture of the head, trunk, and limbs should be evaluated. Abnormalities of the position of the head are frequently associated with disorders of the vestibular system. The head is frequently tilted toward the side with the lesion, whether it be in the labyrinth or in the vestibular nuclei. The postural abnormality may include twisting of the head, twisting of the neck (torticollis), and rotation of the head, neck, and body. Turning of the head (in contrast to tilting) usually indicates cerebral disease.

Deviations in vertebral contour include *scoliosis* (lateral deviation), *lordosis* (ventral deviation), or *kyphosis* (dorsal deviation). These may be caused by abnormal vertebrae or abnormal muscle tone in the paravertebral muscles.

The limbs may be positioned improperly or have abnormal muscle tone. A wide based stance is characteristic of ataxia caused by cerebellar, vestibular, or conscious proprioceptive abnormalities. Proprioceptive deficits may cause the animal to stand with one or more feet knuckled over. Decreased muscle tone from lower motor neuron lesions may produce a variety of abnormal postures of the limb as it is positioned passively. Increased extensor tone from upper motor neuron lesions or cerebellar disease may cause extension of the limb with straightening of the joints. This is most obvious in the pelvic limbs.

Decerebrate rigidity is characterized by ex-

Table 2–4. NEUROLOGIC EXAMINATION FORMS FOR LARGE ANIMALS

VETERINARY MEDICAL TEACHING HOSPITAL
UNIVERSITY OF FLORIDA

NEUROLOGIC EXAMINATION OF LARGE ANIMALS

OUTPATIENT:	STALL NO.:
DATE:	TIME:
CLINICIAN:	CHARGES:
STUDENT:	ACCOUNT:
HISTORY:	

PHYSICAL EXAMINATION:

NEUROLOGIC EXAMINATION

HEAD:
| Behavior: |
| Mental Status: |
| Head Posture: |
| Head Coordination: |

Cranial Nerves:

EYES

	LEFT	RIGHT
Ophthalmic Examination:		
Vision; II:		
Menace; II-VII, Cerebellum:		
Pupils, PLR; II-III:		
Horners; Symp:		
Strabismus; III, IV, VI, VIII:		

FACE
	LEFT	RIGHT
Sensation; Vs, cerebrum:		
Muscle mass, jaw tone; Vm:		
Ear, eye, nose, lip reflex; V-VII:		
Expression; VII:		
Sweating, Symp:		

VESTIBULAR — EAR
	LEFT	RIGHT
Eye drop:		
Nystagmus; resting:		
positional:		
vestibular:		
Hearing:		
Special vestibular:		

TONGUE
	LEFT	RIGHT
Tone, mass, fasciculations; XII, cerebrum:		

PHARYNX, LARYNX
	LEFT	RIGHT
Voice; IX, X:		
Swallow; IX, X:		
Endoscopy:		
Slap test:		

GAIT:
	LEFT FORE	LEFT HIND	RIGHT FORE	RIGHT HIND
Paresis:				
Ataxia:				
Spasticity:				
Dysmetria:				
Total deficit:				
Other:				

NECK & FORELIMBS	LEFT	RIGHT	TRUNK & HINDLIMBS:	LEFT	RIGHT	TAIL & ANUS:	LEFT	RIGHT
Hoofwear:			Hoofwear:			Strength:		
Posture:			Posture:			Muscle Mass:		
Strength:			Strength:			Tone:		
Muscle Mass:			Muscle Mass:			Reflexes:		
Tone:			Tone:			Sensation:		
Reflexes:			Reflexes:			Rectal:		
Sensation:			Sensation:					
Sweating:			Sweating:					

ASSESSMENT

SITE OF LESION(S): General (circle): cerebrum, brainstem, peripheral cranial nerves, cerebellum, spinal cord, peripheral nerves, muscles, skeleton

Specific:

CAUSE OF LESION(S):

PLAN
| DX: |
| RX: |
| EX: |

| SIGNATURE: | DATE: /   / |

From the Veterinary Medical Teaching Hospital, University of Florida.

Table 2–4. NEUROLOGIC EXAMINATION FORMS FOR LARGE ANIMALS *Continued*

VETERINARY MEDICAL TEACHING HOSPITAL
UNIVERSITY OF FLORIDA

LARGE ANIMAL NEONATAL NEUROLOGICAL EXAMINATION

Physical Examination: _____

Temperature: _____
Pulse: _____
Respirations: _____

EVALUATION OF THE HEAD
BEHAVIOR:

Affinity for the mare: _____
Flopping: _____
Flegmen: _____ Odontoprisis: _____ Shivering: _____
MENTAL STATUS: _____ Salivation: _____ Snapping: _____

MENTAL STATUS: _____
HEAD POSTURE AND COORDINATION: _____
CRANIAL NERVES: _____

	RIGHT	LEFT
Ophthalmic Examination:		
Vision (II):		
Menace (II-VII, Cerebellum):		
Pupil Size (II, III, Symp.):		
Pupil Symmetry (II, III, Symp.):		
PLR (II, III):		
Blink to Bright Light (II, VII):		
Strabismus (III, IV, VI, VIII):		
Nystagmus, vestibular (III, IV, VI, VIII):		
Nystagmus, spontaneous (III, IV, VI, VIII):		
Corneal Reflex (V, VII):		
Ear, Eye, & Lip (V, VII):		
Muscle Mass & Jaw Tone (V):		
Smile (V, VII):		
Swallow (IX, X):		
Voice (IX, X):		
Tongue (XIII):		
Endoscopy:		
Slap Test:		

FORELIMBS AND NECK

	RIGHT	LEFT
Cervical-local:		
Cervical-face:		
Muscle Mass:		
Sweating:		
Triceps Reflex:		
Biceps Reflex:		
Ex. Ca. Ra. Reflex:		
Flexor Reflex:		
Crossed Extensor Reflex:		
Babinski Sign:		
Extensor Strength:		
Proprioception:		
Recumbent Extensor Thrust:		

REARLIMBS, TAIL AND ANUS

	RIGHT	LEFT
Panniculus:		
Muscle Mass:		
Sweating:		
Patellar Reflex:		
Cr. Tibial Reflex:		
Gastrocnemius Reflex:		
Flexor Reflex:		
Crossed Extensor Reflex:		
Babinski Sign:		
Extensor Strength:		
Proprioception:		
Recumbent Extensor Thrust:		
Tail:		
Anus:		

PASSIVE TONE: FLEXOR VERSUS EXTENSOR STRENGTH
Forelimb: Heel to elbow, acromion, mid-scapular spine, dorsal scapula. _____
Hindlimb: Minimum distance between Tibial Tuberosity and Third Metatarsus. _____

Neck Movement: _____
Trunk Movement: _____

LIMB POSITION AND PASTERN AXIS:

Normal ≅ 50°   Toe on Ground ⨯ 50°   Toe off Ground ≅ 30°   Toe 1 cm. off Ground < 30°   Fetlock on Ground   Contracted > 50°

EVALUATION OF GAIT AND STRENGTH:

_____

Lesion site(s): _____
Possible etiology: _____
Plan: _____

Signature   Date

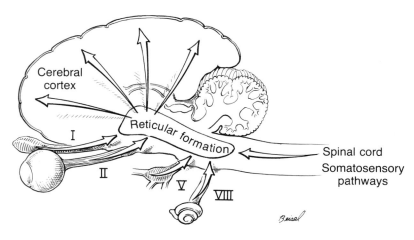

Figure 2–5. The ascending reticular activating system in the brain stem receives sensory information from the spinal cord and the cranial nerves. It projects, through thalamic relays, diffusely to the cerebral cortex, thus maintaining consciousness. (From Oliver JE Jr and Lorenz MD: Handbook of Veterinary Neurologic Diagnosis. Philadelphia, WB Saunders Co, 1983.)

treme extension of all four limbs and the trunk; it is caused by lesions in the rostral brain stem (midbrain or pons). Opisthotonos (extension of the head and neck) frequently accompanies decerebrate rigidity because of damage to the rostral lobes of the cerebellum.

Movement

Method. Abnormal movements such as tremor and myoclonus are evaluated with the animal at rest. If the animal is ambulatory, the various gaits, including at least walking and trotting, turning to the left and right, and backing, are also observed. Walking on a slope and with the head elevated often exaggerates minor gait deficits.

Anatomy and Physiology. The basic neural mechanisms for the control of locomotion are in the spinal cord and brain stem. Stepping centers are located in the C6–T1 and L4–S2 segments of the spinal cord, providing a basis for locomotion. Coordination of all four stepping centers is located in the brain stem. The cerebellum provides a feedback circuit for smooth movement. The cerebral cortex is only necessary for *voluntarily* initiated movements and for fine control. A decorticate animal has relatively normal gaits, although they are not under voluntary control and postural reactions are severely depressed or absent. An animal with a chronic spinal cord transection may have stepping movements, although the limbs will not be coordinated and the movements are not purposeful.[22, 23]

Assessment. Abnormal movements at rest include tremor and myoclonus. *Tremor* is characterized by small, rapid, alternating movements of the head, limbs, or trunk. Tremor may be seen physiologically, such as in fatigue,

fear, or chilling. Drug reactions, muscle disease, and toxins may produce a resting tremor. *Intention tremor* becomes worse as movements are initiated and disappears at rest. Intention tremor is an important sign of cerebellar disease. Severe coarse tremor, which often continues at rest, is seen in many diffuse disorders of myelin.

Myoclonus is a coarse, shocklike jerking of one or more muscle groups. The myoclonus associated with canine distemper encephalomyelitis has been called chorea. However, chorea is defined as irregular, brief, purposeless movements that often move from one part of the body to the other.[1] Distemper myoclonus is constant as to the part affected.

Abnormalities of gait are especially important in neurologic diagnosis of larger animals because postural reactions are difficult to assess. Minimal changes in the gait may be significant. The examiner must become familiar with the normal for the species to be able to detect subtle abnormalities. Most large animals are ambulatory within hours after birth, although they may be incoordinated. Dogs do not generally support weight on all four limbs until the third week. The gait becomes more coordinated in the fourth week after birth. Differentiating neurologic deficits from those caused by musculoskeletal disease is imperative. Neurologic abnormalities of movement include proprioceptive deficits, paresis, spasticity, ataxia, and dysmetria.

Proprioception, or position sense, is the ability to recognize the location of the limbs in relation to the body. At gait, proprioceptive deficits cause ataxia (see also Proprioceptive Positioning under Postural Reactions below).

Paresis is a deficit of voluntary movement. Complete loss of movement is *paralysis*. Terms used to describe paresis include monoparesis (paresis of one limb), hemiparesis (paresis of both limbs on one side of the body), tetraparesis or quadriparesis (paresis of all four limbs), and paraparesis (paresis of the pelvic limbs). The suffix -*plegia* (eg, tetraplegia) denotes complete paralysis. Paresis is caused by a loss of function of the voluntary motor system. It may be in the upper motor neuron (UMN) pathway, which extends from the brain to the spinal cord, or in the lower motor neuron (LMN) pathway, which includes the neuron in the spinal cord or brain stem giving rise to a peripheral spinal or cranial nerve and innervating a muscle. UMN and LMN signs and significance were explained previously.

Spasticity is an increase in tone of the extensor muscles of the limbs, usually caused by an UMN lesion. If the animal is still ambulatory, the limbs are kept straighter than normal with minimal flexion during movements.

Ataxia is a lack of coordination of movements and may be present without paresis or spasticity.[1] Truncal ataxia is a swaying of the body from side to side. Frequently, there is a wide based stance and excessive abduction or adduction of the limbs and swaying of the trunk. The ataxia may be accentuated by turning the animal, in which circumduction or crossing of the limbs occurs. Ataxia may be caused by a lesion in the cerebellum, the vestibular system, or the proprioceptive pathways.

Dysmetria describes movements that are too short (hypometria) or too long (hypermetria). At gait the animal appears to goose-step. Stopping the limb before it reaches the ground causes the animal to lurch from side to side. Dysmetria of the head is most easily seen when the animal tries to eat or drink. Dysmetria is usually a sign of cerebellar or cerebellar pathway disease.

Palpation

Method. Palpation of the skin and musculoskeletal system is a routine part of every physical examination. Whether it is done all at one time or on a regional basis during the examination is not important. Comparison of one side with the other is especially helpful for evaluation of muscles. Rectal examination of large animals is useful to assess sphincters and the urinary bladder.

Assessment. The skin may offer clues to the origin of disease, for example, scars or bruising from trauma. Abnormal wear of nails or hooves

is seen with paresis or proprioceptive deficits. Congenital anomalies of the vertebral column are sometimes associated with abnormal hair patterns; meningoceles may be attached to the skin, creating a dimple. The temperature of the extremities is lowered with arterial occlusion.

The size, tone, and strength of muscles are evaluated. Lesions of the LMN cause atrophy, loss of tone, and reduced strength. Solitary peripheral nerve lesions will produce these signs in the muscles normally innervated by the affected nerve but not in other muscle groups. Generalized peripheral neuropathies will cause similar changes in most, if not all, muscles of the body. LMN lesions produce early, severe atrophy with palpable differences within a week. Disuse atrophy, such as with UMN disorders, is much slower, is less severe, and does not cause a loss of tone or reflexes. Muscle strength is difficult to test. Extensor muscles are probably evaluated best during postural reaction testing. Flexor muscle strength can be assessed with the flexor reflexes.

Palpation of the skeleton may detect alteration in contour, crepitus, abnormal motion, or masses. Animals suspected of undergoing trauma should be palpated carefully. Abnormal motion in the spinal column can produce severe spinal cord compression or laceration. Palpating the spinous processes from the sacrum cranially may reveal alterations in contour. Skull fractures, open fontanelles, and suture lines are often palpable in smaller animals. Peripheral nerve injuries may be associated with fractures of long bones.

In horses, loss of sympathetic innervation of the skin may cause sweating, increased blood flow, and increased skin temperature. Stroking the loins elicits a lordosis, whereas stroking the gluteal region elicits a kyphosis. These movements can be used to assess motility of the vertebral column. Weak horses may buckle when posturing in response to this test.

Postural Reactions

Postural reactions are complex responses involving spinal reflexes and central coordination for normal movement and posture. Because of their complexity, abnormalities in postural reactions do not localize a lesion to one part of the nervous system. However, they are sensitive indicators of abnormality and when combined with other findings are important for diagnosis.

The postural reactions are listed in a sequence that is convenient for examination. Proprioceptive positioning and hopping are among the easiest to use, most reliable, and most sensitive so they should be included in a screening examination (see Table 2–3). The method of testing will be described for small animals with modifications for large animals if necessary.

Proprioceptive Positioning

Method. The foot is knuckled over so that the dorsum is on the floor. The animal should immediately replace the foot in a normal weight-bearing position. Each foot is tested separately (Fig. 2–6). This test may be used on any species. Another method is placing the foot on a piece of cardboard and sliding the cardboard laterally.[19] The animal should replace the limb to a normal position. The latter tests conscious proprioception of the proximal portion of the limb, whereas the former test assesses the distal portion of the limb. The "cardboard method" is not useful in large species. Both tests are not necessarily specific for conscious proprioception. Abnormal posture (eg, wide based stance, crossed feet) is also important to note.

Anatomy and Physiology. Receptors in the joints and muscles detect movements of the limbs. The information is carried to the brain in the dorsal funiculus (thoracic limb) and spinomedullothalamic tract (pelvic limb) through the brain stem to the cerebral cortex.[25] The motor response is initiated in the cerebral cortex and is transmitted to the spinal cord LMN.

Assessment. Proprioceptive positioning is a sensitive test for assessment of central nervous system disease in small animals. Lesions of the sensory cortex will often cause severe deficits of this reaction even when the gait is virtually normal. The proprioceptive pathways in the spinal cord are large fiber systems; they are sensitive to compression. One of the earliest signs of spinal cord compression is loss of proprioceptive positioning. Abnormalities in this reaction are essentially always the result of abnormality in the nervous system. Musculoskeletal disease that causes a severe gait abnormality will not affect this reaction.

Hopping Reaction

Method. The animal is held so that one limb touches the ground (Fig. 2–7). The weight is shifted laterally, forward, and medially. The animal should shift the limb quickly and accurately to support the weight. Hopping medially is difficult for most animals but may elicit subtle abnormalities. Larger animals, such as giant breed dogs, horses, and cows can be assessed by lifting one limb and shifting the weight so that they hop on the opposite limb. Large animals can also be tested by pushing them laterally (the sway reaction), requiring them to step laterally both while standing still and while walking. The pelvic limbs can also be tested by pulling laterally on the tail.

Anatomy and Physiology. The central and peripheral pathways for all of the postural reactions are similar. The sensory input for each of the reactions varies somewhat, but most, such as hopping, are primarily proprioceptive stimuli through skin, muscle, and joint receptors. Sensory input to the cerebral cortex and output from the primary motor cortex are required for accurate performance of the postural reactions. It is important to recognize that gait in animals is not dependent on the cerebral cortex, but postural reactions are. The motor neurons to the muscle of the limb are the final common pathway for the movements.

The hopping reaction is present in the thoracic limbs at 2 to 4 days of age and in the pelvic limbs at 6 to 8 days of age in puppies.

Hopping reactions are sensitive indicators of relatively mild dysfunction. Abnormalities of

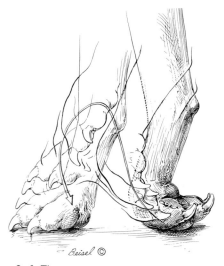

Figure 2–6. The proprioceptive positioning response. Conscious proprioceptive function is tested by placing the dorsal surface of the animal's foot on the floor. The animal immediately should replace it to the normal position. (From Greene CE and Oliver JE Jr: Neurologic examination. *In* Ettinger SJ: Textbook of Veterinary Internal Medicine, 2nd ed. Philadelphia, WB Saunders Co, 1982.)

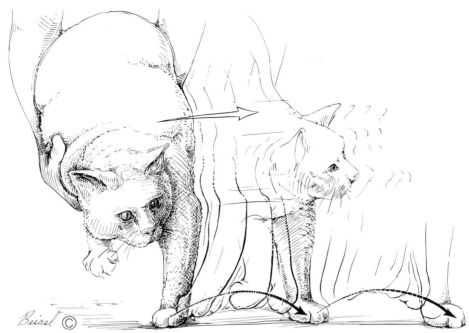

Figure 2–7. The hopping reaction. The normal animal responds to lateral movement of the body by quickly replacing the limb to support weight. (From Greene CE and Oliver JE Jr: Neurologic examination. *In* Ettinger SJ: Textbook of Veterinary Internal Medicine, 2nd ed. Philadelphia, WB Saunders Co, 1982.)

cerebellar regulation of the rate and range of movements are especially apparent on hopping.

Assessment. Slow initiation of the hopping movement suggests a proprioceptive deficit, whereas poor follow-through of the motion is likely to result from a motor system abnormality.[5] Cerebellar lesions will frequently cause inaccuracies in the length of the movement (dysmetria).

An animal with a relatively normal gait with deficits in the hopping reaction has a lesion rostral to the midbrain, usually in the cerebrum.

Wheelbarrowing Reaction

Method. This test can only be done on small to moderate-sized animals. The animal is supported under the abdomen with only the thoracic limbs bearing weight. Moving the animal forward and laterally should cause normal coordinated walking movements. As in all postural reactions, the animal should be maintained in as nearly a normal posture as possible. Elevating the animal's head during wheelbarrowing may accentuate subtle deficits (Fig. 2–8). The position restricts vision, requiring the animal to respond with only proprioceptive information.

It also elicits a tonic neck reaction, which increases extensor tone in the thoracic limbs.

Anatomy and Physiology. Similar to the hopping reaction.

Assessment. Similar to the hopping reaction. Wheelbarrowing is present in puppies by 4 to 5 days of age.

Extensor Postural Thrust Reaction

Method. The animal is supported by the thorax, and the pelvic limbs are lowered to the floor. The normal animal will step caudally to achieve symmetrical support of its weight (Fig. 2–9). As the animal is rapidly lowered to the floor the limbs will extend in preparation for contact. This is a vestibular reaction. It is not reliable enough to be of value in assessing vestibular function, however.

Assessment. Similar to the hopping reaction.

Hemistanding and Hemiwalking

Method. Both limbs on one side are lifted, forcing the animal to stand or walk on the opposite limbs.

Anatomy and Physiology. Similar to the hopping reaction.

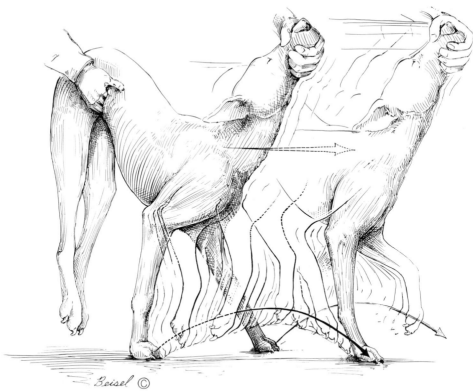

Figure 2–8. Wheelbarrowing with the neck extended. Wheelbarrowing is performed with the pelvic limbs elevated. The body should be in a position as close to normal as possible. The head may be elevated to accentuate abnormalities, as illustrated here. (From Greene CE and Oliver JE Jr: Neurologic examination. *In* Ettinger SJ: Textbook of Veterinary Internal Medicine, 2nd ed. Philadelphia, WB Saunders Co, 1982.)

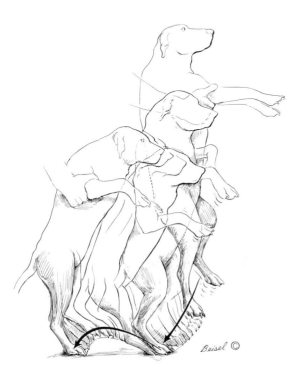

Figure 2–9. The extensor postural thrust reaction. The animal responds by stepping backward when its feet make contact with the floor. (From Greene CE and Oliver JE Jr: Neurologic examination. *In* Ettinger SJ: Textbook of Veterinary Internal Medicine, 2nd ed. WB Saunders Co, 1982.)

Assessment. Similar to the hopping reaction. Wheelbarrowing, extensor postural thrust, hemistanding, and hemiwalking reactions are all used to evaluate the same functions as hopping, except that two limbs are being assessed simultaneously. The size and temperament of the animal are important factors in choosing which of these reactions to assess. Hemistanding and hemiwalking are not usually exhibited by puppies until the third or fourth week of age.

Placing Reactions

Method. The placing reactions are performed first without vision (tactile placing) then with vision (visual placing). The animal is supported under the thorax with the eyes covered. The thoracic limbs are brought into contact with the edge of a table at or below the carpus. The animal should immediately lift the limb and place it in a normal supporting position (Fig. 2–10). Each limb may be tested independently. Restriction of movement of the limb next to the examiner's body may impede the test. Animals that are accustomed to being held may ignore

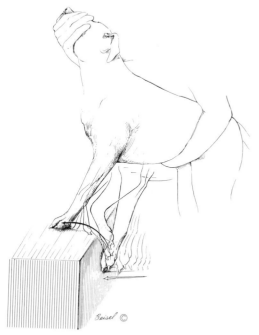

Figure 2–10. The tactile placing reaction is elicited with the eyes covered. When the carpus contacts the edge of the surface, the animal immediately should place its foot on the surface. (From Greene CE and Oliver JE Jr: Neurologic examination. *In* Ettinger SJ: Textbook of Veterinary Internal Medicine, 2nd ed. Philadelphia, WB Saunders Co, 1982.)

the stimulus unless they are held away from the body in a less comfortable position.

Visual placing is tested similarly, but the animal is allowed to see the table and should reach for it before contact is made. This is an excellent test for vision. Lateral visual fields may be assessed by bringing the animal to the table laterally.

Large animals can be tested by leading over steps or curbs.

Anatomy and Physiology. The placing reaction is similar to hopping, except that tactile or visual stimuli are used to induce the reaction. The placing reactions are sensitive indicators of cortical lesions.

Assessment. The interpretation of abnormalities in the placing reaction is similar to that in the hopping reaction except for the difference in sensory input. It is a useful test for vision. Normal tactile placing with a deficit in visual placing indicates a lesion in the visual pathways. Tactile placing is present by 2 to 4 days of age in puppies; visual placing is not present until the fourth week when vision is adequate.

Tonic Neck Reactions

Method. With the animal in a normal standing position its head is elevated, causing a slight extension of the thoracic limbs and flexion of the pelvic limbs. Lowering the head causes slight flexion of the thoracic limbs and extension of the pelvic limbs. Turning the head to one side will cause a slight extension of the ipsilateral thoracic limb and flexion of the contralateral one. The responses are small and easily suppressed by the animal.

Anatomy and Physiology. Activation of sensory receptors in the cervical region initiate these reactions but they are modified by vestibular input. They are components of normal movement. For example, as an animal prepares to jump, the head goes up, and the pelvic limbs flex. Making a turn, an animal plants the ipsilateral thoracic limb to take the turning step.

Assessment. These reactions are not reliable, so interpretation of deficits is not recommended. They are exaggerated in decorticate and decerebrate animals.

Spinal Reflexes

Reflexes are stereotyped responses to stimuli. They require two or more neurons in series, a sensory neuron and a motor neuron, and varying numbers of interneurons. A reflex composed of two neurons is exemplified by the myotatic or stretch reflex. Although the reflex is described simplistically in Figure 2–11, it is really complex. Numerous sensory fibers are activated by the stimulus. The sensory fibers synapse on numerous motor neurons, which in turn cause a contraction of a large group of muscle fibers. In addition, collaterals from the sensory fibers synapse on interneurons, which inhibit motor neurons that innervate antagonistic muscles. Spinal reflexes are modulated by descending pathways and other local synaptic input. However, a spinal reflex does not depend on supraspinal influences and will be present if the sensory and motor nerves and the related spinal cord segments are intact, regardless of the condition of the rest of the CNS.

Most of the spinal reflexes are evaluated with the animal in lateral recumbency. The pelvic limb reflexes are assessed first, followed by the thoracic limb reflexes. The animal is rolled to the opposite side and the process is repeated. It is not possible to test large animals that cannot be put down. Animals with normal postural reactions rarely have deficits in spinal reflexes.

Myotatic or Stretch Reflexes

QUADRICEPS (KNEE JERK, PATELLAR) REFLEX

Method. The animal is placed in lateral recumbency. The pelvic limb is supported under the stifle with the stifle and hock slightly flexed. A plexor is used to percuss the straight patellar ligament. The response should be a brisk contraction of the quadriceps muscle with extension of the stifle (Fig. 2–11).

Anatomy and Physiology. All of the myotatic reflexes are two neuron systems with one synapse (Fig. 2–11). The sensory receptor is in the muscle spindle and is activated by stretching the intrafusal muscle fibers. Both sensory and motor nerves for the quadriceps reflex are in the femoral nerve, which originates from L4–L6 in the dog. Activation of the sensory fiber

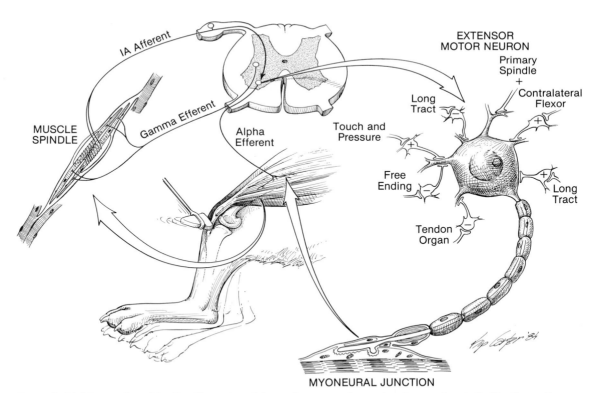

Figure 2–11. Myotatic (stretch) reflex. Percussion of the tendon or muscle stretches the muscle spindle. IA afferent fibers are activated and synapse directly on motor neurons of the muscle. The motor neuron discharges when a threshold level of excitation is reached. The level of excitation of the motor neuron is related to synapses from a variety of sources as illustrated. The impulse travels down the axon (alpha efferent) to the neuromuscular junction, causing a release of acetylcholine. Acetylcholine binds to receptors on the muscle, causing depolarization and contraction of the muscle. Gamma motor neurons maintain tension on the muscle spindle regardless of the state of contraction of the muscle.

initiates a nerve impulse, resulting in a synaptic activation of the motor neuron. If the stimulus is adequate, the motor neuron discharge causes contraction of the muscle.

There are two points of control of the myotatic reflexes. The intrafusal muscle fibers in the neuromuscular spindle are innervated by motor neurons (gamma), which control the degree of stretch of the spindle, allowing for raising or lowering the threshold. In addition, the motor neurons have a variety of segmental and long tract inputs that can facilitate or inhibit their response. The sum of the inputs, facilitatory and inhibitory, establishes the relative excitability of the neuron. Most of the descending tract input is inhibitory. Therefore, if this input is removed, such as occurs in a spinal cord transection, the reflex is released from inhibition and is more excitable than normal. Exaggerated reflexes are indicative of upper motor neuron disease.

Assessment. The quadriceps reflex is the most reliable of the myotatic reflexes. The reflex may be *absent, depressed, normal, exaggerated,* or *exaggerated with clonus.* Clonus means there are multiple muscle contractions in response to one stimulus.

Absent or depressed reflexes indicate a lesion of the sensory or motor nerve composing that reflex arc. The lesion may be in the spinal cord, the spinal nerves, or the specific nerve innervating the muscle. The lesion can involve either the sensory or the motor nerves. Because most lesions causing depressed or absent reflexes involve the motor neuron or the entire nerve, including both sensory and motor neurons, it is usually called a lower motor neuron (LMN) sign. LMN signs are important for localization of lesions (see below).

Normal reflexes indicate that the spinal cord segments, the nerve roots, and the peripheral nerves are intact. A normal reflex does not ensure that the spinal cord cranial to the segmental reflex is intact.

Exaggerated reflexes, with or without clonus, indicate a lesion of the descending pathways cranial to the spinal cord origin of the reflex. In the case of the quadriceps reflex, it means a lesion cranial to L4. This is called an upper motor neuron (UMN) sign. Damage to the descending pathways does not always cause exaggerated reflexes. Reflexes that appear exaggerated with no evidence of paresis should be interpreted cautiously. Variability in the character of the reflex is common. Depressed reflexes are more important for diagnosis.

The quadriceps reflex evaluates the integrity of the L4–L6 spinal cord segments and nerve roots and the femoral nerve. Absent or depressed reflexes usually indicate an LMN lesion. Exaggerated reflexes indicate a UMN lesion cranial to L4.

Myotatic reflexes are difficult to assess in the neonatal dog or cat. They are exaggerated in the calf or foal less than 1 month of age.

CRANIAL TIBIAL REFLEX

Method. The cranial tibial reflex is elicited with the animal in lateral recumbency, as for the quadriceps reflex. The belly of the cranial tibial muscle is percussed just distal to the proximal end of the tibia. The response is flexion of the hock.

Anatomy and Physiology. The cranial tibial muscle is innervated by the peroneal nerve, a branch of the sciatic nerve originating in the L6–L7 segments in the dog.

Assessment. The cranial tibial reflex is not as reliable as the quadriceps reflex. It is not routinely tested unless sciatic nerve injury is suspected. A depressed reflex indicates damage to the L6–L7 spinal cord segments or roots, or the peroneal nerve, but must be interpreted cautiously. The flexor reflex is more reliable.

GASTROCNEMIUS REFLEX

Method. The animal is kept in the same position as for the cranial tibial or quadriceps reflex, and the gastrocnemius tendon is struck just proximal to the tibial tarsal bone. The hock must be flexed to maintain tension on the muscle. The response is a slight extension of the hock.

Anatomy and Physiology. The gastrocnemius muscle is innervated by the tibial nerve, a branch of the sciatic nerve with origin in the L7–S1 segments of the spinal cord in the dog.

Assessment. The gastrocnemius reflex is even less reliable than the cranial tibial reflex and decreased responses should not be considered abnormal. The flexor reflex is more reliable.

EXTENSOR CARPI RADIALIS REFLEX

Method. The animal is maintained on its side to test the reflexes of the thoracic limb. The limb is supported under the elbow with the elbow and carpus flexed. The extensor muscles of the carpus and digits are percussed just distal to the elbow (Fig. 2–12). The response is extension of the carpus. The same reflex can be performed in large animals by percussing the

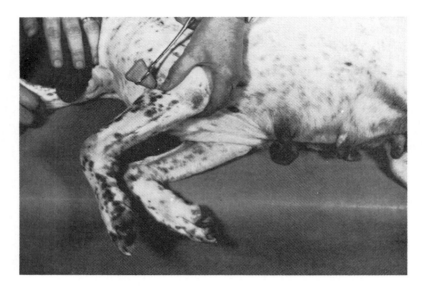

Figure 2–12. The extensor carpi radialis reflex is the most reliable myotatic reflex in the thoracic limb. With the animal in lateral recumbency and the elbow and carpus flexed, the extensor muscle group is percussed distal to the elbow. The response is extension of the carpus. (From Oliver JE Jr and Lorenz MD: Handbook of Veterinary Neurologic Diagnosis. Philadelphia, WB Saunders Co, 1983.)

extensor carpi radialis tendons above the carpus.

Anatomy and Physiology. The extensor muscles are innervated by the radial nerve with origin in the C7, C8, and T1 segments in the dog.

Assessment. The extensor carpi radialis reflex is the most consistent of the myotatic reflexes in the thoracic limb but is not as reliable as the quadriceps reflex. Weak responses must be evaluated cautiously. Strong responses usually indicate a lesion cranial to C7. The reflex is exaggerated in calves and foals less than 1 month old.

TRICEPS REFLEX

Method. The animal is in the same position as for the extensor carpi radialis reflex. The triceps brachii muscle is percussed just proximal to the olecranon.

Anatomy and Physiology. The triceps brachii is innervated by the radial nerve originating from C7, C8, and T1 in the dog.

Assessment. The triceps reflex is difficult to elicit in normal animals. Depressed or absent reflexes are not necessarily indicative of abnormality. Loss of radial nerve function will prevent extension and support of weight on the limb.

BICEPS REFLEX

Method. The animal is held in the same position with the index finger placed over the tendon of the biceps brachii muscle. The finger is percussed producing a flexion of the elbow.

Anatomy and Physiology. The biceps brachii and brachial muscles are innervated by the musculocutaneous nerve originating from C7–C8 in the dog.

Assessment. The biceps reflex is difficult to elicit and should be interpreted with caution. The flexor reflex is easier to evaluate and also assesses the musculocutaneous nerve.

FLEXOR (WITHDRAWAL, PEDAL) REFLEX

Method. The animal is kept in lateral recumbency to test thoracic and pelvic limb flexor reflexes. The limb is extended, and the toe is pinched. The limb should be withdrawn with flexion of the hip, stifle, and hock in the pelvic limb and the shoulder, elbow, and carpus in the thoracic limb (Fig. 2–13). The stimulus should be the least amount required to produce a reflex. If touching the toes causes withdrawal, there is no need to crush them with a hemostat.

Anatomy and Physiology. The stimulus may be to cutaneous or deep receptors, depending on its force. Generally, the stimulus must be noxious (pain producing) to elicit the flexor reflex. Free nerve endings are activated. The nerve impulses pass to the spinal cord and excite interneurons at several segmental levels (thoracic limb, C7–T1; pelvic limb, L6–S2 in the dog). The interneurons activate motor neurons, causing contraction of the flexor muscles of the limb. Simultaneously, the motor neurons that innervate extensor muscles are inhibited to allow the limb to flex (Fig. 2–13).

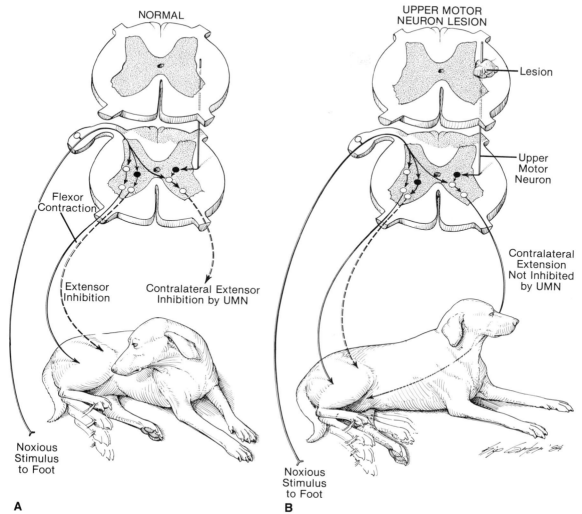

NORMAL

Flexor
Contraction

Extensor
Inhibition

Contralateral Extensor
Inhibition by UMN

Noxious
Stimulus
to Foot

A

**UPPER MOTOR
NEURON LESION**

Lesion

Upper
Motor
Neuron

Contralateral
Extension
Not Inhibited
by UMN

Noxious
Stimulus
to Foot

B

Figure 2–13. Flexor and crossed extension reflexes. A, The animal is positioned in lateral recumbency and a noxious stimulus is applied to a digit. The limb is immediately withdrawn. Sensory fibers enter the spinal cord through the dorsal root to synapse on interneurons. Flexor motor neurons are activated, causing flexion of the limb. Simultaneously, inhibitory interneurons cause relaxation of the antagonistic extensor muscles. Other interneurons cross the spinal cord to activate contralateral extensor muscles—the crossed extensor reflex. B, The crossed extensor reflex is inhibited unless there has been damage to UMN systems. Sensory fibers also project to the brain, causing a conscious awareness of pain and subsequently a behavioral reaction (A). The reflex is not dependent on a behavioral reaction. The behavioral reaction may be absent if sensory pathways are damaged.

The sensory nerves to the digits of the pelvic limb are branches of the sciatic nerve (dorsal surface, peroneal nerve; plantar surface, tibial nerve) and femoral nerve (medial surface, saphenous nerve). The sensory nerves to the digits of the thoracic limb are branches of the ulnar-median (medial and palmar surface) and radial (dorsal and lateral surface) nerves. These areas overlap considerably in the horse and have not been clearly defined in other large animal species.

Assessment. Flexion of the limb indicates that the peripheral nerves and spinal cord segments are intact. Depressed or absent responses indicate a lesion of one of these structures. Unilateral depression of the reflex is usually indicative of a peripheral nerve lesion. Bilateral depression of the reflex is more likely caused by a lesion of the spinal cord segments. The reflex does not require conscious perception of pain. Complete transection of the spinal cord cranial to the origin of the motor neurons will not abolish this reflex. Evaluation of pain sensation will be discussed later.

The flexor reflex is accompanied by a strong crossed extensor reflex in puppies until about 18 days of age and in calves and foals for about 1 month. After that, the response is similar to that in the adult.

EXTENSOR THRUST REFLEX

Method. The animal may be on its side or suspended by the shoulders with the pelvic limbs ventrally. The digits are spread by the fingers with gentle pressure between the pads. The response is extension of the limb.

Anatomy and Physiology. Stretching the digits activates stretch receptors and cutaneous receptors. The result is activation of both flexors and extensors causing rigid extension of the limb.

Assessment. The extensor thrust reflex (not to be confused with the *extensor postural thrust reaction*) is difficult to assess in most animals. It is often exaggerated in animals with UMN lesions.

PERINEAL (BULBOCAVERNOUS) REFLEX

Method. Touch, pinch or pin prick of the perineal region causes a contraction of the anal sphincter and flexion of the tail. Squeezing the bulb of the penis or vulva will produce the same response (Fig. 2–14).

Anatomy and Physiology. Sensory innervation of the perineum is from the sacral spinal cord segments and the pudendal nerve. Motor innervation of the anal sphincter is also in the pudendal nerve. The motor innervation of the tail is in the caudal nerves.

Assessment. The perineal reflex is the best test for the integrity of the sacral spinal cord and cauda equina. The urinary bladder is innervated by the pelvic nerves that originate in the same spinal cord segments, therefore this test is useful for assessing animals with bladder or sphincter dysfunction (see also Chapter 13).

CROSSED EXTENSOR REFLEX

Method. The crossed extensor reflex is a brisk, simultaneous extension of the contralateral limb when a flexor reflex is elicited.

Anatomy and Physiology. The crossed extensor reflex is normal when the animal is standing. Lifting one limb requires increased activity in the contralateral extensor muscles to maintain posture (Fig. 2–13). The reflex is inhibited through descending pathways in recumbent animals.

Assessment. The reflex is considered abnormal in recumbent animals, indicating a lesion of descending pathways from the brain. It is not an invariable sign of severe spinal cord disease, because animals with cervical spinal cord or brain stem lesions may have a crossed extensor reflex yet be ambulatory. It is more likely to be present in animals with chronic lesions.

The crossed extensor reflex is normally evident in puppies until about 18 days of age and in foals and calves until about 1 month of age.

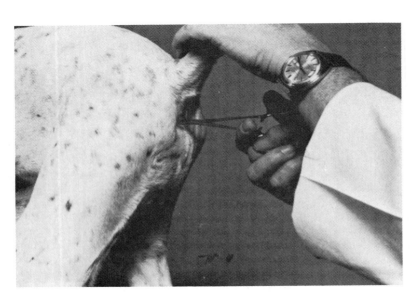

Figure 2–14. The perineal reflex is a contraction of the anal sphincter and a ventral flexion of the tail in response to tactile stimulation of the perineum. (From Oliver JE Jr and Lorenz MD: Handbook of Veterinary Neurologic Diagnosis. Philadelphia, WB Saunders Co, 1983.)

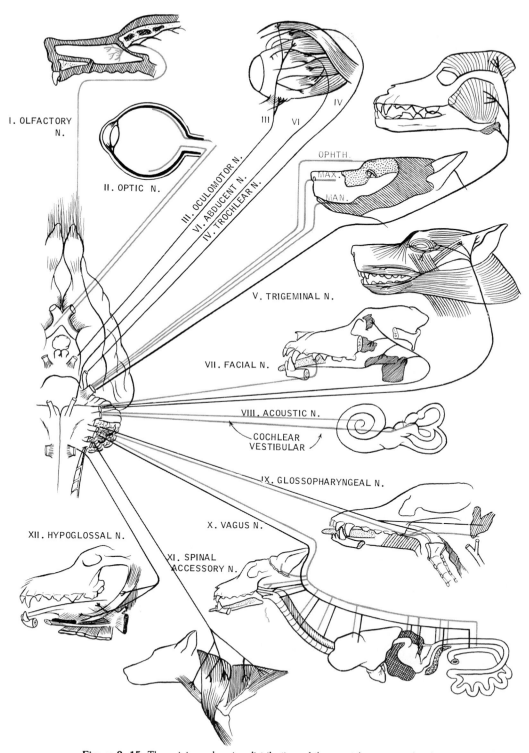

Figure 2–15. The origin and major distribution of the cranial nerves in the dog.

EXTENSOR TOE (BABINSKI) REFLEX

Method. The animal is positioned in lateral recumbency. The pelvic limb is held with the stifle, hock, and digits slightly flexed. A forceps or handle of the plexor is used to stroke down the caudolateral surface of the limb from the hock to the digits. Normal animals will flex the digits or show no reaction. A positive response is extension and fanning of the digits.[10]

Anatomy and Physiology. The extensor toe reflex in animals is not precisely the same as the Babinski reflex in human beings. The Babinski reflex includes elevation of the large toe, which is not present in quadripeds. The extensor toe reflex is not present in normal animals. The spinal reflex arc is not known but is presumed to be a part of the flexor reflex.[6]

Assessment. The extensor toe reflex is evidence of a lesion of descending pathways cranial to L5. It is usually seen in animals with chronic lesions (longer than 3 weeks) with extensor hypertonus and exaggerated myotatic reflexes.

Cranial Nerves

Evaluation of cranial nerves includes both reflex and behavioral tests. An efficient method was described above. Figure 2–15 provides a visual summary of the cranial nerves.

Olfactory Nerve (CN I)

Method. Noxious or pleasurable odors should produce an appropriate behavioral response. Irritating substances, such as ammonia or tobacco smoke, should not be used because they stimulate endings of the trigeminal nerve in the nasal mucosa. Food, alcohol, or cloves have been suggested.

Anatomy and Physiology. Chemoreceptors in the nasal mucosa transmit impulses through axons, which penetrate the cribriform plate to synapse in the olfactory bulb. Neurons in the olfactory bulb send axons to the ipsilateral olfactory cortex. The olfactory cortex, a part of the rhinencephalon, has connections to the limbic system mediating behavior.

Assessment. Evaluation of olfaction is difficult. Complete absence of smell may be detected by the methods described, but less dramatic changes cannot be assessed accurately. Lesions in the nasal passages, such as tumors or infections, are the most common causes of anosmia (loss of olfaction). Electrophysiologic tests for olfaction show promise (see Chapter 5).

Optic Nerve (CN II)

Method. The optic nerve is the sensory pathway for vision and pupillary light reflexes. Tests for vision include observation of the animal as it moves around obstacles, the menace reaction, and the visual placing reaction. Observation of the animal avoiding obstacles is the least reliable method, especially if the animal has other neurologic abnormalities. The menace reaction is a blink in response to a threatening movement aimed at the eye (Fig. 2–16). Each eye can be tested separately. The gesture should not create air currents that might stimulate tactile receptors. The blink response requires

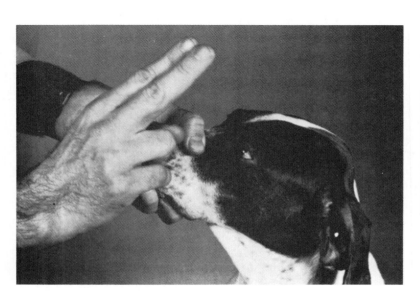

Figure 2–16. The menace reaction is elicited by making a threatening gesture at the eye, which should result in a blink. The examiner must avoid creating wind currents or touching the hairs around the eyes, which will cause a palpebral reflex. (From Oliver JE Jr and Lorenz MD: Handbook of Veterinary Neurologic Diagnosis. Philadelphia, WB Saunders Co, 1983.)

CN VII (facial nerve). An aversive movement of the head may also be seen. The visual placing reaction, described earlier, is an excellent test of vision.

The pupillary light reflex also tests the function of the optic nerve. First, the pupils are examined for symmetry. Resting pupils should be equal in diameter, although slight differences are usually insignificant. Unequal pupil size is called anisocoria. Next, a light is shone in one eye, causing a constriction of the pupil, which is the direct pupillary light reflex. Simultaneously, the pupil of the other eye will constrict, this being the indirect or consensual pupillary light reflex. Each eye should be tested. Constriction of the pupil is mediated by the oculomotor nerve (CN III) (see below).

Anatomy and Physiology. The visual pathway is diagrammed in Figure 2–17. Photoreceptors in the retina are activated by light, initiating action potentials in the various neurons in the retina. Ultimately, the ganglion cells are activated. The axons of the ganglion cells form the optic nerves. Optic nerve fibers traverse the optic chiasm and ascend as the optic tract to synapse in the lateral geniculate nucleus of the

thalamus. Geniculate neurons project to the occipital cortex by way of the optic radiation. In domestic animals, most of the optic nerve fibers cross to the contralateral side in the optic chiasm. In primates, the fibers from the temporal half of the retina remain uncrossed, whereas the fibers from the nasal half of the retina cross. The fibers from the nasal half of the retina cross in all species. In dogs, approximately one half of the temporal fibers cross, for a total of about 75 per cent crossing and 25 per cent remaining on the same side. In the cat, about 65 per cent of the total are crossed. In most herbivores, over 80 per cent are crossed. As a rule, the more lateral the eyes are situated on the head, the more fibers are crossed and the less binocular vision is present. From a clinical perspective, most animals behave as if all of the fibers are crossed. For example, a dog with a lesion of one occipital cortex will appear to be blind in the contralateral eye. Careful testing may reveal some remaining vision in the temporal retina, but it is not easy to verify.

The pathway for the pupillary light reflex is diagrammed in Figure 2–17. Notice that the pathway is the same as for vision through the optic tract but diverges at that point. Optic tract fibers synapse on the pretectal nucleus. Pretectal neurons then synapse on the oculomotor nuclei (parasympathetic nucleus). Most of the fibers in the optic tract are from the contralateral eye. It is reported that the majority of the pretectal neurons cross to the opposite oculomotor nuclei. Hence, the direct pupillary light reflex is slightly stronger (more constriction) than the indirect response.[21] The preganglionic parasympathetic neurons of CN III are located in the rostral portion of the midbrain, ventral to the mesencephalic aqueduct. Fibers of CN III leave the ventral midbrain medial to the crus cerebri, extend across the edge of the tentorium cerebelli, and penetrate the dura mater. CN III is joined by CN IV and CN VI as it runs for a distance in the cavernous sinus before exiting the orbital fissure. Fibers in CN III synapse in the ciliary ganglion ventral to the optic nerve caudal to the globe. Postganglionic fibers in the short ciliary nerves innervate the ciliary muscles and pupillary constrictor muscles.

Sympathetic innervation of the pupil must also be considered when evaluating pupillary light reflexes. Sympathetic nerves innervate the dilator muscles of the pupil. The pathway is generally considered to originate in the hypothalamus (Fig. 2–18). There is a synapse in the

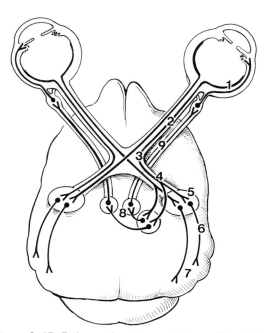

Figure 2–17. Pathways for vision and the pupillary light reflex. 1, Retina or optic nerve; 2, orbit (CN II and CN III); 3, optic chiasm; 4, optic tract; 5, lateral geniculate nucleus; 6, optic radiation; 7, occipital cortex; 8, parasympathetic nucleus of CN III; 9, oculomotor nerve. (The numbers correspond to those in Table 2–5.) (From Oliver JE Jr and Lorenz MD: Handbook of Veterinary Neurologic Diagnosis. Philadelphia, WB Saunders Co, 1983.)

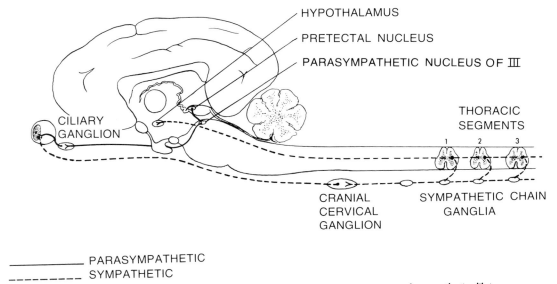

Figure 2–18. The motor pathways to the iris: parasympathetic-constrictor and sympathetic-dilator.

midbrain, the origin of the tectotegmentospinal system.[4] This pathway in the lateral funiculus synapses on the preganglionic sympathetic neurons in the intermediolateral nucleus of the first three thoracic spinal cord segments. The preganglionic axons leave the spinal nerves in the rami communicantes to join the sympathetic trunk. They course cranially as a part of the vagosympathetic trunk to synapse in the cranial cervical ganglion, ventral to the atlas. In the horse this ganglion is in a fold of the guttural pouch. The postganglionic axons follow the internal carotid artery through the tympanooccipital fissure, and through the middle ear in the dog and cat. The axons join the ophthalmic nerve, a branch of the trigeminal nerve (CN V),

and exit the skull through the orbital fissure. They innervate the smooth muscles, glands, and blood vessels of the head and neck to C_2, as well as the dilator muscle of the pupil. These axons are close to the guttural pouch in horses.

Assessment. Both vision and pupillary light reflexes must be tested to establish the location of an abnormality. Figure 2–19 outlines the kind of deficits produced in visual and pupillary light reflex pathways.

The menace reaction and pupillary light reflexes are not reliable until about 4 weeks of age in dogs and cats. The menace reaction is present after about 1 week in large animals, but the pupillary light reflex and blink to light is present in neonates.

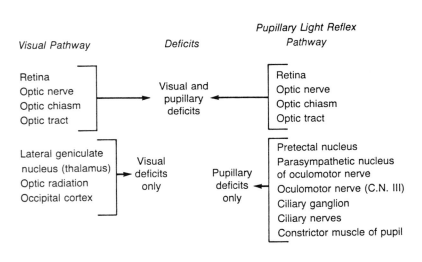

Figure 2–19. Deficits from lesions of the visual and pupillary light reflex pathways. (From Oliver JE Jr and Lorenz MD: Handbook of Veterinary Neurologic Diagnosis. Philadelphia, WB Saunders Co, 1983.)

Table 2–5. SIGNS OF LESIONS IN VISUAL PATHWAYS

Complete Lesion on Right Side	Vision		Resting Pupil		Pupillary Light Reflex	
	Right Eye	Left Eye	Right Eye	Left Eye	Light in Right Eye	Light in Left Eye
1. Retina or optic nerve	Absent	Normal	Slightly dilated	Normal	No response	Both constrict
2. Orbit (CN II and CN III)	Absent	Normal	Dilated	Normal	No response	Left constricted
3. Optic chiasm (bilateral)*	Absent	Absent	Dilated	Dilated	No response	No response
4. Optic tract	Normal	Absent†	Normal	Normal or slightly dilated	Both constrict	Both constrict
5. Lateral geniculate nucleus	Normal	Absent†	Normal	Normal	Both constrict	Both constrict
6. Optic radiation	Normal	Absent†	Normal	Normal	Both constrict	Both constrict
7. Occipital cortex	Normal	Absent†	Normal	Normal	Both constrict	Both constrict
8. Parasympathetic nucleus of CN III (bilateral)*	Normal	Normal	Dilated	Dilated	No response	No response
9. Oculomotor nerve	Normal	Normal	Dilated	Normal	Left constricts	Left constricts
10. Sympathetic nerve	Normal	Normal	Constricted	Normal	Both constrict	Both constrict

The numbers correspond to those in Figure 2–17.
*Unilateral lesions of these structures are rare.
†Possibly loss of sight in left visual field with partial sparing in right visual field.
Modified from Oliver JE Jr and Lorenz MD: Handbook of Veterinary Neurologic Diagnosis. Philadelphia, WB Saunders Co, 1983.

Diffuse lesions of the cerebellar cortex may abolish the menace reaction, although the animal is not blind and has normal palpebral reflexes. The mechanism may be related to increased inhibition of cerebral cortex by the deep cerebellar nuclei.[8] Recent evidence also implicates the deep cerebellar nuclei in the classically conditioned eyeblink response to auditory stimuli.[14] The exact mechanism is still unknown. Some animals with cerebellar disease and a poor menace response do blink in response to a bright light. Other tests for vision, such as placing reactions and visual following, will confirm that vision is present.

Table 2–5 summarizes the combinations of visual and pupillary light reflex abnormalities expected with complete lesions (see also Fig. 2–17). Partial lesions may produce deficits but not a total absence of response. For example, retinal and optic nerve lesions frequently cause blindness with a partial sparing of the pupillary light reflex. By alternating the stimulus, first to one eye and then the other, a slower less complete response will be seen in the affected eye.

Optic tract lesions usually cause minimal pupillary deficits unless both tracts are affected.

Unilateral lesions of the pretectal and parasympathetic nuclei of CN III are rare because the nuclei are only millimeters apart in the brain stem. In addition, there are bilateral projections to both nuclei. Therefore, unilateral signs of oculomotor dysfunction are virtually always caused by lesions of the oculomotor nerve.

Oculomotor Nerve (CN III), Trochlear Nerve (CN IV), Abducent Nerve (CN VI)

These three nerves are considered together because of their common function, movement of the eyeball. The parasympathetic function of CN III, pupillary constriction, is discussed above.

Method. Eye movements are assessed by observing the resting position of the eyes in the orbit and the ability of the animal to follow and by actively eliciting eyeball movement. Sudden movements in the peripheral field of vision may cause the animal to look. Turning the head from side to side and up and down elicits vestibular eye movements (normal nystagmus). The fast beat of the nystagmus will be in the direction of the head movement (Fig. 2–20). Elevation of the head of large animals, and some dogs, will cause a symmetric ventral deviation of the eyeballs. In these animals, the head must be maintained in a normal plane while testing lateral movements.

Anatomy and Physiology. For the anatomy of CN III, see the preceding section, Optic

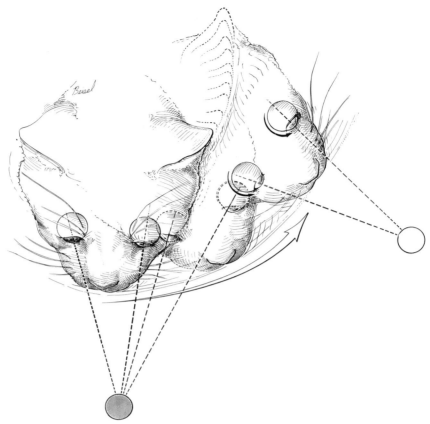

Figure 2–20. Vestibular eye movements are elicited by turning the animal's head from side to side. The eyes will lag behind the head movement and then will rotate to return to the center of the palpebral fissure. Both visual (opticokinetic nystagmus) and vestibular pathways are active in this response, but vestibular pathways predominate and will produce these movements in the absence of vision. (From Oliver JE Jr and Lorenz MD: Handbook of Veterinary Neurologic Diagnosis. Philadelphia, WB Saunders Co, 1983.)

Nerve (CN II). The nucleus of CN III innervating the extraocular eye muscles is just caudal to the parasympathetic nucleus. The peripheral course of the nerve is the same to the orbit. CN III innervates the dorsal, medial, and ventral recti, ventral oblique, and levator palpebrae muscles.

The trochlear nerve (CN IV) originates in the caudal part of the midbrain ventral to the central gray substance in a position similar to the oculomotor nucleus. The axons course dorsally and cross before exiting caudal to the caudal colliculus. They run over the side of the midbrain, extend along the edge of the tentorium cerebelli, and join the oculomotor nerve in the cavernous sinus. The trochlear nerve exits the orbital fissure and innervates the dorsal oblique muscle.

The abducent nerve (CN VI) originates in the rostral medulla ventral to the floor of the fourth ventricle. The axons leave the ventral surface of the medulla lateral to the pyramid. The nerve courses rostrally to join CN III and CN IV in the cavernous sinus. It exits the orbital fissure and innervates the lateral rectus and retractor bulbi muscles.

CN III, IV, and VI function in close coordination to move the eyeballs. The eyes move in concert (conjugate movement), maintaining the same general visual field. Connections among the nuclei of the three nerves, the vestibular nuclei, and voluntary motor centers are made via axons in the medial longitudinal fasciculus (MLF), a small tract in the central part of the brain stem. Turning the head from side to side stimulates the vestibular receptors and, via the vestibular nuclei, activates CN III, IV, and VI through the medial longitudinal fasciculus, producing a normal nystagmus with the fast beat in the same direction as the head movement.

Normal nystagmus can also be produced by visual input, such as watching telephone poles from a moving car. This function is primarily cortical in origin and is difficult to test in animals.

The function of each individual extraocular muscle and of the three cranial nerves has not been definitively established in all domestic animals. Anatomic dissections, muscle and nerve stimulation, and nerve lesions have been used to study the function of these muscles and nerves in the dog.[4a] The function of the recti muscles is as expected from their anatomic location. Obviously, if the eye is in a position other than centered in the palpebral fissure, movements will be different. For example, if the eye is directed dorsally, contraction of the lateral rectus muscle will move the eye ventrally, as well as laterally. For simplicity, it is adequate to assume direct dorsal, ventral, medial, and lateral movements by the respective recti muscles. The oblique muscles do not function in the manner described in human beings. The insertion of these two muscles is close to the equator in animals as compared with a more rostral location in humans. Therefore, they rotate the globe around an anterior-posterior axis through the center of the cornea.

Assessment. Strabismus is an abnormal position of the eyeball. Lesions of CN III, IV, or VI will cause a strabismus to occur in all positions of the head. Definitive studies of all species are not available, but the signs resulting from specific nerve lesions might be presumed to be similar to those occurring in the dog. Oculomotor paralysis causes a ventrolateral strabismus. In addition, there may be a slight ptosis from paralysis of the levator palpebrae muscle and a dilated pupil from loss of parasympathetic neurons. Abducent paralysis causes a medial strabismus and loss of the ability to retract the globe. Trochlear paralysis does not produce a strabismus that is easily detected. The dorsal aspect of the eyeball is rotated laterally. This rotation can be appreciated by examining the eye in species that do not have a round pupil (Fig. 2–21) or by observing the position of the superior retinal vein with an ophthalmoscope. In dogs with experimental lesions of these nerves, the strabismus was present immediately after section of the nerve. Within about 2 weeks, the eyeball returned to a normal resting position in the center of the palpebral fissure. At that time, deficits could be detected only in movements of the eyeball. This finding has been confirmed in clinical cases with chronic lesions.

Strabismus of one eye may also be seen when the head is held in various positions. The most common example is a ventral strabismus in one eye when the head is elevated. Lesions of the vestibular system are usually the cause. It is important to verify the ability of the eye to move in all directions to differentiate vestibular strabismus from the fixed strabismus of a lower motor neuron lesion.

Convergent (medial) strabismus without deficits in eye movements is seen in some animals, especially Siamese cats and Holstein cattle. Divergent strabismus is seen in Jersey cattle. The cats have an abnormal arrangement of the visual pathway rather than an abnormality of CN VI.

The so-called dorsomedial strabismus in cattle with various severe cerebral lesions (eg, polioencephalomalacia) has been attributed to lesions of CN IV. However, this has not been proven.

Conjugate movement of the eyeballs is influenced by the vestibular and cervical proprioceptive (tonic eye movements) systems through the medial longitudinal fasciculus. Lesions of the MLF or vestibular system may cause dysconjugate movements or a lack of normal vestibular nystagmus. Abnormal eye movements have not been reported with lesions of the cervical spinal cord.

Nystagmus at rest is always abnormal. The most common form is alternating fast and slow beats, the so-called jerk nystagmus. It is named by the direction of the fast beat, for example, horizontal nystagmus to the left. Nystagmus is almost always caused by abnormality of the vestibular system (see Vestibular Nerve [CN VIII]). Pendular nystagmus consists of small oscillations of the eyeball that do not have fast and slow components. It is seen in cerebellar disease and is most pronounced as the animal moves the eyes to fix on a new target. Blind animals also may have a pendular nystagmus.

Trigeminal Nerve (CN V)

Method. The trigeminal nerve supplies sensory fibers to the face and motor fibers to the muscles of mastication. Touching or pinching the face with a forceps causes a behavioral reaction in most animals, indicating intact sensation. The sensory fibers for the palpebral and corneal reflexes are in CN V. Animals that are depressed or have decreased sensation will usually respond to stimulation of the nasal mucosa. The three branches of CN V should all be tested (Fig. 2–22). Touching the medial canthus

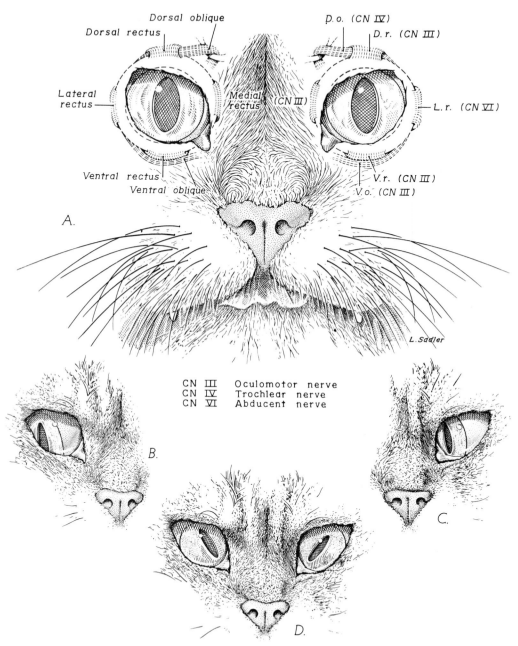

Figure 2–21. Functional anatomy of the extraocular muscles (A). Directions of strabismus following paralysis of the oculomotor (B), abducent (C), and trochlear (D) neurons. (From deLahunta A: Veterinary Neuroanatomy and Clinical Neurology, 2nd ed. Philadelphia, WB Saunders Co, 1983.)

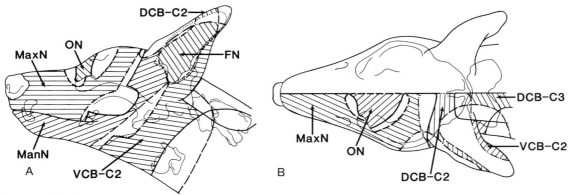

Figure 2–22. Areas of cutaneous innervation of the head that are supplied by one nerve (autonomous zones). DCB–C2, Dorsal cutaneous branch of the second cervical nerve; VCB–C2, ventral cutaneous branch of the second cervical nerve; DCB–C3, dorsal cutaneous branch of the third cervical nerve; FN, facial nerve; MaxN, maxillary nerve, CN V; ManN, mandibular nerve, CN V; ON, ophthalmic nerve, CN V. *A,* Lateral, *B,* dorsal view. (From Whalen LR and Kitchell RL: Electrophysiologic studies of the cutaneous nerves of the head of the dog. Am J Vet Res 44:615, 1983.)

of the eye and eliciting a blink tests the ophthalmic branch. The nasal mucosa is innervated by the maxillary branch. Pinching the skin on the lower lip tests the mandibular branch. Opening the mouth to test jaw tone and palpation of the temporal, masseter, and rostral digastric muscles for atrophy assess the function of the motor branch of the mandibular nerve.

Anatomy and Physiology. The motor nucleus of the trigeminal nerve is located in the pons at the level of the rostral cerebellar peduncle. The cell bodies of the sensory fibers are in the trigeminal ganglion, which is located in the canal for the trigeminal nerve in the petrosal bone. The sensory fibers enter the brain stem on the lateral surface of the pons. The axons course within the brain stem from the pons to the first cervical spinal cord segment as the spinal tract of the trigeminal nerve. The second order neurons are in the pontine sensory nucleus and the nucleus of the spinal tract of the trigeminal nerve, which lies medial to the tract. The pontine nucleus receives fibers from mechanoreceptors. Most of the spinal nucleus transmits nociceptive information. Projections from these nuclei course rostrally to the thalamus associated with the contralateral medial lemniscus. Thalamic neurons project to the cerebral cortex. Axons from the pontine and spinal nuclei also project to the facial nucleus, completing the corneal and palpebral reflex arcs.

Assessment. Lesions of the trigeminal nerve proximal to the separation into its three major branches cause a loss of sensation to the face, loss of corneal and palpebral reflexes, and pa-

ralysis with ultimate atrophy of muscles of mastication.[24] Injury to the branches distal to their separation causes a loss of sensation to the affected area (Fig. 2–22). Discrete lesions of the motor nucleus cause motor deficits without sensory loss. Unilateral motor lesions are difficult to detect until atrophy occurs in 7 to 10 days. Lesions of the spinal tract or nucleus of the trigeminal nerve cause decreased sensation without motor deficits. Nuclear lesions, both motor and sensory, most often will be associated with other signs of brain stem disease.

Bilateral paralysis of the muscles of mastication without loss of sensation is seen in dogs and cats. Animals are unable to close the jaw, preventing prehension of food. Atrophy of the muscles has been reported in a few of these animals, but most recover in 2 to 3 weeks. deLahunta reports that there is a nonsuppurative inflammation of the trigeminal nerve and ganglion.[4] Demyelination was more prominent than axonal degeneration.

In one cat trigeminal neuritis caused severe hyperesthesia of one side of the face. Even light touch caused a reaction expected with severe noxious stimulation. The cat had a nonsuppurative encephalitis with inflammation of the trigeminal nerve.

Lesions of the sensory area of the cerebral cortex or the fibers in the internal capsule cause a decrease in the level of sensation (hypesthesia).[5, 13] If the lesion is unilateral, the contralateral side of the face is less sensitive than the normal side. The animal will usually respond to vigorous stimulation of the nasal mucosa but ignore a hard pinch of the skin. Movements of the facial muscles are normal.

Facial Nerve (CN VII)

Method. The facial nerve innervates the muscles of facial expression and supplies sensory fibers for taste to the rostral two thirds of the tongue. It also innervates the sublingual and mandibular salivary glands, the lacrimal glands, and the stapedius muscle. Facial paralysis is usually apparent because of the asymmetry of the ear, palpebral fissure, lip, and sometimes the nose. The ear may droop if it is normally erect. The palpebral fissure is widened in small animals, and there is no blink in response to a menace or touch. Ptosis is present in large animals. Lifting the head so the nose is vertical reveals asymmetry of the lips. The commissure of the lips on the affected side is lower. The nose is usually deviated away from the affected side in large animals, particularly horses, with only a slight deviation in cats, dogs, and pigs. Electromyography and nerve conduction studies can also be used to substantiate denervation of facial muscles (see Chapter 5).

Taste can be tested by applying a small amount of atropine solution to one side of the tongue with a cotton-tipped applicator. The suspected affected side should be tested first. Normal animals react immediately to the bitter taste. A delayed reaction will be seen as saliva moves the solution to the other side of the tongue.

The Schirmer tear test can be used to assess lacrimation. Functions of the stapedius muscle can be tested electrophysiologically (see Tympanometry and Acoustic Reflex, Chapter 5).

Anatomy and Physiology. The facial motor nucleus is located in the rostral medulla oblongata.[7] The axons course dorsomedially around the abducent nucleus, then turn ventrolaterally to emerge from the medulla ventral to the vestibulocochlear nerve. The facial nerve enters the internal acoustic meatus of the petrosal bone with CN VIII, traverses the facial canal, and exits the skull through the stylomastoid foramen. Branches of the facial nerve innervate the muscles of facial expression (ear, eyelids, cheeks, lips) and the caudal part of the digastric muscle (Fig. 2–23).

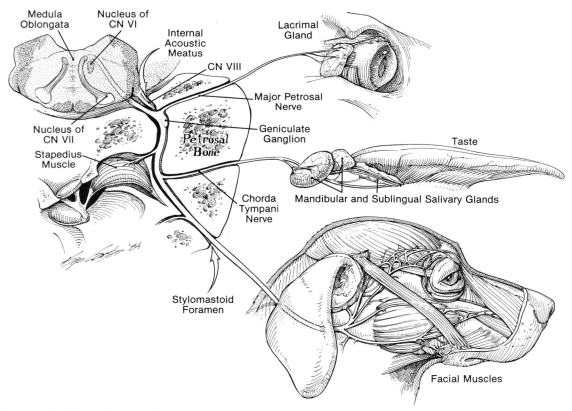

Figure 2–23. The facial nerve originates in the medulla oblongata and enters the internal acoustic meatus of the petrosal bone with the vestibulocochlear nerve (CN VIII). Branches include nerves to the lacrimal glands, stapedius muscle, mandibular and sublingual salivary glands, and sensory fibers for taste. The major component exits the stylomastoid foramen and innervates the muscles of facial expression. Testing for function of the various branches can localize the site of the lesion in facial paralysis.

The facial nerve supplies sensory fibers for taste to the rostral two thirds of the tongue and the palate. These fibers follow trigeminal branches to their terminations. The sensory neuron is in the geniculate ganglion in the petrosal bone. The central terminus is through the solitary tract to the solitary nucleus in the medulla. Projections from the solitary nucleus reach the cortex similarly to the trigeminal afferent pathway. Reflex connections are also present.[4, 7]

A branch of the facial nerve, the chorda tympani, enters the middle ear to innervate the stapedius muscle. Function of this nerve can be assessed with tympanometry (see Chapter 5).

Parasympathetic fibers from the salivatory nucleus in the medulla are also present in the facial nerve. They supply glands in the nasal mucosa, the mandibular and sublingual salivary glands, and the lacrimal glands.

Cutaneous sensory fibers in the facial nerve are distributed to the concave surface of the pinna (see Fig. 2–22).[24]

Assessment. Facial nerve paralysis is usually obvious on initial observation of the animal. Partial lesions causing weak, but not absent, movements can be more difficult to recognize. Drooping of the lip and ear (if normally erect) are usually present in all species (Fig. 2–24). The palpebral fissure is usually widened in small animals because of paralysis of the orbicular eye muscles. Ptosis, possibly resulting from paralysis of the frontalis muscle, is usually seen in large animals.[4] The nose may be pulled toward the normal side, a finding that is more obvious in large animals.

Lesions of individual branches of CN VII with paralysis of some of the facial muscles are more frequent in large animals. Horses restrained on their sides with insufficient padding under their heads are subject to damage to the buccal branches supplying the lips and nose.

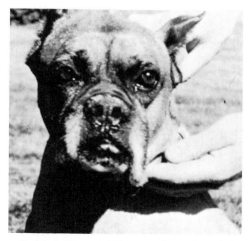

Figure 2–24. A 10 year old boxer with paralysis of the left facial nerve. The sagging lip, widened palpebral fissure, and drooped ear are apparent.

Cattle may injure the palpebral branch while struggling in a stanchion. Damage to the auriculopalpebral branch has been reported in a large breed dog that had a 6 hour surgical procedure while lying on its side.[20]

The location of lesions causing paralysis of all the facial muscles can be estimated by assessing lacrimation, taste, and stapedius muscle function (Table 2–6). Lesions distal to the stylomastoid foramen will affect only the facial muscles (see Fig. 2–23). Lesions in the petrosal bone (eg, inner ear infections) may affect one or all of the functions, depending on the extent of the problem; there are usually vestibular signs, and Horner's syndrome from damage to the sympathetic nerves may be present in small animals. Intracranial-extramedullary lesions will affect all branches of the facial nerve; Horner's syndrome will not be present, and vestibular signs are usually evident owing to the close approximation of CN VIII to CN VII. Intramedullary brain stem lesions affect one or more

Table 2–6. SIGNS OF LESIONS IN FACIAL NERVE

Anatomic Site*	Facial Muscles	Taste	Stapedius Muscle	Lacrimation	Vestibular Signs	Horner's Syndrome	Brain Stem Signs†
Distal to stylomastoid foramen	Abnormal	Normal	Normal	Normal	Normal	Normal	Normal
Petrosal bone	Abnormal	Variable	Variable	Variable	Abnormal	Abnormal‡	Normal
Intracranial-extramedullary	Abnormal	Abnormal	Abnormal	Abnormal	Abnormal	Normal	Variable
Brain stem	Abnormal	Variable	Abnormal	Variable	Variable	Normal	Abnormal

*See Figure 2–23.
†Level of consciousness, abnormality of gait, postural reaction deficits, other cranial nerve signs.
‡In small animals.

of the components of the facial nerve, depending on the location and the size of the lesion. Other brain stem signs such as alteration in the level of consciousness, deficits in proprioception, paresis, and other cranial nerve abnormalities are usually present. Spasms of the facial muscles are seen in early inflammation of CN VII and may also be present in nigropallidal encephalomalacia in horses and in tetanus in all species. UMN lesions appear to cause a paresis of the facial muscles with abnormal grimmacing in some species, especially the horse and dog. Table 2–6 summarizes the signs associated with facial nerve lesions.

Vestibulocochlear Nerve (CN VIII)

The vestibulocochlear nerve has two components: the vestibular division provides information about the orientation of the head with respect to gravity and movement, and the cochlear division mediates hearing.

Method. *Vestibular Division.* Abnormalities of the vestibular system, including the receptors in the inner ear, CN VIII, the vestibular nuclei in the brain stem, the flocculonodular lobes of the cerebellum, and some of the connecting pathways, cause a characteristic group of signs. Most lesions are unilateral. Unilateral vestibular lesions typically cause a head tilt, an asymmetric ataxia, and nystagmus.

The head tilt is usually apparent on initial observation. The head is tilted toward the affected side, with one rare exception (see Assessment). The head, neck, and trunk may be turned toward the affected side. The gait is ataxic, and the animal tends to circle and fall to the side with the lesion. There may be a slight increase in extensor tone contralaterally and a decrease in extensor tone ipsilaterally. The abnormalities in posture are worsened if the animal is lifted from the ground or blindfolded, removing tactile and visual orientation.

Nystagmus is characteristic of vestibular disease. The direction of the nystagmus is that of the fast component. Generally, both eyes are affected, and they move conjugately. The nystagmus may be horizontal, vertical, or rotatory. The examiner should note the direction of the nystagmus in the normal resting position of the head and then with the head extended, flexed, and turned to each side. Changes in the direction of the nystagmus with varying head positions are important in localization. A ventral strabismus may be seen in the eye on the affected side when the animal's head is elevated.

Additional tests of vestibular function can be performed, but they are of little clinical benefit. Various righting reactions may be used to evaluate the animal's ability to correct its posture. In small animals, the pelvis can be grasped firmly and the animal lifted so the thoracic limbs are off the ground. A normal animal will keep the head in a horizontal position. An animal with a vestibular lesion will twist the head and neck to the side with the lesion. In bilateral vestibular disease the animal usually flexes the head.

Postrotatory nystagmus can be used to assess vestibular function, but it too offers little additional information. The animal is held with the head horizontal and the holder rapidly turns 360° ten times and stops. Normal nystagmus is induced while the animal is turning (see Oculomotor Nerve [CN III]). A postrotatory nystagmus occurs in the opposite direction. Normal animals will have three to four beats of nystagmus, with the fast phase opposite the direction of rotation. After 3 to 4 minutes, the test can be repeated in the opposite direction. The ear away from the direction of rotation receives the maximal stimulus. Peripheral lesions will usually cause a decreased response on rotation away from the lesion.

The caloric test is the only method for pure unilateral testing of vestibular function. Unfortunately, negative responses in normal animals are common enough to make this test unreliable. Irrigation of the external ear canal with 50 to 100 ml of ice water for approximately 3 minutes is recommended. A rubber ear syringe, which will not harm the ear in the event of sudden movements, should be used. The ear canal should be free of debris, and the eardrum should be intact. Nystagmus is induced, with the fast phase away from the side being tested. Lesions of the receptors or movement of the head during the test will often prevent a response. It can be of benefit in assessing brain stem function in a comatose animal.

Cochlear Division. Most tests for hearing require a behavioral response from the animal and cannot evaluate each ear independently. Therefore, a responsive, alert animal and bilateral deafness are necessary to detect abnormality. Typical tests include speaking or whistling, clapping the hands, or making some other noise and watching for an alerting reaction. Similar responses may be monitored by electroencephalography or by direct measurement of the respiratory cycle.

The best methods for testing hearing are electrophysiologic. Tympanometry measures impedance changes in the auditory canal, providing information about the middle ear and tympanic membrane, as well as testing hearing. Brain stem auditory evoked responses (BAER) must be recorded on a signal averaging computer. Brain stem auditory evoked response measures electric activity of the brain stem and cerebrum in response to auditory stimuli. (Both of these tests are described in Chapter 5.)

Anatomy and Physiology. *Vestibular Division.* The receptors for the vestibular system are located in the labyrinth of the petrosal bone, the inner ear. The crista ampullaris, the receptor in the three semicircular canals, detects movements of the head. The three canals are at right angles to each other, allowing for detection of motion in any direction. The receptors in the utriculus and sacculus are called maculae. The macula in the utriculus is oriented horizontally, whereas that in the sacculus is oriented vertically. These receptors primarily signal the static position of the head with respect to gravity. Depolarization of the receptor cells generates action potentials in the related vestibular neurons. The bipolar cell bodies of the vestibular neurons are located in the petrosal bone. The vestibular neurons, along with cochlear neurons, leave the petrosal bone through the internal acoustic meatus to enter the brain stem at the cerebellomedullary angle in the rostral medulla. Most of the vestibular neurons terminate in one of the four vestibular nuclei. A few terminate directly in the cerebellum.[3, 7]

The lateral vestibular nucleus projects fibers to the ipsilateral ventral funiculus of the spinal cord as the lateral vestibulospinal tract in the cat. These fibers primarily facilitate ipsilateral extensor muscles and inhibit ipsilateral flexor muscles and contralateral extensor muscles. This is an important pathway for maintenance of normal postural tone in extensor muscles—the antigravity system. The medial vestibular nucleus projects fibers bilaterally to the ventral funiculus of the spinal cord by way of the medial longitudinal fasciculus (MLF). These axons descend as far as the cranial thoracic spinal cord segments. Both the caudal and medial vestibular nuclei send axons to the fastigial nuclei and the flocculonodular lobes of the cerebellum. The rostral, medial, and lateral vestibular nuclei project to the nuclei of CN III, IV, and VI by way of the medial longitudinal fasciculus. This pathway mediates vestibular eye movements. Poorly defined pathways also project to the cerebral cortex by way of the thalamus. Projections to the brain stem reticular formation provide the pathway mediating nausea from vestibular stimulation (motion sickness).

The vestibular system monitors the position of the head and detects movements of the head. The pathways are important in maintaining the posture of the animal and in controlling eye movements.

Assessment. *Vestibular Division.* Abnormal function of any part of the vestibular system may cause alterations in posture, changes in tonus of the muscles of the limbs, and abnormal eye movements.

Differentiating central (brain stem) disease from peripheral (labyrinth) disease is important for therapy and prognosis. Table 2–7 outlines the major differences. The most reliable criterion is the presence or absence of normal postural reactions. Also, diseases affecting the vestibular nuclei almost always will interfere with proprioceptive and motor pathways causing abnormal gait and abnormal postural reactions. During the acute phase of a vestibular syndrome the animal may be so disoriented that reactions are difficult to assess. Generally, with patience, the examiner can hold an animal in an upright position with the toes knuckled to test proprioceptive positioning. It is the most reliable test in small animals. If the results are equivocal and other signs, such as nystagmus, are nondiagnostic, the animal should be reexamined in 24 to 48 hours. Usually, by that time, the animal is more stabilized and an accurate assessment can be made.

An otoscopic examination should be done whenever possible in animals with signs of vestibular disease. The tympanic membrane should be examined to detect middle ear disease. The bulging, opaque, inflamed membrane should be readily distinguished from the normal, translucent membrane. Radiographs of the tympanic bulla may be of benefit (see Chapter 4). Endoscopy of the guttural pouch may reveal blood in traumatic lesions of horses. Tympanometry is useful for assessing the compliance and patency of the tympanic membrane (see Chapter 5).

What has been termed the paradoxic vestibular syndrome may be caused by lesions near the caudal cerebellar peduncles. The signs are similar to those of central vestibular disease, except the head tilt may be contralateral to the side of the lesion. A head tilt in one direction with turning of the head and neck in the opposite direction may also be seen, especially in horses.

Bilateral vestibular disease is relatively rare

Table 2–7. SIGNS OF VESTIBULAR DISEASES

Unilateral Vestibular Disease

Head tilt
Asymmetric ataxia
Falling, rolling
Nystagmus
Positional ventral strabismus

	Peripheral	*Central*
Mental status	Normal	Frequently depressed
Gait	Asymmetric ataxia, may see increased extensor tone contralaterally	Asymmetric ataxia, paresis
Postural reactions	Normal	Abnormal
Cranial nerves	May have deficits in CN VII and Horner's syndrome	May have deficits in CN V, VI, VII, IX, X, or XII
Nystagmus	Horizontal or rotatory, not altered in direction with changes in position of head. Fast phase away from side of lesion	Horizontal, rotatory, or vertical; may change direction with position of head

Bilateral Peripheral Vestibular Disease

Symmetric ataxia, crouching posture with jerky swinging movements of the head
No nystagmus or vestibular eye movements
Deafness

---

but can be perplexing. It is usually caused by bilateral infections of the inner ear but may be idiopathic. The most characteristic signs are jerky, swinging movements of the head, symmetric ataxia, and a lack of vestibular eye movements.

Cochlear Division. Unless the animal is completely deaf, alterations in hearing are difficult to assess. Behavioral responses to sounds may be used (see Method above). Brain stem auditory evoked response (BAER) and tympanometry are the only reliable ways to test for unilateral or partial hearing loss (see Chapter 5).

Glossopharyngeal Nerve (CN IX), Vagus Nerve (CN X)

The glossopharyngeal and vagus nerves are considered together because of their similarities in anatomy and function.

Method. Lesions of these nerves often will cause dysphagia and a weak, or absent, gag reflex. Observation of the pharynx and larynx for symmetry and stimulation of a swallowing response by a tongue depressor (small animals) or nasogastric tube (large animals) are the most reliable tests. Laryngeal paralysis may be observed directly in small animals or with an endoscope in large animals. Cranial nerves IX, X, and XII and the sympathetic nerves may be seen on endoscopy of the guttural pouch in horses. The laryngeal adductor reflex (slap test) is used to assess laryngeal motility in horses. The horse is slapped just behind the withers

while palpating the dorsal larynx or observing the larynx with an endoscope. The response is a contraction of the dorsal laryngeal muscles and adduction of the contralateral arytenoid cartilage and vocal fold. The pathway is through thoracic afferents ascending in the spinal cord contralateral to the stimulus to the nucleus ambiguus. The efferent path is in the vagus nerve through the recurrent laryngeal nerve to the larynx. Lesions anywhere along this pathway cause a decreased or absent response. Laryngeal paralysis usually causes detectable respiratory sounds. Electromyography is useful for evaluating laryngeal paralysis.

Esophageal paralysis usually causes regurgitation. Manometry and radiography are used to assess esophageal function.

The sensation of taste on the caudal one third of the tongue (CN IX) can be evaluated as described for facial nerve (CN VII).

Anatomy and Physiology. The glossopharyngeal nerve carries sensory fibers, including taste, from the rostral pharynx and larynx. These fibers project to the solitary tract and nucleus of the medulla as described for facial nerve (CN VII).

The nucleus ambiguus is a poorly defined motor nucleus in the ventrolateral medulla. Motor nerves from the nucleus ambiguus project through CN IX to the pharynx and palate and through CN X to the pharynx, larynx, and palate. In addition, these motor fibers innervate the striated muscles of the esophagus. The recurrent laryngeal nerves leave the vagus within the thorax and ascend to innervate the cervical esophagus and larynx. CN IX contributes parasympathetic fibers to CN V for innervation of the parotid and zygomatic salivary glands. A major portion of the vagus nerve arises from the parasympathetic vagal nucleus in the medulla, supplying parasympathetic fibers to all of the thoracic and abdominal viscera, except for those in the pelvic canal.

Assessment. Dysphagia, asymmetry of the pharynx or larynx, and a poor swallowing reaction are the most readily detected abnormalities of function of CN IX and X. Any animal with difficulty in swallowing should be considered a rabies suspect until proven otherwise. Caution is necessary in examining these animals. Any diffuse or focally severe forebrain disease can cause UMN dysphagia, particularly in the horse.

Recurrent laryngeal nerve damage or other causes of laryngeal paralysis may be detected by the noisy respiration. Direct observation of the larynx is usually diagnostic. Regurgitation is the most common sign of esophageal paralysis. There are no well-documented signs of loss of vagal innervation to the abdominal viscera in small animals. Poor rumen function and a tendency to bloat are seen in cattle.

Accessory Nerve (CN XI)

Method. The trapezius, sternocephalic, and brachiocephalic muscles may be palpated for atrophy.

Anatomy and Physiology. The accessory nerve innervates the trapezius and parts of the brachiocephalic and sternocephalic muscles. The motor nucleus of the accessory nerve extends from the first to the sixth or seventh cervical spinal cord segment. The nerve fibers extend cranially to exit through the tympano-occipital fissure.

Assessment. Atrophy or loss of function of the trapezius, sternocephalic, and brachiocephalic muscles is indicative of damage to CN XI. Deficits from injury to this nerve rarely are recognized clinically.

Hypoglossal Nerve (CN XII)

Method. The hypoglossal nerve innervates the muscles that protrude and retract the tongue. Each side is innervated independently. Lesions of one hypoglossal nerve will cause paralysis and atrophy of the ipsilateral muscles. When the tongue is protruded, for example, to lick the nose, the tongue will deviate to the paralyzed side. Retraction of the tongue will be weak on the paralyzed side. Rubbing the nose will cause most animals to lick. Strength of retraction may be tested by grasping the tongue.

Anatomy and Physiology. The hypoglossal nucleus is in the caudal medulla. The nerve emerges from the ventral medulla lateral to the pyramids. The hypoglossal nerve traverses the hypoglossal canal to the intrinsic and extrinsic muscles of the tongue and the geniohyoid muscle.

Assessment. Paralysis of the tongue is recognized by the consistent deviation of the tongue to the affected side. Atrophy of the muscle of the tongue is apparent within a week (Fig. 2–25).

UMN lesions, particularly diffuse cerebral disease, cause paresis of the tongue in the horse. It is characterized by dysphagia and protrusion of the tongue but no atrophy. Protrusion of the tongue, with good movement otherwise, has been seen in some dogs with hydrocephalus.

Sensation

Two primary modalities of sensation (excluding special senses) can be assessed in most animals: proprioception and pain. Touch can be evaluated in some animals from some areas of the body, for example, the cornea. However, responses to touch are not consistent enough to be useful in diagnosis. Discrimination of temperature is similarly of no practical use. Proprioception was tested using the postural reaction,

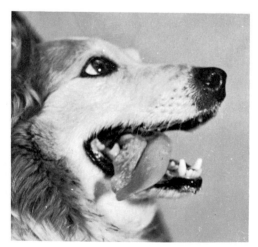

Figure 2–25. A right hypoglossal nerve injury in a dog hit by a car 4 years previously. Notice the atrophy of the right side of the tongue. When it is protruded, the tongue deviates to the injured side. The dog submerges its muzzle to drink.

proprioceptive positioning. This is not purely a sensory test because it requires a motor reaction, but it is the best available.

The other important sensation to be tested is pain. Pain is a subjective experience. The pathways, tests, and interpretation of data regarding noxious stimuli are more properly called nociceptive. However, for simplicity, the term pain will be used.

Pain

Method. There are three components to the examination for pain. First, presence and location of pain are ascertained. Second, whether the animal can perceive superficial pain is determined. Third, if the animal cannot perceive superficial pain from an area of the body, the ability to perceive deep pain is tested.

Painful areas may have been detected from a review of the history or when the animal was palpated. Careful systematic palpation will generally reveal areas of hyperesthesia. Lesions of the nervous system will cause a decrease in sensation distal to the lesion. Therefore, testing is from distal to proximal. The level of a lesion, for example, in the spinal cord, will be marked by a change from decreased to normal sensation, and often by a local painful area as well.

The limbs and trunk are systematically palpated. The objective is to squeeze hard enough to evoke a reaction if the area is painful, but not evoke a reaction if the area is normal. Placing a hand on muscles such as those of the abdomen helps detect the early guarding reactions when a painful area is palpated.

Vertebral pain may also be detected by manipulation. The lumbosacral region is frequently painful when there is cauda equina compression. Direct pressure on the lumbosacral junction will usually elicit a reaction. Extension of the hips also causes pain in this condition through stretching of the sciatic nerve and extension of the sacrum. Flexion, extension, and turning of the neck may be useful in identifying cervical pain.

Superficial, or cutaneous, pain is assessed by pinching or pin pricking the skin. A gentle pinch with a pair of hemostats is preferred. If a needle is used it should be relatively blunt. Two reactions may be elicited. A behavioral reaction, such as crying, biting, turning, or other display of recognition, may be elicited by pinching or pricking any area. A skin twitch, the cutaneous or panniculus reflex, is evoked by stimulation of the trunk between T1 and S1.

Similar responses, as well as cervicofacial responses, can be elicited from the cervical region of the horse. If abnormalities are detected, the boundaries of normal and abnormal responses should be mapped as accurately as possible.

A noxious stimulus that causes a behavioral response is adequate for assessment of deep pain. If superficial pain is present, deep pain is also. If the animal responds to a touch, there is no need to crush a toe. Withdrawal of a limb is a reflex, not a behavioral response, and does not indicate intact sensation beyond the reflex arc. If superficial sensation is absent, squeezing a digit with a hemostat is used to assess deep pain.

Large animals can be incredibly stoic to testing for deep pain. A hemostat can usually be clamped on the neck or trunk of most horses and cattle without unduly upsetting the patient. Therefore, interpretation must be made with caution.

Anatomy and Physiology. Sensory fibers from the viscera, joints, muscles, and skin enter the spinal cord through the dorsal root. The distribution of sensory fibers is relatively consistent within one species and is surprisingly similar in all mammalian species. The strip of skin innervated by one pair of spinal nerves is called a *dermatome* (Fig. 2–3). Each dermatome receives sensory fibers from approximately three roots. Normal peripheral nerves (eg, radial nerve) innervate areas of skin that may correspond to several dermatomes or parts of dermatomes. Areas of skin innervated by only one peripheral nerve are called *autonomous zones* (Fig. 2–26). The autonomous zones have been defined only in the dog[9] and horse.[2a] Proprioceptive fibers ascend in the dorsal funiculus (thoracic limb) or dorsolateral funiculus (pelvic limb) to relay nuclei in the medulla.[25] Fibers for superficial pain synapse in the dorsal horn then project cranially in the lateral funiculi. The majority of these fibers are contralateral, but some are ipsilateral. Fibers for deep pain apparently project cranially on both sides of the spinal cord and have multiple synapses before reaching the brain. This bilateral, multisynaptic, small fiber pathway is resistant to damage.

The cutaneous, or panniculus, reflex is the contraction of the cutaneous trunci muscle in response to a local stimulus of the skin. The sensory pathway is through segmental spinal nerves and the superficial pain pathway. The ascending fibers synapse in the brachial intumesence (C8–T1) with the motor neurons of the lateral thoracic nerve, which innervates the cutaneous trunci muscle (Fig. 2–27). Another

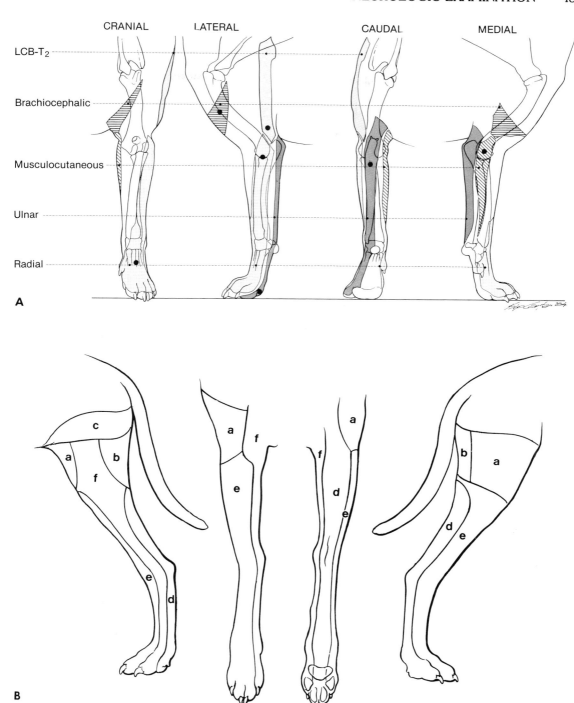

Figure 2–26. A, Cutaneous innervation of the left thoracic limb of the dog. Autonomous zones, areas innervated by only one nerve, are shown, along with recommended sites for testing for sensation (dots). The median nerve does not have an autonomous zone. LCB–T2, lateral cutaneous branch of the second thoracic nerve. B, Approximate cutaneous innervation of the right pelvic limb of the dog. Autonomous zones have not been defined. a, Lateral cutaneous femoral nerve (L3, *L4*, L5); b, caudal cutaneous femoral nerve (L7–S1, *S2*); c, genitofemoral nerve (*L3*, L4); d, tibial nerve (L6, *L7, S1*); e, peroneal nerve (L6, *L7*, S1); f, saphenous nerve (femoral) (L4, *L5*). (A, Based on Kitchell RL et al: Electrophysiological studies of cutaneous nerves of the thoracic limb of the dog. Am J Vet Res 41:61, 1980, and Bailey CS and Kitchell RL: Clinical evaluation of the cutaneous innervation of the canine thoracic limb. J Am Anim Hosp Assoc 20:939, 1984. B, From Oliver JE Jr and Lorenz MD: Handbook of Veterinary Neurologic Diagnosis. Philadelphia, WB Saunders Co, 1983.)

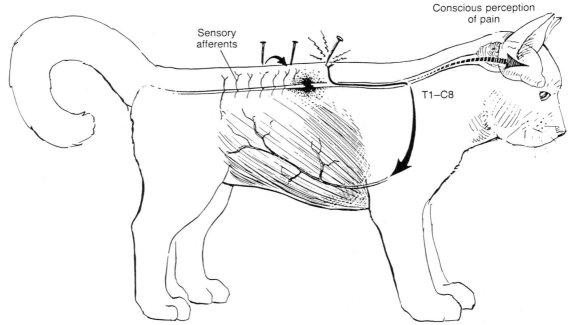

Figure 2–27. The cutaneous (panniculus) reflex is the contraction of cutaneous trunci muscle, producing a skin twitch, from stimulation of cutaneous sensory fibers. (From Greene CE and Oliver JE Jr: Nerologic examination. *In* Ettinger SJ: Textbook of Veterinary Internal Medicine, 2nd ed. Philadelphia, WB Saunders Co, 1982.)

cutaneous reflex, the local cervical reflex, is seen in the horse. The efferent nerves are thought to include CN XI and the segmental cervical nerves.

Assessment. Pain is a psychologic phenomenon and therefore subjective. It is assumed that an animal perceives pain if an escape or attack response is made to a noxious stimulus that the examiner would expect to be painful. An animal is also considered to experience pain if similar reactions are elicited by manipulation or palpation of specific areas but not others. Animals that try to escape or attack regardless of the stimulus should not be automatically considered to be in pain.

Two abnormalities are sought during the sensory examination: loss of sensation and increased sensation. Loss of sensation (hypesthesia, anesthesia) indicates a loss of conduction in sensory pathways (in peripheral nerves, spinal cord, or brain). The area of decreased sensation should be mapped carefully. If the hypesthesia is confined to one limb, the lesion is likely in either a named peripheral nerve or nerve roots (see Figures 2–3 and 2–26 for localization). Lesion of one peripheral nerve should produce hypesthesia in its autonomous zone. Lesion of only one nerve root or spinal cord segment may not produce a detectable deficit because of overlap by other roots in most areas. If the hypesthesia includes the trunk and limbs and is bilateral, the lesion is probably in the spinal cord. Interference with ascending pathways will cause decreased sensation caudal to the level of the lesion. Either the cutaneous reflex or behavioral response, or both, may be used to indicate the level of sensation. The level of normal sensation can be identified on the dermatomal map (see Fig. 2–3) to estimate the level of the lesion. This estimate should be accurate to within three spinal cord segments.

The presence of pain, hyperesthesia, indicates a pathologic change causing increased sensitivity of sensory neurons. The CNS parenchyma has no general somatic afferent nerve endings and hence is not the source of pain. Inflammation of any other tissue can cause pain. In diseases of the nervous system, pain is usually a sign of irritation of the meninges, peripheral nerves, or structures adjacent to the nervous system, such as vertebrae and disks. Localized pain usually reflects a process affecting the distribution of one spinal nerve. If the painful area can be mapped it will generally conform to the patterns of one to three dermatomes (see Fig. 2–3). Some generalized peripheral neuropathies and myopathies and meningeal inflammation cause generalized pain.

Peripheral neuropathies may make the animal hyperreactive to any stimulus. Inflammatory myopathies are characterized by muscles that are painful to deep palpation. Meningitis may cause a poorly localized, generalized pain, but the cervical region is often the most severely affected. Flexion of the neck is likely to cause a painful reaction.

Careful assessment of the boundaries of abnormal sensation can help localize the lesion accurately.

Complete absence of sensation, including deep pain, indicates severe damage to the nervous system. If the signs indicate that the lesion is in the spinal cord, the absence of deep pain should be considered a grave prognostic sign.

LOCALIZATION OF LESIONS

Motor Signs

After the neurologic examination is completed, the thoracic and pelvic limbs should be classified as normal or characterized by LMN or UMN signs (see Table 2–2). Briefly, signs of LMN disease consist of paresis, loss of reflexes, and loss of muscle tone. Signs of UMN disease include loss of voluntary motor activity, increased muscle tone, and normal or exaggerated reflexes. Localization to a region of the spinal cord or brain can be made using these findings in combination with the method in Table 2–8. For example, the presence of UMN signs in both thoracic and pelvic limbs indicates a brain or C1–C5 lesion. Table 2–8 suggests procedures to further localize the lesion. In this case, the cranial nerves should be evaluated to rule out brain stem disease, and the sensory examination should be reviewed for possible signs related to C1–C5.

If the neurologic examination is completed in the sequence previously described, the process of localization is done in stages. Postural reaction testing will indicate deficits in the thoracic limbs, pelvic limbs, or both. If only the pelvic limbs are affected, the lesion is caudal to T2. If both thoracic and pelvic limbs are affected, the lesion is cranial to T2. Deficits in the thoracic limbs with normal pelvic limbs indicate a lesion of C6–T2 gray matter, or more usually outside of the central nervous system.

In each example, spinal reflexes will determine the region affected. For a lesion caudal to T2, LMN signs in the pelvic limbs indicate an L4–S2 lesion. Normal or exaggerated reflexes in the pelvic limbs indicate a T3–L3 lesion.

Similar logic is used in the other examples illustrated in Table 2–8 and summarized in Table 2–9.

Using only the information related to LMN and UMN signs of the limbs it should be possible to localize the lesion to one of the following regions: (1) brain; (2) C1–C5; (3) C6–T2, brachial plexus (thoracic limb); (4) T2–L3; (5) L4–S2, lumbosacral plexus (pelvic limb); (6) S1–S3; (7) Cd1–5.

If LMN signs are present in the limbs, the lesion can be localized further by identifying the muscles affected. Table 2–10 lists the spinal cord segments (roots) and peripheral nerves identified by some of the most commonly tested reflexes. It may be possible to localize the lesion within two to four segments if LMN signs are present.

Spinal cord segments do not correlate directly with vertebral levels. When the spinal cord level is determined, refer to Figure 2–1 for an estimation of the vertebral level.

Sensory Signs

Conscious Proprioception

For purposes of localization, abnormalities of conscious proprioception are interpreted exactly the same as UMN signs. For example, loss of proprioception in the pelvic limbs with normal thoracic limbs indicates a lesion caudal to T2. Spinal nerve or peripheral nerve lesions may cause a loss of proprioceptive positioning, but spinal reflexes will be decreased.

Pain

Hyperesthesia, hypesthesia, and alterations in the cutaneous reflex are useful in localizing lesions, making a prognosis, and, in some instances, narrowing the list of diagnoses.

Many lesions of the spinal cord will cause an area of focal hyperesthesia corresponding to the dermatome of the affected spinal cord segment, a decrease in sensation caudal to the lesion, and a decreased cutaneous reflex caudal to the lesion. Any one of these three findings is useful, but when more than one is present and the levels coincide, confidence in the accuracy of localization increases. Many lesions can be localized to within three spinal cord segments or a named peripheral nerve.

The inability to perceive any painful stimulus, including hard pressure on a bone or joint, is a poor prognostic sign.

Table 2–8. LOCALIZATION OF LESION BASED ON MOTOR FUNCTION

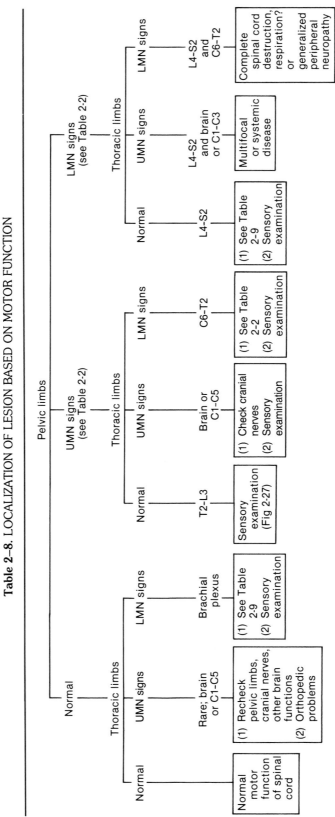

UMN, Upper motor neuron, LMN, Lower motor neuron; C, cervical; T, Thoracic; L, Lumbar; S, sacral spinal cord segments.
Modified from Hoerlein BF: Canine Neurology, 3rd ed. Philadelphia, WB Saunders Co, 1978.

Table 2–9. SIGNS OF LESIONS IN
NERVOUS SYSTEM

Cy1–5	LMN—tail
S1–3	UMN—tail
Pelvic plexus	LMN—anal sphincter, bladder
L4–S1	UMN—tail, bladder, sphincter
Lumbosacral plexus	LMN—pelvic limbs
T3–L3	UMN—pelvic limbs, bladder, sphincter
	LMN—segmental spinal muscles
C6–T2	UMN—pelvic limbs, bladder
Brachial plexus	LMN—thoracic limbs
C1–C6	UMN—all four limbs, bladder
Brain stem	UMN—unilateral or bilateral thoracic and pelvic limbs
	LMN—cranial nerves
Cerebellum	Ataxia, tremor, dysmetria
	Wide based stance
Vestibular system	Turning or circling
	Nystagmus, head tilt
	Ipsilateral weakness
Cerebrum	Behavior, seizures
	Blindness—normal pupils
	Postural reaction changes, contralateral

The presence of pain suggests certain types of diseases. The distribution of the pain may be even more helpful. Pain is one of the cardinal signs of inflammation and is frequently associated with the rapid distortion of tissues. Distortion of tissues, which activates nerve endings, includes distention of bowel; stretching of ligaments, tendons, or muscles; pressure on bone; and other similar change. In neurology, most of the painful problems are caused by spinal cord compressions or inflammatory disease. Inflammations may be meningeal or peripheral nerve. Inflammation of the CNS is not painful, unless the meninges are involved. Spinal cord compression causes pain by distortion of meninges, nerve roots, or surrounding structures such as ligaments, periosteum, or the anulus of the intervertebral disk. Most inflammations are diffuse or multifocal, whereas most compressions are focal.

Localization in Brain

If the lesion is localized to the brain it should be possible to specify one of five regions of the brain or the peripheral vestibular apparatus (Table 2–11).

Cerebrum

The cerebral hemispheres and basal nuclei are included in this classification. The cerebral cortex is the most highly developed part of the nervous system from a phylogenetic point of view. It has a complex organization and numerous specialized functions (Figs. 2–28 and 2–29). However, animals below the level of primates function in many ways quite normally without a cerebrum. Primary deficits that can be detected with lesions of the cerebrum include alterations in behavior and mentation, seizures, abnormal postural reactions with a relatively normal gait, facial hypesthesia, and loss of vision with normal pupillary light reflexes. Focal lesions may produce some of these signs. Unilateral lesions cause contralateral signs.

Compulsive pacing is usually a sign of prefrontal lobe abnormality. If the lesion is unilateral the pacing may be in a wide circle. Circling is not a localizing sign, because it can result from lesions in many areas of the brain. Most often the circling will be toward the side with the lesion, but there are many exceptions. It is preferable to use other findings to localize the lesion.

Table 2–10. SPINAL REFLEXES*

Reflex	Muscle	Peripheral Nerve	Spinal Cord Segments†
Myotatic (stretch)	Biceps brachii	Musculocutaneous	(C6), C7–C8, (T1)
	Triceps brachii	Radial	C7–C8, T1–(T2)
	Extensor carpi radialis	Radial	C7–C8, T1–(T2)
	Quadriceps	Femoral	(L3), L4–L5, (L6)
	Cranial tibial	Peroneal (sciatic)	L6–L7, S1
	Gastrocnemius	Tibial	L6–L7, S1
Flexion (withdrawal)	Thoracic limb	Radial, ulnar, median, musculocutaneous	C6–T2
	Pelvic limb	Sciatic	L6–S1 (S2)
Perineal	Anal sphincter	Pudendal	S1–S2, (S3)

*For the dog; other species may vary slightly.
†Parentheses indicate segments that sometimes contribute to a nerve.

Table 2–11. SIGNS OF LESIONS IN THE BRAIN

	Mental Status	Posture	Movement	Postural Reactions	Cranial Nerves
Cerebral cortex	Abnormal behavior, depression, seizures	Normal	Gait normal to slight hemiparesis (contralateral)	Deficits (contralateral)	Normal (vision and facial sensation may be impaired—contralateral)
Diencephalon (thalamus and hypothalamus)	Abnormal behavior, depression, (endocrine and autonomic)	Normal	Gait normal to hemiparesis or tetraparesis	Deficits (contralateral)	CN II
Brain stem (midbrain and medulla)	Depression, stupor, coma	Normal turning, falling	Hemiparesis to tetraparesis, ataxia	Deficits (ipsi- or contralateral)	CN III–CN XII
Vestibular, central (medulla)	Depression	Head tilt, falling	Hemiparesis (usually ipsilateral), ataxia	Deficits (ipsi- or contralateral)	CN VIII, may also affect CN V and CN VII, nystagmus
Vestibular, peripheral (labyrinth)	Normal	Head tilt	Normal to ataxia	Normal, although may be awkward	CN VIII, sometimes CN VII or Horner's syndrome, nystagmus
Cerebellum	Normal	Normal	Tremor, dysmetria, ataxia	Normal to dysmetria	Normal, may be menace reaction deficit or nystagmus

From Oliver JE Jr and Lorenz MD: Handbook of Veterinary Neurologic Diagnosis. Philadelphia, WB Saunders Co, 1983.

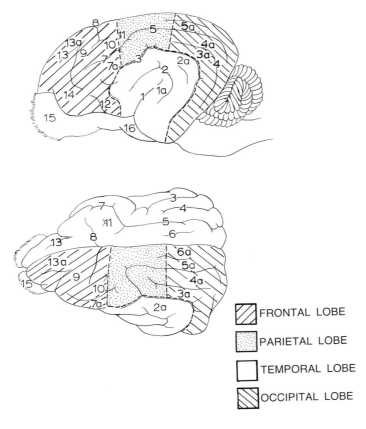

Figure 2–28. Cerebral cortex of the dog. Lobes are approximate. 1, Pseudosylvian fissure; 1a, caudal sylvian gyrus; 2, ectosylvian sulcus; 2a, ectosylvian gyrus; 3, suprasylvian sulcus; 3a, suprasylvian gyrus; 4, ectomarginal sulcus; 4a, ectomarginal gyrus; 5, marginal sulcus; 5a, marginal gyrus; 6, endomarginal sulcus; 6a, endomarginal gyrus; 7, coronal sulcus; 7a, rostral suprasylvian gyrus; 8, cruciate sulcus; 9, precruciate gyrus; 10, postcruciate gyrus; 11, ansate sulcus; 12, presylvian sulcus; 13, prorean sulcus; 13a, prorean gyrus; 14, prorean gyrus; 15, olfactory bulb; 16, piriform lobe.

FRONTAL LOBE

PARIETAL LOBE

TEMPORAL LOBE

OCCIPITAL LOBE

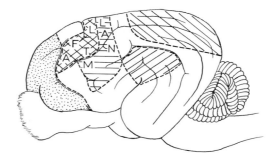

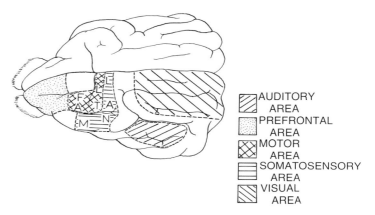

Figure 2–29. Functional areas of the cerebral cortex of the dog. F, Face; A, arm (thoracic limb); M, mouth and tongue; T, trunk; L, leg (pelvic limb); N, nose.

AUDITORY AREA

PREFRONTAL AREA

MOTOR AREA

SOMATOSENSORY AREA

VISUAL AREA

Epileptic seizures usually signify a cerebral abnormality (see Chapter 10).

The key findings in cerebral disease are altered behavior, depression, normal or nearly normal gait with postural reaction deficits, loss of vision with normal pupillary light reflexes, and seizures.

Diencephalon

The diencephalon includes the thalamus and hypothalamus. Anatomically, the diencephalon is part of the brain stem. From a clinical view, it is more like the cerebrum. The thalamus functions as a relay center for the cortex. The hypothalamus is unique and controls the autonomic and endocrine systems of the body.

Lesions of the thalamus generally cause signs similar to lesions of the cerebrum. Hypothalamic dysfunction may produce a variety of autonomic and endocrine disturbances.

The key findings in lesions of the diencephalon are altered behavior; normal or nearly normal gait with postural reaction deficits; loss of vision, usually with normal pupillary light reflexes; autonomic and endocrine dysfunction, such as polyuria, polydipsia, hyperphagia; poor temperature regulation; and altered sleep patterns.

Brain Stem

The brain stem includes the midbrain, pons, and medulla oblongata. The diencephalon, which is a part of the brain stem anatomically, is functionally different. The brain stem is structurally an extension of the spinal cord with some modification to accommodate special groups of neurons.

The locomotor function of quadripeds is located in the midbrain. Normal gait is dependent on this region. Therefore, brain stem disease is usually characterized by an abnormal gait, as well as abnormal postural reactions. This is a significant difference from cerebral and diencephalic lesions. The abnormalities will be UMN in character and will affect all four limbs (tetraparesis) or both of the limbs on one side (hemiparesis), depending on the extent of the lesion.

Lesions of the brain stem that disrupt the connections of the reticular activating system with the cerebral cortex will cause decreased levels of consciousness, ranging from depression to coma.

Cranial nerves III to XII originate in the brain stem. Changes in function of any of these cranial nerves are the best evidence for brain stem disease. If there is a cranial nerve abnormality accompanied by any degree of paresis or loss of mental status, brain stem disease should be suspected. Cranial nerves V and VII have both sensory and motor functions. Peripheral lesions will usually affect both sensory and motor functions. Central lesions often affect either sensory or motor function but not usually both. There are exceptions, however, and the UMN paresis and alterations in consciousness are better indicators of brain stem disease.

The key findings in lesions of the brain stem are abnormal gait and postural reactions, decreased level of consciousness, and, most significantly, cranial nerve abnormalities (CN III–CN XII).

Vestibular System

The vestibular system is concerned with maintenance of posture with respect to gravity and with coordinating eye movements with head movement. The primary diagnostic concern is to differentiate peripheral (labyrinth, receptor, vestibular nerve) disease from central (vestibular nuclei, brain stem) disease.

Unilateral vestibular disease is characterized by an asymmetric ataxia, head tilt, nystagmus, and sometimes falling, rolling, circling, and strabismus. The primary difference between peripheral vestibular disease and central vestibular disease is signs of brain stem disease in the latter. Lesions of the vestibular nucleus will almost invariably affect sensory or motor pathways, causing paresis or postural reaction deficits. Peripheral disease only involves the receptors in the inner ear and does not alter postural reactions. However, in peripheral disease, the performance of postural reactions may seem more awkward because of the loss of balance and disorientation. Paresis will not be present, however. (See Table 2–7 and Vestibulocochlear Nerve [CN VIII] for more details.)

Cerebellum

The cerebellum coordinates movements. It governs the rate and range of voluntary and involuntary movements but does not initiate motor activity. Lesions of the cerebellum cause incoordination without paresis. All of the signs of cerebellar disease are related to alterations in coordination. Dysmetria describes a movement that is too long or too short. Common examples include a goose-stepping gait and sticking the nose too far into the water while trying to drink. Tremor consists of smaller repetitive movements that are also caused by a lack of coordination. In cerebellar disease the tremor is generally worse when the animal initiates a movement (intention tremor). Ataxia describes uncoordinated movements. Cerebellar ataxia is characterized by a wide based stance, dysmetria, and intention tremor. Some degree of abnormal motion of the head should be present to differentiate cerebellar disease from spinal cord disease. Nystagmus may occur in cerebellar disease. It is usually a tremor of the eye without a fast-slow component. The nystagmus is accentuated when the animal shifts its gaze and fixates on a new field.

Diffuse cerebellar disease may cause a deficit in the menace reaction with normal vision and normal palpebral reflexes. The cerebellar nuclei are apparently involved in a conditioned response such as the blink response,[14] and the cerebellum appears to be involved in the menace response. It is important to recognize that an animal with cerebellar disease is not blind in spite of the deficient menace reaction. Otherwise, the visual pathway would be involved, suggesting a more diffuse disease process.

Acute cerebellar lesions, such as may occur in head trauma, cause a completely different clinical picture. Pure cerebellar trauma is unusual because the cerebellum is well protected in the skull. Head injuries are more likely to cause cerebral or brain stem signs. Acute lesions, particularly involving the rostral lobe, cause increased extensor tone of the thoracic limbs, flexion of the pelvic limbs, and opisthotonos. This posture must be differentiated from decerebration (transection of the brain stem near the midbrain or pons), which causes increased extensor tone in all four limbs. Animals with decerebrate posture are usually comatose. Decerebellate animals will be conscious unless there is concomitant brain stem injury.

Lesions of the flocculonodular lobes cause signs of vestibular disease. Lesions near the cerebellar peduncles may cause signs of vestibular disease with the head tilt away from the side with the lesions, so-called paradoxic vestibular disease. (See Vestibulocochlear Nerve [CN VIII] for more details.)

Systemic or Multifocal Disease

When the clinical signs are not consistent with a single focal lesion in the nervous system, the animal has systemic or multifocal disease. Many degenerative and inflammatory diseases will fall into this category. Toxic, metabolic, nutritional, and neoplastic diseases may be multifocal or diffuse in distribution.

Peripheral Spinal Nerve Disease (Monoparesis)

If a monoparesis with LMN signs is found, then specific nerve roots, nerve, group of nerves, or muscles are affected. The origin, distribution, function, and signs with injury are outlined in Tables 2–12 and 2–13. Figure 2–26 illustrates the cutaneous innervation of the limbs. By carefully mapping the distribution of motor and sensory deficits an accurate diagnosis can be made. Figures 14–6 to 14–14, 14–16, and 14–17 demonstrate the primary motor deficit of the various nerve injuries in the dog; specific syndromes affecting peripheral nerves are discussed in Chapter 14. The use of electrodiagnostic tests in assessing peripheral nerve disorders is discussed in Chapter 5.

THE DIAGNOSTIC PLAN

The diagnostic plan must be formulated based on the approach outlined in Table 2–1.

Minimum Data Base. The minimum data base (MDB) is the set of data necessary to solve most problems. The minimum data base can be problem specific, that is, different data are collected on each patient depending on the problem; or it can be the same for all sick patients examined. A data base for small animals with neurologic problems is listed in Table 2–14.

Problems. The problems are identified next. The most common problems associated with diseases of the nervous system are listed in Table 2–15. Appendix I cites the more common diseases causing these problems and a reference to the chapter in which the disease is discussed.

Localization. After identifying the problem, the neurologic examination provides the information necessary to localize the lesion (see Tables 2–8 and 2–11).

Etiology. The signalment and history provide the basic information to identify probable causes of the problem. It is useful to think in general terms first, then focus on specific causes later. A mnemonic is useful as a checklist of mechanisms of disease (Table 2–16). Most of these categories of diseases will have a typical history in terms of onset and progression (see Fig. 2–4). By classifying the animal's problem as to

Table 2–12. NERVES OF THE BRACHIAL PLEXUS*

Nerve	Spinal Cord Segments	Motor Function	Cutaneous Sensory Distribution	Signs of Dysfunction
Suprascapular	C6–C7	Extension and lateral support of shoulder	—	Little gait abnormality, pronounced atrophy of supra- and infraspinatus muscles (sweeny)
Axillary	C6–C7–C8	Flexion of the shoulder	Dorsolateral brachium	Little gait abnormality, decreased shoulder flexor reflex, analgesia on lateral side of limb
Musculocutaneous	C6–C7–C8	Flexion of the elbow	Medial side of the forelimb	Little gait abnormality—weakened flexion of the elbow, analgesia on medial surface of the forelimb
Radial	C6, C7–C8, T1–T2	Extension of the elbow, carpus, and digits	Dorsal surface of paw and dorsal and lateral parts of forelimb	Loss of weight bearing, paw and carpus knuckle over, weakened triceps reflex, analgesia of dorsal surface of paw and forelimb
Median and Ulnar	C8, T1–T2	Flexion of the carpus and digits	Palmar surface of paw, caudal forelimb	Little gait abnormality, slight sinking of the carpus and fetlock, loss of carpal flexion on withdrawal reflex, partial loss of sensation of palmar surface of the paw
Sympathetic†	T1, T2, T3	Dilation of the pupil	—	Miosis, ptosis, and enophthalmia

Numbers in *italics* indicate the major cord segment that forms the peripheral nerve.

*Based on the dog.

†The sympathetic nerve is not considered a part of the brachial plexus; however, its nerve fibers travel along the roots of the brachial plexus as they exit from the vertebral column.

Modified from Oliver JE Jr and Lorenz MD: Handbook of Veterinary Neurologic Diagnosis. Philadelphia, WB Saunders Co, 1983.

Table 2–13. NERVES OF THE LUMBOSACRAL PLEXUS*

Nerve	Spinal Cord Segments	Motor Function	Cutaneous Sensory Distribution	Signs of Dysfunction
Obturator	L4, *L5, L6*	Adduction of pelvic limb	—	Little gait abnormality on normal surfaces; limb may slide laterally on slick surfaces
Femoral	L3, *L4, L5,* L6	Extension of the stifle	Saphenous branch, supplies medial digit and medial surface of limb	Severe gait dysfunction, absence of weight bearing, decreased or absent knee jerk, loss of sensation of medial digit and medial surface or rear limb
Sciatic	L6, *L6, L7; S1, S2*	Flexion and extension of the hip; flexion of the stifle; see tibial and peroneal branches	Caudal and lateral sides of true limb; see tibial and peroneal branches	Severe gait dysfunction; paw is knuckled over but weight bearing occurs; hock cannot be flexed or extended; hip cannot be extended; in more central lesions, hip is flexed and drawn toward the midline; cutaneous desensitization below the stifle, except for areas supplied by the saphenous nerve; absent withdrawal reflex
Peroneal	L5, *L6, L7,* S1, S2	Flexion of the hock, extension of the digits	Dorsal aspect of paw, hock, and distal limb	†Hock is straightened and paw tends to knuckle over; loss of sensation to dorsal aspects of paw, hock, and distal limb; poor hock flexion on withdrawal reflex
Tibial	L5, L6, *L7, S1,* S2	Extension of the hock; flexion of the digits	Plantar surface of the paw	†Hock is dropped; loss of sensation of plantar surface of paw

Numbers in *italics* indicate the major cord segment that forms the peripheral nerve.
*Based on the dog.
†Peroneal and tibial nerve paralysis commonly occur in association with each other. The signs of peroneal nerve damage tend to predominate.
Modified from Oliver JE Jr and Lorenz MD: Handbook of Veterinary Neurologic Diagnosis. Philadelphia, WB Saunders Co, 1983.

onset and course, a small group of probable diagnoses is suggested. The age, species, breed, and sex of the animal narrow the possibilities. Finally, the localization of the process in the nervous system and performance of diagnostic tests will be helpful (Table 2–17).

All of this information should reduce the probable diagnosis to no more than three categories of disease. The best diagnostic tests for each of the major groups of diseases are listed in Table 2–18. There are exceptions within each group, but this table can serve as a guide. It is most important to have a logical approach to

Table 2–14. MINIMUM DATA BASE: NEUROLOGIC PROBLEMS OF SMALL ANIMALS

History
Physical examination
Neurologic examination
Clinical pathology
  CBC
  Urinalysis
  Chemistry profile
    BUN
    SGPT
    Calcium
    Alkaline phosphatase
    Fasting blood glucose
    Total serum protein albumin

Table 2–15. COMMON CLINICAL PROBLEMS INVOLVING THE NERVOUS SYSTEM

Pelvic limb paresis
Tetraparesis, hemiparesis
Ataxia of head and limbs
Disorders of face, tongue, and larynx
Head tilt
Blindness, anisocoria, and abnormal eye movements
Stupor or coma
Seizures and narcolepsy
Behavioral abnormalities
Systemic and multifocal signs
Incontinence

Table 2–16. CHECKLIST OF DISEASE MECHANISMS

D	Degenerative
	Demyelinating
A	Anomalous
M	Metabolic
N	Neoplastic
	Nutritional
I	Inflammatory
	Idiopathic
T	Traumatic
	Toxic
V	Vascular

Table 2–17. DATA USEFUL FOR ETIOLOGIC DIAGNOSIS

Signalment
  Age
  Sex
  Species, breed
  Use
History
  Onset
  Course
  Environment
Examination
  Location and extent of lesion
Diagnostic Aids
  Clinical laboratory profile
  Cerebrospinal fluid examination
  Radiography
  Electrophysiology

Table 2–18. SELECTION OF DIAGNOSTIC TESTS

	Diagnostic Tests	
Disease Category	*Useful*	*Usually Diagnostic*
Degenerative		
Brain	EEG, CSF	Biopsy
Spinal cord	Myelography, CSF	None
Vertebrae	CSF	Radiography, myelography
Demyelinating		
Brain	EEG, CSF	Biopsy
Spinal cord	Myelography, CSF	None
Peripheral nerve	EMG, EDT	Biopsy
Anomalous		
Brain	Examination	Radiography, contrast radiography
Spinal cord	Radiography	Myelography
Vertebrae	Examination	Radiography
Metabolic	History	Clinical laboratory profile
Neoplastic		
Brain	EEG, radiography	Arteriography, scans
Spinal cord	CSF, radiography	Myelography
Peripheral nerve	EDT	Biopsy
Nutritional	History	Radiography
Inflammatory	History, examination	CSF, serology, microbiologic isolation
Traumatic	History, examination	Radiography
Toxic	History	Clinical laboratory profile, toxicologic identification

From Oliver JE Jr and Lorenz MD: Handbook of Veterinary Neurologic Diagnosis. Philadelphia, WB Saunders Co, 1983.

identifying the problem and selecting the diagnostic tests. Chapters 3 through 5 describe these tests in detail.

Appendix I lists the diseases of each species by whether they are acute or chronic and progressive or nonprogressive, with the chapter in which each disease is discussed.

REFERENCES

1. Adams RD and Victor M: Principles of Neurology. New York, McGraw-Hill Book Co, 1977.
2. Blood DC, Henderson JA, and Radostits OM: Veterinary Medicine, 5th ed. Philadelphia, Lea & Febiger, 1979.
2a. Blyth, LL: Personal communication.
3. Chrisman CL: Problems in Small Animal Neurology. Philadelphia, Lea & Febiger, 1982.
4. deLahunta A: Veterinary Neuroanatomy and Clinical Neurology, 2nd ed. Philadelphia, WB Saunders Co, 1983.
4a. Fletcher TF, Purinton PT, and Oliver JE Jr: Unpublished observations.
5. Greene CE and Oliver JE: Neurologic examination. In Ettinger SJ: Textbook of Veterinary Internal Medicine, 2nd ed. Philadelphia, WB Saunders Co, 1983.
6. Hoff HE and Breckenridge CG: Observations on the mammalian reflex prototype of the sign of Babinski. Brain 79:155, 1956.
7. Jenkins TW: Functional Mammalian Neuroanatomy, 2nd ed. Philadelphia, Lea & Febiger, 1978.
8. Kitchell, RL: Misconceptions in neurology. Proc AVNA, NY, 1983.
9. Kitchell RL, Whalen LR, Bailey CS, and Lohse CL: Electrophysiological studies of cutaneous nerves of the thoracic limb of the dog. Am J Vet Res 41:61, 1980.
10. Kneller SK, Oliver JE, and Lewis RE: Differential diagnosis of progressive caudal paresis in an aged German shepherd dog. JAAHA 11:414, 1975.
11. Low DG, Osborne CA, and Finco DR: The pillars of diagnosis: History and physical examination. In Ettinger SJ: Textbook of Veterinary Internal Medicine. Philadelphia, WB Saunders Co, 1975.
12. Mayhew IG: Neurologic evaluation of food producing animals. In Howard JL: Current Veterinary Therapy: Food Animal Practice. Philadelphia, WB Saunders Co, 1981.
13. Mayhew IG and MacKay RJ: The nervous system. In Mausmann RA, McAllister ES, and Pratt PW (eds): Equine Medicine and Surgery, 3rd ed. Santa Barbara, CA, American Veterinary Publications, Inc, 1982.
14. McCormick DA and Thompson RF: Cerebellum: Essential involvement in the classically conditioned eyelid response. Science 223:296, 1984.
15. Oliver JE Jr: Localization of lesions in the nervous system. In Hoerlein BJ: Canine Neurology, 3rd ed. Philadelphia, WB Saunders Co, 1978.
16. Oliver JE Jr: State of the art: Stupor or coma. Proc 2nd ACVIM Forum, Washington, DC, 1984.
17. Oliver JE Jr and Lorenz MD: Handbook of Veterinary Neurologic Diagnosis. Philadelphia, WB Saunders Co, 1983.
18. Osborne CA and Low DG: The medical history redefined: Idealism vs. realism. Proc AAHA 207, 1976.
19. Palmer AC: Introduction to Animal Neurology, 2nd ed. Oxford, Blackwell Scientific Publications, 1976.
20. Renegar WR: Auriculopalpebral nerve paralysis following prolonged anesthesia in a dog. JAVMA 174:1007, 1979.
21. Scaglioti, RH: Neuro-ophthalmology. In Kirk RW: Current Veterinary Therapy VII. Philadelphia, WB Saunders Co, 1980.
22. Shik ML and Orlovsky GN: Neurophysiology of locomotor automatism. Physiol Rev 56:465, 1976.
23. Stein PSG: Motor systems with specific reference to control of locomotion. Ann Rev Neurosci 1:61, 1978.
24. Whalen LR and Kitchell RL: Electrophysiologic studies of the cutaneous nerves of the head of the dog. Am J Vet Res 44:615, 1983.
25. Willis WD and Coggeshall RE: Sensory Mechanisms of the Spinal Cord. New York, Plenum Press, 1978.

Chapter 3

JR Duncan, DVM, PhD
JE Oliver, Jr, DVM, MS, PhD
IG Mayhew, BVSc, PhD

Laboratory Examinations

To establish a diagnosis of a primary neurologic disease, laboratory examination results must be correlated with historical findings and observations from physical, neurologic, and radiologic examinations. Hematologic and serum chemistry findings are seldom diagnostic in primary neurologic disease, but they are often helpful or even essential in the differential diagnosis of diseases that secondarily cause central nervous system signs. Because of its intimate contact with the CNS, cerebrospinal fluid may be altered in many diseases involving the brain and spinal cord. It is, however, usually futile to base a diagnosis solely on CSF findings.

HEMATOLOGY

Hematologic findings associated with neurologic disease are confirmatory at best. An inflammatory-type leukocyte response may or may not be evident in the peripheral blood during inflammatory CNS diseases. Likewise, stress leukograms are inconclusive in both inflammatory and traumatic diseases. Eosinophilia may or may not accompany parasitic diseases.

Polycythemia vera, characterized by an increase in erythrocyte mass and an increase in packed cell volume, hemoglobin concentration, and red blood cell count, may be accompanied by CNS signs caused by the increased viscosity of the blood. Hematopoietic neoplasia involving the CNS may present a leukemic blood picture. Anemia can result in weakness that may modify or exacerbate CNS signs already present. Lead

poisoning has CNS manifestations associated with peripheral blood findings of mild anemia, metarubricytosis, and basophilic stippling.

SERUM CHEMISTRY

Alterations in the concentrations of certain serum constituents that occur secondary to a variety of diseases may be responsible for CNS signs, which may be confused with those caused by primary neurologic diseases. These alterations or diseases include hyperglycemia, hypoglycemia, hypercalcemia, hypocalcemia, hypomagnesemia, uremia, hyperammonemia and hepatic encephalopathy, hyperadrenocorticism, hypoadrenocorticism, hypothyroidism, plasma osmolality disturbances, and acid-base imbalances. Analysis of appropriate serum chemistry parameters is essential for the diagnosis of these diseases. The minimum data base profile will be sufficient to point to many, but others will require a more specific plan for a laboratory diagnosis (see Table 2–14). These diseases are discussed in Chapter 8.

CEREBROSPINAL FLUID

Collection in Small Animals

CSF is obtained by puncture of the cerebellomedullary cistern between the occipital bone and the atlas. Lumbar puncture (L5–L6, L6–L7) is used for myelography, and a sample may be obtained for analysis. However, lumbar puncture is more difficult to perform, and contamination of the sample with blood occurs more frequently. The L7–S1 interspace can be used to obtain fluid from most cats.

The animal should be placed under general anesthesia and intubated to prevent movement. The procedure described is for a right-handed person. The animal is placed in right lateral recumbency near the edge of the table. The area from the occiput to C2, laterally to the ears, is surgically prepared. An assistant holds the head flexed at a right angle to the vertebral column with the nose parallel to the table top. Immediately after positioning, the animal should be observed for adequate ventilation. Excessive flexion of the head is unnecessary and may occlude the airway.

Sterile gloves, two 3 ml syringes, and a 21 gauge, 1.5 inch disposable spinal needle with stylet are needed. Giant breed dogs may require a 2.5 inch needle. The landmarks for puncture are the occipital protuberance and the spinous process of the axis (to identify the midline) and the wings of the atlas. If the following procedure is adhered to the needle and CSF will not be contaminated, and the tap can be performed with maximum safety. The occipital protuberance and spine of the axis (both aseptically prepared areas) should be identified with the index finger and thumb of the left hand. The other three fingers of the left hand are placed on the cranial margin of the wing of the atlas (may not be prepared). Holding the needle by the hub with the notch of the stylet cranially (the notch identifies the bevel of the needle), the needle is inserted on the midline on a line even with the cranial margin of the wings of the atlas. The space between the occipital bone and arch of the atlas can be directly palpated in animals that are not heavily muscled. The first insertion should be through the skin only. Then the needle is directed toward the nose of the animal, maintaining a midline position. As soon as the needle is through the skin, the shaft of the needle is grasped by the index finger and thumb of the left hand. This grasp is not released until the procedure is completed; it prevents motion of the needle during all manipulations. Fascial planes will be felt as they are penetrated. With puncture of the atlantooccipital membrane and dura mater, a loss of resistance is noted; however, this sign is not reliable. The stylet is removed at 2 to 3 mm intervals to observe for flow of fluid, which is the only reliable sign of successful puncture.

If the needle strikes bone, it is withdrawn

slightly and redirected cranially or caudally. If the needle is on the occipital bone, succeeding penetrations in a caudal direction will be slightly deeper because of the angle of the bone. If the needle is on the atlas, the needle will penetrate to the same depth each time, as the arch of the atlas is approximately parallel to the skin. The shaft of the needle is grasped with the index finger and thumb of the left hand at all times.

When fluid flows into the hub of the needle it is carefully aspirated with a syringe. The syringe should not be attached to the needle. Negative pressure usually causes occlusion of the needle and frequently causes hemorrhage. One to 2 ml is collected for laboratory analysis. Using the second syringe one can obtain 1 ml for culture and sensitivity testing, if needed. Both syringes are capped with sterile needles in their covers.

If pressure is to be measured, a three way valve is attached before any fluid is collected. A spinal manometer is attached to the valve, and fluid is allowed to rise in the manometer. The reading is taken at the bottom of the meniscus. Pulsations of the fluid indicate that the needle is patent. The authors do not routinely measure pressure. The additional manipulation may cause blood contamination, and the information obtained is not worth the risk.

If whole blood flows into the needle, the needle should be discarded and another attempt made. If there is blood in the CSF, the procedure is to collect 1 to 2 ml, change syringes, and collect another 1 to 2 ml. The second sample frequently has little or no blood and can be used for analysis, while the first can be used for culture. Continuous bloody CSF may indicate a pathologic condition. Centrifugation will leave a clear supernatant if the blood was a result of the tap.

Collection in Large Animals

The principles of collection of CSF in large animals are the same as those described for small animals. The atlantooccipital or lumbosacral subarachnoid space may be used in all large animals. Atlantooccipital puncture usually requires general anesthesia, except in markedly depressed animals. Fluid should be collected as close to the suspected lesion as possible.

For atlanto-occipital puncture, palpable landmarks include the external occipital protuberance and the cranial borders of the wings of the atlas. The head is flexed at right angles to the neck and the needle inserted on the midline, even with the cranial border of the wings of the atlas and perpendicular to the neck. An 18 to 22 gauge, 3.5 inch spinal needle is used in large patients. In young animals, a 20 gauge, 1.5 inch disposable needle with a plastic hub is recommended.

Lumbosacral puncture may be made in unanesthetized animals, either standing (adults) or in lateral recumbency (smaller animals). Local anesthetic is recommended in horses. A stab incision or 16 gauge needle puncture is made in the skin. Palpable landmarks include the spinous processes of the last lumbar vertebra and the sacrum and the cranial edge of the sacral tuberosities laterally. The needle is inserted on the midline in the depression bounded by these structures. An 18 to 22 gauge needle is used. Length of the needle varies with the size of the animal, ranging from 2.5 inches in smaller animals, to 3.5 inches in ponies and smaller cattle, to 8 inches in most light breed horses. Tail movement and slight response by the patient usually accompany penetration of the dura mater and arachnoid membrane.[7]

Laboratory Examination of Cerebrospinal Fluid

Gross Examination

Normal cerebrospinal fluid is clear and colorless. Red coloration indicates hemorrhage, either iatrogenic or pathologic. The most important laboratory finding in substantiating subarachnoid hemorrhage is the demonstration of erythrocytes or hemoglobin breakdown products in the CSF. Erythrocyte levels of at least 6000/μl are required before the CSF is grossly bloody, and at least 200,000/μl with an appropriate amount of plasma are required for clot formation.

Prior hemorrhage must be differentiated from a traumatic tap. Red tinged CSF that is clear during the latter part of aspiration or fluid that clears on centrifugation suggests a bloody tap. Erythrocytes rapidly degenerate within the CSF; therefore, the demonstration of xanthochromia or crenated erythrocytes is most important in ruling out a traumatic tap.

Xanthochromia is defined as the presence of a yellow-orange pigment in the supernatant of a centrifuged tube of CSF. It is caused by blood pigments, either bilirubin or oxyhemoglobin. Xanthochromia also may occur spuriously with high protein levels (>400 mg/dl). Bilirubin appears in the CSF approximately 48 hours after an episode of bleeding and may persist for up to 3 to 4 weeks. Oxyhemoglobin is derived from lysed erythrocytes, forms in 2 to 4 hours, peaks at 24 to 36 hours, and persists for 4 to 8 days. Xanthochromia is a strong indicator of subarachnoid hemorrhage if it occurs in the absence of icterus or hyperbilirubinemia. Conjugated bilirubin may pass into the CSF from the blood in liver disease. Xanthochromia is associated with trauma, vascular disorders, and infections involving the CNS.

Turbidity of the CSF is usually caused by the presence of cells, usually greater than 500/μl. Microorganisms and protein may contribute to the turbidity.

Protein Concentration

Excessive protein in the CSF may be suggested by the presence of foam following agitation or by a positive urine reagent strip test result for protein (100 mg/dl or more). An increased refractive index may suggest increased protein but may also be caused by cells or other solids. Qualitative screening tests include the Pandy and Nonne-Apelt tests, which are based on the precipitation of globulin by a 10% carbolic acid solution or saturated ammonium sulfate, respectively. These tests are rather insensitive to albumin.

The commonly used biuret method for serum protein determination is too insensitive to measure the milligram quantities of protein found in CSF. The turbidimetric method using trichloroacetic acid is equally sensitive to albumin and globulin and has been used to quantitate total CSF protein.[11] Dye binding methods allow for colorimetric quantitation of small amounts of protein.[17] The ponceau S[14] and Coomassie brilliant blue G-250[1] dye binding methods have been adapted for animal use.

For separation and quantitation of the various protein fractions, electrophoresis and a variety of immunologic techniques have been used. Some of these techniques have been developed for animals using normal CSF,[12] but significant immunochemical testing has not been done in diseased animals.

Most proteins of normal CSF are derived from the blood, and their concentrations are determined by their molecular size and relative permeability of the blood-brain barrier.[4] Normal CSF protein is usually less than 25 mg/dl in the dog and cat; 60 mg/dl in the pig, sheep, goat, and cow; and 100 mg/dl in the horse.

Protein levels in the CSF may be increased in neurologic dysfunctions that affect the permeability of the blood-CSF barrier (eg, meningitis and tumors) or that cause an increase in production of IgG locally within the CNS (eg, certain infectious or inflammatory disorders of the CNS). Measurement of total CSF protein can provide useful information about the presence of a disorder, but quantitation of the various protein fractions may be necessary to differentiate leakage of plasma proteins across the blood-CSF barrier from increased synthesis within the CNS. Comparison of protein values of simultaneous atlantooccipital and lumbosacral collections may aid in localizing a lesion; the location closest to the lesion should have the highest value.

Enzyme Measurement

Enzyme activity has been measured in the CSF to detect CNS damage.[15] The blood-brain barrier is significantly impermeable to enzymes in either direction. Cerebrospinal fluid activity of lactic dehydrogenase (LDH), alanine aminotransferase (ALT), aspartate aminotransferase (AST), and creatine kinase (CK) has been shown to increase in some instances of CNS disease. Although CSF enzymes may be helpful in establishing whether CNS damage has occurred, they do not distinguish between diseases nor do normal values rule out disease.[18]

Neural tissue contains only the BB isoenzyme of CK. This isoenzyme apparently is responsible for the CK activity of normal CSF. In humans, there has been no correlation between the level of CK activity in CSF and the extent, severity, or type of disease. The lesion usually must communicate with the CSF before there is an elevation in CK activity.

Glucose Determination and Other Chemical Analyses

Glucose concentration in the cerebrospinal fluid is dependent on the serum glucose concentration; therefore, CSF glucose analysis should always be done simultaneously with blood glucose determination. CSF levels are usually 60 to 80% of blood levels.[3] Decreased CSF glucose concentration may be associated with bacterial meningitis, in which pyogenic microorganisms and possibly neutrophils utilize glucose and lower the CSF concentration in relation to that of the blood. Cytologic examination and culture are, however, much more reliable means of diagnosing bacterial meningitis.

Levels of CSF electrolytes should also always be measured concurrently with blood electrolytes. Some are normally higher (eg, sodium, chloride, magnesium) and others lower (eg, calcium, potassium) than in the blood.[3] CSF sodium levels may be increased (>160–200 mEq/l) in water deprivation syndrome of swine.[8]

Urea and creatinine levels usually parallel those found in the blood.

Total Blood Cell Count

Determinations must be done soon (within 30 minutes) after collection. Cells degenerate rapidly because the low protein content fails to support them. One side of a hemocytometer counting chamber is charged with well-mixed, undiluted CSF, and the cells within all nine primary squares are counted. The number of cells counted is multiplied by 1.1 to give the total cell count per cubic millimeter. The experienced technologist may be able to differentiate leukocytes and erythrocytes and derive counts of these cell types from the same chamber. Leukocytes are large and granular, whereas erythrocytes are small, refractile, and sometimes crenated.

If leukocytes and erythrocytes cannot be readily differentiated, the cells may be suspended in a diluting fluid (0.2 g crystal violet in 100 ml of a 10% glacial acetic acid solution), which lyses the erythrocytes and stains the leukocytes. This is accomplished with a white blood cell pipet by drawing the diluting fluid to the 1 mark and then drawing CSF to the 11 mark. After mixing and discharging a few drops of the mixture, the other side of the hemocytometer is charged and the nine primary squares counted. Because the CSF has been diluted by a factor of 1.1, the cells counted are multiplied by 1.2 (1.1 × 1.1) to derive a total leukocyte count per cubic millimeter. This count can be subtracted from the total cell count obtained from the other chamber and an erythrocyte count derived.

Often leukocytes are contaminants of the CSF from a bloody tap. Crude methods are used to gain some impression of the effect of this contamination on the actual total white blood cell count. Because leukocytes and erythrocytes are in the blood at a ratio of approximately 1:500, one leukocyte may be subtracted from the CSF white cell count for every 500 erythrocytes present.[5] Other correction formulas take into consideration the peripheral blood leukocyte count. These formulas are usually unreliable and are probably unnecessary because blood contamination of several thousand erythrocytes appears to have little effect on leukocyte numbers and protein concentration.[16]

Differential Cell Count

A differential cell count is indicated with any increase in the nucleated cell count (pleocytosis). Because CSF is relatively cell poor, concentration procedures are necessary to obtain a sufficient number of cells to perform a reliable differential count. These procedures include centrifugation and direct smear, sedimentation, membrane filtration, and cytocentrifugation.

Centrifugation and Direct Smear. The CSF is centrifuged at 1000 rpm for 5 minutes, and the supernatant is removed for chemical analysis. The sediment is resuspended in a drop of homologous serum or 20% albumin to stabilize the cells and prevent drying artifacts, and a smear is made. The smear can be stained with any of the hematologic stains.

Membrane Filtration. Membrane filters with pore sizes of 5 μ can be used for cytologic study.[9] These filters retain on their surface a large percentage of the cells present in the CSF in a morphologic state suitable for differentiation. This procedure gives the best quantitative yield, but cytomorphology is not as well preserved as with sedimentation. A variety of vacuum and filter systems are available. A simple procedure uses a Swinny adapter and small barrel syringe.[7] Up to 1 ml of CSF is fixed immediately after collection in 2 ml of 40% ethanol. The solution is placed in the syringe and allowed to drip through the filter apparatus by gravity or by gentle force with the syringe plunger at the rate of 1 drop per second. The membrane may become plugged if excessive cells or protein is present, but by this time sufficient cells usually have been collected. Excessive pressure causes cellular distortion. The filter is removed and immersed in 95% alcohol for at least 2 minutes. A variety of stains may be used, but because of the prefixation of the cells and the affinity of the membrane for certain stains, the Romanowsky hematologic stains are not appropriate. The quick hematoxylin and eosin stain requires only a few minutes, whereas the more complicated Papanicolaou stain takes longer and requires more solutions.[2] The latter two stains enhance nuclear detail better than other stains; therefore, they are better for neoplastic cells. Cells that are prefixed, as in this procedure, do not expand as much; thus, they are smaller than cells in preparations that are air dried and postfixed. Cells in air dried preparations have less clear nuclear detail.

With the filter technique some cells may become trapped within the pore and cannot be identified. More focusing is necessary because cells will be in slightly different planes on the filter. Improper clearing of the filter will also make identification difficult. Specimens high in protein will have a dark stained background that also makes visualization of cells difficult. The use of prefixed CSF allows a longer period of time between collection and cytologic preparation because degeneration of cells does not occur.

Sedimentation. A variety of glass or plastic cylinders can be used to hold the CSF during cellular sedimentation. The cylinder may be sealed to the slide by first dipping one end in melted paraffin, placing it on a warm slide, and allowing it to dry.[7] Some procedures use a piece of filter paper with a hole the size of the cylinder placed between the slide and cylinder. The cylinder and slide are clasped together with the filter paper serving as a gasket. The filter paper will also absorb the liquid portion of the CSF and allow the cells to settle on the slide.

The cylinder is filled with up to 1 ml of CSF; after 25 minutes, the CSF is aspirated from the chamber, which is dismantled. Excessive CSF is absorbed by absorbent paper and the smear allowed to air dry. Alternatively, the wet smear may be spray fixed before drying. Any hematologic stain may be used. Cells obtained by sedimentation are more expanded and cytoplasmic detail more easily observed. Sedimentation and centrifugation are preferred when dealing with inflammatory or leukemic cells because the cells will appear larger and more cytoplasm will be apparent.[2]

Cytocentrifugation. The advent of the cytocentrifuge gave a reliable, easy method for concentrating cells, but more elaborate equipment was required. The cytocentrifuge allows for concentration of cells onto a small area of a slide similar to the sedimentation method, but the process is accelerated by centrifugation. The final product is a postfixed, air dried preparation with cytologic detail similar to that obtained by sedimentation. This procedure is extensively used in human hospitals and veterinary colleges, but the expense of the cytocentrifuge has limited its use in veterinary practice.

Interpretation. Normal CSF contains less than 5 to 8 cells per μl. These cells are primarily mononuclear and include lymphocytes (60–80%), monocytes, and macrophages. An occasional neutrophil is a normal finding, and piaarachnoid mesothelial cells and ependymal and choroid cells may be rarely observed. It may be difficult to differentiate the monocytoid cells; therefore, the term mononuclear cell has been used for these cells when there is no visible evidence of phagocytosis.

An increase in the total nucleated cell count is referred to as pleocytosis. A mononuclear pleocytosis suggests viral inflammation (Fig. 3–1). An exception is eastern equine encephalomyelitis, which is neutrophilic early and later mononuclear.[5] Some neutrophils are observed in meningoencephalitis caused by feline infectious peritonitis virus. The highest cell counts and protein concentrations are observed with bacterial meningitis (Figs. 3–2 and 3–3). The pleocytosis with bacterial infections is usually neutrophilic, but mononuclear cells predominate in listeriosis.[6] Mycotic and protozoal diseases often have a mixed cell pleocytosis. Eosinophils in varying numbers have been observed in some nonviral inflammations, e.g., cryptococcosis, prototheccosis, and parasitic migrations (Fig. 3–4).

A mild pleocytosis consisting of neutrophils, lymphocytes, and some macrophages may be observed in cerebrovascular diseases.[13] Erythrophagocytosis may also be observed in cerebrovascular diseases (Fig. 3–5). Erythrophagocytosis may also be associated with xan-

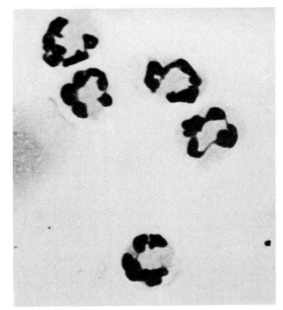

Figure 3–2. Neutrophilic pleocytosis in a case of purulent meningitis in a horse.

thochromia. A mild pleocytosis composed of neutrophils may be noted with trauma or spinal cord compression, particularly if collection is near the site of compression.[13] Degenerative diseases may cause an increase in macrophages,

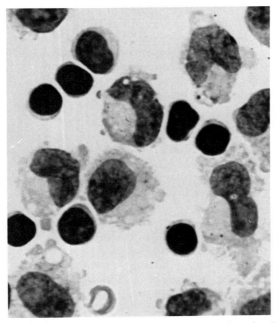

Figure 3–1. Nonsuppurative meningitis in a dog. Small lymphocytes and macrophages are observed.

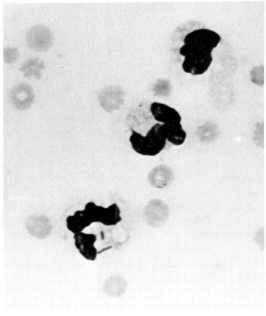

Figure 3–3. Septic meningitis in a cow. Intracellular rods are observed in a neutrophil.

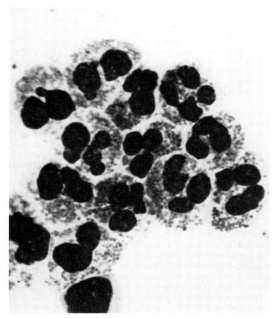

Figure 3–4. Eosinophilic meningitis in a goat suspected to be caused by *Parelaphostrongylus tenus* migration.

lymphocytes, and occasionally some neutrophils. Any destructive process involving the CNS may elicit an inflammatory response that is reflected in the CSF. The cells found initially are erythrocytes and neutrophils, followed within several days by macrophages.[2] Macrophages may have a foamy cytoplasm when lipids and glycoproteins are ingested after myelin destruction. Large foamy macrophages (globoid cells) have been observed in one storage disease.[10] Tumor cells are uncommon in CSF but, when present, usually indicate meningeal invasion (Figs. 3–6 and 3–7). Tumor cells are rarely shed from deep parenchymal lesions.

Usually when a significant pleocytosis occurs, protein concentration in the CSF is increased. In certain instances the protein concentration is increased without an increase in cell count. This is referred to as albuminocytologic dissociation and can be observed with noninflammatory degeneration and necrosis, vascular lesions with hemorrhage and/or transudation, neoplasms, and certain viral diseases.[5] The CSF may be normal in some inflammatory diseases of the CNS.

Microbiology

Occasionally bacterial or fungal organisms may be present in sufficient numbers to be observed on cytologic examination (Fig. 3–8), but usually culture is needed for detection. Cerebrospinal fluid should always be collected aseptically, allowing a portion to be used for

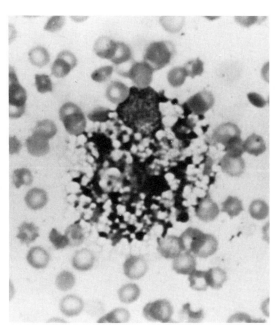

Figure 3–5. A macrophage containing hemosiderin in a case of subarachnoid hemorrhage in a dog.

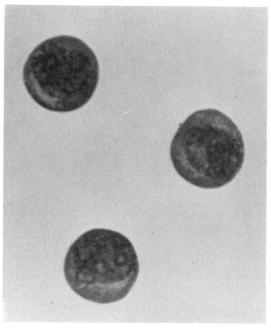

Figure 3–6. Neoplastic lymphocytes from a case of lymphosarcoma involving the meninges in a dog.

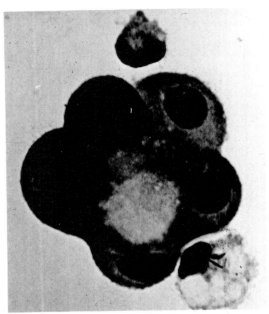

Figure 3–7. A cluster of tumor cells from a case of metastatic mammary adenocarcinoma to the brain in a dog.

culture. Any neutrophilic pleocytosis should cause one to suspect a bacterial meningitis, and the CSF should be cultured. Microbiology texts should be consulted for details about cultural techniques.

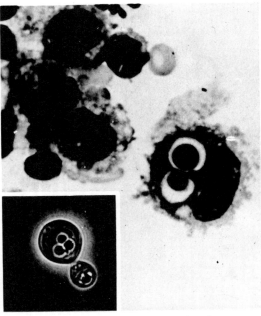

Figure 3–8. A case of cryptococcosis in a dog. *Cryptococcus neoformans* organism in a macrophage. Inset, an India ink preparation demonstrating the organism.

Viral isolation may be attempted from the CSF or blood in cases of suspected viral encephalitis. Serial serum determinations or indirect fluorescent antibody examinations also are used to detect viral disease. Viral antibody also may be detected in the CSF of infected animals. Specific tests for each disease are discussed in Chapter 7.

REFERENCES

1. Barsanti JA and Duncan JR: Determination of the concentration of protein in the cerebrospinal fluid with a new dye-binding method. Vet Clin Pathol 7(3):6, 1978.
2. Bigner SH and Johnston WW: The cytopathology of cerebrospinal fluid. I. Nonneoplastic conditions, lymphoma and leukemia. Acta Cytol 25:335, 1981.
3. Coles EH: Cerebrospinal fluid. *In* Kaneko JJ (ed): Clinical Biochemistry of Domestic Animals. New York, Academic Press, 1980.
4. Cutler RW and Spertell RB: Cerebrospinal fluid: A selective review. Ann Neurol 11:1, 1982.
5. deLahunta A: Veterinary Neuroanatomy and Clinical Neurology, 2nd ed. Philadelphia, WB Saunders Co, 1983.
6. Howard JR: Neurologic disease differentiation. JAVMA 154:1174, 1969.
7. Mayhew IG and Beal CR: Techniques of analysis of cerebrospinal fluid. Vet Clin North Am 10:155, 1980.
8. Osweiler GD and Hurd JW: Determination of sodium content in serum and cerebrospinal fluid as an adjunct to diagnosis of water deprivation in swine. JAVMA 165:165, 1974.
9. Roszel JF: Membrane filtration of canine and feline cerebrospinal fluid for cytologic evaluation. JAVMA 160:720, 1976.
10. Roszel JF, Steinberg SA, and McGrath JT: Periodic-acid Schiff-positive cells in the cerebrospinal cells of dogs with globoid cell leukodystrophy. Neurology 22:738, 1972.
11. Schriever H and Gambino SR: Protein turbidity produced by trichloroacetic acid and sulfosalicylic acid at varying temperatures and varying ratios of albumin and globulin. Am J Clin Pathol 44:667, 1965.
12. Sorjonen DC, Warren JN, and Schultz RD: Qualitative and quantitative determination of albumin, IgG, IgM and IgA in normal cerebrospinal fluid of dogs. J Am Anim Hosp Assoc 17:833, 1981.
13. Vandevelde M and Spano JS: Cerebrospinal fluid cytology in canine neurologic disease. Am J Vet Res 38:1827, 1977.
14. Wilkins RJ: A micro-spectrophotometric method for the determination of protein in CSF. Bull Am Soc Vet Clin Pathol 3:3, 1974.
15. Wilson JW: Clinical application of cerebrospinal fluid creatine phosphokinase determination. JAVMA 171:200, 1977.
16. Wilson JW and Stevens JB: Effects of blood contamination on cerebrospinal fluid analysis. JAVMA 171:256, 1977.
17. Wise BL: The quantitation and fractionation of proteins in cerebrospinal fluid. Am J Med Tech 48:821, 1982.
18. Wright JA: Evaluation of cerebrospinal fluid in the dog. Vet Rec 103:48, 1978.

Chapter 4

DL Barber, DVM, MS
JE Oliver, Jr, DVM, MS, PhD
IG Mayhew, BVSc, PhD

Neuroradiography

GENERAL PRINCIPLES

Scope

Physical and interpretive principles described for the general field of radiography also apply to neuroradiography. Radiographic findings must be correlated with results of other diagnostic techniques as emphasized throughout this text. Radiographic findings characteristic of specific disease processes are presented in chapters covering those diseases.

Equipment

The physical principles of conventional radiographic equipment design, function, and capabilities are well described, and recommendations have been discussed.[9, 27, 109, 143] Equipment for neuroradiography should be superior to that used for general radiography. X-ray generator and tube capacity should be at least 300 mA and 100 kVp. Higher output equipment is preferred. Lower output equipment is functional, but the user must be aware of its limitations and make corresponding adjustments to produce radiographs of diagnostic quality. Because most patients are anesthetized for neuroradiography, short exposure times to limit motion artifact are less critical than in conventional radiography. The x-ray tube should have a good quality beam restrictor, preferably an adjustable collimator with an accurate beam-defining light source instead of a cylinder or cone. Mobility of the x-ray tube is essential for the examination of large animals and preferable in small animal neuroradiography, especially if the tube is mechanically linked to the grid and cassette holder. In small animal work, a floating or motor driven table top adds convenience but is not essential. The combination of tube head and table top mobility provides maximum versatility for small animal neuroradiography. A tilting table is only occasionally of value. A high quality grid should also be part of the system. The grid must be matched to the system because larger patients create more scatter and require greater lead content within the grid. However, this necessitates greater exposure techniques. Aluminum interspaced grids are generally preferable to organic interspaced grids. If the system is adequate, a grid ratio of 10:1 or 12:1 should be used. A Bucky device can be used to eliminate grid lines on the radiograph. However, a good quality, fine line, stationary grid will not result in severely objectionable grid lines and will eliminate many problems encountered with a Bucky system.

The image recording system must match both the x-ray machine capabilities and the requirements of the examination being conducted. The wide spectrum of cassette, screen, and film types and systems is covered in detail elsewhere.[27, 109] For neuroradiography, it is preferable to have both high speed and detail screen-film systems available. The high speed system is adequate in most instances, and the detail system can be used occasionally if finer image detail is required. Newer rare earth screen-film systems can reduce required exposures and can thus extend the capabilities of low output equipment. They may be used routinely to promote radiation safety and extend x-ray tube life. High contrast radiographs are not essential but are usually preferred in neuroradiography. This result is most easily obtained by selecting an appropriate film type to provide a high contrast image. However, it should be noted that a low scale of contrast will provide more latitude in obtaining images of diagnostic quality of thick and thin parts within the same field.

The use of a properly constructed technique chart must be adhered to for consistent radiographs of diagnostic quality. For best results, separate technique charts for different views may be made. Positioning aids are extremely valuable in neuroradiology. These include radiolucent pads or cushions to position the spine or head uniformly, and ties, sandbags, and other devices to maintain positioning. Most patients are placed under general anesthesia for neuroradiography and thus can be adequately restrained with mechanical devices. Accurate and consistent film labeling is important to meet legal requirements, as well as for diagnostic accuracy and convenience. Radiation safety practices should include, as a minimum, the use of leaded aprons and gloves when appropriate, collimation of the x-ray beam to only the area of interest, the use of a personnel monitoring program, chemical restraint of the patient when possible, and the efficient production of diagnostic quality radiographs. The latter can be enhanced by using an accurate technique chart and employing proper darkroom techniques.

General principles of equine neuroradiography are comparable with those described for small animal work. Portable x-ray machines are usually inadequate, and high output mobile equipment is probably a minimum requirement. Larger output, ceiling suspended units are preferable. Initial survey radiographic studies of the skull and cervical vertebrae can be made in the standing, awake animal. Grid channels allow the use of multiple cassettes with the same grid and are thus preferable to grid cassettes. Accurate alignment of the x-ray tube and grid-cassette combination is important. This may be accomplished with a tripod or wall mounted cassette holder before moving the animal into place or with a more elaborate electronic locking system utilizing a ceiling or wall suspended cassette holder. With less accurate alignment methods, a cross-hatched grid (eg, 5:1 focused, cross hatched) may allow more latitude in vertical tube alignment while providing the same scatter cleanup as a higher ratio linear grid (eg, 10:1 linear, focused). Radiography of the recumbent horse with a vertically directed x-ray beam can be performed on a specially constructed table with a built-in grid or Bucky system. More often, a mobile grid channel is used on the floor beneath the recumbent patient. Construction of a cassette tunnel will protect the grid from the weight of the patient and allow easier cassette changing for different views. A leaded sheet on the back of the cassette can be used to absorb backscatter that may fog the radiograph.

Most veterinarians are familiar with conventional radiographic equipment. More specialized techniques are being used with increasing frequency in veterinary medicine, and some of these have specific application in neuroradiography. Survey radiographs and most contrast studies of the head and spine can be made with conventional equipment. An automatic, rapid film changer is necessary for cerebral angiography. Image intensified fluoroscopy is valuable to visualize dynamic changes and to localize structures or lesions. It is a convenient technique to confirm proper injection and dosage in myelography and epidurography. As a localizing tool, fluoroscopy is of value in the percutaneous placement of needles in vertebral bodies or disk spaces either for contrast medium injection (venography, diskography) or for aspiration of material for biopsy or culture. Tomography is a type of body section radiography that produces selective blurring of images of superimposed objects while maintaining relative image sharpness in a preselected plane of interest.[27, 58] It is accomplished by controlled tube-film motion during the exposure. Tomography is especially applicable to neuroradiography because of the complex superimposition of osseous structures at the base of the skull and throughout the vertebral column. Magnification radiography produces a direct enlargement of the radiographic image by using a small focal spot and increasing object-film distance while maintaining a standard tube-film distance.[8, 27] Small anatomic changes may be better visualized by magnification radiography. The technique is most applicable to demonstrate small bone lesions and in combination with cerebral angiography. Additional techniques of nuclear imaging and computed tomography will be discussed more specifically below.

Technique and Interpretation

All neuroradiographic examinations should start with conventional survey radiography. Noting abnormalities on survey radiographs may obviate the need for contrast studies, direct the clinician to the most appropriate diagnostic procedure, and allow adjustment of the exposure technique in anticipation of the addition of contrast medium. Additional views must be made as needed.

One of the most important factors in the production of diagnostic quality radiographs is precise patient positioning. Consistency of precise positioning is essential for familiarity with the appearance of the normal skull and vertebral column. If the appearance of an object in a certain projection is familiar, deviation from this projection will cause a loss of confidence in differentiating normal and abnormal. In addition, subtle lesions may be completely obscured by inadequate positioning (Fig. 4–1). Lastly, precise positioning of the patient is necessary to allow adequate comparison with other references.

Most neuroradiographs are made with the patient under general inhalation anesthesia. Heavy sedation may be adequate for some patients. However, general anesthesia is preferred to decrease motion, to produce muscle relaxation needed for precise positioning, to provide adequate restraint, and to enhance radiation safety practices. General anesthesia also allows one to proceed directly to any necessary contrast studies. Exceptions do exist: Anesthesia should be avoided if medically contraindicated. Anesthesia should also be avoided if patient self protection is important, as in cases of suspected vertebral fracture or luxation. In such cases of instability, unprotected motion during patient manipulation may further traumatize the spinal cord. Anesthesia is also usually unnecessary in many follow-up spinal studies, such as in cases of diskospondylitis.

Interpretation of radiographs should follow a logical, orderly format and should be complete. Thus all body parts included on the radiograph should be evaluated. Knowledge of results of other tests is important but can create a bias that has been shown to lead to overinterpretation of minor, clinically insignificant radiographic variations.[44] Clinical bias can increase the number of true positive, increase the number of false positive, and decrease the number of false negative radiographic interpretations.[41, 44] A knowledge of normal radiographic anatomy is important, but expertise in all the potential variations among species and breeds is difficult to achieve. Thus comparative evaluations are essential, and one may use various reference files or textbooks, although these may be limited in scope.[45, 60, 134, 135, 143] One of the most valuable comparisons available is that of symmetry between right and left sides or between adjacent structures that should be relatively similar in appearance. The latter types of comparative methods further emphasize the importance of precise positioning.

The roentgen sign approach is usually advocated in radiographic interpretation. This provides a logical, descriptive method of communicating radiographic findings. The three classes of roentgen signs are density, geometry, and function. Abnormal density can be either increased or decreased density of an object. Geometry is subdivided into size, shape, number, position, and margination. In neuroradiography, function is subdivided into patency, integrity, and motion. However, a listing of only roentgen signs is of little diagnostic value. Roentgen signs must be considered in the context of differential diagnoses most likely associated with the roentgen signs visualized and the clinical signs observed.

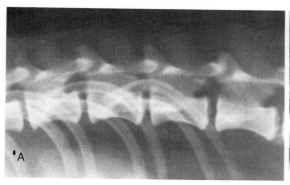 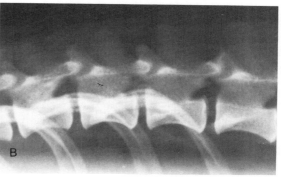

Figure 4–1. Different views of the spine of the same dog that demonstrate the importance of accurate positioning. A, Oblique view. Superimposition of a rib obscures intervertebral foramina at T13–L1. B, True lateral view. Foramina are small and increased density can be seen within the canal over the foramina at T13–L1. Changes were due to disk herniation.

VERTEBRAL COLUMN
AND SPINAL CORD

Small Animal

Survey Radiography

The spinal cord is of low density, is surrounded by bone, and is thus not visible per se on conventional survey radiographs. Without contrast studies, disease of the spinal cord can only be inferred from changes in the vertebral column. Survey radiographs of the spine should be made with the patient under general anesthesia, with the exceptions noted previously. Except in cases of severe vertebral instability, minimum studies should include lateral and ventrodorsal (VD) radiographs made in lateral and dorsal recumbency, respectively. Sectional radiography should be used and is dependent on clinical localization of spinal cord disease. The most common technique is to make initial sectional radiographs of the cervical, thoracolumbar, or lumbosacral vertebrae on longer film and then to make well-collimated, high detail radiographs of any questionable areas that need further assessment. Image geometry is important in explaining the projection of the radiographic image of the spine. Understanding image geometry clarifies the importance of and need for special efforts in patient positioning.

Positioning. Lateral radiographs of the vertebral column should be made with the patient in lateral recumbency with the vertebrae as parallel to the table as possible. In this position, there is a tendency for the cervical and caudal lumbar vertebrae to sag toward the table. This uneven conformation will create uneven, artifactual narrowing of the projected radiographic image of these intervertebral disk spaces and a more en face projection of vertebral end plates. Thus, for the most accurate image projection, these areas of uneven conformation should be supported with radiolucent pads to keep the vertebral column parallel to the table top. The problem is most critical in the cervical area. The number, size, and positioning of the pads will depend on the size and conformation of the individual patient.

The lateral view should also be a true lateral view. Rotational obliquity is minimized by raising or lowering the limbs and sternum so that the ventral midline is the same distance from the table top as is the dorsal midline. In a true lateral view, opposing right and left transverse processes, intervertebral foramina, articular processes, and dorsal rib curvatures should be superimposed. If numerous vertebrae are included in the x-ray field, vertebrae, and especially intervertebral disk spaces at the periphery of the image, will be distorted in accord with the geometry of image projection[42] (Fig. 4–2). End plates of vertebral bodies will be projected more en face rather than in tangent. Thus, for most accurate assessment, additional radiographs with the central axis of the x-ray beam centered over specific areas of concern are often required. These additional radiographs should be well collimated to include only a few vertebrae. The vertebrae should be positioned initially in a relatively neutral position without flexion or hyperextension. Flexed or extended views may be used cautiously as supplemental studies if necessary to document dynamic alterations. Slight traction may be used to assist accurate positioning, but excessive traction should be avoided.

Ventrodorsal radiographs made in lateral recumbency or dorsoventral radiographs made in ventral recumbency are occasionally necessary to minimize manipulation in cases of spinal cord trauma. However, the preferred routine conventional view is a ventrodorsal view made with the patient in dorsal recumbency. This position minimizes vertebrae-film distance and is the easiest for aligning the patient for a true ventrodorsal view without obliquity. Because of the normal kyphotic-lordotic curvatures of the vertebral column, intervertebral disk spaces and vertebral end plates will not be uniformly projected. Disk space evaluation is of less impor-

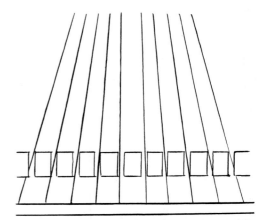

Figure 4–2. Distortion due to the geometry of image projection. Intervertebral disk spaces and vertebrae may be projected inaccurately owing to their location in the periphery of the x-ray beam. More accurate image geometry is obtained nearer the central axis of the beam. (Based on Douglas SW and Williamson HD: Principles of Veterinary Radiology. Baltimore, Williams & Wilkins Co, 1963.)

tance on the ventrodorsal view because most disk space lesions are better seen on lateral views. Cervical intervertebral disk spaces and end plates can be seen better on the ventrodorsal view by using a 5 to 10° caudal-to-cranial tube angulation. A similar concept may be applied to the lumbosacral disk space, but the angle is more variable, depending on pelvic traction and positioning. In narrow, deep-chested breeds of dogs, large differences in body part thicknesses between thoracic and lumbar regions and between cranial cervical and cranial thoracic regions may necessitate different radiographic exposure techniques for these sections.

Oblique views are occasionally of value, especially in the cervical region. With the patient in dorsal recumbency the ventrum is obliqued approximately 45° away from the vertically directed x-ray beam. These views will allow isolated projection of intervertebral foramina and articular processes from C2–C3 through C7–T1 without the superimposition of structures normally encountered on the standard lateral view. With the ventrum obliqued to the right, the left intervertebral foramina will be seen. The right intervertebral foramina will be appreciated best with the ventrum obliqued to the left. Both right and left oblique views should be made for comparison. These views are apparently of most value following a normal cervical myelogram to help diagnose intraforaminal and lateral disk extrusions causing nerve root compression.[47] The odontoid process of C2 is obscured by the superimposed lateral processes of C1 on a true lateral view. Slight obliquity (20°) from the true lateral view will separate lateral processes of C1 to allow visualization of the odontoid process.

Normal Appearance. It is not possible to detail all of the normal radiographic anatomic features and variations of the vertebral column because of differences in species, breed, and age. For those unfamiliar with the normal radiographic anatomy, the value of comparison is again stressed. Survey radiographs are included as examples (Fig. 4–3), and general points of emphasis will be noted. In general terms of roentgen signs, vertebrae are of bone density and intervertebral disk spaces and foramina are of soft tissue density. The vertebral formula for dogs and cats is C7:T13:L7:S3:Cdx. Vertebrae and disk spaces vary in size and shape in the different regions. Vertebrae are positioned in a smooth, continuous alignment with relatively gradual curvatures. Bone contour of vertebrae should be smooth and sharply marginated.

The first and second cervical vertebrae are unique in shape. Vertebral bodies of C2–C7 appear relatively long and thin, and spinous processes are short at C3 and gradually lengthen through C7. Intervertebral disk spaces are relatively large and uniform from C3–C4 through C6–C7. The disk spaces at C2–C3 and C7–T1 may be slightly narrower than other cervical disk spaces. Articular processes are large and tend to obscure intervertebral foramina on the lateral view. Transverse processes of C6 have unique large plates directed ventrolaterally.

Vertebral bodies of the thoracic region tend to be shorter and squared in appearance compared with those of the cervical region. Long spinous processes slope caudally and gradually shorten to T10 and then remain equal in height. Spinous processes of T9 and T10 have a marked caudal slope, and those of T11–T13 are more vertically oriented. Articular processes are positioned more dorsally and joint spaces aligned more horizontally, allowing better visualization of intervertebral foramina. At T10–T11 articular processes change alignment to be more dorsally positioned, vertically oriented joints that are more characteristic of the lumbar vertebrae. Rib heads and dorsal rib curvatures may be superimposed over the vertebral canal to varying degrees. Intervertebral disk spaces are uniformly narrow throughout the thoracic region T1–T10. The disk space at T10–T11 is often the narrowest, and spaces at T11–T12 and then T12–T13 become wider and more comparable to lumbar spaces.

Vertebral bodies elongate and enlarge again through the lumbar area. The seventh lumbar vertebra is shorter than L6. Spinous processes are relatively large and vertically oriented, except for L7, which has a short spinous process. Joint spaces of articular processes are located dorsal to the vertebral canal and are oriented vertically. Intervertebral foramina are easily seen, relatively large, and radiolucent. Accessory processes may be projected over intervertebral foramina from T11–T12 through L5–L6. Intervertebral disk spaces are relatively large and uniform but may appear to narrow slightly caudally owing to positioning. The disk space at L7–S1 is normally wedge shaped, being narrower dorsally than ventrally.

The sacrum consists of three fused vertebrae, and all aspects of sacral radiographic morphology progressively decrease in size moving caudally. The sacrovertebral angle is the dorsal angle created at the point of intersection of lines drawn parallel to the dorsal margins of the lumbar and sacral vertebral bodies on the lateral

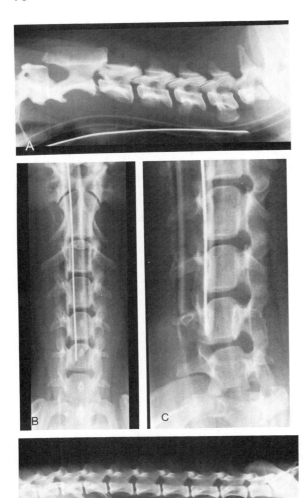

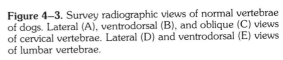

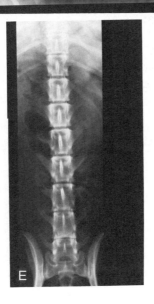

Figure 4–3. Survey radiographic views of normal vertebrae of dogs. Lateral (A), ventrodorsal (B), and oblique (C) views of cervical vertebrae. Lateral (D) and ventrodorsal (E) views of lumbar vertebrae.

radiograph. The angle is variable, depending on the degree of stress applied at the lumbo-sacral junction during positioning.

Interpretation of Abnormalities. Characteristic radiographic abnormalities of specific diseases are described in subsequent chapters. The reader is also referred to articles on the principles of radiographic interpretation of osseous structures.[127] Evaluation of the radiographs must be complete, even though there may be clinical bias.

A logical starting point is to count the number of vertebrae in the section being radiographed to help ascertain any anomalies of segmentation. Next, the radiograph should be evaluated for alignment of vertebral bodies and the vertebral canal. The vertebral canal should be further assessed for changes in size, shape, and density. Each intervertebral disk space and intervertebral foramen must be evaluated for changes in size, shape, and density. This is best accomplished by comparing each space with those immediately cranial and caudal to it. Vertebral bodies, pedicles, laminae, and processes must be further assessed for changes in density and geometry. Morphology and density of vertebral end plates are especially important to note. Articular processes should be evaluated, as well as relative size of the joint spaces. This is especially important in the lumbar region in conjunction with assessment of intervertebral disk spaces and foramina. Lastly, one should make special note of any asymmetry of structures that may be used as surgical landmarks. For example, on a thoracolumbar study, one must always remember to evaluate the last pair of ribs on the ventrodorsal view.

Congenital malformations of vertebrae occur commonly in animals but are less frequently of clinical significance (see Chapter 6). Radiographic findings in vertebral anomalies have been summarized.[108] Fusion anomaly (block vertebrae) causes complete or partial fusion of two or more vertebrae. If only partial fusion occurs, a persistent partial disk space may be visible and may cause abnormal angulation of the vertebral column. Spinous processes may also fuse independently of vertebral bodies. Hemivertebrae are due to incomplete ossification or union of ossification centers of vertebral bodies. The two major types recognized are butterfly and cuneiform vertebrae. Butterfly vertebrae are visible on the ventrodorsal radiograph and are recognized by a midsagittal cleft caused by lack of fusion of the two lateral ossification centers of the vertebral body (see Fig. 6–11). Cuneiform vertebrae are wedge

shaped, with a base that is wider than the narrower apex. If the base is the dorsal or ventral portion of the vertebral body, the anomaly is seen best on the lateral view with the narrower apex directed ventrally or dorsally, respectively. If the base is lateral with the apex directed contralaterally, the anomaly is best seen on the ventrodorsal view. Vertebrae that are adjacent to such an anomalous segment are also frequently altered in shape to correspond to the anomalous vertebra. Kyphosis, lordosis, or scoliosis may result from such anomalies. In the thoracic region, corresponding rib anomalies may also be present. Vertebral remodeling with spondylosis may occur concurrently with such anomalies. Spina bifida is a defect caused by the failure of fusion of the two lateral ossification centers that form the vertebral arch.[108, 147] Variations in appearance are dependent on degrees of fusion or ossification defects. The anomaly is most commonly seen on the ventrodorsal view. In its mildest form, the defect appears as a sagittal splitting of the spinous process with two bone densities on either side of midline, which represent ununited arches. With more severe defects, the spinous process may be absent and the defect may extend across the width of the vertebral arch. Myelography is necessary to document any associated neural or meningeal anomalies (see Fig. 6–7).

Transitional vertebrae occur at junctions of major divisions of the vertebral column and assume characteristics of the adjacent segments.[108] Thus, transitional vertebrae occur at the cervicothoracic, thoracolumbar, lumbosacral, and sacrocaudal junctions. The transition may occur in either direction, usually involves dorsal laminae and processes, and infrequently involves vertebral bodies. At the cervicothoracic junction, the most common anomaly is the presence of unilateral or bilateral ribs on C7. The rib may be hypoplastic or equal to the normal first rib in size and shape. Transitional anomalies are more common at the thoracolumbar junction, and the shift may be in either direction. The ribs of T13 may be replaced unilaterally or bilaterally with thick transverse processes fused to the vertebral body. Conversely, L1 may have unilateral or bilateral ribs that articulate with the vertebral body instead of normal transverse processes. Incomplete ossification of the last pair of ribs may occur unilaterally or bilaterally. At the lumbosacral junction, L7 may fuse with the sacrum unilaterally or bilaterally with a large wing replacing the normal transverse process(es) of L7. Conversely, S1 may have transverse processes instead of normal alae. Such lumbosacral anomalies are best seen on the ventrodorsal view and may cause scoliosis if unilateral. Additional sacral anomalies may include segmentation of normally fused sacral segments or sacrocaudal vertebral fusion. More complex congenital anomalies can occur throughout the vertebral column. Vertebral malformations in the Manx cat appear to relate primarily to sacral dysgenesis or agenesis and spina bifida, as well as anomalies of the spinal cord and meninges[76, 88] (see Fig. 6–8).

One of the most common indications for vertebral radiography in dogs is for the diagnosis and localization of intervertebral disk herniation or protrusion (see Chapter 12). Disk degeneration and herniation have been well described.[65, 121] The partial protrusion of type II disk disease may be difficult to see on survey radiographs. The protruded disk is usually of soft tissue density, is localized to the floor of the vertebral canal, and is not necessarily associated with a narrowed intervertebral disk space. Thus myelography is frequently necessary for radiographic diagnosis. Survey radiography has a much higher yield in demonstrating changes of disk herniation associated with type I disk disease. The recognition of intervertebral disk calcification in situ is of little clinical value, as a high percentage of chondrodystrophoid disks calcify. The major radiographic findings of disk herniation are narrowed intervertebral disk spaces, small intervertebral foramina, and narrowed diarthrodial joint spaces, as seen on the lateral view (Fig. 4–4A). The disk space may be uniformly narrowed or wedge shaped with narrowing more prominent dorsally. A disk may degenerate, dehydrate, and narrow without herniation of the nucleus pulposus.[108] Where visible, intervertebral foramina may be small owing to shifting of adjacent vertebrae closer together in association with the narrowed disk space. Craniocaudal narrowing of diarthrodial joint spaces, as seen on the lateral view, may have a similar basis. This is only of radiographic value in the caudal thoracic and lumbar regions and is usually a supplementary rather than a primary finding. Herniated disk material may produce increased density within the vertebral canal (Fig. 4–4B). If the material is not heavily calcified, it will be harder to see. If the material is at the level of the intervertebral foramina, it will produce increased density over the foramina and be easier to identify. If heavily calcified material herniates as a mass, it will be readily seen as a calcific nodule within the vertebral canal. However, if the calcific material spreads out over a larger area, it will again be more difficult to see. Some significance has been placed on intervertebral disk spaces without calcification if adjacent disks are heavily calcified in situ. This finding may imply disk herniation but is of little value in specific diagnosis, except if previous radiographs of the same patient demonstrated calcification in situ of a disk that is currently void of that calcific density. It should also be noted that disk calcification in situ does not exclude that disk as a possible source of a current herniation because some calcified material may remain in the disk space. Chronic herniation may eventually cause sclerosis and eburnation of vertebral end plates and spondylosis. In the attempt to localize current or acute disk herniation radiographically, it is extremely important to correlate results of radiographic and clinical neurologic examinations. Radiographs should be made of the entire section of the vertebral column that could be implicated in the neurologic findings observed. Previous episodes of neurologic problems and surgery, such as fenestration, are important points in assessing the significance of radio-

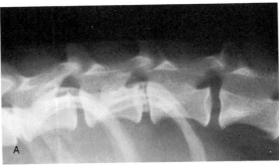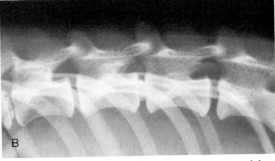

Figure 4–4. A, Disk herniation at T13–L1. There is slight narrowing of the intervertebral disk space, foramina, and facet joint spaces at T13–L1. These changes are best appreciated by comparing the space being evaluated with those immediately cranial and caudal to it. Also note the calcified material remaining in the intervertebral disk space at T13–L1. B, Disk herniation at T12–13. Note the increased density of intervertebral foramina at T12–T13 compared with other foramina.

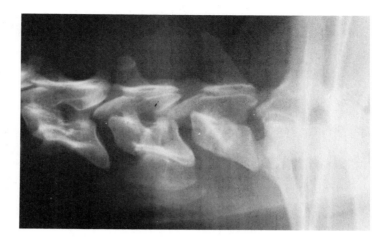

Figure 4–5. Severe cervical spondylopathy in a Doberman pinscher with malformation and displacement of C7.

graphic findings. Disk herniations may not be detected on survey radiographs, they may appear to be multiple, or the radiographic and neurologic findings may not agree. Myelography is necessary in each of these situations.[149] However, if myelography is not diagnostic and there is a strong suspicion of cervical nerve root compression, oblique views of the cervical vertebrae can demonstrate intraforaminal and lateral disk extrusions.[47]

Cervical vertebral malformation/malarticulation is a well-described condition of certain breeds of dogs that appears to be quite complex and variable in radiographic appearance and severity[36, 133, 145, 152] (see Chapter 6). Major findings on survey radiographs are subluxation of vertebrae, angular deviation, deformity of vertebrae, hyperostosis of vertebral laminae, and bony stenosis of the cranial or caudal orifice of vertebral foramina (Fig. 4–5). Significance of angular deviation (unless severe) is difficult to define because a considerable degree of cervical mobility is present in normal dogs.[31, 152] Asymmetry and periarticular remodeling of articular processes may occur. Hansen's type II disk protrusion and hyperplasia of ligamentous and other soft tissue structures may occur and project into the vertebral canal to cause spinal cord compression. Myelography is essential to document the site and degree of spinal cord compression and to identify the specific cause (whether it be soft tissue structures, disk protrusion, or bone encroachment into the vertebral canal). Myelography is also essential if surgery is contemplated because myelography may often demonstrate that spinal cord compression is present or even more severe at sites different from those suspected based on survey radiographs. Lumbosacral spondylopathy may occur with similar findings of vertebral displacement, stenosis, disk herniation, and soft tissue hypertrophy.[37, 118]

Both infections and malignant neoplasms of vertebrae tend to cause changes in bone structure described as aggressive bone lesions. Aggressive bone lesions are likely to produce a mixture of osteolytic and osteoproductive changes. Cortical erosion and irregular, active bone production are characteristic findings in aggressive bone lesions, and there may be an associated soft tissue component. Benign bone lesions tend to be well demarcated, are more smoothly marginated, and cause slow remodeling of bone rather than erosion through cortical barriers. Osteochondroma is the most common benign tumor affecting vertebrae and may be multiple. Primary malignant vertebral tumors are usually aggressive in appearance, are monostotic in origin, tend not to cross the intervertebral disk space, and may have an associated paravertebral soft tissue mass. Multiple myeloma and lymphosarcoma more typically produce purely osteolytic lesions, usually without periosteal response, and may be polyostotic. Tumors metastatic to vertebrae frequently are carcinomas from primary prostatic, mammary, pulmonary, and renal sites.[21] Radiographic recognition of these tumors probably occurs relatively late in the disease process. Earlier recognition may be achieved with increased use of radionuclide bone scanning. Neoplasia of nervous tissue elements may not produce survey radiographic abnormalities.[101, 153] With larger, slowly expanding masses, one may see remodeling of vertebrae causing focal enlargement of the vertebral canal or an intervertebral foramen (Fig. 4–6). Recognition of these tumors is dependent often on myelography.[123]

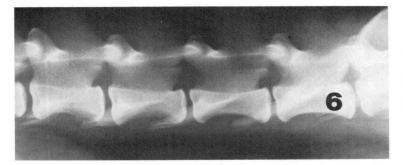

Figure 4–6. An expansile lesion within the vertebral canal has caused enlargement of the vertebral canal from mid L4 through L5–6. Remodeling has caused thinning of vertebral laminae and bodies. (6 = body of L6.)

Diskitis is an infection of the intervertebral disk and is rarely recognized radiographically. Radionuclide scanning with ^{67}Ga has been shown to be of diagnostic value in humans with diskitis.[23] Diskospondylitis is an infectious process of the intervertebral disk and adjacent vertebral body and has been well described in dogs[16, 75, 93] (see Chapter 7). The earliest radiographic lesion appears to be a focal osteolytic defect in the vertebral end plate (Fig. 4–7A). More commonly, diskospondylitis is identified as an aggressive lesion with extensive erosion of adjacent vertebral end plates and bodies (Fig. 4–7B). Irregular, active bone production is often present around the periphery of the vertebral body, and there may be sclerosis within the body. The vertebral body may be shortened, the disk space may be narrowed, and adjacent vertebrae are usually involved. The lesion may occur at one or multiple sites. Spondylitis is inflammation of a vertebral body.[83] Although spondylitis may extend into an intervertebral disk, origination of the infection in the vertebral body usually causes a more uniform involvement of the body compared with diskospondylitis, in which the infection starts in the disk and extends into the body. Radionuclide bone scans may be more sensitive in the diagnosis of diskospondylitis and spondylitis than is radiography.[61, 87]

Trauma to the vertebral column can produce fracture or luxation of vertebrae (see Chapter 11). Vertebral luxation of articular processes with concurrent rupture of the anulus fibrosus is not common. When luxation is present, associated chip fractures, fractured processes, or vertebral body fractures are also usually present.[108] More commonly, vertebral fractures involve fractures through the vertebral body. Compression fractures cause shortening of the vertebral body with little change in alignment. Slight overriding may occur, and subtle breaks in the cortex may be observed. Oblique fractures may occur through the vertebral body and be associated with severe displacement of fracture fragments. Fractures of the body with displacement are often associated with luxation of the diarthrodial joints. Physeal fractures can also occur in immature animals. Dorsal and transverse processes may be fractured alone or in combination with vertebral body fractures.

Atlantoaxial subluxation causes instability at C1–C2 and allows abnormal flexion with dorsal displacement of the cranial portion of the body

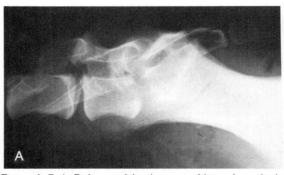

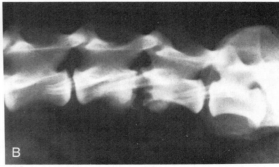

Figure 4–7. A, Diskospondylitis has caused lysis of vertebral end plates at L7–S1. Results of blood and urine cultures were negative, but *Staphylococcus aureus* was cultured from a fluoroscopically guided, percutaneous aspirate of the disk space. B, Diskospondylitis has caused lysis of vertebral end plates and active bone production at L5–L6. Slight vertebral displacement is also present owing to instability.

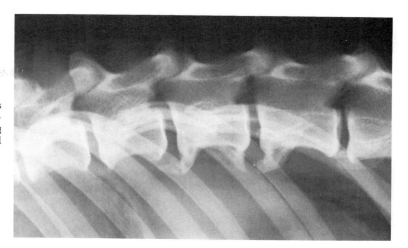

Figure 4–8. Spondylosis deformans is the smoothly marginated, curved, ventral bone production present in varying degrees at T11–12, T12–T13, and T13–L1.

of C2 into the vertebral canal (see Chapter 6). The syndrome may be due to agenesis of the dens, hypoplasia of the dens, nonunion of the dens with C2, fracture of the dens from the body of C2, or rupture of ligaments that secure the dens to the floor of the vertebral canal in C1.[7, 117] This syndrome should first be assessed radiographically by projecting the dens in a nonstressed view. This is best accomplished with a lateral oblique radiograph, in which architecture of the dens may be seen. The dens may also be seen on ventrodorsal views of the vertebrae or a rostrocaudal open mouth view of the skull. However, care must be taken not to further traumatize the spinal cord. Instability is best documented on a true lateral view made with slight flexion in the awake patient. Increased mobility at C1–C2 is confirmed by displacement of the body of C2 dorsally and cranially into the vertebral canal and by an increased distance between the arch of C1 and the cranial tip of the spinous process of C2.

Degenerative changes of vertebrae are recognized most often as incidental findings, usually without clinical significance (see Chapter 6). Spondylosis deformans is the formation of osteophytes that originate from ventral or lateral margins of vertebral end plates and project across intervertebral disk spaces. They range in size from small to large, are smooth and sharply marginated, and have a characteristic curve with the concavity toward the disk (Fig. 4–8). Lateral osteophytes may appear to project into the vertebral canal on lateral views, but the ventrodorsal view confirms their lateral location. Bone production is usually more prominent ventrally and, if extensive, may extend the length of vertebral bodies and also interdigitate with osteophytes from adjacent vertebrae. Ex-

tensive confluent bone production may be analogous to ankylosing hyperostosis.[151] Nerve root compression could be possible from extensive lateral bone production, but spinal cord compression would be unlikely. Vertebral osteophytes may also occur secondary to conditions such as instability, disk degeneration, trauma, and diskospondylitis. Degenerative joint disease of true synovial joints may be inferred from chronic, osteoproductive remodeling of articular processes. On the lateral view, this may be difficult to differentiate from benign, chronic bone production on the midline between adjacent arches and spinous processes.[108] Differentiation requires good quality ventrodorsal radiographs. Dural ossification may produce sharply marginated, linear, calcific densities within the vertebral canal.[108] These are usually best seen in the cervical and lumbar vertebral canal just dorsal to the floor of the vertebral canal (Fig. 4–9). They are usually easier to see in large breed dogs, in which they are located more dorsally off the floor of the canal. The dorsal margin of the vertebral body may be confused with dural ossification on lateral oblique radiographs.

Systemic loss of bone density due to a variety of metabolic conditions may occasionally be noted in vertebrae. Although osteoporosis, or osteopenia, may affect the entire skeleton, radiographic changes may be most pronounced in vertebrae. Radiographic changes include thin cortices, decreased bone radiopacity, and end plates that stand out in comparison with decreased radiopacity of vertebral bodies. Such changes are most often associated with systemic disorders of calcium and phosphorus metabolism. Hyperparathyroidism (primary and secondary nutritional, and renal), pseudohyperpar-

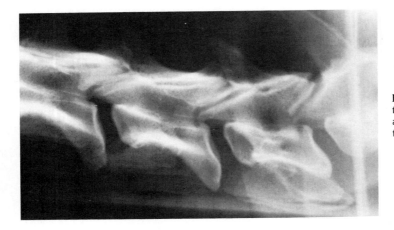

Figure 4–9. Dural ossification causes the thin, linear, calcific density in the ventral aspect of the vertebral canal from C4 through C7.

athyroidism, and hypercorticism are the most common causes. However, many other diseases may be considered. Hypervitaminosis A in cats can also cause osteoporosis (see Chapter 8). However, the predominant finding is spondylosis of the cervical vertebrae.[29, 132] Early lesions may be subtle and involve only the first few cervical vertebrae. More severe or progressive disease can produce extensive, confluent spondylosis of cervical and thoracic vertebrae with involvement of articular processes. The disease may progress to cause complete fusion of the entire vertebral column and also affect appendicular long bones and joints.

Myelography

Myelography is radiography following the introduction of a contrast medium into the spinal subarachnoid space. Myelography is used in veterinary medicine to outline the contour of the spinal cord because it is not visible per se on conventional radiographs. Indications for myelography in veterinary medicine have been reviewed.[2, 12, 149] Myelography is of value in patients with transverse (localized) myelopathies that produce a change in contour of the spinal cord, such as intervertebral disk herniation, vertebral canal stenosis, neoplasia, and hematoma. The technique is useful to supplement survey radiography if findings on survey radiographs are inconclusive or do not correspond with clinically observed neurologic abnormalities. Myelography is helpful in defining the location and extent of spinal cord diseases prior to surgical intervention and thus may also aid in determining prognosis.

Contrast Media. The medical literature on myelographic contrast media is extensive. The ideal contrast medium should provide good contrast, be nontoxic, persist within the subarachnoid space long enough to complete the study, flow freely and be miscible with cerebrospinal fluid to produce uniform distribution, be readily absorbed, and be inexpensive. The ideal contrast medium does not yet exist. Much of the clinical literature on myelography relates to the technique in humans. However, anatomic and procedural differences between humans and animals limit much comparative information. Contrast media can be subdivided into negative and positive contrast media. Negative contrast media such as air may be applicable in the cervical region of humans in combination with tomography. However, gas provides insufficient contrast in the small subarachnoid space of animals.

Many positive contrast media have been used experimentally and clinically in animals. The initial agent in common use was ethyl iodophenylhundecylate (Pantopaque, Myodil), an iodized, radiopaque oil. This agent provided good contrast but had poor flow characteristics and tended to break into droplets, producing a nonuniform column. Immediate toxicity was minimal, but the agent caused acute and chronic leptomeningitis.[69, 74, 146] The contrast medium was removed from the subarachnoid space following myelography in humans, but this is not possible in animals. Thorium dioxide had better flow characteristics but was radioactive and proved to be toxic.[66, 70, 141] Methiodal sodium (sodium iodomethanesulfonate [Skiodan, Abrodil, Kontrast U]) is an aqueous, iodinated contrast medium that replaced iodophenylhundecylate as the myelographic agent of choice in veterinary medicine. Extensive studies were performed both experimentally and clinically in dogs. This contrast medium did have both acute and chronic toxicity but was often used by mixing lidocaine with the contrast medium.[24, 55, 56, 124] Many other agents such as methylglucamine iothalamate and meglumine iocarmate have been tried but proved unacceptable.[1, 28, 124] Most iodinated, water soluble contrast media used are ionic media that are hypertonic compared with CSF. Current research is being directed at nonionic, water soluble contrast media that can deliver similar iodine opacity at osmolality values comparable with those of CSF.[5, 107] Metrizamide was the first such agent in clinical use and is currently the myelographic contrast medium of choice.[11, 54, 100, 137] Metrizamide has been shown to be relatively safe in practice and lacks significant long-term toxic effects.[85] However, metrizamide is not the perfect myelographic contrast medium because it is associated with a high frequency of short-term adverse effects, cannot be autoclaved, is inconvenient to prepare, and is relatively expensive.[3, 10, 28, 85] Continued work is being directed toward evaluating less toxic and heat stable nonionic media such as iopamidol and iohexol, which may eventually replace metrizamide.[13, 43, 85]

Metrizamide is a triiodobenzamido derivative of glucose.[107] It is a water soluble, nonionic, iodinated contrast medium that has less neurotoxicity than previously used contrast media and good miscibility and flow characteristics in the subarachnoid space. Metrizamide may be purchased as a pharmaceutical grade agent (Amipaque) in sterile, preweighed, single dose vials. Different sizes are available, yielding different volumes and different concentrations of sterile solution when reconstituted. These volumes may be appropriate for some patients. Reconstitution is relatively convenient. The medium has a short shelf life for clinical use, as storage of the reconstituted solution may increase neurotoxicity.[2] Amipaque is relatively expensive. More commonly, metrizamide is purchased as a generic, analytic grade powder. Preweighed aliquots are placed in rubber stoppered test tubes and maintained in a desiccator. Because metrizamide is unstable in solution, reconstitution should immediately precede use. Reconstitution of 0.42 g/ml of sterile water or 0.005% bicarbonate diluent will produce a solution with 170 mg of iodine per milliliter, which has an osmolality of 0.3 mol kg^{-1}. Metrizamide is not heat tolerant, thus it cannot be autoclaved. Instead, the solution is aspirated from the tube into a syringe with a filter straw to remove any large, undissolved particles. This solution is then passed through a 0.22 μm disposable filter, through a sterile stopcock, and into the final syringe. This technique is thought to be less expensive but is time consuming and laborious.

Technique. There is great variability in techniques described for myelography. Pretreatment with diazepam (Valium) has been recommended.[11, 137] Phenothiazine derivatives and neuroleptic drugs should be avoided because they lower the epileptogenic threshold. General anesthesia is necessary, and the most common technique is to induce anesthesia with thiobarbiturate (Surital) and to maintain a surgical plane of anesthesia with halothane (Fluothane), nitrous oxide, and oxygen. Survey radiographs are made and evaluated, and technical factors are adjusted as needed. The site for subarachnoid puncture is surgically prepared. Analysis of CSF should precede myelography if the differential diagnosis includes meningitis. Myelography is contraindicated in meningitis because contrast medium injection could disseminate an infection and it exacerbates the inflammatory process. Most variations in technique are variations in spinal needle placement. Possibilities include cervical injection for total myelography, cervical injection for only cervical myelography, lumbar injection for only thoracolumbar myelography, and lumbar injection for total myelography in either lateral or ventral recumbency. It has been recommended that the injection be made as close to the suspected lesion as possible.[54] The techniques of subarachnoid puncture are described in Chapter 3. Advisability of CSF removal prior to injection is arguable. Although it may decrease the pressure induced by the addition of contrast medium, it may also result in a higher concentration of medium in the subarachnoid space.

For injection into the cisterna magna, the head must be elevated to promote caudal flow of the medium. Experience varies considerably on the incidence of subsequent seizures and the consistency of caudal flow of the medium with cisternal injections.[3, 11, 54, 100] In the authors' experience, cisternal injection is associated with inconsistent caudal flow and a higher incidence of seizures. Thus all our myelograms are performed via lumbar injection.

The needle is preferably placed at L5–L6 in either the ventral (transmedullary approach) or dorsal subarachnoid space. Needle penetration of the spinal cord does produce histologic damage of the cord, but little clinical significance is documented.[12] Palpation of the needle against the floor of the vertebral canal does add a sense of security as to needle placement. Operator confidence in dorsal space injection can be gained if the injection is made during fluoroscopic observation. The needle bevel should be directed cranially, and the needle should be connected to the syringe with a flexible extension tube to avoid unnecessary movement of the needle. The connecting tube should first be filled with contrast medium to avoid injection of air bubbles. The smallest syringe possible should be used to make back pressure easier to feel. Contrast medium should be injected slowly.

The dose needed is variable for different sites, and an absolute dosage based solely on body weight or crown-rump length appears inconsistent.[142] Generally 0.3 ml/kg of body weight is adequate to fill the subarachnoid space to the mid-to-cranial thoracic region following lumbar injection or to fill the cervical region following cisternal injection. A dose of 0.45 to 0.50 ml/kg of body weight is usually adequate to fill the cervical region following a lumbar injection. Volume of the connecting tube must be accounted for in medium preparation. Insufficient dosage may occur with significant epidural spillage, which appears to occur more often in larger dogs. If inadequate dosage occurs, the patient must be positioned to promote flow of the contrast medium. One should try to prevent contrast medium from entering the cranium. Even though this may appear to be prevented on radiographs, it has been shown with computed tomography that all myelograms result in some medium within the subarachnoid space of the cranium regardless of injection site and patient positioning.[130] With a lumbar injection and the patient in lateral recumbency, dosage is most accurately monitored with fluoroscopy. For cervical myelography, injection should be terminated when contrast medium is visualized at about C3 with fluoroscopy, as this usually demonstrates the entire cervical spine on subsequent radiographs. An additional value of fluoroscopy is the ability to make spot radiographs during the injection. In some patients, severe spinal cord pressure attenuates the subarachnoid space so that it is not visible on subsequent radiographs and is best seen during the injection.

The needle should be removed following injection and radiographs made soon thereafter. The head should be elevated as soon as possible. In humans, migration of medium into the cranium is retarded by hyperextension of the head, even with the table tilted to lower the head for cranial flow of the medium. This position is maintained until the patient can be placed in an upright position. This technique deserves evaluation in veterinary medicine. Metrizamide will provide diagnostic detail for up to 1 hour following injection and is eventually excreted by the kidneys.[2, 11, 100]

Aftercare and Complications. Recovery is usually uncomplicated following metrizamide myelography. The head should be elevated until recovery is complete. Spontaneous muscle action potentials and motor unit potentials may occur immediately after injection but do not persist for more than 5 minutes.[90] Apnea may occur if injection is too rapid.[2] The most common complications are focal or generalized tonic-clonic seizures.[3, 11] Seizure incidence varies in different reports and appears to be independent of observable intracranial contrast medium.[3] Seizures may be delayed for as long as 12 hours after myelography. Incidences up to nearly one third have been reported in dogs.[3] Seizures appear to be most frequent in larger dogs, with the use of larger doses, and with cisternal injection.[3] If surgery immediately follows myelography, then prolonged anesthesia may lessen the incidence of seizures. Seizures are most commonly treated with diazepam; pentobarbital may be used if necessary. Infrequent complications include malignant hyperthermia and transitory depression or worsening of original clinical signs.[3, 154] The latter may be due to manipulation of the vertebrae during radiography. Vomiting, hyperesthesia, pyrexia, and death have also been reported following metrizamide myelography.[3, 154] The primary complications in humans are headache and nausea.[28, 64] Pleocytosis with a predominance of neutrophils can occur in CSF 24 hours after metrizamide myelography.[26] Clinical experience is limited with myelography in the cat. However, technique, dosage, and incidence of seizures are probably similar to those in the dog.[2]

Normal Appearance. Because the spinal subarachnoid space is thin in animals, there is usually inadequate opacification of the entire sheath of contrast medium as it encircles the spinal cord. Contrast medium is best visualized as a thin column at the periphery of the sheath where the x-ray beam strikes the edges of the contrast sheath tangentially. Thus the dorsal and ventral spinal subarachnoid spaces are visualized on the lateral view, and the right and left spaces on the ventrodorsal view (Fig. 4–10).

The column of contrast medium should be relatively uniform throughout its course, with the following exceptions. There may be slight narrowing of the ventral column directly over

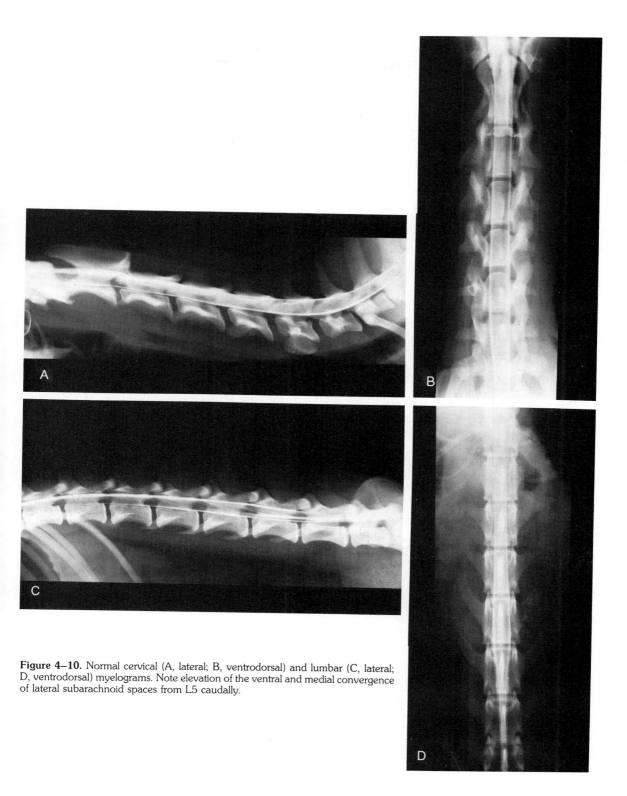

Figure 4–10. Normal cervical (A, lateral; B, ventrodorsal) and lumbar (C, lateral; D, ventrodorsal) myelograms. Note elevation of the ventral and medial convergence of lateral subarachnoid spaces from L5 caudally.

intervertebral disk spaces. This is especially prominent in older dogs and at C2–C3. The ventral column is often narrower than the dorsal column, especially in the thoracolumbar region. Flexion of the vertebrae may also cause thinning or attenuation of the ventral column. Occasionally, the ventral subarachnoid space does not fill well in the mid-to-caudal thoracic region. The dorsal column is larger in the cranial cervical region, especially through C1 and C2. Slight dorsal column enlargement may also be seen in the caudal cervical and cranial thoracic regions. Columns of contrast medium should be parallel on both views, with slight divergence due to spinal cord widening at the cervical and lumbar enlargements. The cervical enlargement is generally at the C6–C7 vertebral level and the lumbar enlargement is at the L4–L5 vertebral level, but they are variable in location. Both appear more prominent on the ventrodorsal view. The subarachnoid space (myelographic columns) appears to fill the entire vertebral canal in small dogs and cats but appears relatively smaller compared with the size of the vertebral canal in large breed dogs. This is especially pronounced in the caudal cervical region of large dogs, where the ventral column may be more elevated from the ventral margin of the canal in neutral and hyperextended positions. As the spinal cord terminates, one may see longitudinal striations of the cauda equina. Narrowing of the spinal cord begins at L5 as the columns gradually deviate away from margins of the vertebral canal. The ventral column gradually rises and lateral columns converge medially to produce a single column, which may be inconsistently seen through the sacral canal. However, myelography is an unreliable technique to evaluate the vertebral canal caudal to L6.

Artifacts may be created during myelography. Filling of lumbar vertebral venous sinuses is occasionally seen with lumbar injection. A more common artifact with lumbar injection is epidural leakage or partial epidural injection. Contrast medium in the epidural space produces an uneven column that is sometimes superimposed over and sometimes separated from the subarachnoid column. With large amounts of epidural contrast medium, the medium may flow out nerve root sheaths and be visible on the lateral view as opaque nodules in the intervertebral foramina and on the ventrodorsal view as linear striations extending outward from the intervertebral foramina. A large amount of epidural medium may compromise myelographic interpretation. If this occurs, it has been sug-

gested that several minutes of caudal abdominal compression with an elastic wrap will increase blood flow through vertebral sinuses and enhance removal of epidural medium.[2] Occasionally the myelogram must be repeated. Leakage of contrast medium back into the needle tract occurs with both lumbar and cisternal injections but appears to cause no clinical or diagnostic problems. Occasionally the central canal is opacified during lumbar injection without other evidence of cord disruption. This may be attributable to leakage of medium through the needle tract during a transmedullary approach.

Interpretation of Abnormalities. Interpretation of myelograms is dependent primarily on recognition of changes in size, shape, and position of the spinal subarachnoid space. These changes, in turn, demonstrate alterations in spinal cord contour and reflect the origin and severity of compressive lesions of the cord. Correlation of both lateral and ventrodorsal views is essential to understand the three dimensional nature of spinal cord morphology. Focal lesions of the spinal cord are usually classified as being extradural, intramedullary, or intradural-extramedullary in origin.[110, 140, 144] Lesions are categorized on the basis of characteristic patterns observed on myelograms.

Extradural mass lesions within the vertebral canal cause deviation of the subarachnoid space away from the bony margin of the canal in at least one view. This usually causes attenuation or thinning of the subarachnoid space and narrowing of the spinal cord at this site. With small focal extradural masses, there may be no other changes. With larger masses, the spinal cord may be displaced away from the extradural mass and the subarachnoid space on the opposing side may be narrowed (Fig. 4–11). As the cord is pushed against the opposite side of the canal, it may be flattened against the bony margin, and this will appear as a corresponding focal widening of the cord on the orthogonal view. The most common cause of an extradural mass lesion is protrusion of disk material into the vertebral canal. Other causes include tumor, hematoma, and projection of hypertrophied ligaments into the vertebral canal. Narrowing of the spinal cord from opposing directions produces an hourglass narrowing of the cord. In the caudal cervical spine of large dogs such a change may be due to combinations of vertebral malformation, ligamentous hypertrophy, and disk protrusion. Circumferential stenosis produces an hourglass narrowing of the cord on all views. Flexed and extended lateral views of the cervical vertebrae during myelography are im-

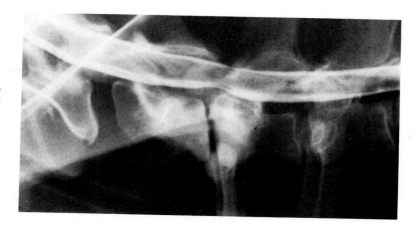

Figure 4–11. Extradural mass at C7–T1. The ventral subarachnoid space is elevated and thinned over C7–T1. The spinal cord is pressed dorsally, causing thinning of the dorsal subarachnoid space.

portant in large breed dogs because of variability in the appearance of extradural lesions (Fig. 4–12). Hypertrophy of the interarcuate ligament may produce an extradural compression with the neck in extension, but the dorsal subarachnoid space may appear normal during flexion. Focal hypertrophy of the dorsal longitudinal ligament may produce an extradural mass over the disk space that is also accentuated with extension and minimized with flexion. The ventral extradural mass produced by dorsal disk protrusion in these breeds will be accentuated with flexion but minimized with extension.

Intramedullary lesions that cause enlargement of the spinal cord usually produce uniform circumferential enlargement, causing outward deviation and attenuation of the subarachnoid space that appears the same on all views (Fig. 4–13). Size and length of such lesions are quite variable. Differential diagnoses include spinal cord edema and neoplasia. Tumors are most often relatively focal. Edema can be focal or extend the length of several vertebrae. If the

compression is severe enough, the subarachnoid space will not be visible because the pressure prevents retention of contrast medium at this site. Thus one may see an area with total absence of contrast medium.

The classic intradural-extramedullary mass lesion is one that appears as a filling defect located within the subarachnoid space (Fig. 4–14). If small, such a lesion may appear as an air bubble encircled by contrast medium. However, most lesions are larger and cause focal narrowing of the spinal cord. A filling defect may still be present on the same view, but often the filling defect may not be totally outlined by the contrast medium. Instead, the contrast column may appear to widen up to the margin of the lesion. If the lesion is compressive, the spinal cord may appear narrowed on one view and widened on the other view with associated thinning of the subarachnoid space. The origin of this type of lesion may be difficult to define, and such lesions may appear as extradural masses.

Compressive lesions may occasionally be se-

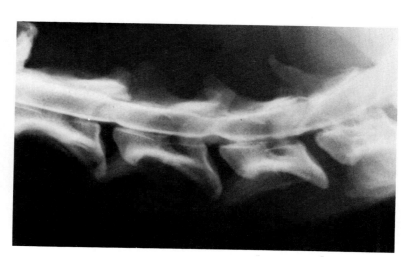

Figure 4–12. Dorsal and ventral extradural compression at C4–C5 demonstrated on a fully extended lateral view. The ventral lesion was less severe and the dorsal lesion was not visible with the spine in neutral and flexed positions. Similar but less severe changes are present at C3–C4.

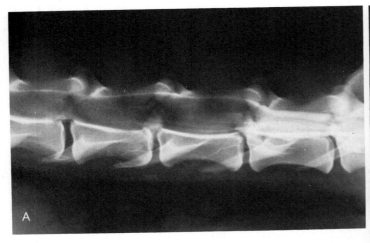

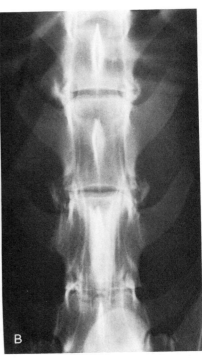

Figure 4–13. Intramedullary mass that caused outward deviation and thinning of contrast columns. A, Lateral view. B, Ventrodorsal view. Myelographic injection was at L6–L7, and there is contrast medium present in both subarachnoid and epidural spaces. Only the caudal margin of the mass at L5–L6 is outlined well. Same dog as in Figure 4–6.

vere enough to completely block the subarachnoid space. Myelography only outlines one end of the lesion, and increased resistance may be felt during lumbar injection. Malacia of the spinal cord occasionally causes an irregular or patchy accumulation of contrast medium within the spinal cord (Fig. 4–15). The central canal may fill with contrast medium owing to spinal cord malacia, misplaced injection, leakage into the needle tract during transmedullary spinal puncture, and some congenital anomalies.

Epidurography

Epidurography is spinal radiography following the introduction of a contrast medium into the spinal epidural space. Air and oil based and aqueous contrast media have been used in humans and animals. The current contrast medium of choice is metrizamide, which appears to be safe and nonirritating.[22, 86] Because of complications of myelography prior to development of metrizamide, epidurography was

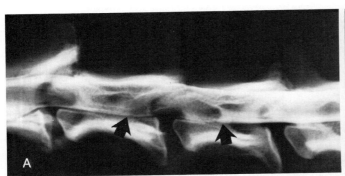

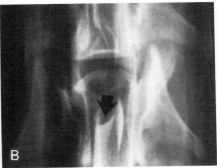

Figure 4–14. Intradural-extramedullary mass at C3–C4. A, On the lateral view, the mass produces an oval filling defect within the subarachnoid space, with cranial and caudal limits noted by arrows. B, On the ventrodorsal view, the mass is not completely outlined but still produces widening of the subarachnoid space, with a characteristic filling defect at its caudal margin (arrow).

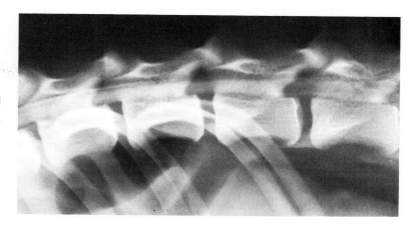

Figure 4–15. Myelogram of a dog with diffuse contrast medium opacification of the spinal cord due to extensive myelomalacia.

evaluated as a technique for the diagnosis of spinal cord lesions.[89] This indication has not been widely accepted, especially in view of advances made in myelography. However, myelography is of limited value caudal to the termination of the spinal cord in animals. This is because the subarachnoid space moves away from the lateral and ventral margins of the vertebral canal caudal to L5–L6. Thus techniques other than myelography are used to evaluate compressive lesions within the vertebral canal from L6 caudally. The two techniques for this purpose are epidurography and vertebral sinus venography. Artifacts are occasionally noted with venography, and epidurography is easier to perform and produces minimal patient trauma.[86, 118] For these reasons the authors prefer epidurography over venography.

Technique. The patient is placed under general inhalation anesthesia. Survey radiographs are made and evaluated, and technical factors are adjusted as necessary. The animal may be placed in either lateral or ventral recumbency. The authors prefer lateral recumbency, especially if the injection is to be monitored with fluoroscopy. The site of puncture should be surgically prepared. A short spinal needle is passed into the vertebral canal at S3–Cd1, but any vertebral junction from S3 through the first few caudal vertebrae can be used.[46] The needle is passed to the floor of the vertebral canal, and the bevel is directed cranially. The syringe is connected to the needle with a flexible extension tube filled with contrast medium. The extension tube minimizes unnecessary movement of the needle and allows the operator's hands to be moved away from the x-ray beam. Even in normal dogs there is poor correlation between the extent of cranial flow of contrast medium and the dose injected.[46] An initial dose of 0.15 ml/kg of body weight has been recom-

mended.[46] Fluoroscopy can be used to ascertain that the medium is within the vertebral canal. Radiographic exposure is made just prior to the termination of injection. Additional contrast medium should be injected for each additional view. Subsequent doses of 0.10 ml/kg of body weight have been recommended.[46] Although two views are recommended, the lateral view appears to provide the most diagnostic information. A dorsoventral view with the animal in sternal recumbency allows the exposure to be made with the needle in place during injection. Flexed and extended lateral views may also be of value. The technique appears to be safe, and adverse effects have not been noted.[22, 46]

Normal Appearance. Epidurography does not produce the well-defined, linear contrast columns seen with myelography (Fig. 4–16A). The contrast column may be relatively wide and nonuniform in density. On the lateral view, the contrast column gradually narrows from the cranial part of L7 to the caudal part of S1 and then tapers more dramatically through the sacrum.[46] Varying degrees of slight dorsal deviation may be seen at the level of intervertebral spaces. Undulations and irregular pooling may be due to epidural fat. The dorsoventral view is usually more difficult to evaluate. Linear striations and filling defects may be due to nerve roots and are more apparent on the dorsoventral view than on the lateral view. Contrast medium may follow nerve roots through intervertebral foramina even in normal animals.

Interpretation of Abnormalities. Abnormalities of lumbosacral epidurography must be closely correlated with other neurologic findings of the cauda equina. Abnormality of the epidurogram may appear as a focal indentation of the contrast column (Fig. 4–16B). These areas may also be associated with abrupt thinning of the contrast column. Such lesions could be due

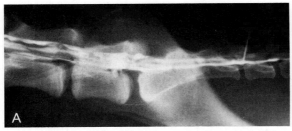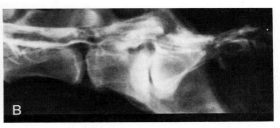

Figure 4–16. A, Normal lumbosacral epidurogram. Note the slight dorsal deviation of the ventral contrast column over intervertebral disk spaces and irregular pooling of contrast medium. B, Abnormal lumbosacral epidurogram. There is pronounced dorsal deviation and thinning of the ventral contrast column at L7–S1 that was due to dorsal protrusion of disk material.

to focal mass type lesions such as disk protrusions, tumors, or hypertrophied ligaments projecting into the vertebral canal. More symmetric stenosis of the vertebral canal may produce a more symmetric narrowing and deviation of the contrast column. Some lesions within the vertebral canal may produce complete obstruction to flow of the contrast medium. Such lesions may be associated with an increased resistance to injection and greater loss of contrast medium out of the vertebral canal. Venous opacification may occur.

Vertebral Venography

Vertebral venography is radiography of the vertebral column following opacification of vertebral venous plexuses with positive contrast medium. An understanding of anatomy and blood flow dynamics through this region is important. Of primary concern is opacification of the ventral internal vertebral venous plexuses. For cervical studies, contrast medium can be injected into the angularis oculi, nasal, or facial veins with simultaneous compression of external jugular veins. This technique can produce vertebral venous sinus opacification to T1 or T2.[31] Opacification of lumbar vertebral veins can be accomplished by a variety of techniques. Owing to the current practicality and value of myelography throughout the spine cranial to L6, most venographic studies are directed at diseases of the caudal lumbar and lumbosacral vertebral canal. Ventral internal vertebral venous plexuses are in close apposition with dorsal surfaces of vertebral bodies and intervertebral disks. Because these vessels have thin walls and are easily collapsed, compressive lesions within the vertebral canal may be reflected in abnormal patterns of opacification of these vessels.

Anatomic and hemodynamic considerations have led to use of various techniques to fill these vessels with contrast medium. Most techniques make use of the fact that, with compression or occlusion of the caudal vena cava, the vertebral venous plexuses become the principal route for return of blood from the caudal part of the body.[148] Initial studies were accomplished by ligation of the caudal vena cava.[148] One clinical approach is to pass an occluding, balloon (thrombectomy) catheter via femoral venotomy into the caudal vena cava to the midlumbar level.[92] A second angiographic catheter is passed to the caudal lumbar level from the contralateral femoral vein. A radiograph is made 10 seconds after injection of 10 to 15 ml of contrast medium. Filling of venous radicals peripheral to the vertebral canal may tend to obscure the internal vertebral venous plexuses. An alternate and less invasive technique is to compress the caudal vena cava by application of external abdominal compression and to inject contrast medium into a pelvic limb vein.[97] This technique can opacify the vertebral venous plexuses up to T11. This technique is said to demonstrate slight compressive lesions but may be of more value in excluding rather than localizing compressive lesions. The more commonly used techniques involve the injection of contrast medium into the intraosseous vascular system (transosseous venography) of the vertebral body of Cd4 or L7.[17, 105] These appear to be the most frequently accepted techniques and will be described in more detail. Selective catheterization of the median sacral vein via a transjugular approach has been used in dogs to study vascular anatomy and hemodynamics.[91] Technical difficulties and variations in vascular anatomy limit clinical usefulness of the technique.

Technique. The transosseous technique is performed as follows.[105] The patient is placed under general inhalation anesthesia and positioned in lateral recumbency. The tailhead is prepared for surgery. A 16 or 18 gauge bone marrow biopsy needle is placed into the marrow cavity of the body of Cd4. Placement and subsequent monitoring of injection are facilitated by fluoroscopy. Bone marrow should be aspirated to confirm proper placement of the needle. A water soluble, iodinated contrast medium such as meglumine iothalamate is used. The syringe and a flexible extension tube filled with contrast medium are connected to the needle, and a test injection of 2 ml is made during fluoroscopic observation. Caudal abdominal compression is applied as for compressive excretory urography. Doses of 6 ml and 8 ml are used for medium-sized and large dogs, respectively. The radiographic contrast medium is manually injected rapidly. Radiographic exposure is made during injection of the last 1 to 2 ml of medium. The patient is repositioned and reinjected for the ventrodorsal view.

An alternate technique involves percutaneous placement of a 16 gauge caudal needle into the vertebral body of L7 from a ventrolateral approach ventral to the ilium.[17] Slight variations in the technique of injection have been noted. Heparinized saline may be injected first to flush vascular channels of the marrow cavity. An extension tube is used to inject 10 ml of contrast medium. A lateral radiograph is made as the last 1 ml is being injected. An infrequently used technique involves injecting into a spinous process.[120] Magnification techniques are recommended in humans and may be applicable in small animals.[59]

Potential contraindications include infection at the site of injection, medical contraindications for general anesthesia, and a known history of hypersensitivity to contrast media. Most complications appear to relate to improper techniques that result in nondiagnostic studies.[17, 105] Epidural injection, local perivertebral extravasation of contrast medium, and inadequate abdominal compression can cause loss of definition of venous plexuses, inadequate volume of medium to fully identify plexuses, or excess medium accumulation in the extravertebral circulation. Placement of the bevel of the needle within the center of the medullary cavity is important. The injection may be compromised if the tip of the needle is against cortical bone. Extravasation into the epidural space can occur if the tip of the needle enters the vertebral canal or if excessive injection pressure is used. Multiple needle entries create holes that allow perivertebral accumulation of contrast medium. The approach to L7 has the potential of damaging the sixth lumbar spinal nerve.

Normal Appearance. Internal ventral vertebral venous plexuses are demonstrated on the lateral view more consistently than on the ventrodorsal view. On the lateral view (Fig. 4–17A), the plexuses appear as relatively large vessels that lie along the ventral vertebral canal. They are in close apposition with the ventral margin of the vertebral canal in the midportions

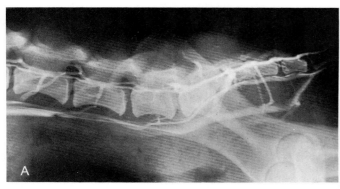
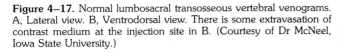
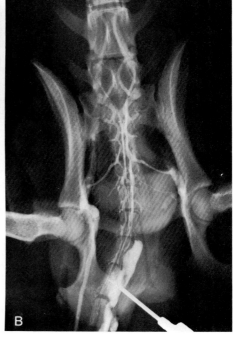

Figure 4–17. Normal lumbosacral transosseous vertebral venograms. A, Lateral view. B, Ventrodorsal view. There is some extravasation of contrast medium at the injection site in B. (Courtesy of Dr McNeel, Iowa State University.)

of the vertebral bodies. Slight to prominent dorsal elevation of these vessels occurs over intervertebral disks, causing the vessels to be superimposed over intervertebral foramina. On the ventrodorsal view (Fig. 4–17B), the vessels have regular undulations as right and left plexuses approach the midline over the vertebral bodies and then deviate laterally to the periphery of the vertebral canal at the level of the intervertebral disk. There is gradual, symmetric curvature between medial and lateral points. Occasionally the plexuses cranial to the lumbosacral junction may fail to fill with contrast medium on the ventrodorsal view with the injection in Cd4.[105] With injection in L7, sacral plexuses are filled by reflux. This reflux may not occur with injection into L6.[17]

Interpretation of Abnormalities. Abnormalities of the internal ventral vertebral venous plexuses include narrowing, displacement, and obstruction. Differences in the pattern and severity of abnormality are due to differences in origin and severity of the lesion. For example, dorsal protrusion of disk material at L7–S1 would be expected to cause dorsal elevation and possible thinning of the vessel at this site. Most common diagnoses with this technique relate to mass lesions and stenotic lesions of the lumbosacral vertebral canal. Poor results may be seen with venography following laminectomy owing to adhesions and scarring within the epidural space.[105]

It is generally believed that venography is a sensitive technique because it usually detects lesions that are present. However, false positive results have also been seen as contrast medium flowed through extravertebral veins without filling intravertebral venous plexuses in dogs that did not have obstruction of the lumbosacral vertebral canal.[118] Additional problems relate to inconsistencies seen on ventrodorsal views of normal dogs and inconsistencies associated with compression of the caudal vena cava.

Diskography and Disk Aspiration

A needle may be placed into the nucleus of an intervertebral disk. Diskography is radiography following injection of contrast medium into the disk space. Conversely, the technique may be used to aspirate material from a disk (or vertebral body) for subsequent culture and sensitivity testing (or microscopic examination). The initial technique of diskography in humans used a posterior approach through the vertebral canal into the nucleus of a disk.[98] The disk is much smaller in dogs than in humans, and the dorsal approach would appear to provide the wrong angle for consistent entry into the disk. A lateral or dorsolateral approach was recommended to preclude penetration of the spinal cord and to avoid creating a needle tract in the dorsal anulus, where most disks herniate.[57] The technique was difficult without surgical exposure. However, the dorsolateral and lateral approaches would appear to have potential to damage nerve roots and extravertebral venous channels, especially in the cervical region. Thus the authors prefer to use a ventrolateral approach beneath the transverse processes with the needle directed dorsomedially. The technique can be performed with a percutaneous approach and with fluoroscopic guidance, thus obviating the need for surgical exposure.

The patient is placed under general inhalation anesthesia and positioned in lateral recumbency. A large area over the entry site is prepared for surgery. A sterile radiopaque marker (small needle) is placed at the potential area of needle penetration of the skin. Accuracy is evaluated fluoroscopically. A small skin incision is made if the technique is performed for aspiration. A spinal needle with stylet is usually adequate to enter the disk. However, specialized needles may be needed to biopsy bone or penetrate large spondylotic areas. The needle is advanced toward the disk of concern using palpable landmarks and periodic, intermittent fluoroscopic observation. Passage of the needle through the anulus is associated with increased resistance that is felt during advancement of the needle. The needle tip should be centrally located in the disk space. A **C** arm fluoroscopic system would be of further advantage.

For diskography, the needle is connected to an extension tube and syringe containing a water soluble, organic, iodinated contrast medium such as meglumine iothalamate. In the normal disk, resistance to injection is great, and the disk will accommodate only 0.1 to 0.5 ml of medium.[12, 57] Fluoroscopic monitoring during injection can be used to confirm that medium is injected and that it is injected into the proper site. Contrast medium in a normal disk should appear as a small, sharply marginated nodule centered in the nucleus pulposus (Fig. 4–18). Irregular filling defects may be due to gas bubbles from the needle or nonuniform distribution of the medium. Abnormal findings may include the ability to inject larger volumes with less resistance and abnormal location of contrast medium.[30, 155]

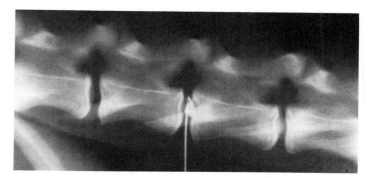

Figure 4–18. Lumbar diskogram in a normal dog. The needle is still in place.

The technique of fluoroscopically guided percutaneous aspiration has more value than diskography in veterinary medicine. Percutaneous skeletal biopsy may be an accurate technique for the confirmation or exclusion of cancer and inflammatory diseases.[111] Percutaneous biopsy of vertebral bodies is a widely practiced and safe procedure in humans, as is percutaneous aspiration of disk spaces in patients with suspected diskospondylitis.[6, 111, 131] In patients with suspected diskospondylitis, percutaneous aspiration offers a direct means to obtain material for bacterial culture and sensitivity testing as compared with the more indirect approach of bacterial culture of blood and urine and the invasive method of open biopsy.[6, 131] Such a technique may be of most value in patients with diskospondylitis in which cultures of blood and urine are negative or contradictory, and in cases that do not respond to medical therapy based on results of blood and urine cultures (Fig. 4–7A). The authors have used this technique on several dogs with cervical, lumbar, and lumbosacral diskospondylitis. Although the technique appears to be a viable one, there are insufficient case numbers to confirm its true value.

Equine

Survey Radiography

Radiographs can be made of segments throughout the equine vertebral column for a variety of neurologic and musculoskeletal problems. Evaluation of thoracic, lumbar, and sacral abnormalities can be accomplished with high output, dedicated systems.[80, 82] However, most neuroradiographic studies in the horse are concerned with the cervical vertebrae. These studies can be readily performed with more conventional equipment and thus will be the focus of this section. Readers are referred elsewhere for specific information on radiography of the thoracic, lumbar, and sacral vertebral regions.[78, 79, 81]

Technique. Lateral survey radiographs of the equine cervical vertebrae are preferably made in the conscious, standing horse. Care must be taken in alignment of the x-ray beam and grid-cassette system. Methods have been discussed above. Rare earth screen-film systems are of special value for the caudal cervical vertebrae. The examination is essentially limited to studies in a relatively neutral position because flexed and extended views require general anesthesia. The initial study is often used as a screening procedure that may adequately demonstrate some fractures, anomalies, and infectious lesions of vertebrae. The entire cervical vertebral column can be evaluated with better technical control with the animal under general anesthesia. However, with large, muscular horses, true lateral alignment can be more difficult than alignment in the standing animal. Lateral radiographs can be made in the flexed, neutral, and extended positions. Ventrodorsal radiographs can be made of the C1–C5 cervical region. For lateral radiographs, the same geometric principles apply as previously described. The vertebrae should be maintained parallel to the grid-cassette and perpendicular to the central axis of the x-ray beam. Rotational obliquity should be minimized as much as possible. Positioning for flexed and extended views is aided by using rope ties to move the thoracic limbs caudally and to maintain positioning of the head to produce the appropriate stress.[112, 125] The neck is radiographed in sections using overlapping fields to include the entire cervical region from the base of the skull to T1. This may require two or three radiographs for each position. The ventrodorsal view is made with the animal in dorsal recumbency and is usually limited to the first few vertebrae. This is usually a supplemen-

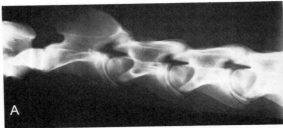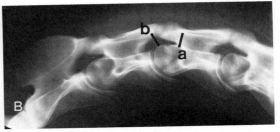

Figure 4–19. Normal survey radiographs of the cervical vertebrae of a horse. A, Neutral lateral view. B, Flexed lateral view. Sites for measuring the minimum sagittal diameter (a) and the minimum flexion diameter (b) are noted.

tal view that is obtained as indicated rather than as part of a standard protocol.

Normal Appearance. Radiographs of a normal equine cervical vertebral column are presented in Figure 4–19. There are seven cervical vertebrae, and C1 and C2 have characteristic unique morphology. The contour of the cranial vertebral notch of C2 varies considerably and may form a true foramen, especially in adult horses after the ligament ossifies to complete a bony foramen. The dens is separated by a physis from the cranial epiphysis of the body of C2 in immature animals. Morphology of C3 through C5 appears relatively similar. C6 is slightly shorter than C5, and C7 is shorter yet. There usually are a pair of ventral processes present on C6 that can be helpful landmarks. In a small proportion of thoroughbred horses at least one or, more often, both these ventral processes will be transposed onto C7 and, less frequently, onto C5. Ossification centers may be visible at the tips of transverse processes and, more prominently, on the caudal aspect of the ventral processes of C6. Curvatures of the vertebral column are relatively smooth, with gradual changes in alignment of vertebrae, but will vary depending on the stress of positioning. Dorsal

and ventral margins of the vertebral canal within each vertebra should be approximately parallel.[125]

Extensive work has been performed to define normal ranges of various dimensions of the cervical vertebrae in horses.[103] Of various measurements possible, the most significant ones on survey radiographs are measurements of sagittal diameters of the vertebral canal. The minimum sagittal diameter (MSD) of the vertebral canal is measured at the narrowest point between dorsal and ventral margins of the vertebral foramen within each vertebra. The minimum flexion diameter (MFD) is the minimum sagittal diameter of the vertebral canal measured between adjacent vertebrae at each cervical intervertebral space with the vertebrae flexed. Landmarks for the minimum flexion diameter correspond to the dorsal surface of the cranial epiphysis of one vertebral body and the dorsal rim of the caudal orifice of the vertebral foramen of the next cranial vertebra. Although ranges are reported for these measurements, the most significant values appear to be minimum values. The values most often referred to are listed in Table 4–1. It is also noted that the values listed are direct measurements rather than relative

Table 4–1. MINIMUM VALUES OF EQUINE CERVICAL VERTEBRAL AND MYELOGRAPHIC MEASUREMENTS

Body Weight	Minimum Sagittal Diameter (MSD) (mm)					
	C2	C3	C4	C5	C6	C7
Under 320 kg	20.8	18.1	16.7	17.3	18.3	19.8
Over 320 kg	22.1	18.5	17.7	18.7	19.0	22.2
	Minimum Flexion Diameter (MFD) (mm)					
		C2-C3	C3-C4	C4-C5	C5-C6	C6-C7
Under 320 kg		19.3	13.4	13.2	16.1	21.6
Over 320 kg		22.8	15.6	14.8	17.9	28.5
	Minimum Flexed Dural Sagittal Diameter (MDD) (mm)					
		C2-C3	C3-C4	C4-C5	C5-C6	C6-C7
Under 320 kg		11.3	9.0	9.9	11.9	17.3
Over 320 kg		12.9	10.5	10.8	11.4	17.6

From Mayhew IG, Whitlock RH, and deLahunta A: Spinal cord disease in the horse: Electromyographic and radiographic studies. Cornell Vet 68 (Suppl 6):44, 1978.

values. Measurements may be influenced by geometric magnification factors during radiography. Thus measurements may be better made on radiographs obtained with the patient under anesthesia where the degree of magnification is more controlled and uniform.

Interpretation of Abnormalities. Principles of radiographic interpretation of abnormalities of the equine cervical vertebrae are comparable with those described above. However, in addition to the diagnoses of fractures, anomalies, and infections, there is a complex syndrome called cervical vertebral malformation (see Chapters 6 and 17).[102, 103] Survey radiographic findings of vertebral canal stenosis, enlarged caudal epiphyseal plates, caudal extension of the dorsal aspect of the caudal vertebral orifice, proliferative remodeling of articular processes or vertebral bodies, and angular deformity of adjacent vertebrae contribute to the diagnosis.[103, 125] Obvious narrowing of the vertebral canal may be evident, and objective (measured) values for vertebral canal diameters less than those listed in Table 4–1 are likely to indicate stenosis of the vertebral canal. However, myelography is necessary to confirm the presence of compressive myelopathy.

Cervical Myelography

Myelography is being used with increasing frequency in the diagnosis of equine cervical myelopathies. Historical considerations of myelographic contrast media are comparable with those described above. Until the development of metrizamide, myelography in the horse usually was a terminal procedure. Since the first reports appeared on the clinical use of metrizamide in horses, subsequent reports have further described the use, effects, and value of metrizamide myelography.[15, 112, 125, 138]

Technique. Differences in technique are described, but general principles are similar.[15, 112, 125] Pretreatment is variable. Phenylbutazone may be used, and drugs that may potentiate seizures should be avoided. General anesthesia is induced with glyceryl guaiacolate and sodium thiamylal and maintained with halothane and oxygen. The patient is placed in lateral recumbency, positioning and restraint devices are applied, and survey radiographs are made and evaluated. The head and neck should then be elevated after being placed on a rigid plywood sheet. Aseptic cisternal puncture is made with an 18 gauge spinal needle. A volume of spinal fluid equal to about half the anticipated volume of metrizamide to be injected is removed. Me-

trizamide is prepared by the technique previously described. Slight variations have been described that utilize 0.42 to 0.45 g of metrizamide per milliliter of diluent. Diluent may be sterile distilled water with or without the addition of sodium bicarbonate and xylocaine. The dose used may be approximately 50 ml for horses over 320 kg and 25 ml for horses under 320 kg of body weight. The contrast medium is injected slowly over several minutes through an extension tube with the bevel of the needle directed caudally. The head should be elevated an additional 5 minutes. Insertion of a spinal needle in the lumbosacral subarachnoid space as a drain facilitates caudal movement of contrast medium. Radiographs are then made in the various positions described. Recovery should be in a padded stall with close monitoring.

Most complications described appear to be mild reactions that may persist for about 24 hours.[15, 112] Fever (102–106°F), depression, muscle fasciculations, and head and neck jerking are commonly described. Transient worsening of the patient's condition may occur. Following myelography, CSF may be cloudy and xanthochromic and may contain increased levels of protein, white blood cells, and erythrocytes.[112] A mild, sterile, suppurative meningitis is present on microscopic examination.[112]

Normal Appearance. Normal cervical myelograms are presented in Figure 4–20. Leakage of contrast medium may occasionally be seen at the puncture site. The columns of contrast medium are usually adequately visualized throughout the cervical region but may be more difficult to visualize caudal to C6 on the lateral view and caudal to C5 on the ventrodorsal view. Opacification usually persists long enough to allow performance of a diagnostic study. The appearance of contrast columns has been described.[112, 125] On the ventrodorsal views, right and left contrast columns are uniform and symmetric when visible, although subtle widening of the total column may be evident at intervertebral levels. On lateral views, the dorsal and ventral columns are of equal width through C1 and C2. The dorsal column is generally wider than the ventral column through the remainder of the cervical region. The dorsal column is also relatively uniform in width. In the neutral position, the dorsal column may be slightly narrowed at each cranial vertebral orifice and slightly wider at each caudal vertebral orifice. A similar pattern with slight variations is present with full extension. In the flexed position, the dorsal column is narrowed slightly at inter-

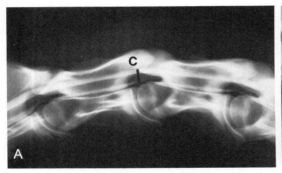
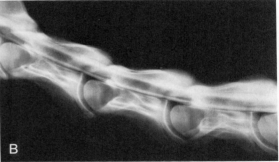

Figure 4-20. Normal equine cervical myelograms. A, Flexed lateral view. B, Extended lateral view. A site for measuring the minimum flexed dural sagittal diameter (c) is noted.

vertebral spaces. Excessive flexion, particularly in smaller horses, can result in obliteration of the dorsal and ventral contrast columns. The ventral column is also relatively wide in neutral and fully extended positions. In the neutral position the ventral column may be slightly narrowed at each caudal vertebral orifice and slightly widened at each cranial vertebral orifice. A similar pattern with slight variations is present in full extension. In the flexed position there is pronounced thinning of the ventral column, associated with a dorsal excursion of the cranial epiphyses of vertebrae. Thinning of the ventral column occurs at all intervertebral spaces from C2-C3 through C6-C7 but is most pronounced over the spaces at C3-C4 and C4-C5. The minimum dural sagittal diameter during flexion (MDD) is measured at each intervertebral space.[103] Minimum normal values are listed in Table 4-1.

Interpretation of Abnormalities. Principles of extradural, intramedullary, and intradural-extramedullary myelographic patterns apply.

However, for practical purposes, almost all cervical myelographic lesions recognized in horses are extradural compressive lesions. In addition, most such lesions are recognized as dorsoventral compression on lateral views (Fig. 4-21). The major difficulty is separation of normal contour variations of the contrast column from abnormalities. In areas where the contrast columns are severely narrowed dorsally and ventrally, lesions are usually visible in all of the lateral positions and frequently correlate with narrowing of the vertebral canal. In some cases, narrowing of the contrast columns may only be visible on one of the lateral positions. Thus the entire series is usually recommended. Subjective evaluation is usually adequate in patients with severe compressive myelopathy. Measured values less than those listed in Table 4-1 may increase confidence in diagnosis of more subtle lesions.[103] Development of reference ranges for different techniques and facilities in neutral, flexed, and extended views is recommended.

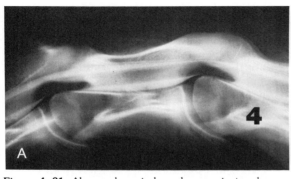
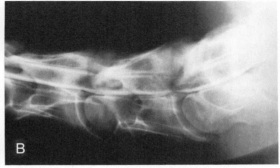

Figure 4-21. Abnormal cervical myelograms in two horses. A, Flexed lateral view. The minimum flexed dural sagittal diameter was small, and there is spinal cord compression with associated thinning of the dorsal subarachnoid space at C3-C4. The thin radiopaque line over cranial articular processes of C4 is an artifact. 4 = C4. B, Extended lateral view of C5, 6, 7. There is narrowing of the spinal cord with thinning of the subarachnoid space at C6-C7. There is vertebral osteoarthritis at C5-C6, and particularly at C6-C7, with prominent bone production and hypertrophy of soft tissue structures.

BRAIN AND SKULL

Small Animal

Survey Radiography

Neural elements of the skull are not visible on survey radiographs. Without the use of special procedures, neuroradiographic diagnosis is based indirectly on recognition of osseous abnormalities of the skull. Survey radiography of the skull is generally unrewarding for most diseases of the brain. The yield of neuroradiographic studies is greatly increased if radiographs are made to specifically evaluate well-defined areas of the skull following characterization of localized diseases by other neurologic examination techniques. For example, radiographic examination of the tympanic bullae is often performed following localization of disease to the peripheral vestibular system. More specialized techniques such as contrast radiography, nuclear imaging, and computed tomography are necessary to further evaluate many lesions of the brain. Bony structure of the skull is complex, and radiographic lesions may be very subtle or difficult to project. Consulting published references is valuable.[60, 134] A prepared skeletal specimen of the skull is of additional benefit for both positioning and interpretive reference. This section will discuss areas of the skull of neurologic importance but will not deal with nasal, mandibular, and dental radiography.

Positioning. Accurate positioning is important in radiographic examination of the skull. General anesthesia is essential to provide restraint, allow accurate positioning, and enhance radiation safety practices. Heavy sedation may be used if general anesthesia is medically contraindicated. Radiolucent positioning pads and restraint devices are necessary. Extra care must be taken to ensure accurate labeling of views, and supplemental labels should be used to identify specific areas projected. Multiple views are available to evaluate the skull, and detailed information for these views and their variations is described elsewhere.[31, 104, 109, 143] Not all radiographic views of the skull are used routinely because many views adequately project only specific localized areas of the skull. The initial radiographic examination usually includes the lateral and ventrodorsal (or dorsoventral) views. Clinical information must be used to select additional views needed for a specific radiographic study.

The lateral view of the skull is made with the animal in lateral recumbency (Fig. 4–22A). The head is positioned so that the median plane is parallel to the cassette and perpendicular to the central axis of the vertical x-ray beam. Correct positioning usually requires radiolucent padding under the nose and mandible. An oral speculum to hold the mouth open may help prevent rotational obliquity and avoid superimposition of coronoid processes of the mandible over the skull. Either the ventrodorsal (Fig. 4–22B) or dorsoventral view may be used as the second routine view. It may be easier to obtain symmetric positioning in some animals by using the dorsoventral view. Pressing the mandibles against the table top assists in positioning the head symmetrically. In other animals, the ventrodorsal view made in dorsal recumbency may be easier to obtain. In either view, the hard palate should be parallel to the cassette. The skull will appear slightly different on the two views owing to differences in the geometry of projection. The ventrodorsal and dorsoventral views of the skull serve primarily as complements to the lateral view, but many lesions are further evaluated and often better visualized on selected additional views.

Oblique views can be made to better visualize each tympanic bulla (Fig. 4–22C). The animal is positioned in lateral recumbency, and the head is rotated to elevate the ventral aspect so that the sagittal plane is obliqued about 20° from the plane of the cassette. As an example, this can produce a left 20° ventral–right dorsal oblique view.[143] The mouth should be closed. This view will project the dependent tympanic bulla and contralateral frontal sinus. The opposite view should be made for comparison, and care must be taken to produce comparable positioning. Oblique views of frontal sinuses are best made with rotation of the head in the opposite direction to project the dependent frontal sinus, such as with a left 20° dorsal–right ventral oblique view. Frontal sinuses can be evaluated on the same radiograph by using a frontal or rostrocaudal view for the frontal sinuses. The animal is positioned in dorsal recumbency with the neck flexed so that the bridge of the nose and hard palate are perpendicular to the cassette and parallel to the central axis of the vertical x-ray beam. The beam is directed between the eyes. Isolated projection of frontal sinuses can be obtained only in breeds with prominent frontal bones. An additional frontal view, the frontooccipital view, is described as a rostral 20° dorsal–caudoventral oblique view of the cranium (Fig. 4–22D). Positioning is comparable with that for the rostrocaudal view, but

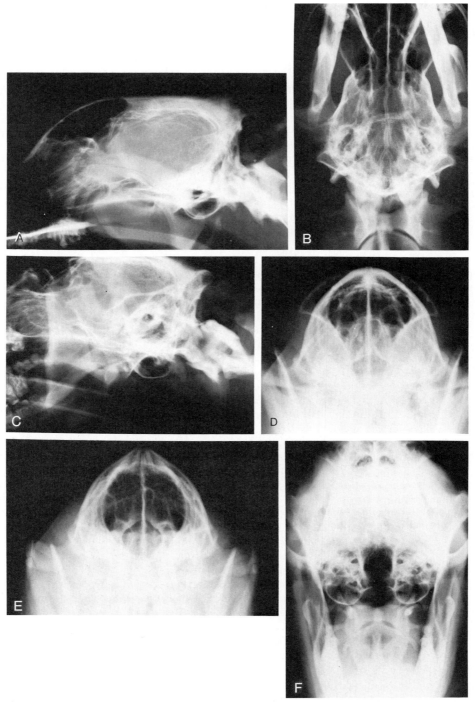

Figure 4–22. Radiographic views to evaluate the skull should include at least the lateral (A) and ventrodorsal (B) views. The left 20° ventral–right dorsal oblique view (C) projects the right tympanic bulla in an isolated manner. A corresponding view is obtained for the opposite bulla. Note the good visualization of the dens with this degree of obliquity. The rostral 20° dorsal–caudoventral oblique view (D) is made for a frontal projection of the cranial cavity. Superimposition of large frontal sinuses may occur. Note the good visualization of lateral walls of the neurocranium. The rostral 30° dorsal–caudoventral oblique view (E) is made to best visualize the foramen magnum. The rostral 30° ventral–caudodorsal open mouth view (F) is made primarily for bilateral tympanic bullae visualization. Also note visualization of the dens.

the neck is flexed so that the bridge of the nose is 20° from the vertically oriented central axis of the x-ray beam and 70° from the vertebral column. This position provides a frontal view of the neurocranium with minimal superimposition of other structures. This view can also project lateral walls of the cranial cavity and portions of the zygomatic arches and coronoid processes of the mandible. The foramen magnum can be visualized on this view, but greater flexion to 30° to 45° from vertical may be more appropriate (Fig. 4–22E). The foramen magnum may also be best visualized by maintaining the nose directed vertically and perpendicular to the cassette.[104] The x-ray tube is angled 30° from vertical, and the beam is directed midway between the orbits. A basilar view is described as a rostral 30° ventral–caudodorsal open mouth view (Fig. 4–22F). With the patient in dorsal recumbency, the nose is directed vertically, and the mouth is opened about 60°. The vertically directed x-ray beam bisects this open mouth angle. Slight variations may be needed in the angle of the hard palate from the vertical axis. Ears must be pulled laterally and moved from the field of interest. The tongue should be centered on midline, extended, and secured to the mandible with the endotracheal tube. This view is used primarily to evaluate tympanic bullae. It is occasionally difficult to perform and to maintain symmetry in positioning. Thus the lateral oblique views of the tympanic bullae may be more often used. The basilar view can also provide good visualization of the odontoid process. However, the odontoid process is more often evaluated by other views. Depending on variations in angles of projection, the basilar view may be of value to visualize bones and foramina of the base of the neurocranium in the diagnosis of basilar skull fractures.[31]

Normal Appearance. A complete description of the radiographic anatomy of the normal skull of dogs and cats is not possible in this section. Numerous sources are available for comparative reference.[60, 134, 143] Extreme variations exist in the shape and size of the skull among species and breeds. However, the basic radiographic appearances are sufficiently similar to allow adequate comparison to a standard once one learns to recognize key diagnostic areas. One should also use the bilateral symmetry of the normal skull as a key diagnostic feature.

Bony structures immediately adjacent to neurologic structures of concern must be thoroughly evaluated. These include the neurocranium surrounding the brain, the osseous base of the skull, the petrous temporal bone and the tympanic bullae, the osseous cerebellar tentorium, the foramen magnum, and the occipitoatlantal articulation. In very young animals, radiolucencies of sutures between different bones are normal. Sutures usually close by 3 weeks of age, and fontanelles close as animals approach maturity.[12] The tympanic bullae should be thin walled, rounded, smoothly margined, relatively radiolucent within, and bilaterally symmetric. Density within the tympanic bullae may vary slightly, depending on the amount of soft tissue superimposition. The foramen magnum may vary greatly in shape and size among breeds of dogs.[60, 150] The transverse diameter is usually the widest dimension, but in some skulls the vertical dimension may be the largest. Primary differences are in the degree of dorsal extension that appears more prominent in toy breeds of dogs. In some dogs, the supraoccipital bone may be thin just dorsal to the foramen magnum.[119, 150] This area may appear radiolucent on radiographs and thus simulate dorsal extension of the foramen magnum. The size, shape, and relative density of the neurocranium should be noted. The cranial cavity generally corresponds to the form and size of the neurocranium, especially in breeds with small frontal sinuses and relatively effaced superficial crests.[60] One must also thoroughly evaluate those areas surrounding the neurocranium that may occasionally be associated with neurologic diseases. These include frontal sinuses, orbits, ethmoid turbinates, zygomatic arches, and soft tissues surrounding the skull.

Interpretation of Abnormalities. Because of the complexity of structures of the skull, interpretation of skull radiographs must necessarily be biased, based on results of other neurologic examination techniques. However, this does not preclude the need for a thorough examination of all parts included on the radiographs. Bone lesions should be characterized as to their aggressive or nonaggressive appearance and as to their focal or diffuse nature. Focal lesions of the neurocranium may be osteolytic, osteoproductive, or a mixture of the two. Osteosarcomas are the most common primary malignant tumors of the calvaria and are primarily osteoproductive in appearance. Osteomas are the most common benign tumors of the calvaria and are usually well-margined, nonaggressive, osteoproductive lesions. Meningiomas may cause lytic changes in the bone or may cause increased bone density owing to periosteal reaction or mineralization of the tumor. Multiple myelomas may produce multifocal, discrete, osteolytic lesions of the calvaria. Aggressive lesions may also be caused by osteomyelitis, and extension to or from the nasal, ethmoid, and frontal sinus areas may occur.

Exudate or hyperplastic tissue of chronic otitis externa may occlude the normally radiolucent ear canal. Changes are better assessed by physical examination than by radiography. Dystrophic mineralization may be seen. Chronic otitis media and interna may cause thickening of the wall of the tympanic bulla and sclerosis of the petrous temporal bone. If exudate is present in the middle ear, fluid may be present within the tympanic bulla. Osteomyelitis and neoplasia can cause an aggressive lesion of the tympanic bulla.

Fractures of the skull are easiest to visualize if fracture fragments are displaced. However, many skull fractures are small, linear, fissure fractures without displacement and are difficult to visualize. Such fractures appear as linear, or curvilinear, radiolucent lines and may require excellent quality radiographs, multiple views, and careful evaluation for recognition. Basilar skull fractures are especially difficult to diagnose. Brain trauma can also readily occur without the presence of skull fractures (see Chapter 11).

Diffuse decreased bone density of the skull may occur with systemic diseases that cause diffuse decreased skeletal density such as hyperparathyroidism (see Chapter 8). Changes may be most pronounced in the neurocranium, but interpretation is quite subjective. Craniomandibular osteopathy can produce local or diffuse increased bone density. This disease affects primarily the petrous temporal bone around the tympanic bullae and the mandible. The calvaria may be diffusely thickened and sclerotic in some cases. Hypovitaminosis A may cause thickening of cranial bones in growing dogs.

Size and shape changes of the neurocranium may be due to primary bone malformation or secondary to changes of the brain within the cranial cavity. As an example, occipital dysplasia is a developmental malformation of the occipital bone with an enlarged foramen magnum[119] (see Chapter 6). Slight to marked enlargement of the foramen magnum may be present, with the major defect occurring in the dorsal occipital border. However, normal breed variation noted previously makes radiographic diagnosis difficult and necessitates close correlation with clinical signs.[60, 150] Other anomalies such as shortening of C1 may occur in some cases.[108] Hydrocephalus may cause enlargement of the cranial cavity (see Chapter 6). The neurocra-

nium may be domed and thinned, and sutures and fontanelles may remain open. The appearance of the inner tables of the neurocranium is quite variable and does not provide an accurate diagnostic criterion. The skull may also be radiographically normal in patients with hydrocephalus. Conversely, the neurocranium may be misshapen owing to decreased volume of brain segments. The occipital bone may be flattened in dogs with agenesis of the cerebellar vermis, and cats with a grossly hypoplastic cerebellum may have decreased size of the caudal fossa visualized on the lateral view.

Cerebral Angiography

Cerebral angiography is rapid, sequential radiography of the skull following injection of a positive contrast medium into the arterial circulation of the brain. Radiographs are made to follow contrast medium opacification of arterial, capillary, and venous phases of circulation. The technique can provide detailed radiographic images of vascular structures, and thus cerebral angiography has been the technique of choice for years to demonstrate most mass lesions and vascular abnormalities of the brain. The only specific contraindication to cerebral angiography is a known history of anaphylactic reaction to the contrast medium. General contraindications may relate to general anesthesia, the relatively long and invasive nature of the procedure, and cost-risk-benefit considerations. Cerebral angiography requires the use of a rapid film changer, and fluoroscopy is necessary for one approach. Magnification techniques greatly enhance small vessel visualization, and subtraction techniques may be of considerable value. General principles of angiographic technique should be understood and adhered to.

Technique. Various techniques have been described to perform cerebral angiography in dogs. The two major techniques are catheterization of either an internal carotid artery or a vertebral artery. The most common technique involves selective catheterization of the internal carotid artery. Premedication with corticosteroids for 24 to 48 hours prior to the procedure may help prevent cerebral edema.[32] The patient is placed under general inhalation anesthesia, and vital signs are monitored closely throughout the procedure. The neck is surgically prepared, and a cut-down is performed to expose the common carotid artery. If unilateral localizing signs are present, one should approach the artery on the same side as the suspected lesion. Blunt dissection is used to trace the artery rostrally to its division into the internal and the external carotid arteries. The internal carotid artery is recognized by the unique carotid bulb at its origin. The occipital artery originates from the external carotid artery just past this bifurcation. A 3 to 4 Fr, end-hole, soft catheter is placed into the common carotid artery by either arteriotomy or a modified Seldinger technique using a needle, guide wire, and catheter replacement procedure.[139] Using digital manipulation, the catheter is advanced rostrally into the internal carotid artery. Fluoroscopically guided catheter advancement techniques are possible but require considerable expertise.[77, 139] Normal physiologic flow patterns should be maintained.[35, 62, 139] Thus the catheter is not tied in place with encircling ligatures or clamps. Sutures may be placed to seal the arteriotomy site around the catheter. The catheter should not be so large or be advanced so far as to totally occlude the lumen of the internal carotid artery. Although not usually performed, temporary occlusion of the contralateral common carotid artery during injection will favor more complete filling of the arterial circle of the brain and most of the major intracerebral vessels on both sides of the brain.[35]

A second technique involves catheterization of a vertebral artery via a femoral approach.[34, 126] With the patient under general anesthesia, the medial aspect of the thigh is aseptically prepared. The catheter is introduced into the femoral artery by arteriotomy or by percutaneous puncture using the Seldinger technique. A 4 to 5 Fr, open-end catheter and guide wire are advanced cranially under fluoroscopic control. The catheter is advanced into and through the aorta to the origin of the left subclavian artery. By using appropriate manipulation, the tip of the catheter is advanced into a vertebral artery (usually the left) at least to the level of the C3–C4 intervertebral space or preferably to the C1–C2 interspace.[62, 126]

The choice between internal carotid and vertebral artery techniques may be determined by clinical localization of the suspected disease process. The vertebral artery technique appears to provide the most consistent visualization of all vessels of concern but may occasionally fail to adequately fill rostral and middle cerebral arteries.[31, 126] Thus the vertebral artery technique is most beneficial in evaluating structures supplied by the caudal cerebral artery and branches of the basilar artery. The internal carotid artery technique is most valuable for assessing structures supplied by the rostral and middle cerebral arteries because the caudal

cerebral artery and the basilar artery and its branches may be inconsistently filled.[31, 35] General principles of angiography must be understood for either technique. Important points include frequent flushing of the catheter with heparinized saline or small amounts of contrast medium to retard formation of thrombi, use of appropriate angiographic catheters of good quality with smooth tips, avoidance of excessive trauma to vessels being catheterized, and avoidance of occluding vessels being injected.

Although work has been done with many contrast media, meglumine iothalamate has been preferred for cerebral angiography because of its lower neurotoxicity compared with other ionic, water soluble, organic iodide media.[106] Contrast media can cause a variety of physiologic and toxic changes. Local effects of contrast media on an organ appear to depend on the type, volume, and concentration of the contrast medium and the contact time in the organ.[139] Osmolality and lipid solubility of the anionic component may be of specific concern in neurotoxicity.[106] It has been shown in humans that newer nonionic contrast media such as metrizamide are associated with less pain and decreased change of capillaries and the blood-brain barrier.[63, 129] This is associated with decreased toxicity and edema of neural tissue.[63] Thus it seems likely that agents such as metrizamide may become the preferred agents for cerebral angiography. Newer nonionic media such as iohexol and iopamidol may be less toxic than metrizamide.[63]

Extreme variations in dosage and injection techniques have been described. Manual injection from either approach is adequate, and automated power injectors are not required. However, automated injectors are of value to deliver precise doses at specified physiologic flow rates.[62, 139] Excessively high doses are severely neurotoxic.[40, 77] A general dose of 1 to 4 ml would seem appropriate for internal carotid artery injection, depending on the size of the patient.[35, 62, 139] Larger doses may increase filling of contralateral vessels. For vertebral artery injection, 3 to 8 ml may be the optimum smallest dose.[62, 126] Larger doses may be required if the catheter tip is positioned caudal to C3–C4. However, more caudal positioning of the catheter and injection of larger doses may increase the risk of damaging the spinal cord supplied by branches from the vertebral artery.[38, 126] Injection rate is also important. Injection into the internal carotid artery of 1 ml over 3 seconds may approach physiologic flow.[35] Manual injection using a small syringe is usually performed at a moderate rate. This injection rate will usually produce good filling around to the contralateral rostral cerebral artery and occasionally to the contralateral middle cerebral artery. Excessive injection rates may alter flow patterns (see below). The vertebral artery injection can also be performed manually over 2 to 3 seconds.[126] The potential for spinal cord damage should be considered.

Different radiographic exposure sequences have been used. Principal components of the cerebral angiogram are the arterial, capillary, and venous phases, and all phases should be evaluated. The arterial phase will persist as long as contrast medium is being injected. However, flow is rapid enough that arteries may be void of contrast medium within 0.5 second after termination of injection.[35] Larger, major vessels are of primary concern, and these are best visualized before filling of all the smaller arteries and the capillary network. Thus the earliest radiographs of the arterial phase are of most value, and these are best obtained by starting sequential exposures just prior to initiation of injection. During this early phase, two films per second may be adequate, but three or more films per second are preferred. This rapid rate does not need to be continued throughout the series, and one exposure per 1 to 2 seconds is usually adequate after the first 2 seconds. The series should be carried through the capillary phase, and delayed films should be made during or after the venous phase. Timing is variable, but the venous phase is usually best visualized several seconds following injection. The pri-

mary purpose of these later films is not to evaluate veins themselves but to identify persistence of contrast medium opacification in some focal lesions after the remainder of the brain has been cleared. The sequence must be repeated for both lateral and ventrodorsal views because biplane capabilities are rarely available in veterinary medicine.

As with any angiographic procedure, cerebral angiography can potentially cause vascular trauma. Injection via the vertebral artery will cause a mild increase in the rate and depth of respiration and has the potential of inducing spinal cord damage.[38, 126] Large volumes of more neurotoxic media injected into the internal carotid artery can cause severe convulsions, respiratory embarrassment, and death.[40, 77] Less severe reactions include slight muscle tremors of the head and neck. A 0.34% fatality rate and a 2.1% complication rate have been noted in humans following cerebral angiography, with motor deficiency being a prevalent finding.[48] Reactions are fewer and less severe with meglumine iothalamate and with low volumes.[63]

Normal Appearance. Detailed studies describe vascular anatomy of cerebral circulation, anatomic relationships of vessels with segments of the brain, and hemodynamics of internal and external cerebral anastomoses.[34, 35, 45, 60] Major arteries that should be evaluated include internal carotid, rostral cerebral, middle cerebral, caudal communicating, caudal cerebral, rostral cerebellar, basilar, and basilar branch arteries. Other vessels can also be visualized, but the ability to specifically identify many of the

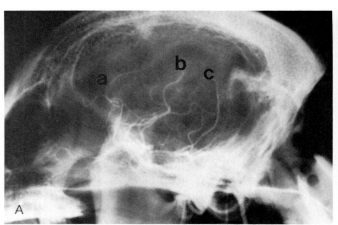
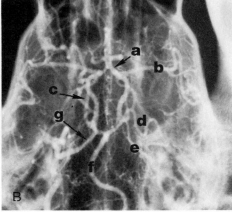

Figure 4–23. Normal arterial phases of magnified cerebral angiograms following internal carotid artery injections. A, Lateral view. Rostral (a), middle (b), and caudal (c) cerebral arteries are filled bilaterally. Caudal communicating and basilar arteries are also visible. B, Ventrodorsal view. There is good bilateral filling of rostral cerebral (a), middle cerebral (b), caudal communicating (c), caudal cerebral (d), and rostral cerebellar (e) arteries. The basilar (f) and right internal carotid (g) arteries are also noted. (B courtesy of Dr J Gomez, University of California, Davis.)

smaller arteries is greatly dependent on the quality of the radiographic technique. One should at least be able to identify most of the major arteries of intracranial circulation. The lateral view is probably the most valuable for clear visualization of cerebral vessels (Fig. 4–23A). The ventrodorsal view is better for assessing bilateral symmetry and vascular anatomy at the base of the brain (Fig. 4–23B). Variations can occur in normal cerebral angiograms. Rostral cerebral arteries may not be filled from vertebral artery injection.[32, 126] Injection into an internal carotid artery may not fill caudal cerebral and more caudal arteries and may not opacify contralateral arteries well.[32, 35] Excessive injection volumes or rates may cause considerable opacification of extracerebral vessels owing to reflux around the catheter into the external carotid artery or owing to shunting through various anastomoses between internal and external circulations. This problem is avoided with vertebral artery injection.

Interpretation of Abnormalities. Bilateral symmetry is important, but slight differences may not be significant unless they correlate with other findings. Variations in symmetry may also be due to variations in positioning. Individual arteries should be evaluated for changes in size, shape, course, patency, and integrity. Failure to fill some arteries may be dependent on technique, and emboli may occur because of poor catheterization technique. Primary vascular diseases such as arteriovenous malformations or fistulas may occur but are rare. Such lesions produce focal enlargement of vessels and early filling of veins. Mass lesions may cause displacement of vessels (Fig. 4–24). Well-vascularized masses such as certain tumors may have irregular, tortuous small vessels within the mass. Retention of contrast medium may occur in some masses after contrast medium has cleared

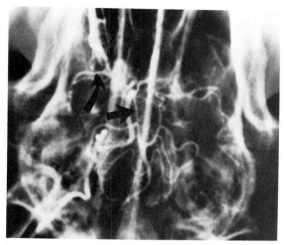

Figure 4–24. Abnormal cerebral angiogram made with a 105 mm spot camera. On this ventrodorsal view, the right caudal communicating artery (straight arrow) is displaced medially. The right middle cerebral artery (curved arrow) has a wide arc compared with the course of the left middle cerebral artery. Changes were due to a meningioma located at the base of the brain on the right and extending into the right hemisphere of the brain.

from normal portions of the brain and passed on through the venous system. This may be recognized as a momentary residual focal area of opacity (Fig. 4–25).

Ventriculography

Cerebral ventriculography is radiography of the skull after the introduction of contrast medium into the cerebral ventricular system. The technique is used primarily to evaluate size, shape, and position of ventricles and rarely to evaluate patency of interventricular communications. Thus ventriculography is used primarily in patients suspected of having hydrocephalus. The technique can be used to diagnose mass

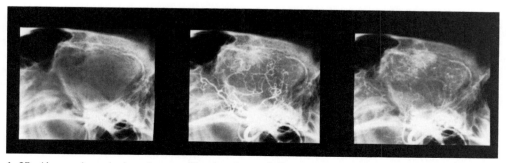

Figure 4–25. Abnormal cerebral angiogram. The first frame (left) was made prior to injection. Note the progressive opacification and retention of contrast medium in a large area at the rostrodorsal aspect of the cranial cavity during sequential exposures (center, right). The lesion was a large meningioma.

lesions of the brain that may displace, distort, or project into the ventricles, but mass lesions are better evaluated by techniques such as cerebral angiography, nuclear imaging, or computed tomography. Ventriculography is relatively safe and effective if performed properly but does pose some hazard to the patient.[71, 116] Thus risk-benefit considerations are important in assessing the potential value of information to be gained. Ventricles are filled most commonly by the technique of direct needle puncture of lateral ventricles. Pneumoencephalography is a technique used to fill the ventricular system by the injection of negative contrast medium into the spinal subarachnoid space. Procedures have been described in dogs using either lumbar or cisternal injection techniques,[71] but pneumoencephalography is rarely used in veterinary medicine.

Technique. Unless medically contraindicated, corticosteroids should be administered for 24 to 48 hours prior to the study to decrease the risk of cerebral edema that may be caused by trauma to the brain.[116] The patient is placed under general anesthesia. Vital signs must be monitored closely throughout the procedure because ventriculography can cause apnea.[116] A moderate degree of hyperventilation may help prevent cerebral edema.[116] The patient is placed in ventral recumbency, and the dorsum of the head is prepared for aseptic surgery. A special head holding device allows easy manipulation of the patient, provides easy access to the cranium, and helps prevent inadvertent compression of jugular veins[115] (see Fig. 16–1). Radiographs are made with a horizontal beam when this device is used. The technique is usually performed bilaterally. Penetration sites of the skull are 0.5 to 1.0 cm from midline, midway between a line drawn through the lateral canthus of the eyes and a parallel line through the external occipital protuberance. The technique must be aseptic, and penetration must be lateral to midline to avoid penetration of the dorsal sagittal sinus. Stab incisions are made through the skin and temporal muscles at the injection sites. If large open fontanelles are present, needles may be inserted through the lateral margins of the fontanelles. If fontanelles are closed, a small Steinmann pin in a hand chuck is used to penetrate the bone to the inner table of the skull. A 22 gauge, 1.5 inch, short beveled spinal needle with stylet is used to penetrate the inner table of the skull. This technique creates a tight fit with little motion of the needle during the procedure. One needle is inserted slowly in a ventral direction parallel to midline to the estimated depth of the lateral ventricle. The stylet is removed, and external jugular veins are compressed if necessary to increase CSF pressure. The needle should be withdrawn slowly until fluid appears in the hub. The needle should not be advanced without the stylet in place and should not be aspirated with a syringe. The second needle should then be placed in the other lateral ventricle. Enough CSF is collected for analysis, and the pressure on jugular veins is released. The opposite needle should be left open during injection of contrast medium to prevent a sudden increase in intraventricular pressure. For pneumoventriculography, 2 to 4 ml of air is injected into one ventricle and then the other. The procedure should be stopped if changes occur in pulse or respiration and continued only when they return to normal.

Air is the safest and most commonly used contrast medium for cerebral ventriculography using the technique described above. However, air will usually not fill the entire ventricular system. If ventricles are dilated, a horizontal x-ray beam is required, and multiple positions of the skull can be used to move the air bubble around the periphery and document the limits of the lateral ventricles. If ventricular dilation is moderate to severe, one does not usually need to outline the complete ventricle, and often a single lateral view may suffice. A vertically directed x-ray beam may be misleading if the entire ventricular volume is not replaced in pneumoventriculography. The small air bubble will appear centrally located in the fluid volume of the ventricle and will not truly outline the margin between the ventricle and brain tissue. If horizontal beam capabilities are not available, then the entire ventricle must be filled with contrast medium. This should not be done with gas in moderate to severe cases of hydrocephalus. Positive contrast media can also be employed in ventriculography. Positive contrast media can be used with a vertically directed x-ray beam, can provide good contrast, and can demonstrate patency of the mesencephalic aqueduct. Small volumes of positive contrast media that are freely miscible with CSF can outline the entire ventricular system. Iophendylate has been used but is not reabsorbed and can cause a chronic granulomatous meningitis.[69, 72] Ionic water soluble media such as meglumine iothalamate cause acute toxicity.[4, 22] Newer nonionic media such as metrizamide or iohexol may prove preferable.[113]

Lateral views are the most valuable to evaluate ventricular size. If the ventricles are of

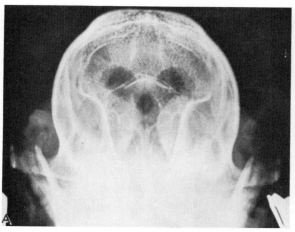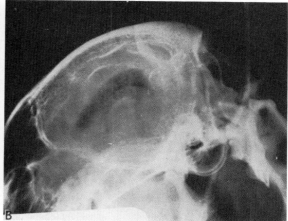

Figure 4–26. A pneumoventriculogram of a normal dog. A, Frontal view. B, Lateral view. Air is present in lateral ventricles and a portion of the third ventricle. (From Oliver JE Jr and Lorenz MD: Handbook of Veterinary Neurologic Diagnosis. Philadelphia, WB Saunders Co, 1983.)

normal size, additional comparative views are necessary. A rostral 20° dorsal–caudoventral (frontal) view is probably better and makes the air easier to visualize than does a dorsoventral view. All three views may be of value with positive contrast ventriculography.

Morbidity of ventriculography is relatively low if the technique is performed properly. Laceration of a vein or venous sinus can occur using an improper site for needle placement. Inappropriate needle movement during the procedure can lacerate the brain. Sudden changes in intracranial pressure can cause cardiac and respiratory difficulties. If too much fluid is removed from an enlarged ventricle, ventricular collapse and subdural hematoma can occur. Positive contrast media may cause meningitis or postoperative hypersensitivity to external stimuli.[4, 72]

Normal Appearance. In the normal animal, pneumoventriculography will outline most of the lateral ventricles and may demonstrate part of the third ventricle (Fig. 4–26). Ventricular anatomy is more completely visualized with positive contrast media because the entire ventricular system may be opacified (Fig. 4–27). Anatomy of the ventricles of dogs has been described.[45, 52] Lateral ventricles can be relatively large even in normal animals. They are bilaterally paired cavities on each side of the cerebral hemispheres and are divided into a rostral horn, a body, and a caudal (temporal) horn. The rostral horn has an extension into the olfactory bulb, which is rarely seen on a ventriculogram. The caudal horn curves ventrally and laterally around the caudal margins of the thalamus. The third ventricle is an unpaired, median cavity that is ventral and medial to the lateral ventricles. The third ventricle surrounds the interthalamic adhesion, which on the lateral view produces a round filling defect within the third ventricle. The mesencephalic aqueduct is a narrow tube through the midbrain that extends from the caudal end of the third ventricle to the rostral end of the fourth ventricle. The fourth ventricle is a tubular cavity directed rostrocaudally with laterally directed processes at its caudal aspect. The fourth ventricle communicates with the subarachnoid space through the lateral apertures and caudally with the central canal of the spinal cord. There is some variation in radiographic appearances of shape, size, and filling of various segments of the ventricular system.

Interpretation of Abnormalities. Ventriculography is used primarily to diagnose hydrocephalus. Diagnosis is dependent on enlargement of lateral ventricles and thinning of brain substance dorsal to the ventricles (see Fig. 6–4). However, in less severe cases, the technique usually does not differentiate whether thinning of the brain is secondary to ventricular enlargement or ventricular enlargement is secondary to cerebral atrophy. Slight ventricular enlargement may occur with aging owing to senile cerebral atrophy. Recognition of narrowing or obstruction of ventricular pathways requires use of positive contrast media. Mass lesions of the brain may displace ventricles. The direction of displacement may aid in localization of the

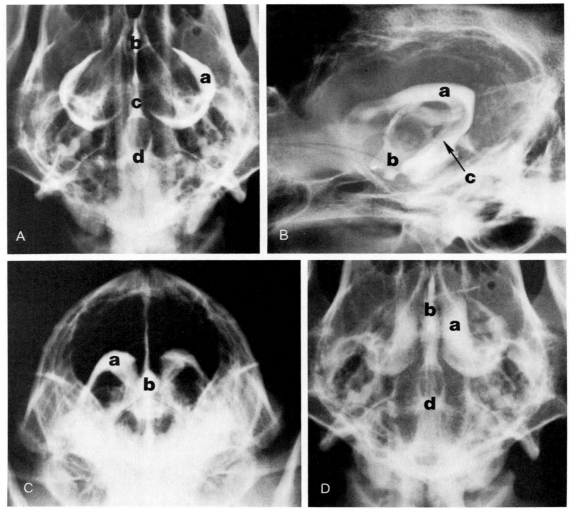

Figure 4–27. Positive contrast ventriculogram of a normal dog made following injection of 2 ml of 60% meglumine iothalamate. Radiographs were made in the following sequence. A, Dorsoventral; B, lateral; C, frontal; D, ventrodorsal views. Structures that can be visualized include the lateral ventricles (a), third ventricle (b), mesencephalic aqueduct (c), and fourth ventricle (d).

mass. Small masses originating at the surface of the ventricle, such as a choroid plexus papilloma, may project into the lumen of the ventricle.

Cavernous Sinus Venography

Cranial sinus venography is radiography of the head following injection of contrast medium into the venous system of the skull. Techniques include cavernous sinus venography and dorsal sagittal sinus venography.[114] Dorsal sagittal and transverse sinuses can be visualized by dorsal sagittal sinus venography. This technique re-

quires surgical exposure and catheterization of the rostral end of the dorsal sagittal sinus. The technique is inconvenient, carries potential serious risk, and is rarely indicated or used in veterinary medicine. The same vessels may be visualized during the venous phase of cerebral angiography, although not as well as with venography. Cavernous sinus venography is a more commonly used technique and will be described in detail below. Cavernous sinus venography is a technically easy and safe procedure. It is used to evaluate structures of the orbit and on the floor of the middle cranial fossa by opacification of veins of the orbit and sinuses and veins of the base of the cranial vault.[96, 114]

Technique. The patient is placed under general inhalation anesthesia, survey radiographs of the skull are made, and exposure technique is established. The patient is placed in ventral recumbency and positioned for a dorsoventral radiograph of the skull. Dorsal nasal, or preferably angularis oculi, veins are used as sites of injection. Injection may be made through a needle puncture, but catheterization is preferred. Flexible extension tubes are helpful and allow hands to be moved farther from the x-ray beam. Better vascular filling is more consistently obtained with bilateral injection. External jugular veins are compressed during injection. A total of 5 to 10 ml of intravenous contrast medium such as meglumine iothalamate is equally divided between catheters. Rapid injection is accomplished manually, and the radiograph is made as the last milliliter of contrast medium is injected. Occlusion of facial veins may decrease opacification of the extracranial venous system but is of variable value.[114] The lateral venogram is of infrequent value, and usually only the dorsoventral view is obtained.

Normal Appearance. Cavernous sinus venography will opacify veins of the orbit and ventral venous sinuses and veins of the cranial vault and those as far caudal as vertebral venous plexuses of the cranial thoracic vertebrae.[31] Normal anatomy and radiographic appearance have been described.[45, 114] Figure 4–28A illustrates a normal dorsoventral cavernous sinus venogram. Unilateral injection cannot be expected to produce bilateral filling. The study is compromised primarily by inadequate compression of external jugular veins, which would favor opacification

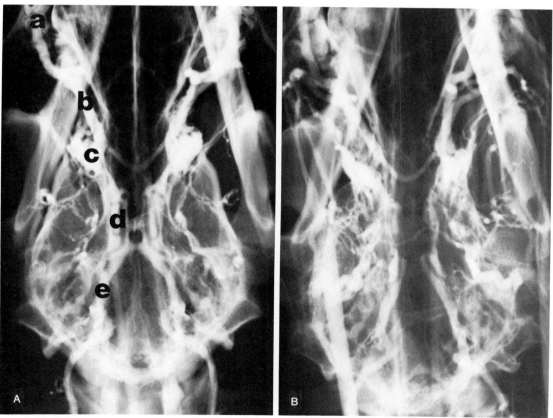

Figure 4–28. A, Normal dorsoventral cavernous sinus venogram. Note bilateral filling of angularis oculi veins (a), ophthalmic veins (b), orbital plexuses (c), cavernous sinuses (d), and ventral petrosal sinuses (e). The anastomoses of right and left ophthalmic veins and rostral and caudal intercavernous sinuses are also well visualized. The latter two structures may not always be present. Linear filling defects in the cavernous sinuses are due to internal carotid and anastomotic arteries. The pituitary gland is located just rostral to the rostral intercavernous sinus. B, Abnormal dorsoventral cavernous sinus venogram. There is lack of filling of rostral and caudal intercavernous sinuses, which may be a normal variation. Cavernous sinuses are incompletely filled. Linear filling defects of internal carotid and anastomotic arteries are not present because of incomplete filling of cavernous sinuses. The lesion was a large adenoma of the pituitary gland.

of extracranial venous drainage. Special note should be made of flow patterns, bilateral symmetry, and identification of ophthalmic veins, orbital plexuses, and cavernous sinuses. Rostral and caudal intercavernous sinuses are usually but not always present.

Interpretation of Abnormalities. The diagnosis of abnormalities is dependent primarily on incomplete filling of segments of the intracranial venous system due to adjacent mass lesions. Such lesions may displace and compress segments of the venous system, producing incomplete or absent filling (Fig. 4–28B).

Cisternography and Optic Thecography

The structures on the ventral surface of the brain can be outlined by injecting positive contrast medium into the subarachnoid space and allowing it to flow into the cranial cavity.[95] The subarachnoid space extends along the optic nerves, hence they may be outlined with this technique.

Technique. Metrizamide (3–6 ml), in the same concentration as described for myelography, is injected into the subarachnoid space at the cerebellomedullary cistern with the dog in lateral recumbency. The dog is rolled to ventral recumbency and the head is lowered (table tilted to 30° from horizontal) for 6 minutes. Dorsoventral radiographs of the skull are taken within 2 minutes. In an experimental series of eight dogs, there were no seizures or other complications.[95]

Normal Appearance. The sheath of the optic nerve is outlined from the optic chiasm to the sclera (Fig. 4–29). The subarachnoid basal cisterns are opacified, outlining the pituitary gland, the basilar arteries, internal carotid arteries, and rostral cerebellar arteries. The caudal communicating arteries and rostral and middle cerebral arteries are outlined less consistently.

Interpretation of Abnormalities. Mass lesions on the floor of the cranium have been demonstrated with this technique. In one case a meningioma rostral to the optic chiasm was seen that was not visible using cavernous sinus venography. Mass lesions near the arterial circle should be outlined.

Nuclear Imaging (Scintigraphy)

Concepts of nuclear imaging have been briefly reviewed, and detailed textbooks are available.[10, 14, 67] Nuclear images (scintigrams) are two dimensional, pictorial representations

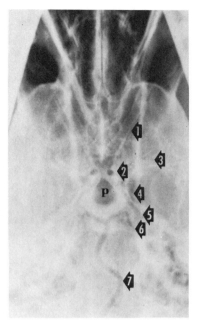

Figure 4–29. Dorsoventral radiograph of the skull of a dog after injection of metrizamide in the subarachnoid space. Structures outlined include p, pituitary gland; 1, optic nerves; 2, internal carotid artery, with the optic chiasm rostromedial to it; 3, middle cerebral artery; 4, caudal communicating artery; 5, caudal cerebral artery; 6, rostral cerebellar artery; and 7, basilar artery. (From Lecouter RA, Scagliotti RH, Beck KA, and Holliday TA: Indirect imaging of the canine optic nerve, using metrizamide [optic thecography]. Am J Vet Res 43:1424, 1982.)

of the distribution of systemically administered radiopharmaceuticals. Distribution of radiopharmaceuticals within the body occurs by various physiologic processes, depending on the radiopharmaceutical used. Most distribution processes are organ specific rather than disease specific. Scintillation detectors are used to record activity and geometry of distribution of the administered radiopharmaceutical and to create a representative image on film. Nuclear imaging provides information based primarily on physiologic principles, and architectural resolution is not directly comparable with radiography, in which fine image detail is dependent primarily on anatomic principles.

A rectilinear scanner is an imaging system with a small detector that moves systematically over an area of interest, collecting information point by point. Images produced are usually the same size as the object being scanned and can thus be compared directly with radiographs of the object. Rectilinear scanners became available in veterinary medicine in the early 1970s and were used for a variety of research, as well as clinical, studies. However, because the scanning procedure was slow, general anesthesia was required and the technique was limited in clinical use. A scintillation (gamma) camera is an imaging system with a large, stationary detector that encompasses a larger field of view. The resultant image is reduced, and multiformat capabilities are usually available. Image acquisition is much more rapid, and thus general anesthesia is only occasionally needed. Nuclear imaging using scintillation cameras has thus become a valuable diagnostic technique in veterinary medicine. Cost of equipment and knowledge of and licensing for radionuclide use usually limit scintigraphy to veterinary schools. Many veterinary schools currently have nuclear imaging capabilities, and arrangements with research or other facilities can occasionally be made to perform studies on individual patients.

Brain scanning is thought to be based on integrity of the blood-brain barrier.[14, 67] Radiopharmaceuticals enter the brain substance only when the blood-brain barrier is damaged. Thus the normal brain appears as an area of relatively low activity compared with surrounding structures that contain higher vascular activity. Radionuclide brain scanning is a relatively sensitive, convenient, noninvasive, and nontraumatic technique to identify many focal lesions of the brain.[19]

Technique. The radionuclide used for a conventional brain scan is technetium-99m (^{99m}Tc) because of its short physical half life (6 hours), its appropriate gamma ray emission (140 keV), its ready availability, and availability of appropriate localizing pharmaceuticals. Brain scans can be performed with ^{99m}Tc in its ionic form as ^{99m}TcO$_4$ (pertechnetate). However, active accumulation by the choroid plexus and salivary glands requires pretreatment with potassium perchlorate, and thus most brain scans are not performed with pertechnetate. The pharmaceuticals diethylenetriaminepentaacetic acid (DTPA) and gluceptate are both acceptable and commonly used, although there may be some preference for gluceptate.[128] Both agents are excreted by the kidneys, producing relatively rapid clearance of blood activity. An exact dosage has not been established in veterinary medicine; the dose may vary from about 7 to 20 mCi, depending on the size of the patient, from cats to large dogs. Lower doses enhance radiation safety but require longer time periods to accumulate data. The radiopharmaceutical is injected intraveneously. A small volume of high specific activity is required for sequential dynamic flow studies of carotid and cerebral perfusion. However, the value of this technique has not been documented in veterinary medicine, and most studies consist only of delayed static scans. Heavy sedation or general anesthesia is required for brain scans because of the relatively longer times required to accumulate data compared with most other scans. Seizure potentiating drugs must be avoided. The scintillation detector is most often equipped with a low energy, all purpose parallel hole or converging collimator for brain scans. Dorsal and both left and right lateral views should be included as part of the standard protocol. A caudal view has been described and may be occasionally of value.[20, 84] Images may first be made at 20 to 30 minutes following injection, as some lesions may be visible this early. However, lesions may not be visible until 2 to 4 hours after injection, and thus delayed scans are essential.[51, 68] Generally 300,000 to 500,000 counts may be collected for each view. A greater number of counts can increase resolution but take longer to accumulate. General anesthesia provides the restraint necessary to collect more counts without patient motion. The dorsal and first lateral views should be made to a predetermined count. The opposite lateral view can be made to a predetermined count or to the time required for the first lateral view.

Normal Appearance. If a flow study is performed, activity of common carotid arteries and the skull should be noted to progress in a bilaterally symmetric pattern. On delayed scans there should be a relatively void or inactive area in the region of the brain (Fig. 4–30A). On the dorsal view in the dog, it has been shown that the entire area of inactivity is not due solely to the brain but also includes temporal and masseter muscle mass.[20] This area of inactivity on the dorsal view may appear shaped as a tulip.[20] However, this shape is variable, depending on the breed and angulation of the detector. On the lateral view, the inactive area more closely approximates the shape of the cranial cavity. Similar normal patterns are present in the cat, except that the area of the brain appears more rounded. In both species, areas of activity represent activity within the vascular pool. Thus the nasal area may appear relatively active owing to the vascularity of the nasal mucosa. The eyes may appear as round areas of relative inactivity compared with surrounding regions of activity.

Interpretation of Abnormalities. Focal lesions of the brain may cause focal damage of the blood-brain barrier.[14, 67] This may allow the

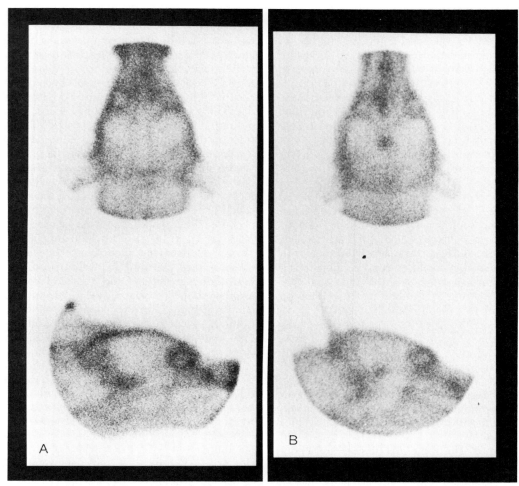

Figure 4–30. A, Dorsal and right lateral views of a normal brain scan in a dog using ⁹⁹ᵐTc-gluceptate. Radiopharmaceutical activity is distributed throughout the blood pool, leaving the cranial cavity and muscle mass around the neurocranium relatively void of activity. B, Dorsal and right lateral views of an abnormal brain scan in a dog using ⁹⁹ᵐTc-gluceptate. There is focal accumulation of radiopharmaceutical activity centrally located on the dorsal view. The abnormality is more difficult to see on the lateral view because it is located at the floor of the cranial cavity. The lesion was a chromophobe carcinoma of the pituitary gland.

radiopharmaceutical to enter the brain or lesion and thus create a focal area with increased activity (hot spot) compared with the relative inactivity of surrounding normal brain substance (Fig. 4–30B). Most focal lesions are best visualized on the dorsal view but should be confirmed and correlated with findings on lateral views. Lesions of the tips of the frontal lobes may be difficult to separate from normal caudal nasal activity. Lesions at the base of the skull may be difficult to identify on lateral views but may be well visualized on the dorsal view. Most positive brain scan findings in veterinary medicine appear to be attributable to tumors.[39, 84] However, degenerative and inflammatory le-

sions have been recognized in animals.[84] Considerable experience in humans has demonstrated the value of radionuclide brain scans for various types of lesions, as well as defined limitations of the technique.[67] In veterinary medicine, current inability to specify the causes of recognized lesions may improve with increased experience in pattern recognition and correlative studies.

Computed Tomography

Computed tomography is the method of constructing images of internal structures of an object by computer analysis of absorption patterns of x-rays utilizing multiple projections. This creates a cross-sectional image of the object with capabilities of differentiating soft tissue densities that cannot be perceived on a conventional radiograph. The physics and computer concepts of computed tomography are complex, and equipment design and construction are improving rapidly. Basic physics is described in textbooks and articles and briefly explained in the veterinary literature.[8, 27, 73]

Equipment consists of data production, analysis, and display devices. Information is produced by an x-ray tube that revolves around an object placed in the center of the rotation circle. The x-ray beam is collimated to a narrow fan shape a few millimeters wide and broad enough to cover the width of the object. Exposure is made as the x-ray tube rotates around the object. Intensity of the altered x-ray beam is quantitated by radiation detectors rather than recorded on film. Thus data collected are quantitative data of beam intensity emerging from the object following narrow beam, rotational exposure. The narrow cross-sectional layer of the object is divided into thousands of smaller blocks, and a computer is used to determine attenuation coefficient values, or computed tomographic numbers, for each block. A gray scale image is constructed by converting these numbers to shades of black, white, or gray.

Images are displayed on a monitor and recorded on film.

Computed tomography is unique because of quantitative results, computer analysis, and an adjustable gray scale image. Conventional radiography cannot be used to perceive differences in opacity of less than 5 to 7%.[27, 73] The brain itself is not visible at all because of surrounding and superimposed bone. Computed tomography can produce a thin cross-sectional image of the brain in which it is possible to visualize differences in soft tissue opacities as little as 0.5%. Some lesions may be further accentuated by using intravenous contrast media.[33] Computed tomography is widely utilized in evaluation of many brain diseases in humans. Equipment and maintenance costs have limited purchase of computed tomographic equipment in veterinary medicine, and most animal patients have been studied at human medical institutions. The technique is well established in humans and appears to have value in animals[49, 50, 94, 99] (Figs. 4–31 and 4–32). As used equipment is becoming available, a few veterinary schools are obtaining computed tomographic equipment. Future reports may document the practicality, use, and value of computed tomography in veterinary medicine compared with other diagnostic techniques. Such studies are being evaluated in humans.[136]

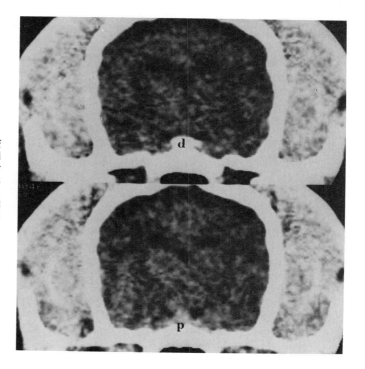

Figure 4–31. Computerized tomographic scan of a dog at the level of the oval foramen. The lateral and third ventricles are the darker structures near the center. d, Dorsum sellae; p, hypophyseal fossa and pituitary gland. (From Fike JR, Lecouter RA, and Cann CE: Anatomy of the canine brain using high resolution computed tomography. Vet Rad 22:236, 1981.)

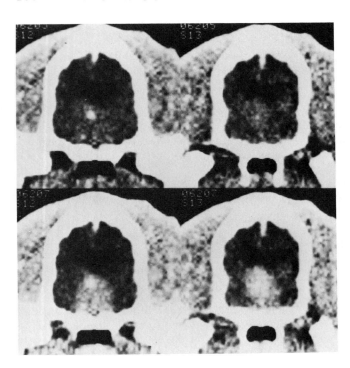

Figure 4–32. Computerized tomographic scans of an 8 year old male boxer dog with a brain tumor. Precontrast scans (top) show an increased density in the midbrain region (gray area) with focal areas of high density contained within this area. Postcontrast scans (bottom) show a non-uniform enhancement of this region. The lateral ventricles are enlarged on both the pre- and postcontrast scans. (From Fike JR, Lecouter RA, Cann CE, and Pflugfelder CM: Am J Vet Res 42:275, 1981.)

Equine

Comments concerning small animal survey radiography of the calvarium are entirely appropriate to large domestic animals. Techniques and reference radiographs are published for the horse.[108, 109, 135]

The density of the calvarium, the thickness of soft tissues of the head, and complexities of the bones and suture lines of the neurocranium all help to make accurate interpretation of radiographs of the head of large animal patients difficult. Indeed, even radiographic confirmation of overt fractures of the skull can be impossible. Comparison with radiographs of comparable, normal animals taken under the same conditions is suggested.

Apart from suspected head trauma, one of the more frequent indications for skull radiographs in horses is the evaluation of cases of vestibular syndrome. Lateral, ventrodorsal, and various oblique views of the base of the skull, temporal bones, and stylohyoid bones can assist in defining bony lesions that are associated with syndromes of vestibulocochlear and facial nerve disease in horses.[18, 122]

Profound, congenital, internal hydrocephalus in newborn foals can be substantiated with plain survey radiographs of the skull. In addition, ultrasonography has been used to assist in defining the extent of attenuation of cerebral tissue in such cases.[53]

REFERENCES

1. Ackerman N and Corwin LA: Myelography with MP 2032-NMG meglumine iocarmate. J Am Vet Radiol Soc 16:174, 1975.
2. Adams WM: Myelography. Vet Clin North Am (Small Anim Pract) 12:295, 1982.
3. Adams WM and Stowater JL: Complications of metrizamide myelography in the dog: A summary of 107 clinical case histories. Vet Radiol 22:27, 1981.
4. Albert RA: Canine Ventriculography and Encephalography. Thesis (MS), Auburn University, Auburn, AL, 1967.
5. Almén T: Experience from 10 years of development of water-soluble nonionic contrast media. Invest Radiol 15:(Suppl) S283, 1980.
6. Armstrong P, Chalmers AH, Green J, and Irving JD: Needle aspiration/biopsy of the spine in suspected disc space infection. Br J Radiol 51:333, 1978.
7. Bailey CS and Holliday TA: Diseases of the spinal cord. In Ettinger SJ: Textbook of Veterinary Internal Medicine. Philadelphia, WB Saunders Co, 1975, p 401.
8. Barber DL: Imaging: Radiography—II. Vet Radiol 22:149, 1981.
9. Barber DL and Lewis RE: Guidelines for Radiology Service in Veterinary Medicine. Schaumburg, IL, American Veterinary Medical Association, 1982.
10. Barber DL and Roberts RE: Imaging: Nuclear. Vet Radiol 24:50, 1983.

11. Bartels JE, Braund KG, and Redding RW: An experimental evaluation of a non-ionic agent Amipaque (metrizamide) as a neuroradiologic medium in the dog. J Am Vet Radiol Soc 18:117, 1977.

12. Bartels JE, Hoerlein BF, and Boring JG: Neuroradiology. *In* Hoerlein BF: Canine Neurology, 3rd ed. Philadelphia, WB Saunders Co, 1978, p 103.

13. Bassi P, Cecchini A, Dettori P, and Signorini E: Myelography with iopamidol, a nonionic water-soluble contrast medium: Incidence of complications. Neuroradiology 24:85, 1982.

14. Baum S and Bramlet R: Basic Nuclear Medicine. New York, Appleton-Century-Crofts, 1975.

15. Beech J: Metrizamide myelography in the horse. J Am Vet Radiol Soc 20:22, 1979.

16. Bennett D, Carmichael S, and Griffiths IR: Diskospondylitis in the dog. J Small Anim Pract 22:539, 1981.

17. Blevins WE: Transosseous vertebral venography: A diagnostic aid in lumbosacral disease. Vet Radiol 21:50, 1980.

18. Blythe LL, Watrous BJ, Schmitz JA, and Kaneps AJ: Vestibular syndrome associated with temporohyoid joint fusion and temporal bone fracture in three horses. JAVMA 185:775, 1984.

19. Boucher BJ and Sear R: A summary of results of radioisotope brain scans on a large series of patients. Br J Radiol 53:1174, 1980.

20. Brawner WR Jr: Static and Dynamic Radionuclide Brain Imaging in the Normal Canine: Technique and Appearance. Thesis (PhD), Auburn University, Auburn, AL, 1981.

21. Brodey RS, Reid CF, and Sauer RM: Metastatic bone neoplasms in the dog. JAVMA 148:29, 1966.

22. Bromage PR, Bramwell RSB, et al: Peridurography with metrizamide: Animal and human studies. Radiology 128:123, 1978.

23. Bruschwein DA, Brown ML, and McLeod RA: Gallium scintigraphy in the evaluation of disk-space infections: Concise communication. J Nucl Med 21:925, 1980.

24. Bullock LP, and Zook BL: Myelography in dogs using water-soluble contrast mediums. JAVMA 151:321, 1967.

25. Campbell RI, Campbell JA, Heinburger RF, et al: Ventriculography and myelography with absorbable radio-opaque medium. Radiology 82:286, 1964.

26. Carakostas MC, Gossett KA, Watters JW, and MacWilliams PS: Effects of metrizamide myelography on cerebrospinal fluid analysis in the dog. Vet Radiol 24:267, 1983.

27. Christensen EE, Curry TS, and Dowdy JE: Introduction to the Physics of Diagnostic Radiology, 2nd ed. Philadelphia, Lea & Febiger, 1978.

28. Chrzanowski R: The contrast media used for myelography. Eur J Neurol 21:194, 1982.

29. Clark L: Hypervitaminosis A: A review. Aust Vet J 47:568, 1971.

30. Cloward RB and Buzoid LI: Diskography: Technique, indications and evaluation of the normal and abnormal intervertebral disc. Am J Roentgenol 68:552, 1952.

31. Conrad CR: Radiographic examination of the central nervous system. *In* Ettinger SJ: Textbook of Veterinary Internal Medicine. Philadelphia, WB Saunders Co, 1975, p 333.

32. Conrad CR and Oliver JE Jr: Cerebral angiography. *In* Ticer JW: Radiographic Technique in Small Animal Practice. Philadelphia, WB Saunders Co, 1975, p 278.

33. Davis JM, Davis KR, Newhouse J, and Pfister R: Expanded high iodine dose in computed cranial tomography: A preliminary report. Radiology 131:373, 1979.

34. DeLaTorre E, Mitchell OC, and Netsky MG: Anatomic and angiographic study of the vertebral-basilar arterial systems in the dog. Am J Anat 110:187, 1962.

35. DeLaTorre E, Netsky MG, and Meschan I: Intracranial and extracranial circulations in the dog: Anatomic and angiographic studies. Am J Anat 105:343, 1959.

36. Denny HR, Gibbs C, and Gaskell CJ: Cervical spondylopathy in the dog—a review of thirty-five cases. J Small Anim Pract 18:117, 1977.

37. Denny HR, Gibbs C, and Holt PE: The diagnosis and treatment of cauda equina lesions in the dog. J Small Anim Pract 23:425, 1982.

38. DiChiro G: Opinion: Unintentional spinal cord arteriography: A warning. Radiology 112:231, 1974.

39. Dijkshoorn NA and Rijnberk A: Detection of brain tumors in dogs by scintigraphy. J Am Vet Radiol Soc 18:147, 1977.

40. Dorn AS: A standard technique for canine cerebral angiography. JAVMA 161:12, 1972.

41. Doubilet P and Herman PG: Interpretation of radiographs: Effect of clinical history. Am J Roentgenol 137:1055, 1981.

42. Douglas SW and Williamson HD: Principles of Veterinary Radiography, 2nd ed. Baltimore, Williams & Wilkins Co, 1972.

43. Drayer B, Warner MA, Sudilovsky A, et al: Iopamidol vs. metrizamide: A double blind study for cervical myelography. Neuroradiology 24:77, 1982.

44. Eldevik OP, Dugstad G, Orrison WW, and Haughton VM: The effect of clinical bias on the interpretation of myelography and spinal computed tomography. Radiology 145:85, 1982.

45. Evans HE and Christensen GC: Miller's Anatomy of the Dog, 2nd ed. Philadelphia, WB Saunders Co, 1979.

46. Feeney DA and Wise M: Epidurography in the normal dog: Technique and radiographic findings. Vet Radiol 22:35, 1981.

47. Felts JF and Prata RG: Cervical disk disease in the dog: Intraforaminal and lateral extrusions. JAAHA 19:755, 1983.

48. Field JR, Robertson JT, and DeSaussure RL: Complication of cerebral angiography in 2000 consecutive cases. J Neurosurg 19:775, 1962.

49. Fike JR, LeCouteur RA, and Cann CE: Anatomy of the canine brain using high resolution computed tomography. Vet Radiol 22:236, 1981.

50. Fike JR, LeCouteur RA, Cann CE, and Pflugfelder CM: Computerized tomography of brain tumors of the rostral and middle fossa in the dog. Am J Vet Res 42:275, 1981.

51. Fink-Bennett D, Uppal TK, and Wesolowski DP: Tc-99m glucoheptonate brain scintigraphy: A clinical comparison between one- and two-hour delayed images: Concise communication. J Nucl Med 23:17, 1982.

52. Fitzgerald TC: Anatomy of the cerebral ventricles of domestic animals. Vet Med 56:38, 1961.

53. Foreman JH, Reed SM, Rantanen NW, et al: Congenital internal hydrocephalus in a quarterhorse foal. J Equine Vet Sci 3:154, 1984.

54. Funkquist B: Myelographic localization of spinal cord compression in dogs: A comparison between cisternal and lumbar injections of metrizamide "Amipaque" in diagnosing and locating spinal cord compression. Acta Vet Scand 16:269, 1975.

55. Funkquist B: Thoracolumbar myelography with water-soluble contrast medium in dogs. 1. Technique of myelography, side effects and complications. J Small Anim Pract 3:53, 1962.

56. Funkquist B, and Obel N: Effect on the spinal cord of subarachnoid injection of water-soluble contrast medium. Excerptum Acta Radiol 56:449, 1961.

57. Garrick JG and Sullivan CR: A technique for performing discography in dogs. Proc Mayo Clin 39:270, 1964.

58. Geary JC: Veterinary tomography. J Am Vet Radiol Soc 8:32, 1967.

59. Gershater R and Holgate RC: Lumbar epidural venography in the diagnosis of disc herniations. Am J Roentgenol 126:992, 1976.

60. Getty R: Sisson and Grossman's The Anatomy of Domestic Animals, 5th ed. Philadelphia, WB Saunders Co, 1975.

61. Gilday DL, Paul DJ, and Paterson J: Diagnosis of osteomyelitis in children by combined blood pool and bone imaging. Radiology 117:331, 1975.

62. Gomez JA: Personal communication.

63. Grainger RD: Intravascular contrast media—the past, the present, and the future. Br J Radiol 55:1, 1982.

64. Grainger RG, Kendall BE, and Wylie IG: Lumbar myelography with metrizamide. A new nonionic contrast medium. Br J Radiol 49:996, 1976.

65. Hansen H-J: A pathologic-anatomical study on disc degeneration in dog. Acta Orthop Scand Suppl II: 1952.

66. Hansen H-J, Olsson S-E, and Fankhauser R: Spät-schäden am rückenmark durch thorotrast myelographie beim hund. Schweiz Arch Tierheilkd 108:351, 1966.

67. Heck LL, Gottschalk A, and Hoffer PB: Static and dynamic brain imaging. In Gottschalk A and Potchen EJ (eds): Diagnostic Nuclear Medicine. Baltimore, Williams & Wilkins Co, 1976, p 278.

68. Hilts SV: Brain imaging—what should we be doing? Clin Nucl Med 1:26, 1976.

69. Hoerlein BF: Canine Neurology, 2nd ed. Philadelphia, WB Saunders Co, 1971.

70. Hoerlein BF: Intervertebral Disc Protrusion in the Dog: A Clinical and Pathological Study. Thesis (PhD), Cornell University, Ithaca, NY, 1952.

71. Hoerlein BF and Petty MF: Contrast encephalography and ventriculography in the dog—preliminary studies. Am J Vet Res 22:1041, 1961.

72. Horwitz NJ: Positive contrast ventriculography—critical evaluation. J Neurosurg 13:388, 1956.

73. Hounsfield GN: Computerized transverse axial scanning (tomography). Part I. Description of system. Br J Radiol 46:1016, 1973.

74. Howland WJ and Curry JL: Pantopaque arachnoiditis. Acta Radiol 5:1032, 1966.

75. Hurov L, Troy G, and Turnwald G: Diskospondylitis in the dog: 27 cases. JAVMA 173:275, 1978.

76. James CCM, Lassman LP, and Tomlinson BE: Congenital anomalies of the lower spine and spinal cord in manx cats. J Pathol 97:269, 1969.

77. James CW and Hoerlein BF: Cerebral angiography in the dog. Vet Med 55:12, 1960.

78. Jeffcott LB: Disorders of the thoracolumbar spine of the horse—a survey of 443 cases. Equine Vet J 12:197, 1980.

79. Jeffcott LB: Radiographic appearance of equine lumbosacral and pelvic abnormalities by linear tomography. Vet Radiol 24:201, 1983.

80. Jeffcott LB: Radiographic examination of the equine vertebral column. Vet Radiol 20:135, 1979.

81. Jeffcott LB: Radiographic features of the normal equine thoracolumbar spine. Vet Radiol 20:140, 1979.

82. Jeffcott LB: Technique of linear tomography for the pelvic region of the horse. Vet Radiol 24:194, 1983.

83. Johnston DE and Summers BA: Osteomyelitis of the lumbar vertebrae in dogs caused by grass-seed foreign bodies. Aust Vet J 47:289, 1971.

84. Kallfelz FA, deLahunta A, and Allhands RV: Scintigraphic diagnosis of brain lesions in the dog and cat. JAVMA 172:589, 1978.

85. Kendall B, Schneider A, Stevens J, and Harrison M: Clinical trial of iohexol for lumbar myelography. Br J Radiol 56:539, 1983.

86. Kido DK, Schoene W, Baker RA, and Rumbaugh CL: Metrizamide: Epidurography in dogs. Radiology 128:123, 1978.

87. Kirchner PT and Simon MA: Current concepts review: Radioisotopic evaluation of skeletal disease. J Bone Joint Surg 63A:673, 1981.

88. Kitchen H, Murray RE, and Cockrell BY: Animal model for human disease. Spina bifida, sacral dysgenesis and myelocele. Animal model: Manx cats. Am J Pathol 68:203, 1972.

89. Klide AM, Steinberg SA, and Pond MJ: Epiduralograms in the dog: The uses and advantages of the diagnostic procedure. J Am Vet Radiol Soc 8:39, 1967.

90. Knecht CD, Hathcock JT, and Redding RW: Immediate effects of metrizamide myelography on electromyographic findings in dogs. Am J Vet Res 43:2042, 1982.

91. Koblik PD and Suter PF: Lumbo-sacral vertebral sinus venography via transjugular catheterization in the dog. Vet Radiol 22:69, 1981.

92. Koper S and Mucha M: Visualization of the vertebral canal veins in the dog: A radiological method. J Am Vet Radiol Soc 18:105, 1976.

93. Kornegay JL and Barber DL: Diskospondylitis in dogs. JAVMA 177:337, 1980.

94. LeCouteur R, Fike JR, Cann CE, and Pedroia VG: Computed tomography of brain tumors in the caudal fossa of the dog. Vet Radiol 22:244, 1981.

95. LeCouteur RA, Scagliotti RH, Beck KA, and Holliday TA: Indirect imaging of the canine optic nerve, using metrizamide (optic thecography). Am J Vet Res 43:1424, 1982.

96. Lee R and Griffiths IR: A comparison of cerebral arteriography and cavernous sinus venography in the dog. J Small Anim Pract 13:225, 1972.

97. Lindblad G, Ljunggren G, and Olsson S-E: On spinal cord compression in the dog: An angiographic study. Adv Small Anim Pract 3:121, 1962.

98. Lindbloom K: Technique and results of diagnostic disc puncture and injection (discography) in the lumbar region. Acta Orthop Scand 20:315, 1950–1951.

99. Loden D, Norton D, Wolfe LH, and Ford RB: Diagnosis of intracranial lesions by computerized tomography in three dogs. JAAHA 19:303, 1983.

100. Lord PF and Olsson S-E: Myelography with metrizamide in the dog: A clinical study on its use for the demonstration of spinal cord lesions other than those caused by intervertebral disk protrusions. J Am Vet Radiol Soc 17:42, 1976.

101. Luttgen PJ, Braund KG, Brawner WR Jr, and Vandevelde M: A retrospective study of 29 spinal tumors in the dog and cat. J Small Anim Pract 21:213, 1980.

102. Mayhew IG, Watson AG, and Heissan JA: Congenital occipitoatlantoaxial malformations in the horse. Equine Vet J 10:103, 1978.

103. Mayhew IG, Whitlock RH, and deLahunta A: Spinal

cord disease in the horse: Electromyographic and radiographic studies. Cornell Vet 68 (Suppl 6):44, 1978.

104. McNeel SV: Radiology of the skull and cervical spine. Vet Clin North Am (Small Anim Pract) 12:259, 1982.

105. McNeel SV and Morgan JP: Intraosseous vertebral venography: A technique for examination of the canine lumbosacral junction. J Am Vet Radiol Soc 19:168, 1978.

106. Melartin E, Tuohimaa PJ, and Dabb R: Neurotoxicity of iothalamates and diatrizoates. I. Significance of concentration and cation. Invest Radiol 5:13, 1970.

107. Metrizamide: A non-ionic water-soluble contrast medium: Experimental and preliminary clinical investigations. Acta Radiol Suppl 335, 1973.

108. Morgan JP: Radiology in Veterinary Orthopedics. Philadelphia, Lea & Febiger, 1972.

109. Morgan JP and Silverman S: Techniques of Veterinary Radiography, 3rd ed. Davis, CA, Veterinary Radiology Associates, 1982.

110. Morgan JP, Suter PF, and Holliday TA: Myelography with water-soluble contrast medium: Radiographic interpretation of disc herniation in dogs. Acta Radiol (Suppl) 319:217, 1972.

111. Murphy WA, Destouet JM, and Gilula LA: Percutaneous skeletal biopsy 1981: A procedure for radiologists—results, review, and recommendations. Radiology 139:545, 1981.

112. Nyland TG, Blythe LL, Pool RR, et al: Metrizamide myelography in the horse: Clinical, radiographic, and pathologic changes. Am J Vet Res 41:204, 1980.

113. Oftedal S-I: Intraventricular application of water-soluble contrast media in cats. Acta Radiol (Suppl) 335:125, 1973.

114. Oliver JE Jr: Cranial sinus venography. J Am Vet Radiol Soc 10:66, 1969.

115. Oliver JE Jr: Principles of canine brain surgery. Anim Hosp 2:73, 1966.

116. Oliver JE Jr and Conrad CR: Cerebral ventriculography. In Ticer JW: Radiographic Technique in Small Animal Practice. Philadelphia, WB Saunders Co, 1975, p 271.

117. Oliver JE Jr and Lewis RE: Lesions of the atlas and axis in dogs. JAAHA 9:304, 1973.

118. Oliver JE Jr, Selcer RR, and Simpson S: Cauda equina compression from lumbosacral malarticulation and malformation in the dog. JAVMA 173:207, 1978.

119. Parker AJ and Park RD: Occipital dysplasia in the dog. JAAHA 10:520, 1974.

120. Parker AJ, Park RD, and Stowater JL: Traumatic occlusion of segmental spinal veins. Am J Vet Res 35:857, 1974.

121. Pettit GD (ed): Intervertebral Disc Protrusion in the Dog. New York, Appleton-Century-Crofts, 1966.

122. Power HT, Watrous BJ, and deLahunta A: Facial and vestibulocochlear nerve disease in six horses. JAVMA 183:1076, 1983.

123. Prata RG: Diagnosis of spinal cord tumors in the dog. Vet Clin North Am 7:165, 1977.

124. Radberg C and Wennberg E: Late sequelae following myelography with water-soluble contrast media. Acta Radiol 14:Fasc 5, 1973.

125. Rantanen NW, Gavin PR, Barbee DD, and Sande RD: Ataxia and paresis in horses. Part II. Radiographic and myelographic examination of the cervical vertebral column. Compend Contin Educ 3:S161, 1981.

126. Rising JL and Lewis RE: Femorovertebral cerebral angiography in the dog. Am J Vet Res 33:665, 1972.

127. Roberts RE: Radiographic examination of the muscu-loskeletal system. Vet Clin North Am (Small Anim Pract) 13:19, 1983.

128. Rollo FD, Cavalieri RR, Born M, et al: Comparative evaluation of ^{99m}TcGH, ^{99m}TcO$_4$, and ^{99m}TcDTPA as brain imaging agents. Radiology 123:379, 1977.

129. Rosenberg FJ, Romano JJ, and Shaw DD: Metrizamide, iothalamate, and metrizoate: Effects of internal carotid arterial injections on the blood-brain-barrier of the rabbit. Invest Radiol 15:Suppl S275, 1980.

130. Sackett JF, Strother CM, and Quaglieri CE: Metrizamide—CSF contrast medium: Analysis of clinical application in 215 patients. Radiology 123:779, 1977.

131. Schajowicz F and Derqui HJC: Puncture biopsy in lesions of the locomotor system. Review and results of 4050 cases, including 941 vertebral punctures. Cancer 21:531, 1968.

132. Seawright AA, English PB, and Gartner RJW: Hypervitaminosis A of the cat. Adv Vet Sci Comp Med 14:1, 1970.

133. Selcer RR and Oliver JE Jr: Cervical spondylopathy—wobbler syndrome in dogs. JAAHA 11:175, 1975.

134. Shebitz H and Wilkens H: Atlas of Radiographic Anatomy of the Dog and Cat, 3rd ed. Philadelphia, WB Saunders Co, 1978.

135. Shebitz H and Wilkens H: Atlas of Radiographic Anatomy of the Horse, 3rd ed. Philadelphia, WB Saunders Co, 1978.

136. Siberstein EB: New perspectives on the relationship of radionuclide and CT brain imaging. Appl Radiol March-April:35, 1981.

137. Stowater JL and Kneller SK: Clinical evaluation of metrizamide as a myelographic agent in the dog. JAVMA 175:191, 1979.

138. Stowater JL, Kneller SK, and Froelich PS: Metrizamide myelography in two horses. Vet Med Small Anim Clin 73:117, 1978.

139. Suter PF: Cerebral angiography in the dog: Technique, complications, and indications. Proc 39th Ann Meet AAHA 39:536, 1972.

140. Suter PF, Morgan JP, Holliday TA, and O'Brien TR: Myelography in the dog: Diagnosis of tumors of the spinal cord and vertebrae. J Am Vet Radiol Soc 12:29, 1972.

141. Taylor DC: The pathological effects of thorotrast myelography in the dog. J Comp Pathol Therapeut 68:213, 1958.

142. Thrall DE, Lewis RE, Walker MA, et al: The basis for dosing water soluble myelographic medium for lumbar administration: Body weight or crown rump length. J Am Vet Radiol Soc 16:130, 1975.

143. Ticer JW: Radiographic Technique in Veterinary Practice, 2nd ed. Philadelphia, WB Saunders Co, 1984.

144. Ticer JW and Brown SG: Water-soluble myelography in canine intervertebral disk protrusion. J Am Vet Radiol Soc 15:3, 1974.

145. Trotter EJ, deLahunta A, Geary JC, and Brasmer TR: Caudal cervical vertebral malformation-malarticulation in Great Danes and Doberman pinschers. JAVMA 168:917, 1976.

146. Wilson JW, Bahr RJ, Leipold HW, and Guffy MM: Acute leptomeningeal reaction to subarachnoid injection of ethyl iodophenylhundecylate in dogs. JAVMA 169:415, 1976.

147. Wilson JW, Kurtz HJ, Leipold HW, and Lees GE: Spina bifida in the dog. Vet Pathol 16:165, 1979.

148. Worthman RP: The longitudinal vertebral venous sinuses of the dog. II. Functional aspects. Am J Vet Res 17:349, 1956.

149. Wortman JA: Radiographic diagnosis of intervertebral disc diseases in the dog: A comparison of non-contrast and myelographic studies. Proc 41st Ann Meet AAHA 41:698, 1974.
150. Wright JA: A study of the radiographic anatomy of the foramen magnum in dogs. J Small Anim Pract 20:501, 1979.
151. Wright JA: A study of vertebral osteophyte formation in the canine spine. II. Radiographic survey. J Small Anim Pract 23:747, 1982.
152. Wright JA: The use of sagittal diameter measurement in the diagnosis of cervical spinal stenosis. J Small Anim Pract 20:331, 1979.
153. Wright JA, Bell DA, and Clayton-Jones DG: The clinical and radiological features associated with spinal tumors in thirty dogs. J Small Anim Pract 20:461, 1979.
154. Wright JA and Clayton-Jones DG: Metrizamide myelography in sixty-eight dogs. J Small Anim Pract 22:415, 1981.
155. Wrigley RH and Reuter RE: Canine cervical discography. Vet Radiol 25:274, 1984.

Chapter 5

Electrophysiologic Diagnosis

Section 1   *R W Redding, DVM, PhD*

ELECTROENCEPHALOGRAPHY

THE PRODUCTION OF THE ELECTROENCEPHALOGRAM

If electrodes are placed on the scalp of the dog over an area in which the cerebral hemispheres are near the surface, one can record, with appropriate amplifiers and writing instruments, oscillations of electric potential that arise from the cerebral cortex. This activity consists of alterations in electrical potential from 3 to 300 microvolts (μV) recurring at frequencies of 0.5 to 40 hertz (Hz). A recording of such activity is called the electroencephalogram (EEG).

Action potentials, variable resting potentials, excitatory postsynaptic potentials (EPSP), and inhibitory postsynaptic potentials (IPSP) occur in the cerebral cortex. It is doubtful that synchronization of action potentials could account for much of the EEG activity. The variable resting potentials of cortical neurons are a result of excitatory postsynaptic and inhibitory postsynaptic potentials. The slow time course of such potentials is compatible with those of the EEG. The reticular activating system (RAS) is the major afferent system to the cerebral cortex and probably influences the frequency and amplitude of the EEG via the thalamus. The EEG frequency has rhythmic activity, suggesting a pacemaker source. It is believed that the thalamus utilizing oscillating neuronal circuits is responsible for the rhythmicity.

The EEG recorded from the scalp is an algebraic summation of the variable resting potentials of cortical neurons, excitatory postsynaptic potentials, inhibitory postsynaptic potentials, and possibly action potentials of cortical neurons and their processes.[19, 24, 26, 30, 38, 49, 60, 69] The variations in rhythmicity, frequency, and amplitude are a result of subcortical influence. The normal EEG of newborn and adult horses has been reported.[51a]

INSTRUMENTS AND RECORDING TECHNIQUE

The Electroencephalograph

The electroencephalograph is an electronic device that amplifies and graphically records potential alterations from the cerebral cortex. Many types of amplifier-recording systems are commercially available. It is beyond the scope of this text to discuss the various instruments in detail. All the devices consist of a lead system, preamplifiers, amplifiers, and a pen-writing galvanometer. The amplifiers are designed to give an amplification of approximately one million times. This is necessary because the magnitude of the voltages from the surface of the scalp ranges from 3 to 300 μV. All EEG machines available have incorporated a reference signal that can be used to standardize the channels of the machine simultaneously. The usual standardization signal is 50 μV. The amplifiers are adjusted so that the standardization signal causes a deflection on the vertical scale of the galvanometer of 10 mm for animal electroencephalography. With this standardization, the range of voltage available from the surface of the scalp will be accurately recorded without distortion caused by the limits of the galvanometer. Some animals with thick skulls and heavy musculature may require an EEG amplifier with increased sensitivity to reflect the actual cortical potentials.

Electrodes

An electroencephalogram obtained without harm to the patient is necessary for evaluation of the physiologic status of the cerebral hemispheres in an animal suspected of having a cerebral disorder. Several types of electrodes that are available for use in humans have been used on animals with varying degrees of success. None of them has been found to be completely satisfactory. Such electrodes are Reymond tripods, silver disk electrodes, and needle electrodes. The electrode must be attached easily, must be secured to the skin over the cranium, and must have a low stable resistance. None of the aforementioned types meets all these criteria when used on the dog. The electrode found to be most suitable is a small copper battery or alligator clamp that grasps a portion of the skin firmly and securely. It makes good electric contact with the skin when used with electrode gel to assure the best conduction of the electric impulses generated by the cerebral cortex.[60] Needle electrodes are more suitable in small animals because of the close proximity of the electrodes on the scalp. The electrode resistance is usually high, 35,000 to 50,000 ohms. This high resistance may cause undesirable baseline fluctuations; however, the EEG recorded is readable.

Technique of Applying Electrodes

It is not necessary to clip the hair from the head of the animal. To assure good electric contact with clamp electrodes, the scalp is first defatted by being rubbed vigorously with acetone or alcohol. To prevent pain when the electrode clamps are applied to the skin over the scalp, it is necessary to infiltrate the skin and subcutaneous tissue at the point of application of the electrode with a long-acting local anesthetic solution such as 0.5% lidocaine (this diluted concentration is sufficient for local anesthesia but will not produce toxic side reactions when absorbed). When infiltrating the subcutaneous tissue with the local anesthetic solution, it is convenient to infiltrate also the skeletal musculature of the head immediately under the point of application of the electrode, to eliminate the muscle potential artifact that might otherwise be recorded during electroencephalography.

After the skin and skeletal muscle have been anesthetized, the electrode gel is applied and rubbed into the area in which the electrodes are to be attached. It is necessary to make certain that the adjacent areas treated with electrode gel do not come in contact with each other, as this will cause a shorting of the circuit. The gel is applied, and the skin is grasped with the electrode and squeezed tightly. The resistance should be checked between the adjacent electrodes to assure good electric contact. A resistance of 10,000 ohms or less is desirable for recording the EEG with clamp electrodes.

Electrode Placement

There are various methods called montages for electrode placement on the scalp. Each montage has its own merits, and each individual electroencephalographer has his or her own frame of reference for detecting abnormalities. No one method is perfect, and the best aspects of each should be utilized in electroencephalography.

A suitable electrode arrangement for recording the EEG of the dog consists of two electrodes on the frontoparietal areas, two over the occipital areas, and one over the vertex. A ground electrode is also necessary. This may be attached to the skin over the external occipital protuberance (Fig. 5–1). With these five electrode recording points it is possible to record the following: the four areas of the cerebral hemispheres against the vertex lead as a common reference; transoccipital leads; transfrontal leads; left hemispheric leads, occipital to frontal; and right hemispheric leads, occipital to frontal. When an eight channel EEG recording system is used, one can record simultaneously all these leads.

The advantage of referential recording (vertex leads) is an undistorted display of the shape of the potential changes; it is used to record potentials that have wide distribution. Bipolar linkages (hemispheric, transfrontal, and transoccipital) distinguish potentials between the electrodes so that localized circumscribed potentials can be easily identified. The disadvantage of bipolar recordings is that widely distributed potentials are distorted. By simultaneously recording the referential and bipolar leads on an eight channel machine, the advantages of each

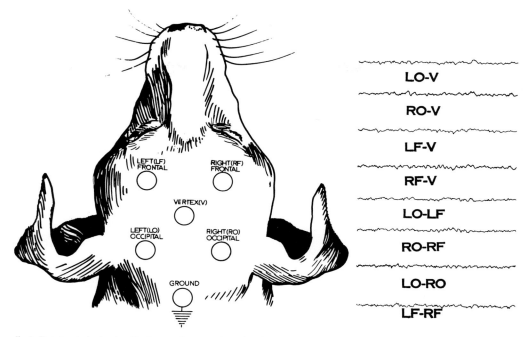

Figure 5–1. Points of electrode attachment for recording the electroencephalogram. Recordings obtained from a combination of the lead points are shown on the right.

montage are compared and used for clinical evaluation.

Restraint of the Patient

It is desirable to restrain the patient without the use of any chemical agent, because any such agent causes alteration of cortical activity. One type of restraint is mechanical. The thoracic limbs are bound together with tape, as are the pelvic limbs. The eyes are covered to prevent visual stimuli from affecting the cortical potentials. It is also desirable to decrease auditory perception by placing a large pledget of cotton in each external auditory canal, and it is essential to obtain the recording in an environment free of noise and at a temperature at which the animal neither shivers nor pants. With the aforementioned restraint, an assistant holds the animal in a lateral recumbent position or the animal may be secured to a table with a seat belt type strap. When so restrained, most patients struggle for only a short time, then relax so that a recording may be made. Some patients actually doze or sleep for a short period if the room is quiet and dark. This is useful for the interpretation of the record, as abnormalities frequently are displayed when the animal is relaxed. Another form of physical restraint that

may be used on small uncooperative animals is the restraint bag—a flexible plastic bag filled with tiny polyurethane balls. The restraint bag is molded around the animal, leaving the head exposed, and the air is exhausted using a vacuum, causing the bag to solidify and securely restrain the patient. A run of approximately 20 minutes usually is sufficient for most clinical cases. Figure 5–2 A–C shows a typical recording obtained from a normal adult dog when alert, relaxed, and in light sleep.

Other methods of restraint have been proposed. Klemm[37, 38, 45, 47] prefers to use barbiturate anesthesia. Herin et al.[29] utilize gallamine triethiodide, a skeletal muscle paralyzing agent, and artificial respiration during the recording of the EEG.

Approximately 10% of the animals resist mechanical restraint to the degree that a clinically useful EEG is not obtainable. The author has found that giving the dog etchchlorvynol (Placidyl) by mouth in a dose of 10 to 20 mg/lb (20–40 mg/kg) body weight 45 minutes prior to attempting a recording will result in sufficient relaxation to obtain a diagnostic EEG. The animal tends to drift into a light sleep. However, arousal can be accomplished easily by an auditory or tactile stimulus, so that one can obtain both awake and light sleep recordings for interpretation.

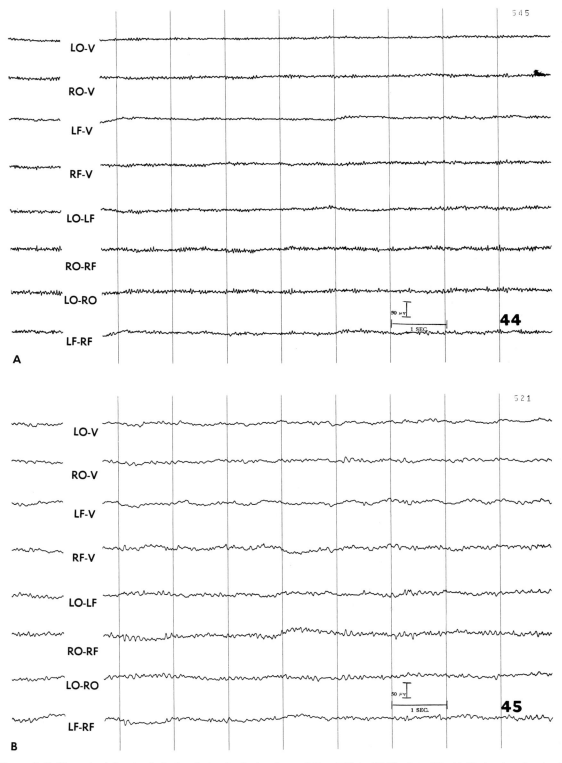

Figure 5–2. Normal adult animal. A, An alert animal, showing activity of 15 to 30 Hz, 3 to 10 μV. B, A relaxed animal, showing activity of 5 to 15 Hz, 10 to 25 μV. C, An animal in light sleep, showing activity of 3 to 15 Hz, 10 to 80 μV.

Illustration continued on opposite page

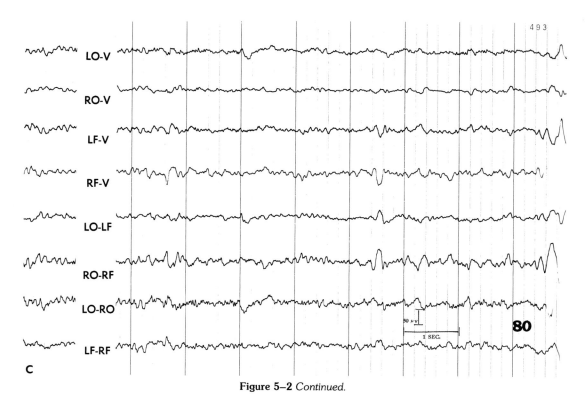

493

LO-V

RO-V

LF-V

RF-V

LO-LF

RO-RF

LO-RO

50 μV

1 SEC.

80

LF-RF

C

Figure 5–2 *Continued.*

CANINE BREED DIFFERENCE IN RECORDING

Some breeds of dogs, such as the boxer and hound, have heavy musculature over the portion of the scalp from which the EEG is to be recorded. In these animals, it is difficult to obtain good recordings, especially of the occipital areas. Increasing the gain of the amplification system when using scalp electrodes may aid in obtaining a diagnostic EEG tracing. Some species of dogs have a rather large and extensive frontal sinus, which may extend over a portion of the frontal cortex and interfere with the recordings being made over the frontoparietal area. Care must be taken to assure proper placement of the electrode so that it does not overlie a frontal sinus.

PHYSIOLOGIC STATES AFFECTING THE ELECTROENCEPHALOGRAM

It should be appreciated that cortical electric activity is influenced by physiologic variables. The age of the patient must be known, along with the state of consciousness at the time the recording is made.[8, 22, 52, 60]

Age of the Individual

The stage of maturation of the cerebral cortex and other subcortical structures of the central nervous system influences the EEG pattern.[6, 8, 22, 25, 38, 52, 60, 64, 72] In the young animal, from birth to approximately 7 days, little cortical activity is seen. Random bursts of 5 to 10 Hz activity with voltages of approximately 25 μV may be seen. There is no correlation between the two hemispheres in this burst of activity. When the animal is approximately 3 weeks of age, the pattern has developed to a medium voltage potential of low frequency. The medium voltage–low frequency pattern gradually matures during puppyhood and adolescence, progressing to an adult alert pattern of approximately 10 to 30 Hz with a voltage of approximately 5 to 15 μV. This pattern is acquired by about 22 to 30 weeks of age, depending on sex and breed. The basis for this change to an adult pattern is not well understood, but it is probably due to increased arborization of a dendritic network and myelinization of the tracts within the central nervous system. The light sleep pattern of a mature animal is shown in Figure 5–2C. Figure 5–3 A–C shows the typical pattern at

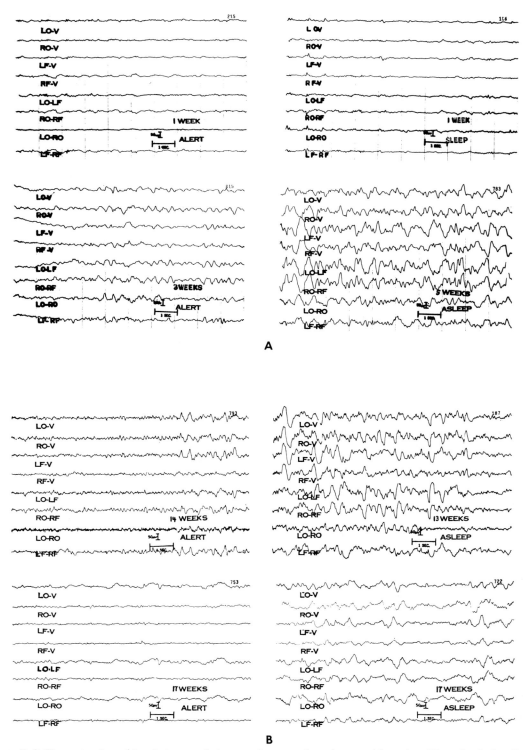

Figure 5–3. The maturation of the electroencephalogram of a puppy from the age of 1 week to 52 weeks. A, 1 to 5 weeks; B, 13 to 17 weeks; C, 22 to 52 weeks. The "alert" electroencephalogram is shown on the left side of the illustration and the "somnolent" on the right.

Illustration continued on opposite page

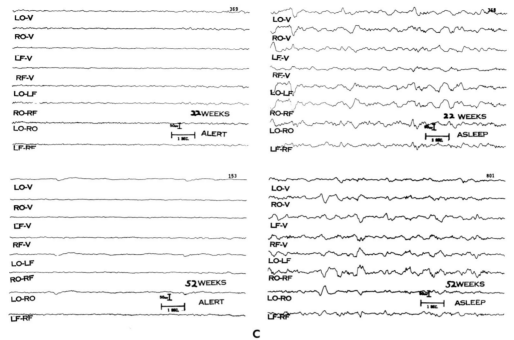

C

Figure 5–3 *Continued.*

various age levels in both the alert and sleep states.

During the maturation process, the waveforms change considerably, and some of the normal frequencies and amplitudes seen are similar to, if not indistinguishable from, those symptomatic of disease. It becomes obvious that the age of the animal must be known in evaluating a tracing, so that a normal recording at a specific age will not be misinterpreted as a disease process pattern.

The Level of Consciousness

The EEG is markedly influenced by the level of consciousness.[22, 52, 56, 60] Awareness produces a high frequency–low voltage pattern. A relaxed but not somnolent state produces a higher voltage–lower frequency pattern. Drowsiness is characterized by an even slower frequency and higher voltage; light sleep (a continuation of drowsiness) by frequencies of 4 to 6 Hz and voltages of 75 to 100 μV. Deep sleep is characterized by very high voltage, 150 to 200 μV and slow frequency discharge, 1 to 3 Hz. Deep sleep patterns are seldom recorded under clinical examination conditions.

ARTIFACTS

Electroencephalographic tracings of the patient may contain artifacts[36, 60] that may, if improperly interpreted, lead to an erroneous diagnosis of a disease that the animal does not have. *Muscle potentials*, especially over the occipital areas, are frequently encountered (Fig. 5–4). These muscle potentials may be mistaken for high voltage spikes thought to originate in the occipital cortex. Occasionally, electrodes placed over the frontal sinuses show no activity or little activity (Fig. 5–4). This should not be mistaken for a disease state in which very low voltages are encountered.

Ear movements cause a shift in the baseline of the recording made adjacent to that ear (Fig. 5–4). Eyeblinks and eyeball movements are frequently seen in the frontal recordings. They may be unilateral or bilateral (Fig. 5–4).

Licking, chewing, and swallowing movements cause a characteristic overall baseline shift (Fig. 5–4).

Many dogs of the toy breeds shiver periodically and produce characteristic oscillations of the baseline (Fig. 5–4).

Electrodes having poor contact with the skin or those having poor electric contacts in the

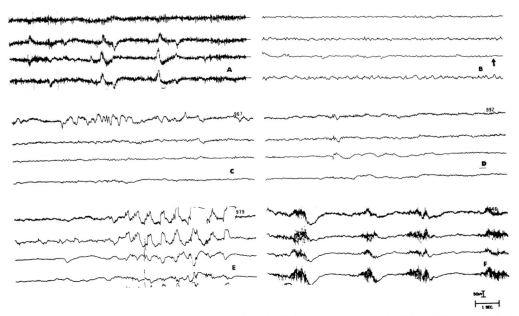

Figure 5–4. Artifacts seen in electroencephalogram of the dog. A, Skeletal muscle with potentials. B, Electrode indicated by arrow placed at edge of frontal sinus. Note reduced voltage compared with lower tracing of opposite side. C, Upper tracing indicates movement of the left ear. D, Eyelid blinks followed by eyeball movement. E, Licking, chewing, and swallowing movements. F, Shivering with muscle potentials in bursts.

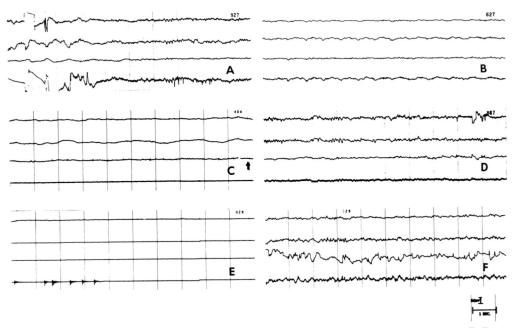

Figure 5–5. Artifacts seen in EEG recording of the dog. A, Loose electrode wire causing spikelike activity. B, Panting: note the rhythmic one cycle per second waves in the second and fourth tracings. C, Electrocardiogram in tracing indicated by arrow. D, Alternating current interference can be seen in the lower tracing. E, Microphonic tube in amplifier. F, Noise in one amplifier due to defective connection evident in third tracing.

wiring show rapid shifts in the baseline or spikelike discharges. These should not be mistaken for spiking activity originating in the cerebral cortex (Fig. 5–5). Canine choreiform movements may cause the entire body or a portion of the body to shift slightly during each spasm. This spasm will cause a baseline shift in the recording.

A common artifact that may simulate slow wave activity is that produced by *panting*, which is readily recognized by simultaneous observation of the animal and the recording (Fig. 5–5).

The electrocardiogram (ECG) may be seen as a rhythmic spikelike activity in the tracing and should not be mistaken for spikes that originate in the cerebral cortex. This artifact may appear because the reference electrode is applied to the ear, or the animal may have a *wet haircoat*. The identification of this artifact can be confirmed by simultaneously recording the ECG on one channel of the EEG machine.

Interference due to alternating current is occasionally encountered, and the use of a shielded room or a cage may be necessary to eliminate it completely. Modern EEG machines adequately reject 60 Hz interference. The typical pattern of alternating current interference is shown in Figure 5–5.

Noise originating within the channels or wiring of the EEG itself present difficulties. Such noise may originate in the amplifier or be due to a poor wiring connection within the circuit (Fig. 5–5).

THE NORMAL ELECTROENCEPHALOGRAM

The definition of normality is difficult to state, because it depends on the method of restraint used to make the recording (chemical or physical restraint). Each method of restraint influences the type of recording obtained. In addition, the frequency and amplitude vary from one animal to another and from one breed to another. For example, thin skulled animals (such as the Chihuahua) show relatively higher voltages and slower frequencies than do heavy skulled, heavy muscled animals (such as the boxer).

The interpreter of the EEG must have a clear mental picture of what is considered normal before he or she can interpret the tracing with any degree of accuracy. Figure 5–2 A–C shows normal EEG obtained without chemical re-

straint. Electroencephalograms are reported in frequency and amplitude, with the frequency on the abscissa and the amplitude on the ordinate of the graph. An adult alert pattern is approximately 8 to 38 Hz, with voltages from 3 to 15 μV.

Once the patterns seen in an electroencephalographic tracing have been learned, visual analysis of the electroencephalogram becomes a relatively simple task of recognition. To gain proficiency in interpreting electroencephalograms, practice is necessary. The sample tracings in this chapter will provide the reader with some concept of normality and abnormalities.

THE ELECTROENCEPHALOGRAM IN DISEASE

The EEG may be used in clinical medicine as one more diagnostic aid in evaluating the patient's neurologic status.[10–13, 17, 21, 23, 36, 38, 55, 57, 58, 60, 62, 67] In diseases of the cerebral hemispheres and in generalized metabolic disturbances, the EEG pattern is altered. The interpreter of an EEG must have a clear mental picture of the normal pattern variations that will serve as a reference for comparison with EEG from animals with suspected brain disease. The patient's age and state of awareness must be taken into consideration when one evaluates such records. In general, the abnormal record shows excessively slow or excessively fast activity for the physiologic state under which the recording was made. The records may demonstrate focal abnormalities of various types such as spiked discharges, paroxysmal bursts of either slow or fast activity, or generalized slowing with the greatest slowing over specific areas.

Some general conclusions concerning abnormalities can be stated. The most fundamental is that disease causes changes in either amplitude or frequency and occasionally in both. Of the two changes, amplitude changes are the most dramatic indicator of disease. Frequency changes, on the other hand, are relatively more reliable. The following is a list of conclusions formulated by Klemm and Hall[44] that relate to animal electroencephalography:

1. Low voltage–fast activity (LVFA) and spikes indicate an ongoing irritative process due to a variety of causes.

2. High voltage–slow waves (HVSA), if persistent, indicate death of many neurons due to a variety of causes.

3. LVFA and HVSA are not pathognomonic

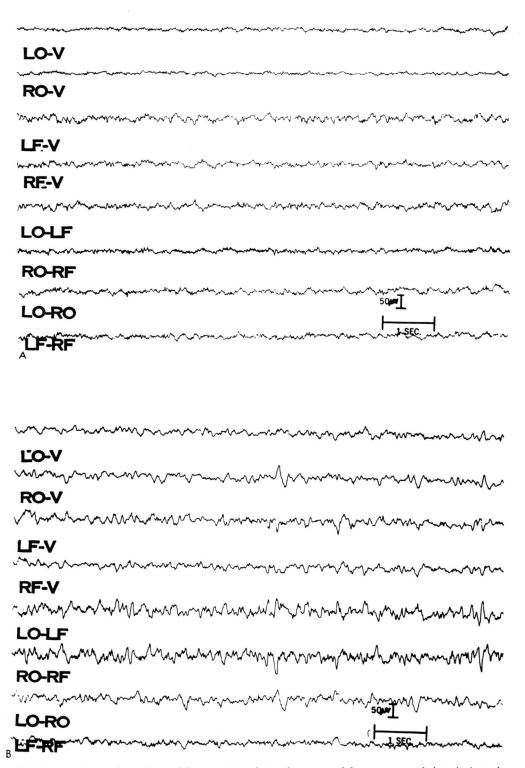

Figure 5–6. A series of recordings obtained from a patient during the course of distemper encephalitis. A, Animal presented for examination because of anorexia and depression—early encephalitis. B, Five days after first EEG recording—transition from early to acute stage. C, Seven days after first EEG examination—acute stage of encephalitis. Two weeks after C, clinical recovery was complete. D, Two weeks after clinical recovery—beginning of late encephalitis pattern.

Illustration continued on opposite page

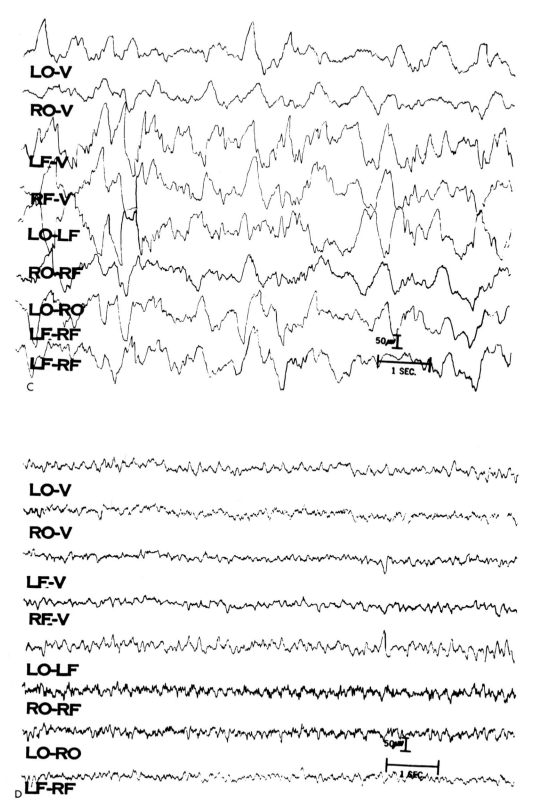

Figure 5–6 *Continued.*

of any given disease but are suggestive of several diseases.

4. Local EEG abnormalities indicate a cortical rather than a subcortical lesion.

5. Common causes of local cortical lesions are vascular disorders (infarct), hemorrhage, an early tumor, or focal necrosis.

6. Generalized EEG abnormalities can indicate that a lesion is either generalized in the cortex or focal subcortically.

7. Common causes of generalized lesions are infections, trauma, space occupying lesions (tumor, hydrocephalus), or idiopathic epilepsy.

8. Cerebral recordings during illness can indicate the effectiveness of therapy in altering the progress of the disease process.

Low voltage–fast activity and high voltage–slow activity are not necessarily characteristic of specific diseases. However, abnormal brain wave activity is useful in indicating what kind of disease process is involved and whether it is acute or chronic and improving or regressing. Acute inflammatory diseases such as canine distemper encephalitis cause low voltage–fast activity and spikes in the initial stages. As the disease progresses, the pattern converts from low voltage–fast to high voltage–slow, on which there may be superimposed fast activity. On the other hand, high voltage–slow wave activity is produced by various degenerative diseases such as trauma, vascular disorders, and hydrocephalus. Tumors generally show abnormally slow waves with occasional spikes in the area on which the tumor is encroaching. If the tumor is deeply located, it will cause generalized slow wave activity and occasionally some superimposed spikes.

The electroencephalographic abnormalities just described can occur throughout any area of the cerebral cortex, or they may be localized at a few points and detectable by proper electrode placement. If the abnormality is localized, the lesion is also localized and most probably in the cerebral cortex. Most EEG recordings are obtained from the cortical tissue, and lesions in one area of the cortex will cause local EEG abnormalities. If the lesion is below the cortex, the EEG abnormality will most likely appear in several areas of the cortex because the subcortical brain tissue sends projecting fiber tracts to scattered areas on the cerebral cortex.

Knowledge of the focal or diffuse nature of EEG abnormalities suggests certain conclusions about potential causes of encephalopathies. Focal brain damage can be caused by vascular disorders, such as small infarcts or hemorrhages, an early tumor, or a focal necrosis of hematogenous origin. In dogs and cats, focal brain damage appears to be relatively rare, except in cases of trauma. Diffuse brain damage, however, is often seen in the dog and cat and is usually caused by viral, protozoan, fungal, or bacterial infections and by space occupying lesions located deep within the diencephalon. To follow the course of any encephalopathy, it is important to make serial recordings of the EEG, because such recordings can indicate whether the disease is progressing, resolving, or remaining unchanged. In addition, the effectiveness of therapy is easily evaluated by serial recordings.

Inflammatory Diseases

Distemper Encephalitis

Perhaps one of the most useful tools in the diagnosis of encephalitis[10, 11, 21, 23, 45, 57, 58, 60, 62, 67] is the electroencephalogram. What appears to be encephalitis on clinical observation may be proved beyond doubt when the EEG is obtained from the animal. Early encephalitis is characterized by a 3 to 5 cycle pattern on which is superimposed a 20 to 30 cycle spike discharge. An acute case of encephalitis is characterized by slow, 2 to 3 Hz activity with voltages of approximately 100 to 200 μV. Late encephalitis is characterized by 4 to 7 Hz with voltages of 10 to 15 μV. The pattern is relatively consistent, and can be altered for only a few seconds[61] by either auditory or visual stimulation, after which it returns to the characteristic pattern for that stage of the disease. Because the slowing takes on a character somewhat similar to that of sleep, one must be certain of the stage of awareness when interpreting the record. However, with experience there is little difficulty in differentiating the two.

Residual slow wave activity of the EEG is present in postencephalitic patients for as long as 1 year after clinical recovery. The clinical signs of recovery can be correlated with lessening of slow wave activity and the return to normal frequencies. Persistent abnormal slow wave activity is frequently associated with seizures; therefore its presence can be helpful in the differential diagnosis of seizures. Figures 5–6 and 5–7 show sequential recordings from a case of distemper encephalitis, from the early stages of the disease to complete clinical recovery. Residual slow wave activity was still present 6 months after recovery. Occasional seizures were seen in this case and were controlled with anticonvulsant drugs.

Chronic Encephalitis

Occasionally a confirmed case of encephalitis fails to show the progression of changes just described under distemper encephalitis. This is more commonly seen in older dogs and has been termed old dog encephalitis. Repeated sequential EEG tracings show an almost consistent medium voltage–slow wave activity. The pattern does not change over months of time. The dog frequently has seizures that are difficult to control with medication. In addition, the animal may show generalized depression. Distemper inclusion bodies may be found in these cases.

Other Encephalopathies

There are many histopathologic classifications of other confirmed cases of encephalopathies. They include panencephalitis, meningoencephalitis, poliomeningoencephalomyelitis, encephalomalacia, meningoencephalomyelitis, polioencephalitis, and encephalomyelitis. There are no specific patterns for any one of these. They all show abnormal slow wave activity with superimposed fast waves or paroxysmal discharges. The voltages vary from medium to high, 25 to 150 µV.

Brain Abscesses

Brain abscesses (Fig. 5–8 A and B) frequently show localized slow wave activity on which there may be superimposed spikes indicating the focus of the infectious process.

Leukodystrophy

Electroencephalographic studies from three dogs afflicted with globoid cell leukodystrophy have been reported by Fletcher.[20] Electroencephalographic abnormalities seen in this disease consist of generalized cerebral hemispheric asymmetry, asymmetric spindling and spikes, excessive high voltage–low frequency activity, and a decrease in EEG arousal to auditory stimuli. Apparently the EEG is a useful diagnostic tool in the early stages of globoid cell leukodystrophy because it can reveal diffuse cerebral hemisphere disorders before they are identified clinically.

Seizure Disorders

One of the most common reasons for electroencephalographic examination is to determine the cause of seizures.[58, 60] Among the many causes of seizural activity are encephalitis, hydrocephalus, post-traumatic lesions, brain tumors, vascular disorders, metabolic diseases, toxins, and bacterial infections. The waveforms seen with these disturbances have been or will be discussed. The following are additional seizure disorders yielding abnormal EEG findings.

Psychomotorlike Epilepsy. Psychomotorlike epilepsy EEG tracings reveal bursts of medium slow wave activity and are frequently associated with behavior changes of a paroxysmal nature (Fig. 5–9).

Absence Epilepsy. In humans, typical spike and wave patterns are characteristic of absence attack. Less frequently, a comparable electroencephalographic pattern is seen in dogs (Fig. 5–10). This pattern is usually associated with the absence type of seizural activity in which the animal has a transient loss of contact with reality and may show minor motor signs.

Tonic-Clonic Epilepsy. Tracings recorded from physically restrained animals are disappointing because the pattern typically seen in human tonic-clonic epilepsy is seldom, if ever, obtained. The pattern seen in humans consists of high voltage–high frequency activity with frequent spikes. Klemm[45] has reported high frequency–high voltage spikes in animals with tonic-clonic epilepsy when using barbiturate anesthesia to activate abnormal foci. Apparently, chemical restraints may be necessary to activate abnormal, tonic-clonic epileptic seizural activity that may be recorded on the EEG.

Idiopathic Epilepsy. Idiopathic epilepsy frequently occurs in the dog and has familial tendencies. The interictal EEG pattern is usually nondiagnostic. Occasionally, however, paroxysmal spindles will be recorded. Figure 5–11 is a tracing from a dog with idiopathic epilepsy showing the spindle-type waveforms. This particular pattern is also recorded when the animal shivers. Careful observation of the patient is necessary during the recording period to be sure that the spindle waveform is not an artifact.

Emotional Disorders. Turbes and Jobe[71] have studied the EEG changes in emotional disorders of the dog and cat. Of 83 dogs studied, 51 showed some dysrhythmia, with the major abnormality being recorded in the temporooccipital regions and usually consisting of abnormal slow wave activity. However, no specific pattern was related to any one individual behavior problem. Electroencephalographic tracings obtained by the author from animals with abnormal behavior have been disappointing in that few abnormalities were seen.

Text continued on page 128

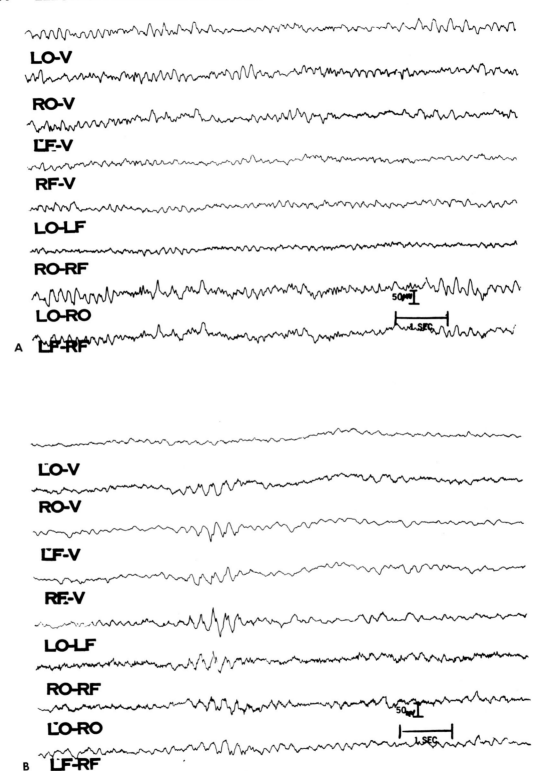

Figure 5–7. Same patient as in Figure 5–6. A, Two months after clinical recovery. B, Four months after clinical recovery—genesis of the burst of 4 Hz activity unknown. C, Five months after clinical recovery. D, Six months after clinical recovery with some residual 6 Hz, low voltage activity present. Some muscle artifact seen in occipital areas.

Illustration continued on opposite page

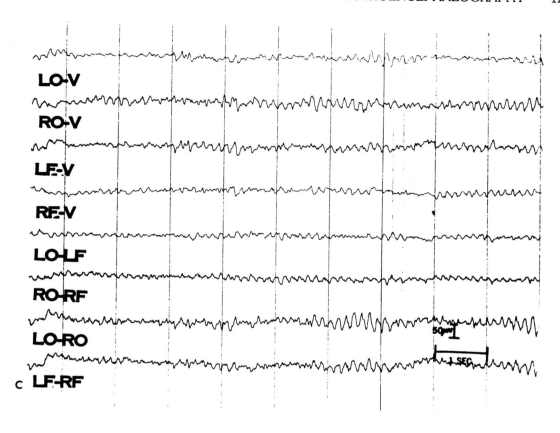

LO-V

RO-V

LF-V

RF-V

LO-LF

RO-RF

LO-RO

c LF-RF

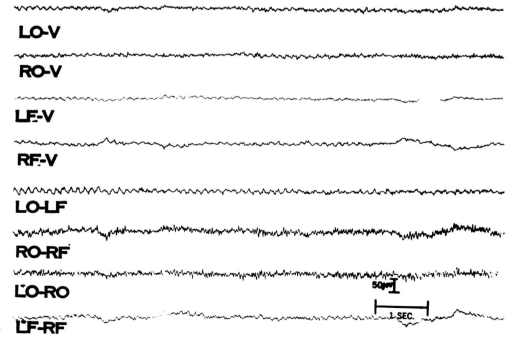

LO-V

RO-V

LF-V

RF-V

LO-LF

RO-RF

LO-RO

D LF-RF

Figure 5–7 *Continued.*

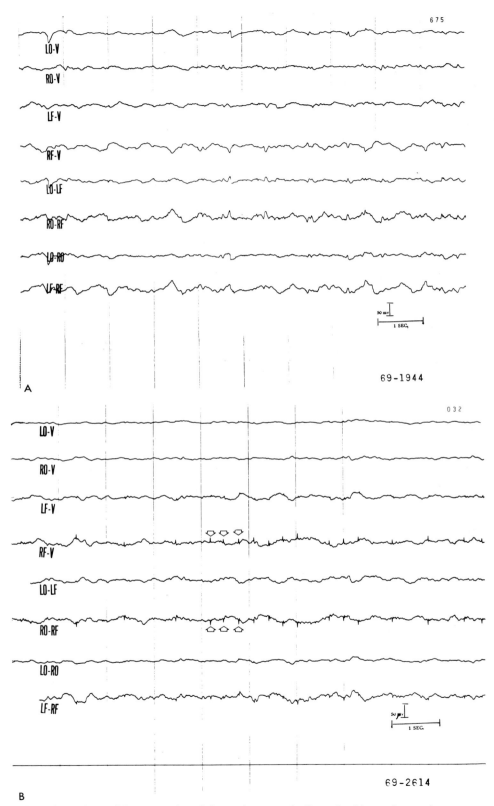

Figure 5–8. Recordings obtained from animals with brain abscesses. A, Generalized low voltage—slow wave present. B, Focal spike activity (arrows) is seen. The brain abscess followed an infection of the right eye.

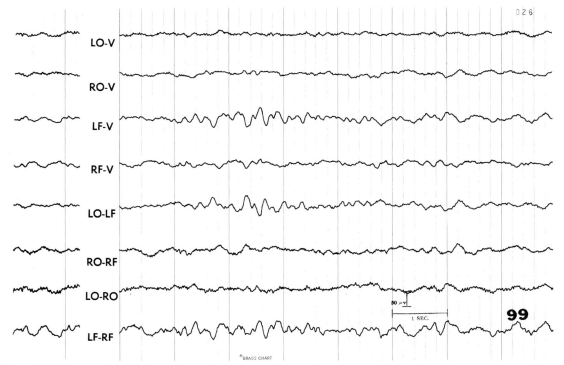

Figure 5–9. Tracing obtained from a dog with a periodic behavior change signaled by signs of fear followed by aggression. Note that paroxysm shows waves in the left frontal lead.

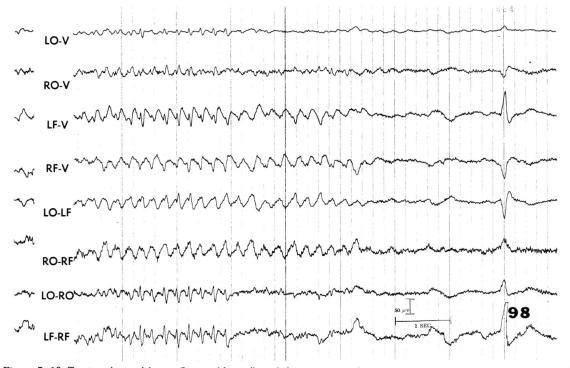

Figure 5–10. Tracing obtained from a 3 year old poodle with frequent signs of a transient loss of contact with reality signaled by staring. Note the spike and waveforms that last for approximately 3 to 4 seconds. The animal did not show abnormal clinical signs at the time of the tracing.

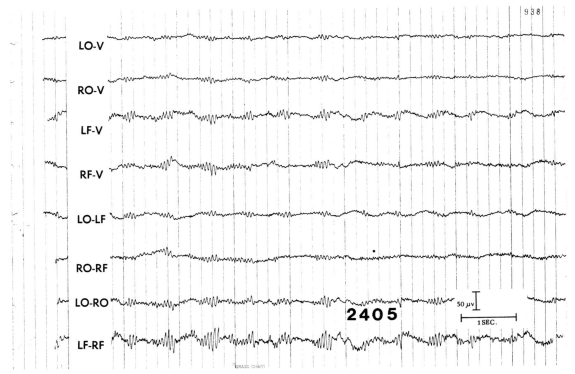

Figure 5–11. Tracing obtained from a 1½ year old poodle with a history of idiopathic epilepsy. The spindle formation is marked. Many idiopathic epileptics have the same waveform but less frequently.

Cerebral Trauma

Cerebral trauma results from head injuries, and the abnormality varies depending on the degree of injury to the brain tissue (Fig. 5–12 A–B). Damage to the cerebral hemispheres, especially to the more superficial portions, is more accessible to EEG examination. Recordings made immediately following cerebral trauma (mild concussion) show characteristic low voltage–slow waves at first, but these are rapidly replaced by high voltage–slow waves. If a lesion is localized, focal high amplitude activity is produced by the damaged tissue. Occasionally the high voltage–slow wave activity is accompanied by a high frequency component riding on the slow wave activity in the area of damage. Structures in the posterior fossa may also be damaged by head injuries. EEG recordings of animals with posterior fossa damage may not show any gross abnormality; some slowing, however, may be noted and is probably associated with damage to the reticular activating system in the rostral portion of the brain stem that influences the thalamic or diencephalic structures.

In localized brain damage, the focal electric high voltage activity may not be seen at first. Instead, there is generalized slowing, indicative of the general brain edema, which gradually disappears and allows the focal damaged area to persist and to be demonstrated electroencephalographically. The focal abnormality may persist for weeks or even months. The damaged area may act as a focal point for epileptic seizures that occur 3 to 5 months following the injury.

Head injuries may also cause vascular lesions, such as cerebral hemorrhage or subdural hematoma. One might suspect that cerebral hemorrhage would result in a localized abnormality, but it has been the author's experience that it is difficult to establish a localized abnormality using an electroencephalogram in cerebral hemorrhage following trauma. In subdural hematomas, the pattern may show generalized high voltage–slow wave activity as shown in Figure 5–13. Occasionally random spiking is seen in subdural hematomas.

Cerebral Edema

Generalized cerebral edema, usually associated with head trauma, results in generalized

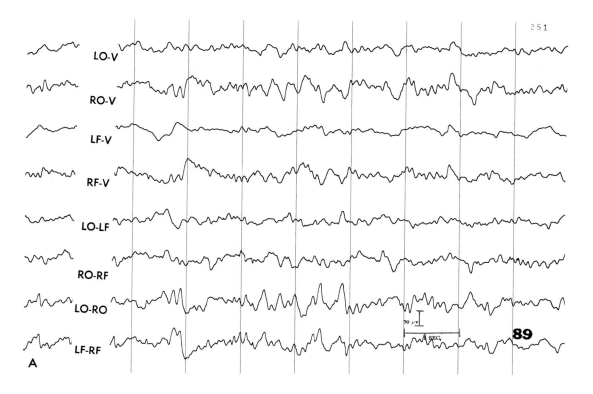

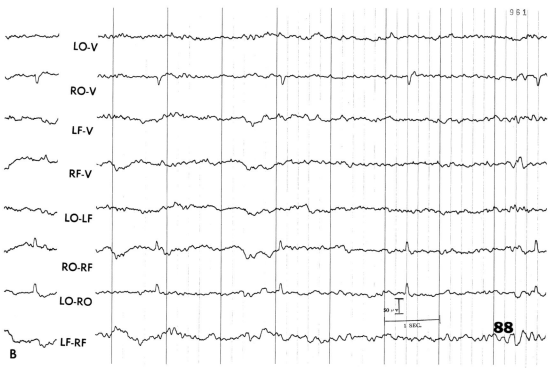

Figure 5–12. Electroencephalograms obtained from patients suffering from various head injuries and resultant cerebral trauma. A, Animal had been dropped on its head 4 days prior to presentation. B, Animal was hit by a basketball 5 days before tracing was made.

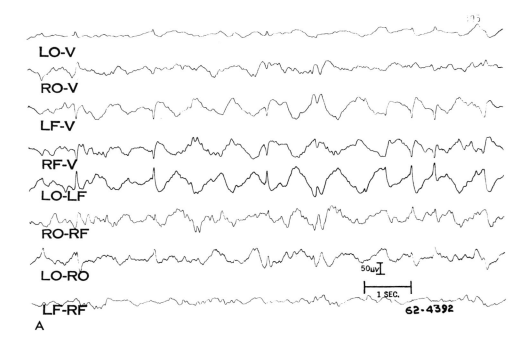

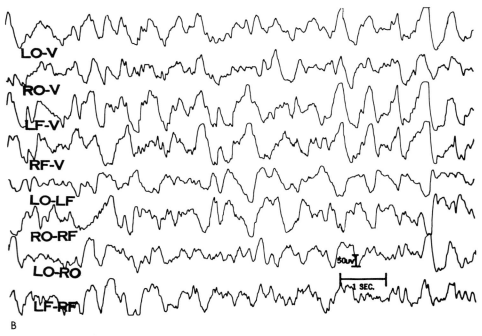

Figure 5–13. A, The animal from which this recording was made had a massive subdural hematoma over the frontoparietal region. B, Recording obtained from an animal with a massive diffuse subdural hematoma (confirmed at necropsy).

slow wave activity, which gradually disappears and is replaced by normal patterns, if there is no residual brain damage. Localized cerebral edema is difficult to detect electroencephalographically. Experimental studies in which localized edema was produced failed to demonstrate any electroencephalographic abnormalities, although the local edema was as large as 3 cm in diameter and 2 to 3 cm deep.[68]

Hydrocephalus

Hydrocephalus, like distemper encephalitis, is easily diagnosed through the use of the electroencephalogram and can be confirmed by radiographic studies.[36,55,60] Of all the abnormalities involving the cerebral cortex, hydrocephalus shows the greatest variety of changes in both frequency and amplitude. The spectrum ranges from high frequency–medium-to-high voltage to low frequency–high voltage. The electroencephalograms presented in Figure 5–14 demonstrate this wide range.

Hydrocephalus may be congenital or acquired and may be the result of cerebral injury. This is especially true of the toy breeds. The presence or absence of an open fontanel is not a good index for the diagnosis of hydrocephalus. Animals with a closed fontanel frequently show hydrocephalus-type patterns.

This author suspects that the different patterns seen in hydrocephalus may be related to the development of increased intraventricular pressure. In those EEG tracings that show high voltage–relatively fast activity (50–150 μV, 5–8 Hz), the early, rapid development of pressure is seen. Those tracings that show slower activity and even higher voltages (1–5 Hz, 100–200 μV) are related to cortical thinning as a result of a relatively long period of pressure development. There is also another pattern, consisting of higher frequencies and spikelike waveforms, that appears to be related to acquired hydrocephalus usually associated with previous cerebral trauma (Fig. 5–15).

Lissencephaly

Lissencephaly, an abnormality of cerebral cortical development frequently seen in the Lhasa apso breed, is characterized by irregular random slow waves with a marked lack of symmetry between comparable cortical areas (Fig. 5–16).

Vascular Disorders

Vascular lesions of the cerebral hemispheres are relatively common in humans and are accompanied by dramatic signs such as motor paralysis and sensory deficits. The signs of vascular disorders may occur in dogs and cats; however, the clinical signs are relatively less dramatic if they are superficial. It is probably that the so-called strokelike syndrome seen in dogs in which there is a hemiparesis may be associated with a vascular lesion of the basal nuclei or internal capsule. Electroencephalographic examinations of animals with hemiparesis and a strokelike syndrome have been generally unremarkable. The brain waves appear to be relatively normal and have relatively good symmetry. In a few instances, abnormal low voltages may be seen in one hemispheric lead, but this is not the common observation. The use of the electroencephalogram in the diagnosis of cerebral vascular accidents (CVA) appears to be limited in veterinary medicine. In one confirmed case of a CVA of the caudate nucleus in a dog with quadriplegia and mental depression generalized random slow waves were visible (Fig. 5–17).

Metabolic Diseases

Hepatoencephalopathy. Hepatoencephalopathy is characterized electroencephalographically by medium to fast frequencies of 5 to 20 Hz and medium voltages of 15 to 50 μV. Figure 5–18 is a tracing obtained from an animal in the latter stages of the disease.

Hypothyroidism. In hypothyroidism, the electroencephalogram shows extremely low voltage–medium frequency activity (Fig. 5–19). The voltages are generally so low that they are difficult to measure when the standard recording technique of 50 μV/cm is used.

Hypocalcemia. Hypocalcemia in dogs shows persistent rhythmic discharges of low voltage, 20 to 25 Hz activity.[33] Some spindling of the discharges may be seen.

Other metabolic diseases have not been studied sufficiently in veterinary medicine to establish the EEG patterns.

Toxins

Chlorinated Hydrocarbons. Chlorinated hydrocarbon intoxication frequently results in a high frequency–low voltage activity that is gen-

Text continued on page 136

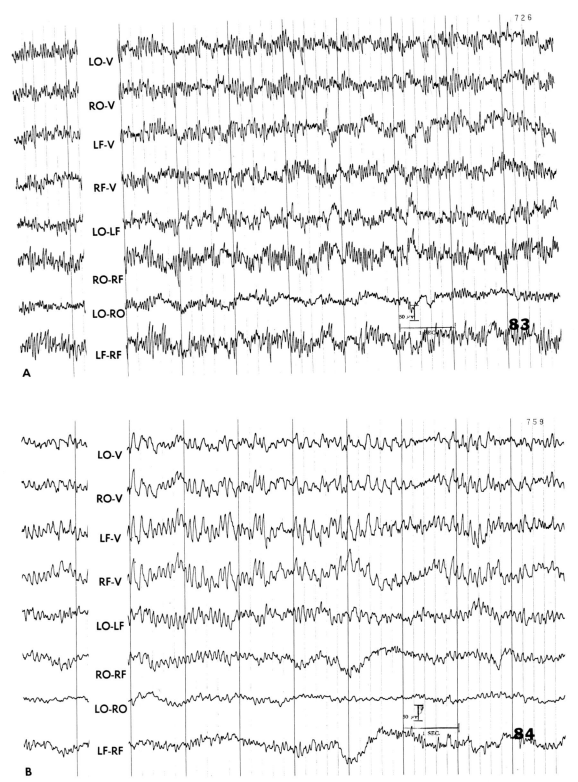

Figure 5–14. Electroencephalographic patterns seen in hydrocephalus. (From Redding RW and Knecht CD: Neurologic examination. *In* Ettinger SJ: Textbook of Veterinary Internal Medicine. Philadelphia, WB Saunders Co., 1975.)

Illustration continued on opposite page

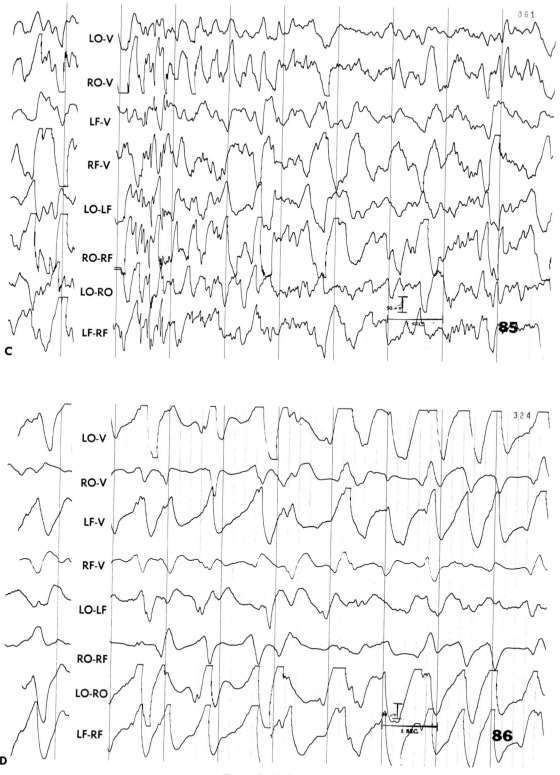

Figure 5–14 *Continued.*

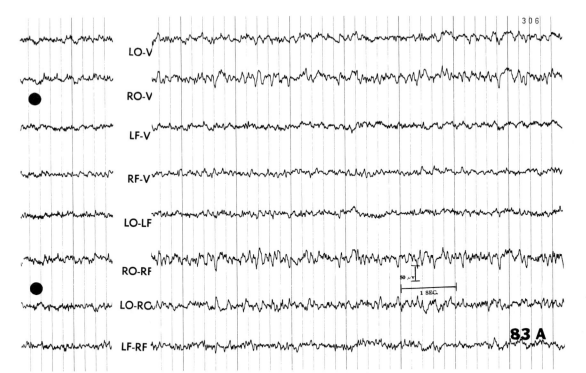

Figure 5–15. Pattern obtained from a dog with hydrocephalus associated with previous cerebral trauma. The patient had been attacked by a larger dog about 1 week before the recording was made. The EEG findings suggested a diagnosis of concussion with localized damage over the left occipital area, and possible hemorrhage. (From Redding RW and Knecht CD: Neurologic examination *In* Ettinger SJ: Textbook of Veterinary Internal Medicine. Philadelphia, WB Saunders Co, 1975.)

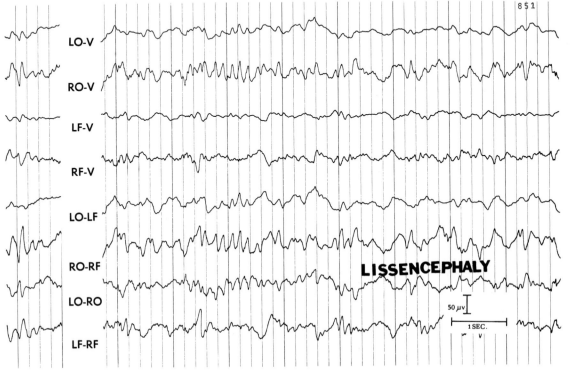

Figure 5–16. Tracing obtained from a 1 year old Lhasa apso showing signs of blindness, abnormal aggressive behavior, syncope, and seizures. The gross and histopathologic diagnosis was lissencephaly.

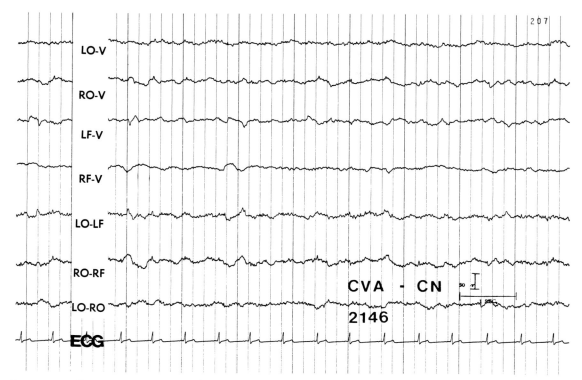

Figure 5–17. Tracing of an 8 year old Labrador retriever that had a sudden onset of quadriplegia and depression. The waveforms are random and slow. An ECG artifact is confirmed by simultaneous recording of the electrocardiogram. Necropsy examination showed a rupture of the arteries with hemorrhage in the caudate nucleus.

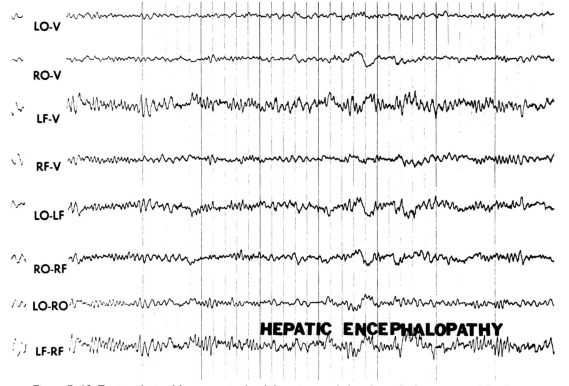

Figure 5–18. Tracing obtained from an animal with hepatic encephalopathy in the latter stages of the disease.

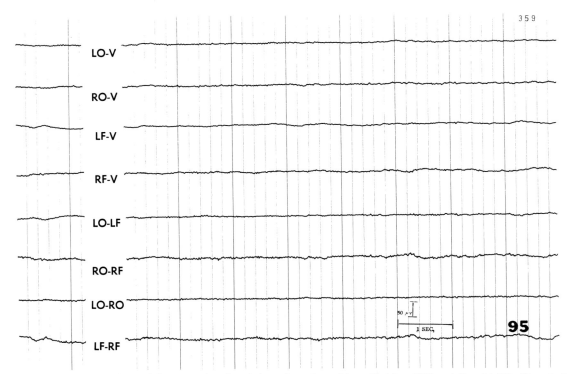

Figure 5–19. Tracing obtained from an animal with hypothyroidism. (From Redding RW and Knecht CD: Neurologic examination. *In* Ettinger SJ:Textbook of Veterinary Internal Medicine. Philadelphia, WB Saunders Co, 1975.)

eralized in nature and not specifically diagnostic for a particular agent.

Organophosphate Poisoning. The electroencephalogram in organophosphate intoxication also shows high frequency–low voltage activity and is not specifically diagnostic.

Lead Toxicosis. Lead toxicosis shows an encephalitic pattern characterized by paroxysmal high voltage–medium frequency waves superimposed on the encephalitic pattern.[46] In severe lead toxicosis very high voltage slow waves are seen intermittently.

Neoplasia

The changes in the EEG associated with brain tumors are a result of the reaction of the electrically active brain tissue to the growing mass; the tumor itself is electrically silent. The site of the tumor influences the recording. If it is deep within the brain and remote from the recording electrodes, the abnormalities seen are minimal and tend to be diffuse; if it is near the surface, marked abnormalities may be seen; if it is deep and located on the midline, generalized abnormal slow waves are seen in both hemispheres (Fig. 5–20 A–D); if it is more superficial and unilateral, the record shows localized slowing of greater magnitude.

In general, tumors produce slow activity with high voltages. Occasionally, there are bursts of high frequency activity superimposed on the slow wave activity. In some cases, high frequency spiking is the predominant feature. In the dog, it is possible to demonstrate midline tumors that influence both hemispheres and to localize unilateral hemispheric tumors if they involve the occipital, parietal, or frontal areas. With the techniques now available, it is not possible to demonstrate temporal tumors unless they are large enough to produce abnormalities of other associated structures.

Other Infections

Invasion of the brain by organisms such as *Blastomyces dermatitidis, Toxoplasma gondii,* and *Cryptococcus neoformans* gives rise to ab-
Text continued on page 141

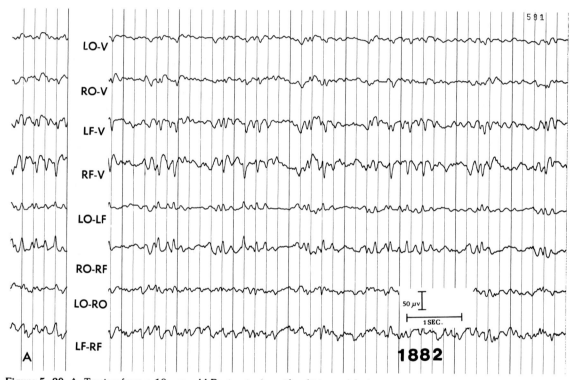

Figure 5–20. A, Tracing from a 10 year old Boston terrier with a history of Jacksonian-type seizures starting on the left side and eventually including the entire body. Note the sharp wave originating in the right frontal region. An oligodendroglioma involving the right frontoparietal cortex was found at necropsy.

Illustration continued on following page

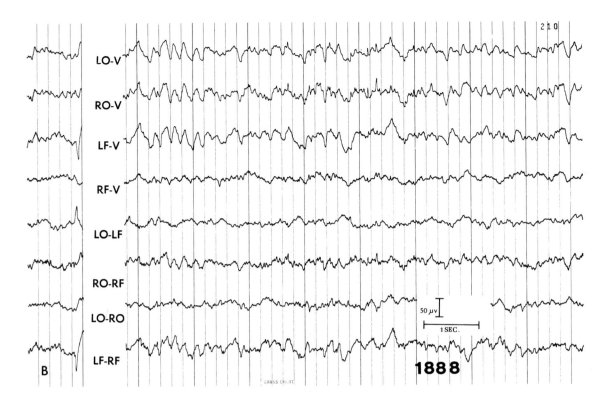

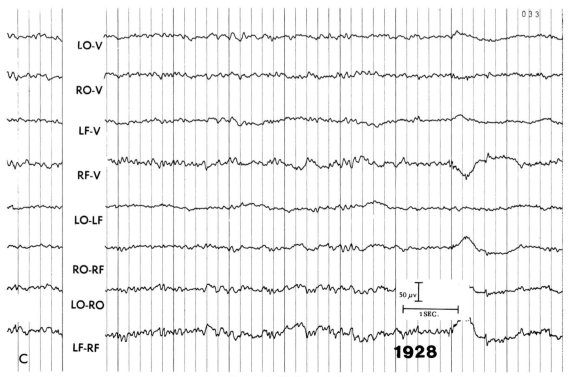

Figure 5–20 *Continued.*

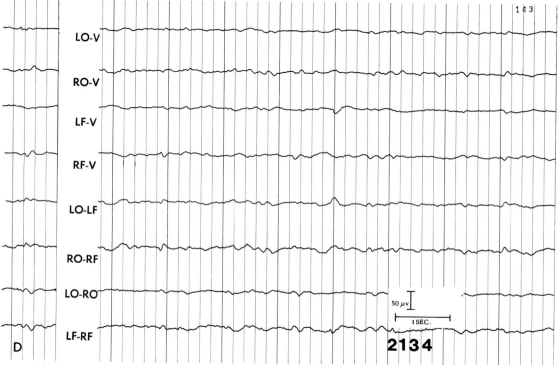

Figure 5–20 *Continued.* B, Tracing from a 5 year old Boston terrier that had become suddenly blind. Note the generalized slowing and paroxysmal 5 Hz discharges. Some spikes are also evident. An oligodendroglioma involving the left caudate nucleus and protruding into the lateral ventricle was found at necropsy. C, Tracing obtained from a 4 year old poodle with tonic-clonic seizures. Note generalized, random, medium to slow waves, 5 to 12 Hz, 10 to 30 µV. A hemangioblastoma of the midbrain and upper medulla was found at necropsy. D, Tracing obtained from a 6 year old Great Dane with a history of blindness and ataxia. At the time of the EEG recording the animal was severely depressed. Note the generalized random slow waves in all leads. The animal did not respond to auditory or tactile stimulation. A diffuse cerebral astrocytoma was found at necropsy.

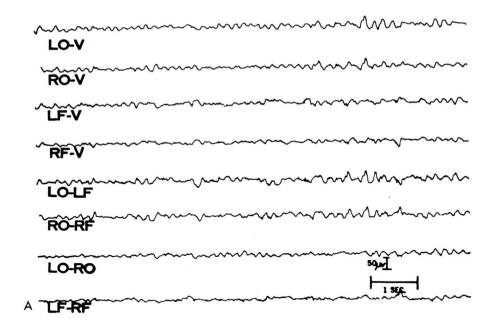

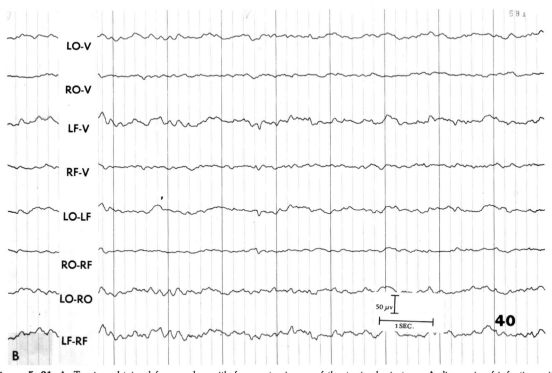

Figure 5–21. A, Tracing obtained from a dog with frequent seizures of the tonic-clonic type. A diagnosis of infection with *Toxoplasma gondii* was made at necropsy. B, Tracing obtained from a 3 year old Afghan hound with a severe uveitis and postorbital abscess of the left eye. The animal developed depression and seizures. Note the asymmetry of leads and slow waves in the left frontal area. A diagnosis of blastomycosis was made at necropsy. C, Tracing obtained from a dog with generalized seizures and depression. Note the irregular random waveforms. A diagnosis of cryptococcosis was made at necropsy.

Illustration continued on opposite page

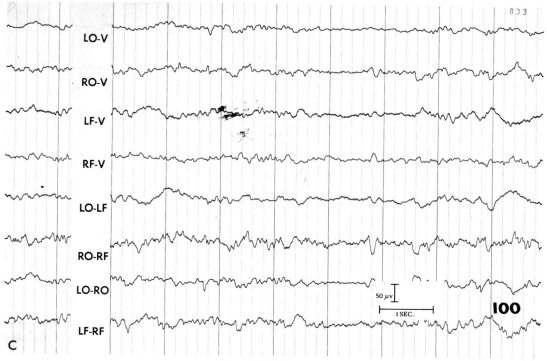

Figure 5–21 *Continued.*

normal EEG patterns. The patterns are not diagnostic for the specific infection, but are suggestive of brain damage (Fig. 5–21).

ELECTROENCEPHALOGRAPHIC AUDIOMETRY

A dog's hearing ability is difficult to determine. Clinical tests used to ascertain whether a dog can hear consist of auditory stimuli produced by loud noises, high and low pitched whistles, and spoken words or commands familiar to the dog. If the dog hears these sounds, it may respond by changing posture or by moving its head, eyes, and ears in the direction of the sound. If the dog is unresponsive to these sound stimuli, it is assumed to be deaf. However, disinterest, distraction, temperament, depression, pain, and other unrelated conditions can prevent the dog's reacting to the sounds and commands. The final decision as to whether a dog can hear or not is an arbitrary one at best.

Electroencephalographic audiometry may be used to determine if the animal can hear and, if so, in what frequency range. This technique is based upon the *arousal (alerting) phenomenon,* a generalized response that is not specific for any type of stimulus. Sounds may act as a stimulus to alert the cerebral cortex and thereby make it possible to determine if the animal hears.

EEG tracings are obtained while the animal is in a relaxed state. During the recording period, sudden periodic auditory stimuli are elicited. The normal animal shows an increase in frequency and a decrease in voltage on the EEG. The most prominent feature of the recording is, however, a movement artifact at the time of the stimulus application. This movement artifact signals the reception of the sound by the animal. It is assumed that, if no change in the EEG and no movement artifact are seen, the animal cannot hear. The range of hearing can be determined if a variable frequency audiogenerator and a high frequency electrostatic loudspeaker are available. Using such equipment, the author has found an upper frequency range of hearing in a group of 25 dogs to be from 32 to 52 kHz. In clinical cases of suspected deafness, the dogs either were found to be totally deaf or had an upper limit of hearing at 12 kHz. Figure 5–22 A–D shows a typical arousal response seen on EEG tracings.

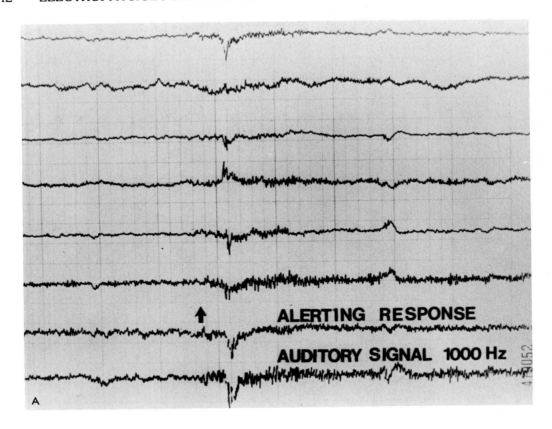

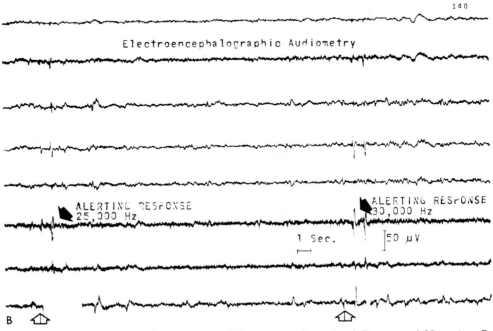

Figure 5–22. A, Typical arousal (alerting) response seen following an auditory signal. Paper speed 30 mm/sec. B, Alerting response seen at both 25 and 30 kHz (arrows) auditory signals. Paper speed 6 mm/sec.

Illustration continued on opposite page

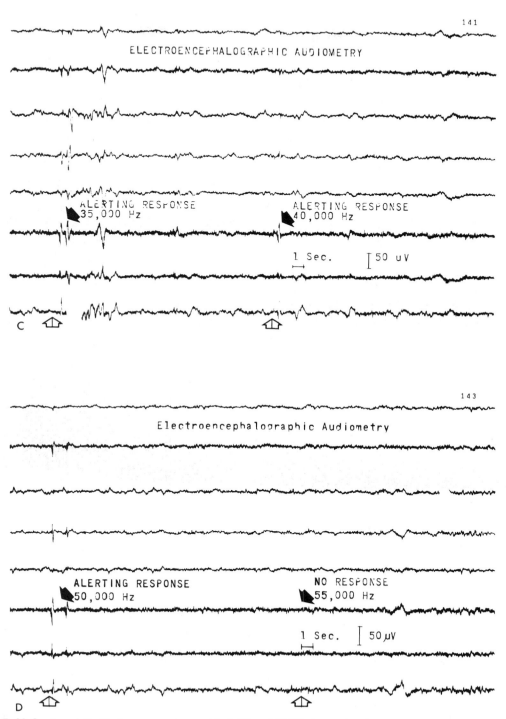

Figure 5–22 *Continued.* C, Alerting response seen at both 35 and 40 kHz (arrows) auditory signals. Paper speed 6 mm/sec. D, Alerting response seen at 50 kHz but not at 55 kHz, indicating that the limit of auditory acuity was between these frequencies. Paper speed 6 mm/sec.

ELECTROENCEPHALOGRAPHIC ANESTHESIA MONITORING

Electroencephalography is of value to an anesthesiologist and surgeon because the EEG correlates with the levels of depression produced by the anesthetics and the stages of anesthesia. In addition, it may serve as an indicator of generalized cerebral hypoxia and give evidence of localized impairment of cerebral blood supply.

Various anesthetic agents, both alone and in combinations, produce slightly different patterns; however, they all cause generalized slow wave activity and reduced voltages in deeper levels of anesthesia.

REFERENCES

1. Bagedda G.: The electroencephalogram as an aid to the topographical diagnosis of a cerebral lesion in a puppy: Neurosurgical treatment and the postoperative EEG: Clinical course. J Small Anim Pract 13:185, 1972.
2. Bagedda G and Arru E: Electroencephalography to assess brain damage before undertaking surgery on dogs. Clin Vet 94:373, 1971.
3. Bartels KE: Surgical implantation of electroencephalographic electrodes in the dog. Am J Vet Res 37:83, 1976.
4. Beaver BVG and Klemm WR: Electroencephalograms of normal anesthetized cats. Am J Vet Res 34:1441, 1973.
5. Blauch BS and Cash WC: A brief review of narcolepsy with presentation of two cases in dogs. J Am Anim Hosp Assoc 11:467, 1975.
6. Brass W: Über electroencephalographische Untersuchungen beim Hund. Dtsch Tieraerztl p 242, 1959.
7. Brechner WL, Walter RD, and Dillon JB: Practical Electroencephalography for the Anesthesiologist. Springfield, IL, Charles C Thomas, 1962.
8. Charles MS and Fuller JL: Developmental study of the electroencephalogram of the dog. Electroencephalogr Clin Neurophysiol 8:645, 1956.
9. Cooper R, Osselton JW, Shaw JC: EEG Technology, 2nd ed. London, Butterworths, 1974.
10. Croft PG: The EEG as an aid to diagnosis of nervous diseases in the dog and cat. J Small Anim Pract 3:205, 1962.
11. Croft PG: Conditions affecting the central nervous system in small animals. J Small Anim Pract 6:261, 1965.
12. Croft PG: Use of the electroencephalogram in small animal medicine. Proc R Soc Med 58:548, 1965.
13. Croft PG: Fits in dogs: A survey of 260 cases. Vet Rec 77:438, 1965.
14. Croft PG: The use of electroencephalographs in the detection of epilepsy as a hereditary condition in the dog. Vet Rec 80:712, 1968.
15. Croft PG: Electroencephalography and space occupying lesions in small animals. J Small Anim Pract 13:175, 1972.
16. Cunningham JG: Canine seizure disorders, JAVMA 158:589, 1971.
17. deLahunta A and Cummings JF: The clinical and electroencephalographic features of hydrocephalus in three dogs. JAVMA 146:954, 1965.
18. Elsberry DD: Computer processing of electroencephalographic data. Am J Vet Res 33:235, 1972.
19. Elul R: Specific site of generation of brain waves. Physiologist 7:125, 1964.
20. Fletcher TF: Electroencephalographic features of leukodystrophic disease in the dog. JAVMA 157:190, 1970.
21. Florio R and Lapras M: Variations de l'électroencephalogramme dans l'épilepsie du chien: Déductions cliniqués et thérapeutiques. Rev Méd Vét 114:674, 1963.
22. Fox MW: Postnatal development of the EEG in the dog. J Small Anim Pract 8:71, 1967.
23. Fox MW and Stone AG: An electroencephalographic study of epilepsy in the dog. J Small Anim Pract 8:703, 1967.
24. Fromm GH and Bond HW: The relationship between neuron activity and cortical steady potentials. Electroencephalogr Clin Neurophysiol 22:159, 1967.
25. Gedoll SH: Quantitative determination of hearing to audiometric frequencies in the electroencephalogram. Arch Otol 55:597, 1952.
26. Gibbs FA and Gibbs EI: Atlas of Electroencephalography, vol 1–3. Reading, MA, Addison-Wesley Pub Co 1958, 1959, 1964.
27. Hatch RD, Currie RB, and Grive GA: Feline electroencephalograms and plasma thiopental concentrations associated with clinical states of anesthesia. Am J Vet Res 31:291, 1970.
28. Herin RA: Induction technique changes and electroencephalographic body temperature, and pupillary light reflex studies in dogs anesthetized with electric current. Am J Vet Res 25:739, 1964.
29. Herin RA, Purinton PT, and Fletcher TF: Electroencephalography in the unanesthetized dog. Am J Vet Res 29:329, 1968.
30. Hill D and Parr G: Electroencephalography. New York, The MacMillan Co, 1963.
31. Hughes RR: An Introduction to Clinical Electroencephalography. Bristol, John Wright and Sons, Ltd, Stonebridge Press, 1961.
32. Kaleb P, Rotztocil V, and Kalab Z: Blockage of myopotentials by means of chlorpromazine during electroencephalographic examination of dogs. Acta Veterinaria Bron 44:69, 1975.
33. Katherman, AE: Electroencephalographic Changes Associated with Canine Hypocalcemia. Thesis. University of Minnesota, 1982.
34. Kiloh IG and Osselton JW: Clinical Electroencephalography, London, Butterworths, 1966.
35. Klemm WR: Attempts to standardize veterinary electroencephalographic techniques. Am J Vet Res 29:1895, 1968.
36. Klemm WR: Electroencephalograms of anesthetized dogs and cats with neurologic diseases. Am J Vet Res 29:337, 1968.
37. Klemm WR: Subjective and quantitative analysis of the electro-encephalograms of anesthetized normal dogs—control data for clinical diagnosis. Am J Vet Res 29:1267, 1968.
38. Klemm WR: Animal Electroencephalography. New York, Academic Press, 1969.
39. Klemm, WR: Electroencephalography in small animal medicine. Southwest Vet 22:92, 1969.
40. Klemm WR: Applied Electronics for Veterinary Medicine and Animal Physiology. Springfield, IL, Charles C Thomas, 1976.

41. Klemm WR and Hall CL: Electroencephalographic "seizures" in anesthetized dogs with neurologic diseases. JAVMA 157:1640, 1970.
42. Klemm WR and Hall CL: Electroencephalograms of anesthetized dogs with hydrocephalus. Am J Vet Res 32:1859, 1971.
43. Klemm WR and Hall CL: Electroencephalographic pattern abnormalities in dogs with neurologic disorders. Am J Vet Res 33:2011, 1972.
44. Klemm WR and Hall CL: Current status and trends in veterinary encephalography. JAVMA 164:529, 1974.
45. Klemm WR and Mallo GL: Clinical electroencephalography in anesthetized small animals. JAVMA 148:1038, 1966.
46. Knecht CD, Crabtree J, and Katherman A: Clinical, clinicopathologic and electroencephalographic features of lead poisoning in dogs. JAVMA 175:196, 1979.
47. Knecht CD, Kazmierczak K, and Katherman A: Effects of succinylcholine on the EEG of dogs. Am J Vet Res 41:1435, 1440, 1980.
48. Laidlaw J and Stanton JB: The EEG in Clinical Practice. Edinburgh, E and S Livingstone, Ltd, 1966.
49. Li CI, McLinnan H, and Jasper HH: Brain waves and unit discharges in cerebral cortex. Science 116:656, 1952.
50. Lucas EA, Powell EW, and Murphree OD: Hippocampal theta in nervous pointer dogs. Physiol Behav 12:609, 1974.
51. Miller MH and Polisor LA: Audiology Evaluation of the Pediatric Patient. Springfield, IL, Charles C Thomas, 1964.
51a. Mysinger PW, Redding RW, Vaughn JT, et al.: Electroencephalographic patterns of clinically normal, sedated, and tranquilized newborn foals and adult horses. Am J Vet Res 46:36, 1985.
52. Pampiglione G: Development of Cerebral Function in the Dog. Washington, DC, Butterworth, Inc, 1963.
53. Parker AJ, Marshall AE, and Sharp JG: Study of the use of evoked cortical activity for clinical evaluation of spinal cord sensory transmission. Am J Vet Res 35:673, 1974.
54. Prynn RB and Redding RW: The EEG continuum with methoxyflurane and halothane anesthesia. Am J Vet Res 29:1913, 1968.
55. Prynn RB and Redding RW: Electroencephalogram in occult canine hydrocephalus. JAVMA 152:1651, 1968.
56. Redding RW: A simple technique for obtaining an electroencephalogram of the dog. Am J Vet Res 25:854, 1964.
57. Redding RW: Application of electroencephalography in small animal medicine. Proc AAHA 230, 1968.
58. Redding RW: Diagnosis and therapy of seizures J Am Anim Hosp Assoc 5:79, 1969.
59. Redding RW and Colwell RK: Verification of the significance of canine electroencephalograms by comparison with electrocorticogram. Am J Vet Res 25:857, 1964.
60. Redding RW and Knecht CD: Atlas of Electroencephalography in the Dog and Cat. New York, Prager Scientific, 1984.
61. Redding RW, Prynn B, and Colwell RK: The phenomenon of alternate sleep and wakefulness in the young dog. JAVMA 144:605, 1964.
62. Redding RW, Prynn B, and Wagner JL: Clinical use of the electroencephalogram in canine encephalitis. JAVMA 148:141, 1966.
63. Rogers, D: Canine Electroencephalographic Audiometry. Senior seminar, Auburn University, Auburn, AL, 1970.
64. Rougier G and Faure J: Potentiels bioeléctriques du chien éveillé et normal recueillié sur le crâne. J Physiol (Paris) 12:716, 1950.
65. Ruckenbush Y: L'électroencephalogramme normal du chien. Rev Méd Vét 114:119, 1963.
66. Sandove MS, Becka D and Gibbs FA: Electroencephalography for Anesthesiologists and Surgeons. Philadelphia, JB Lippincott Co., 1967.
67. Schweingruker R, Ketz F, and Frankhauser R: Zu Frage der genuinen Epilepsie beim Hund. Psychiat Neurol 143:65, 1962.
68. Sims M and Redding RW: The use of dexamethasome in the prevention of cerebral edema in dogs. J Am Anim Hosp Assoc 11:439, 1975.
69. Spehlmann R: EEG Primer. Amsterdam, Elsevier/North-Holland Biomedical, 1981.
70. Tonuma F: Electroencephalography with barbiturate anesthesia in the dog. Can Vet J 8:181, 1967.
71. Turbes CC and Jobe D: EEG studies on emotional disorders of the cat and dog. Personal communication, 1973.
72. Ventruroli M: L'electroencefalogramma normale del cane. Clin Veterinaria 85:252, 1962.
73. Weiderholt WC: Electrophysiologic analysis of epileptic beagles. Neurology 24:149, 1974.
74. Zook BC, Carpenter JL, and Roberts RM: Lead poisoning in dogs. Occurrence, source, clinical pathology and electroencephalography. Am J Vet Res 33:903, 1972.

Section 2

John M Bowen, DVM, PhD

ELECTROMYOGRAPHY

Electrodiagnostic testing (EDT) was introduced into veterinary medicine in 1949[1] and involves evaluation of the response of the skeletal muscles to electric stimulation. Because of limitations of electronic instrumentation for recording electric activity of muscles, electromyography (EMG) did not begin to develop as an independent field until 1944 and was not introduced into veterinary medicine until 1967,[6] although it had been used previously in animal research.[29] The clinical application of EDT, EMG, and nerve conduction velocity (NCV) measurement as objective diagnostic aids in veterinary neurology has expanded rapidly.[8, 14, 23] An understanding of interrelationships of the peripheral nervous system, central nervous system, and striated muscles is essential to effective clinical application of electrodiagnostic testing and electromyography. A comprehensive report on many aspects of EMG has been edited by Desmedt.[17]

Muscles under voluntary control are innervated by nerve fibers arising from motor neuron cells in the ventral horns of the spinal cord and in certain cranial nerve nuclei. These neurons are called lower motor neurons and are excited or inhibited by impulses from upper motor neurons or sensory neurons (Fig. 5–23). The sensory neurons of special importance are associated with muscle spindles, which are receptors that are sensitive to changes in muscle length (Fig. 5–23). The degree of sensitivity of a muscle spindle to stretch is influenced by the activity of small motor neurons (gamma efferents) supplying the muscle fibers within the spindle. When excitation exceeds a threshold value in the motor neuron cell, an impulse is initiated in the axon and is conducted peripherally to the nerve terminals at a velocity dependent on the diameter of the axon.

The nerve terminals are located on the surface of muscle fibers and constitute the prejunctional component of the neuromuscular junction. Each muscle fiber usually has only one neuromuscular junction. Entrance of the nerve impulse into the nerve terminal results in the release of acetylcholine (excitation-secretion coupling), which diffuses across the neuromuscular junction to the postjunctional or end plate membrane, where it effects localized depolarization of the muscle cell. If this localized depolarization or end plate potential is of suprathreshold amplitude, muscle action potentials are initiated and conducted from the end plate region to the ends of the muscle fiber. In transit, the muscle action potential triggers the mechanical response (excitation-contraction coupling).

One lower motor neuron innervates a fixed number of muscle fibers. This neuron and the muscle fibers it supplies constitute a motor unit (Fig. 5–23). The size of a motor unit in terms of the number of muscle fibers innervated decreases as refinement of muscle movements increases in the various muscles of the body.

Thus, the extraocular muscles have small motor units (about 3 muscle fibers) and antigravity muscles have large motor units (about 1000 muscle fibers). The size of a motor unit potential is influenced by the number of muscle fibers in a motor unit. Small motor units are recruited first and tend to fire at low frequencies, whereas larger motor units are recruited with increased effort and tend to fire at higher frequencies. Fibers composing a motor unit are intermingled with those of as many as 30 other motor units. Electromyographic activities of slow contracting motor units (type I muscle fibers) and fast contracting motor units (type II muscle fibers) differ,[66] firing of the former being better sustained than that of the latter.

A deficit in motor function can result from alterations in input to a lower motor neuron, as in upper motor neuron disease, or it can result from pathologic change at any of several points in the motor unit itself, i.e., the ventral horn cell, ventral root, peripheral nerve, nerve terminals, and muscle fibers (Fig. 5–23). When attempting diagnosis of a condition involving a deficit in motor function, it is important that the level at which the disorder arises be determined. The first approach should always be a standard neurologic examination (see Chapter 2). It is the object of this section to describe electrodiagnostic and electromyographic testing procedures that can serve as valuable adjuncts to the neurologic examination.

The purpose of electrodiagnostic testing of peripheral nerves is to demonstrate the presence, absence, reduction, or abnormality of the contractile response of a muscle to electric stimulation of either the muscle itself (direct stimulation method) or its motor nerve (indirect stimulation method). An important advantage is that subject cooperation is not necessary. The purpose of electromyography is to demonstrate quantitative or qualitative alterations in the electric activity of a muscle in the resting state,

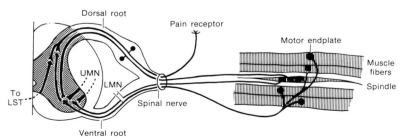

Figure 5–23. Organizational interrelationships among upper motor neurons (UMN), lower motor neurons (LMN), sensory afferent fibers of the dorsal root, striated muscle fibers, and muscle spindle. Understanding factors controlling or influencing these interrelationships is important in the clinical applications of EDT and EMG. Input to LMN arises from reflexes such as the myotatic or stretch reflex, which involves the muscle spindle. In addition, sensory input to higher centers via the lateral spinothalamic tract (LST) can result in input to LMN via UMN. The LMN provide innervation to four striated muscle fibers (motor unit size is four) and to the muscle spindle.

following either direct or indirect electric stimulation, or during either voluntary or reflex activation. In addition, EMG provides a means of evaluating nerve conduction velocity and nerve terminal conduction time.

PERIPHERAL NERVE ELECTRODIAGNOSTICS

If the neurologic examination indicates the need for further information on the state of innervation of a muscle or muscles, EDT or EMG should be employed. Firm guidelines have not been established for choosing between the two methods. Often a survey evaluation of peripheral nerves with EDT will aid the electromyographer in planning the EMG examination. When the individual performing the EDT or EMG does not also perform the neurologic examination, the results of this examination should be reviewed, noting particularly the duration of the disorder and its location. The presence of any volitional movement of the involved region should be noted, and the region should be palpated during movement to determine the degree of muscle tone, contractile activity, and atrophy present. If the disorder is not bilateral, the symmetric, normal muscles can be examined from a comparative standpoint. Anesthetics or tranquilizers may be administered prior to EDT. Clinical concentrations of these agents will not influence electrically induced motor responses examined in EDT but will suppress or abolish sensory responses that sometimes provide additional information that is helpful in reaching a final diagnosis. Equipment requirements for performance of peripheral nerve EDT include a source of electric stimuli (stimulator) and the electrodes for application of the stimuli to a nerve or muscle. The stimulator may consist simply of a flashlight battery.[1] For more extensive EDT evaluations, an electronic stimulator (Fig. 5–24) specifically for EDT or EMG should be used.[8, 9, 11]

Electrodes

For electrodiagnostic testing two electrodes are needed for stimulation of a nerve or a muscle. Either needle or surface electrodes may be used. Excitable tissues are most responsive to electric current flow at the negative electrode. Denervated muscle is best stimulated with electrodes having large surface areas.

Procedure

Sites selected for application of electrodiagnostic testing of peripheral nerves depend on the nature of the deficit in motor function and its location. Commonly used sites of stimulation are shown in Figure 5–25, and a listing of innervation of various muscles is provided in Tables 5–1 and 5–2. A suitable site is a motor point or any point along the course of a motor nerve that is accessible to electric stimulation.[1, 59] A motor point is located in the region of a muscle where its motor nerve enters or in a region that has a high density of nerve terminals. The nerve terminals are usually localized in a fairly narrow band that passes trans-

Figure 5–24. Stimulator for electrodiagnostic testing. Controls enable regulation of the amplitude, duration, and frequency of the rectangular stimulus pulses. Important accessories include a stimulus isolation unit (top left) and constant current unit (top right). When this stimulator is a component of an electromyograph, it is used also for inducing evoked potentials and for determining nerve conduction velocities.

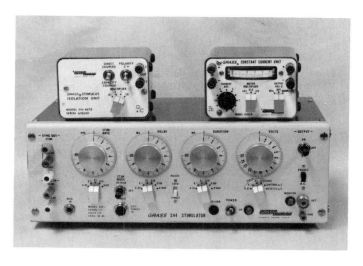

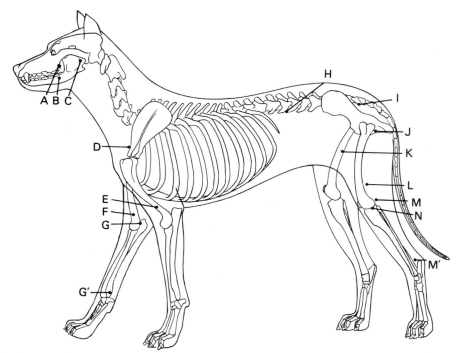

Figure 5–25. Anatomic localization of sites for stimulation of the principal nerves examined in electrodiagnostic testing. A and B, Dorsal and ventral buccal branches of the facial nerve—unilateral movement of the lips. C, Masseteric branch of the trigeminal nerve—masseter muscle contraction and closure of the mouth. D, Suprascapular nerve—contraction of the supraspinatus and infraspinatus muscles. E, Radial nerve—extension of the elbow, carpus and digits. F, Median nerve—flexion of the carpus and digits. G, Ulnar nerve—flexion of the carpus and digits. G', Ulnar nerve—flexion of the digits. H, Spinal nerves—movements of the muscles of the chest and abdomen. I, Coccygeal nerves—movement of the tail. J, Ischiatic nerve—extension of the hip and flexion of the stifle joints and combined effects of tibial and peroneal nerve stimulation. K, Femoral nerve—extension of the stifle joint. L, Ischiatic nerve (use caudal approach)—combined effects of tibial and peroneal nerve stimulation. M, Tibial nerve (use caudal approach)—extension of the hock and flexion of the digits. M', Tibial nerve—flexion of the digits. N, Peroneal (fibular) nerve—flexion of the hock and extension of the digits.

versely across the muscle at about the midpoint of the muscle fibers.

Response to electric stimulation of the motor nerve in the absence of nerve or muscle disease is a brisk contraction of the muscle. Deviations from this type of response should be noted. If a laboratory stimulator is available, chronaxy measurements and strength-duration curves can be determined. Chronaxy is defined as the minimum pulse duration required to produce a just-minimal contraction of a muscle that is stimulated at its motor point with a pulse strength that is twice rheobase. In practical terms rheobase is the threshold voltage required to induce a response with pulse duration greater than 100 msec. For normally innervated muscles, chronaxy is about 0.1 msec. Values exceeding 1 msec are considered abnormal. Strength-duration (S-D) curves are prepared by plotting on the ordinate (Y axis) the strength of the stimulus required to induce a just-minimal

contractile response to a motor point stimulation at various pulse durations, and on the abscissa (X axis) the pulse duration, which is varied from 0.05 to 100 msec. Chronaxy is one point on the strength-duration curve. The strength-duration curve reflects the degree of innervation of a muscle; curves differ characteristically for muscles that are fully innervated, partially denervated, or completely denervated because nerve fibers are excited by shorter duration pulses than muscle fibers. Chronaxy values and strength-duration curves for muscles of dogs[61] and cats[37] have been reported. EDT abnormalities have been noted in myotonic goats.[12]

Interpretation of Results

Electrodiagnostic testing of peripheral nerves has its greatest value in diagnosing disorders of

Table 5–1. INNERVATION OF MUSCLES OF THE THORACIC LIMB*

Root	Nerve	Muscle
C1–C6	Spinal accessory (external branch)	Trapezius Brachiocephalicus
C7–C8	Thoracodorsal	Latissimus dorsi
C6–C7	Suprascapular	Supraspinatus Infraspinatus
C7 (C6, C8)†	Axillary	Deltoideus Teres minor
C7	Musculocutaneous	Biceps brachii
C6–C8	Ventral thoracic	Superficial pectoral
C7–C8, T1–T2	Radial	Triceps Extensor carpi radialis Extensor digitorum communis Extensor digitorum lateralis Extensor carpi ulnaris Supinator
C8, T1–T2	Median	Pronator teres Flexor carpi radialis Flexor digitorum superficialis Flexor digitorum profundus
C8, T1–T2	Ulnar	Flexor carpi ulnaris Flexor digitorum profundus Interossei

*Based on the dog.
†Sometimes involved.

Table 5–2. INNERVATION OF MUSCLES OF THE PELVIC LIMB*

Root	Nerve	Muscle
L6–L7	Cranial gluteal	Tensor fasciae latae Gluteus medius Gluteus profundus
L7, S1–S2	Caudal gluteal	Gluteus superficialis
L4–L6	Femoral	Sartorius Vastus lateralis Rectus femoris Vastus medialis
L5–L7, S1–S2	Ischiatic	Biceps femoris Semitendinosus Semimembranosus
L5–L7, S1–S2	Peroneal	Tibialis cranialis Extensor digitorum longus Peroneus longus
L5–L7, S1–S2	Tibial	Gastrocnemius Flexor digitorum superficialis Flexor digitorum profundus Interossei
L4–L6	Obturator	Pectineus Gracilis Adductor
S1–S3	Pudendal	External anal sphincter External urethral sphincter

*Based on the dog.

lower motor neurons and in establishing functional integrity of nerves and muscles suitable for compensatory grafting in motor nerve disorders.[28, 33] When a lower motor neuron has been damaged to the extent that functional innervation of a muscle is no longer present, the following results will be obtained with EDT:

1. Absence of response to stimulation of the motor nerve normally supplying the muscle. This applies to all points proximal to the injury immediately after damage occurs. Because degeneration migrates peripherally following nerve damage, the nerve terminals and thus the motor point will retain their excitability for 3 to 21 days, depending on the distance between site of nerve injury and affected muscle as influenced by species and age of the animal. At the time of nerve terminal degeneration, an abrupt reduction in excitability or increase in threshold occurs and the motor point disappears. An increase in threshold may occur in normally innervated muscles when edema is present and when the size and volume of a muscle have been reduced, as in disuse atrophy. The latter can readily be distinguished from denervation atrophy by EDT.

2. Chronaxy greater than 1 msec.

3. Strength-duration curves typical of denervated muscle. Strength-duration curves are not as sensitive as EMG for detecting early evidence of reinnervation, but they may give earlier evidence of denervation following nerve injury than EMG, as lack of response to nerve stimulation will precede onset of abnormal electromyographic activity. In muscles exhibiting partial denervation, intermediate changes will be present and are often difficult to evaluate without strength-duration curves or electromyograms.

In some cases, a deficit in motor function is caused by factors other than lower motor neuron disorders. In these cases, EDT demonstrates the presence of normal lower motor neuron function, which indicates the presence of a lesion at other sites, such as upper motor neurons or joints. Additional information on animal EDT is provided elsewhere.[11]

ELECTROMYOGRAPHY

Electromyography (EMG) permits visual, graphic, and audio evaluation of the electric activity of striated muscles. The evaluation may be quantitative or qualitative and provides information that, when combined with the results of the neurologic examination, frequently is the determining factor in reaching a diagnosis. It is particularly helpful when clinical signs are modified by pain, upper motor neuron disease, and compensatory actions of synergistic muscles. In addition, the prognosis is aided by evaluation of results of serial electromyographic examinations. The instrument used to record the electric activity of muscle is the electromyograph.

The Electromyograph

The electromyograph can be purchased commercially with all components installed in a single console (Fig. 5–26), or components can be purchased individually and arranged in a manner suitable to the electromyographer. The latter unit is termed a hybrid electromyograph and is often less expensive than the commercial electromyograph. However, operation of a hybrid electromyograph is often less convenient,

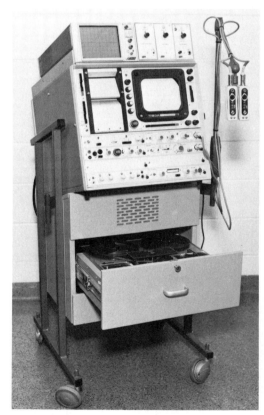

Figure 5–26. A two channel, direct recording electromyograph, which includes (top to bottom) a storage oscilloscopic display, fiberoptic graphic recorder, calibrated oscilloscopic display, stimulator, amplifiers, audio monitor, and tape recorder. Electrodes are connected to the arm at right, which can be extended toward the patient. Not shown is a Polaroid camera. (Model TE-4, TECA Corporation, White Plains, NY.)

although performance characteristics may be excellent. Components of an electromyograph are shown in Figure 5–27. The essential elements are the amplifier, oscilloscope, and loudspeaker system. The electromyograph amplifier is a high impedance, high gain, and low noise differential amplifier that has three input terminals: positive, negative, and ground. A signal applied symmetrically to both positive and negative terminals is rejected. This is referred to as common mode rejection and is useful in attenuating 60 Hz interference from nearby power lines. Because a motor unit potential is applied asymmetrically to the electrodes, a potential difference will exist between positive and negative input terminals. The potential difference will be amplified by a high quality electromyograph amplifier at least 50,000 times as much as common mode interfering signals.

A system of electric filters should be included in the electromyograph amplifier. Two filters are needed, one to attenuate frequencies lower than electromyographic signals and one to attenuate frequencies higher than electromyographic signals. For good fidelity recording of electromyographic signals, the lower and upper cutoff frequencies should be 2 Hz and 10 kHz, respectively. In clinical EMG some reduction in signal fidelity is acceptable. Thus, when low and high frequency interference is a problem, the low cutoff frequency may be raised to 15 Hz and the high cutoff frequency may be lowered to 3 kHz.

The electromyograph oscilloscope provides a visual display of electromyographic signals. Because a motor unit potential has a duration of only a few milliseconds, the low inertia of the electron beam of the oscilloscope can follow the rapid voltage variations, whereas the pen of a mechanical oscillograph (as in an electroencephalograph) cannot follow these rapid changes. Fiberoptic graphic recorders have frequency responses compatible with clinical evaluation of electromyographic signals (Fig. 5–26).

Electromyographic signals can be converted into sounds with the aid of an audio amplifier and loudspeaker. Audio monitoring of these signals is time saving to the electromyographer because it aids positioning of the electrodes without requiring observation of the oscilloscope display. In addition, sounds of different types of electromyographic signals are characteristic (Table 5–3) and often the signal is more readily identified by ear than by eye. The electromyophone is an inexpensive instrument designed specifically for audio evaluation of electromyographic signals (Fig. 5–28).

Permanent records of electromyograms can be prepared by photographing the oscilloscope display of the signal with a Polaroid or 35 mm camera synchronized with the oscilloscope sweep or by recording the signal on magnetic

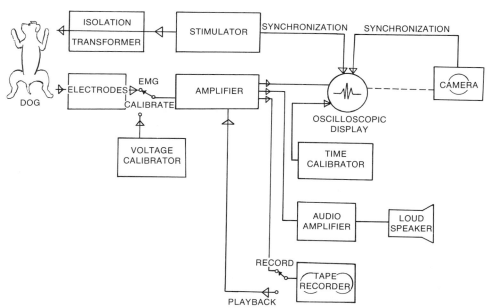

Figure 5–27. A schematic diagram of a complete instrumentation system for electromyography in the dog. (Adapted from Rogoff JB and Reiner S: Electrodiagnostic apparatus. *In* Licht S (ed): Electrodiagnosis and Electromyography, 2nd ed. Baltimore, Waverly Press, 1961.)

Table 5–3. CHARACTERISTIC SOUNDS OF ELECTROMYOGRAPHIC ACTIVITY

EMG Activity	Sound
Normal Muscle	
Resting	
Electrode insertion	No added sounds when electrode is released
Non–end plate region	Electric "silence"
	(background low level hissing; amplifier noise)
End plate region	Moderately loud hissing
Nerve activity	High pitched hissing
Contracting (minimal effort)	
Single motor unit potentials	Sharp, single cracking or popping that ceases with relaxation
Contracting (maximal effort)	
Many motor unit potentials	Loud blast without single sounds that decreases in intensity and then ceases with relaxation
Abnormal Muscle	
Resting (denervation >5 days)	
Insertion activity	Loud crackling that decreases after 1 to several minutes
Fibrillation potential	Rain on a tin roof or frying eggs
Positive potentials	Varies from a musical tone or a sound like an idling outboard motor to roar of diving airplane
Fasciculation potentials	Sharp crackling or popping not associated with effort
Bizarre high frequency discharge	Banjo-like twang
Contracting (immediate postdenervation effort)	
Complete denervation	
No motor unit potentials	No change with effort
Partial denervation	
A few motor unit potentials	Response similar to normal minimal effort pattern even though a maximal effort is attempted
Reinnervation	
Miniature motor unit potentials	Rough, rasping, cracking, or popping sound that has a higher pitch than normal motor unit potential sound
Giant motor unit potential	Very loud rasping or popping sound
Myotonia (tap electrode)	Diving airplane or revving motorcycle (sound may wax and wane)
Interference	
ECG	Dull thumping that follows pulse rate
60 Hz	Hum or buzz

tape (Fig. 5–27). The development of the storage oscilloscope has been of great value in EMG because it permits retention of the display of single or multiple sweeps for many minutes. This procedure reduces photographic expenses. Inexpensive cassette magnetic tape recorders can be used to record the audio signal, but accurate recording of individual electromyographic potentials for detailed configurational analysis requires a high quality audio tape recorder or, preferably, an instrumentation quality tape recorder with a bandwidth similar to that for the electromyographic amplifier. Photographs and magnetic tape records are useful for evaluation of the progression or regression of a disease process at subsequent examinations. The instrumentation quality tape recorder also permits replay at a reduced speed, which may enable preparation of records on a mechanical oscillograph or may enhance the comprehensiveness of computer analysis of electromyograms by providing a relative reduction in speed of the signal.

A stimulator and a stimulating electrode system must be added to the electromyograph if evoked potentials and nerve conduction velocities are to be evaluated. The stimulator should be the laboratory type (see Fig. 5–24) and should have circuitry that triggers the oscilloscope sweep and, after a variable delay, transmits the stimulus pulse, so that the display contains both the stimulus artifact and the evoked potential. In addition, an external trigger input should be available for synchronizing the stimulator and thereby the oscilloscope with the action of a percussion hammer or camera shutter. Electrode systems will be discussed below.

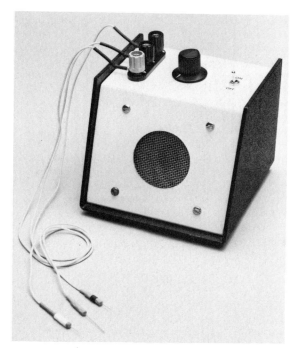

Figure 5–28. An electromyophone. This is an inexpensive instrument for audio evaluation of electromyographic activity. The unit is battery operated, making it portable for easy use on small or large animals.

phy. The oscilloscopic display can be synchronized through the delay line circuitry to trigger on a specific part of a motor unit potential, but the actual display of the potential will be delayed by a preset interval, which is usually between 1 and 10 msec. The effect is an apparent "freezing" of the position at which a repetitively occurring potential appears on the display. A moderately stable, low frequency motor unit potential activity is needed for effective use of a delay line.

Telemetry offers a method of transmitting electromyographic data from an animal to a remote receiver without interconnecting wires. This represents a significant advantage when working with mobile, unanesthetized animals.[4, 54] Some telemetry amplifiers require only two electrode inputs rather than three. Telemetry is especially useful in reducing electric interference problems in large animal EMG because recordings from these species are often done under conditions of wet bedding and nearby electric interference generators that enhance such problems.

Digital computers have been used to perform various types of analyses of electromyographic data either on line or off line by tape recorder replay. Analyses include identification and determination of characteristics of motor unit potentials,[57] identification and counting of fibrillation potentials and positive sharp waves,[10] and determination of the frequency spectra for interference patterns.[3] For identification and characterization of electromyographic potentials, an analog-to-digital sampling rate of about 8 kHz is needed. Computer analyses can aid in enhancing speed and accuracy of diagnostic interpretation of electromyograms.

Other electronic devices for use in electromyography include integrators, delay lines, telemetry systems, and digital computers. Integrators have output signals that are related to the total electromyographic activity. The signal is easily evaluated visually (Fig. 5–29) and can be calibrated to provide a continuous quantitative measure of total electromyographic activity. Several types of integrators are used in EMG. One type provides a running average (Fig. 5–29); another type produces a series of pulses, the number of pulses per unit time being proportional to the electromyographic activity.[62]

Delay lines are useful in capturing motor unit potentials for visual examination and photogra-

Electrodes

Three electrodes are required for recording electromyograms with a differential amplifier.

Figure 5–29. Electric activity recorded from the right pectineus muscle during sustained stretch produced by maximal abductive tension. The arrows indicate onset and cessation of tension. A marked decrease in amplitude of the electromyogram (EMG) and integrated electromyogram (IEMG) occurred before release of tension. The hip dysplasia was grade II. (From Bowen IM: Electromyographic analysis of reflex and spastic activities of canine pectineus muscles in the presence and absence of hip dysplasia. Am J Vet Res 35:661, 1974.)

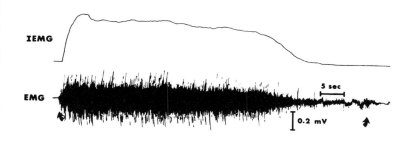

These electrodes are referred to as the active, reference, and ground electrodes and are connected to the positive, negative, and ground input terminals, respectively. With this arrangement of electrode connections, an upward deflection on the oscilloscope display indicates that the active electrode is positive relative to the reference electrode, and a downward deflection indicates that the active electrode is negative relative to the reference electrode. Some electromyographers prefer the reverse of these connections, which leads to a downward deflection for a positive change in potential. To serve as a stable reference, the reference electrode should be positioned over an electrically inactive tissue such as bone or tendon. In animal EMG, surface electrodes may be employed, but better results are obtained with needle electrodes. The monopolar and concentric needle electrodes are the most commonly used types (Fig. 5–30). The monopolar needle electrode is an excellent choice for veterinary clinical EMG, especially when working with small animals. The concentric electrodes function better with large animals. A monopolar active electrode consists of a 25, 37, or 50 mm, 28 gauge needle,* insulated with Teflon except for the very tip (Fig. 5–30). Tips should be examined frequently and the electrodes discarded (or used for EDT) when fraying of insulation is apparent and the exposed tip exceeds about 0.5 mm. Occasional sharpening of the tip on a fine abrasive stone is desirable. Teflon is an excellent material for insulation of the needle electrode because it lacks tissue toxicity and because it creates an extremely smooth, slippery surface that seems to minimize pain associated with passage of the needle through the skin and subcutaneous tissues. Such electrodes are usually well tolerated by unanesthetized animals. A monopolar electrode of this design records evoked potential activity from a spheric volume of muscle tissue with a radius of about 2 cm from the electrode tip and fibrillation potential and motor unit potential activity from a volume of muscle having a radius of about 1 mm. A 12 mm, 26 gauge uninsulated needle electrode† serves as a reference electrode for combination with a monopolar active electrode. The ground electrode consists of either a needle electrode, the same as used for the reference electrode, or a large surface electrode coated with electrode paste.

*Types MF25, MF37, and MF50, Teca Corporation, White Plains, NY.
†Type RE12, Teca Corporation, White Plains, NY.

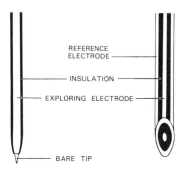

Figure 5–30. Diagrams of a monopolar needle electrode (left) and a concentric needle electrode (right).

In a concentric needle electrode, the active and reference electrodes are combined in a single unit (Fig. 5–30). The active electrode is represented by the tip of an insulated wire sealed into the barrel of a 24 to 30 gauge hypodermic needle. The shaft of the needle serves as the reference electrode. The concentric electrode samples the electric activity of a volume of muscle tissue with a radius of about 0.7 mm.[58] Because of the proximity of the active and reference electrodes in a concentric electrode, interference (60 Hz) is better rejected by the differential amplifier than for monopolar electrodes. The concentric electrode is especially valuable when conducting electromyographic examinations on large animals under conditions conducive to electric interference problems. The concentric electrode induces more pain on insertion than the monopolar electrode, but only one insertion is necessary. A ground electrode must also be used with a concentric electrode.

Both monopolar and concentric electrodes will be displaced by muscle movement. This may physically damage the electrodes, as well as preclude recording of the desired electromyographic signals. To record activity associated with muscle contraction, manual fixation of the limb is desirable. An alternative approach that minimizes the problem of electrode displacement is to implant fine wire hook electrodes in the muscle.[2] The procedure for implantation is easy and requires a small gauge hypodermic needle. Fine wire electrodes are frequently used in kinesiologic studies.[60] Needle and wire EMG electrodes should be sterilized before use, and the insertion sites should be cleansed with antiseptic.

Stimulating needle electrodes used in EMG are identical to those previously described for use in EDT in that approximately 5 mm of the needle tip is free of insulation. Long electrodes (200 mm) may be needed in large animals.[52]

Focal myopathic changes produced by needle electrode insertion have no permanent effects, but can lead to misinterpretation of muscle histophathology when an insertion tract is present in the biopsy.[19] Therefore, biopsies should be obtained from areas not subjected to needle electrode insertion.

Procedure

Knowledge of both the anatomy of the skeletal muscles and peripheral nerves and the types of electric activity associated with various nerve and muscle diseases is essential to performance of a diagnostically useful electromyographic examination. The results of a neurologic examination, including EDT if performed, should be reviewed before application of EMG. It is important that the history indicate as definitively as possible the time elapsed since onset of the neurologic problem. Each examination must be tailored to the specific neurologic problem. Thus, a routine examination procedure cannot be established for EMG as for ECG or EEG. Furthermore, interpretation of the results is influenced by a number of factors operative during the examination, so interpretation should be done at the time of the examination. The results of each step of an examination often determine the nature of subsequent steps.

Preparation of the animal for an electromyographic examination includes (1) warming of the region to be examined with a heat lamp or heating pad if the tissue temperature is subnormal, (2) application of an antiseptic to the skin overlying the muscle to be examined with needle electrodes, and (3) administration of general anesthetics or tranquilizers if indicated. General anesthesia is usually required for determination of nerve conduction velocity and for identification of localized denervation activity in the paraspinal muscles when this is obscured by motor unit potential activity caused by tensing of these muscles. In other types of electromyographic examinations, general anesthesia is best avoided because it does suppress voluntary induction of motor unit potential activity. However, a light plane of general anesthesia will not suppress motor unit potential activity in muscles that can be activated by withdrawal or stretch reflexes.[10] Fractious or frightened animals may be tranquilized, but muscle tension or tremors noted when these animals are not treated with a tranquilizer may

aid evaluation of motor unit potential activity. Selection of a recumbent or standing position for examination of the unanesthetized animal will depend on whether resting or contracting muscle activity is to be evaluated.

Ground and reference electrodes are positioned first and then the active electrode is inserted into the belly of the muscle, care being taken to avoid nerves or vessels. To reposition the active electrode, the tip should be withdrawn to a subcutaneous level and then reinserted into the muscle at a new angle. Evaluation of a muscle can best be accomplished by dividing the region surrounding the point of insertion of the needle into quadrants. Each quadrant is sampled at two or three different levels of insertion.[16] This procedure must be varied to conform with the dimensions of the muscle being tested. Large muscles are best divided into halves or thirds horizontally and/or vertically and each subdivision examined as described previously. Insertion of a stomach tube will aid in examination of the striated musculature of the esophagus with needle electrodes that are inserted through the skin of the neck. Excessive needle insertions may lead to high serum creatine phosphokinase (CPK) levels.[18] Blood samples for determination of CPK levels should be obtained prior to a needle electromyographic examination.

The time required for an electromyographic examination varies from a few minutes for a single muscle to an hour or more for detailed evaluation of many muscles and determination of conduction velocities of several nerves. Except for effects on CPK levels, aftereffects of needle electromyographic examinations are negligible and signs of tenderness at insertion or stimulation sites are rarely observed.

Various report forms have been devised for describing the results of an electromyographic examination. The Mayo Clinic form provides a suitable model.[27] The report should include a summary of the significant findings of the needle electrode examination, the nerve conduction velocity values, and the electromyographer's interpretation of these results. Anatomic diagrams such as prepared by Thomson and Bowen[59] are useful for direct notation of findings. The types of errors that appear in electromyographic examination reports have been summarized.[31]

Electric Activity of Skeletal Muscle

Electric activity of muscle recorded with needle electrodes during an electromyographic examination can be divided into four types, as follows: (1) activity associated with electrode insertion or movement, (2) spontaneous activity of the resting muscle, (3) activity associated with voluntarily or reflexively induced muscle contractions, and (4) activity induced by electric stimulation of motor nerves. Abnormality of the electric activity is defined by its presence or absence, alterations in its configuration, and its repetition rate. A composite diagram of normal and abnormal electric activity is presented in

Figure 5–31, and the sounds associated with this activity are described in Table 5–3. No electromyographic waveform can be considered pathognomonic of a specific disease entity. The standard terminology* for human electromyograms is used in this discussion of animal electromyograms.

---

*Terminology of Electromyography. Subcommittee Report. JA Simpson, Chairman, Electroencephalogr Clin Neurophysiol 26:224, 1969.

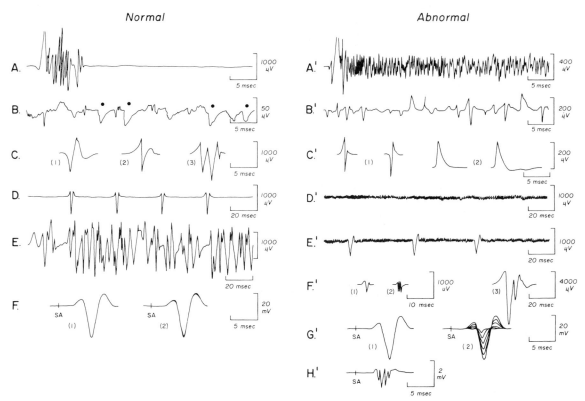

Figure 5–31. Composite diagram of major types of electromyograms encountered in clinical examinations. It is important to note the calibration values for each electromyogram.

Normal Activity: A, Brief burst of activity associated with needle electrode insertion, followed by electric silence soon after electrode movement stops. B, End plate noise encountered when the electrode up is positioned in the end plate region. The dots indicate probable individual miniature end plate potentials. C, Motor unit potentials recorded from (1) the end plate region, (2) the non–end plate region of a muscle, and (3) a polyphasic motor unit potential. D, Repetitive firing of a single motor unit. E, Interference pattern associated with the high frequency discharge of several motor units during maximal sustained voluntary effort. F, Evoked potentials: (1) response to a single stimulus and (2) superimposition of six responses induced at a frequency of 30/sec. (SA, stimulus artifact.)

Abnormal Activity: A′, Prolonged burst of activity associated with needle electrode insertion into a muscle 8 days after denervation. B′, Denervation activity after disappearance of insertion activity. C′, (1) Fibrillation potentials recorded from non–end plate and end plate regions and (2) positive sharp waves without and with a slow terminal negative phase. D′, Attempted use of a completely denervated muscle reveals only background denervation activity. E′, Attempted use of a partially denervated muscle reveals the repetitive firing of a single motor unit in addition to the background denervation activity. F′, (1) Small and (2) polyphasic motor unit potentials that are noted during reinnervation and (3) a giant motor unit potential associated with a chronic neuronopathy. G′, Evoked potentials in a myasthenia gravis–like syndrome: (1) response to a single stimulus and (2) lack of superimposition of six responses induced at a frequency of 30/sec because of a progressive reduction in amplitude. H′, Polyphasic evoked potential such as that frequently noted in polyradiculoneuritis.

Activity Associated with Electrode Insertion or Movement. Insertion of a needle electrode into a normally innervated muscle initiates a brief burst of electric activity that includes a large baseline deflection and monophasic and polyphasic potentials of variable amplitude and duration (Fig. 5–31A). The burst of activity ends soon after cessation of needle movement. This response can be reinitiated after insertion by pressing or tapping on the electrode, but again it is of brief duration and terminates almost as soon as the needle stops moving. When needle insertion is followed by prolonged discharge of electric activity (Fig. 5–31A′), response of the muscle fibers to mechanical injury by the electrode reflects cellular hyperirritability and is considered abnormal. In a denervated canine muscle, increased insertion activity becomes noticeable on the fourth or fifth day postdenervation (Fig. 5–32). This activity is especially prominent from the eighth to tenth days; thereafter it declines in duration and intensity (Fig. 5–32). The duration of insertion activity usually does not exceed 3 minutes in denervated muscle of the dog.[29] Increased insertion activity slightly precedes onset of fibrillation activity in a denervated muscle.

Potentials associated with insertion activity in denervated muscles usually measure 100 to 650 μV in amplitude, 1.9 to 4.1 msec in duration, and 50 to 200 per second in frequency.[29] Positive sharp waves may be greater than 1 mV in amplitude in insertion activity. Sound associated with insertion activity is described in Table 5–3.

Spontaneous Activity of the Resting Muscle. Normal resting muscle lacks electric activity as soon as the electrode has attained a stable position in the muscle (Fig. 5–31A). Normal muscles are said to be "electrically silent" because of the absence of an audible signal from the loudspeaker of the electromyograph (see Table 5–3). Exceptions are noted if the tip of the exploring electrode lies within the end plate region from which end plate noise is recorded (Fig. 5–31B) or adjacent to a nerve from which nerve action potentials are recorded. End plate noise represents the summation of miniature end plate potentials and consists of low amplitude (3-60 μV), negative discharges that are continuous at frequencies up to 600 to 1000 Hz.[67] This activity is normal and should not be confused with fibrillation activity. The sound associated with end plate noise differs from that associated with fibrillation activity and nerve action potentials (see Table 5–3).

Spontaneous activity, termed preinnervation infantile activity, has been recorded from the muscles of human fetuses but not from muscles of canine fetuses.[6]

Several days after denervation of a striated muscle, spontaneous, randomly occurring potentials can be recorded (Fig. 5–31B′). These potentials are termed fibrillation potentials (FP) and represent the action potential of a single muscle fiber, or in some instances several muscle fibers. Fibrillation potentials usually arise in the end plate region of the muscle fiber[30] as the result of an instability in the membrane potential. The time of onset of fibrillation potentials after denervation varies according to species. In the rat, onset takes 2 to 3 days; in the cat and dog (Fig. 5–32), 5 days; and in people, 16 days.[20] Time of onset in large animals has not been evaluated, but it appears to be between 12 and 16 days. As a general rule in mammals, the smaller the size of the animal, the earlier is the onset and the greater the

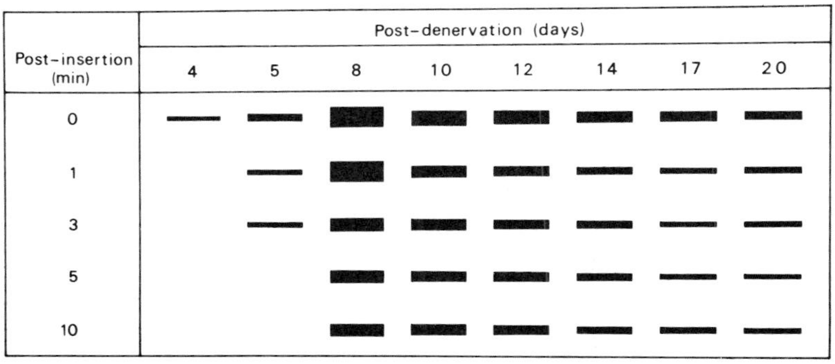

Post-insertion (min)	Post-denervation (days)							
	4	5	8	10	12	14	17	20
0	—	—	▬	▬	▬	▬	▬	▬
1		—	▬	▬	▬	▬	—	▬
3		—	▬	▬	▬	▬	▬	—
5			▬	▬	▬	—	—	
10			▬	▬	▬	—	—	

Figure 5–32. Electromyographic activity associated with denervation includes insertion activity and fibrillation potentials. In denervated dog muscle this activity begins on the fourth day after denervation, becomes more prominent on the fifth day, and peaks on the eighth day. Insertion activity decreases with time after insertion of the needle electrode. The bars are a schematic representation of actual magnitude of activity appearing on an electromyograph display. (Adapted from Inada S, Sugano S, and Ibaraki T: Electromyographic study on denervated muscles in the dog. Jap J Vet Sci 25:327, 1963.)

intensity of fibrillation activity. In addition, the shorter the distance along a nerve from the site of nerve injury to the muscle it innervates, the earlier the onset of fibrillation activity.[38] Atrophy begins before fibrillation potentials can be recorded, and a 50% reduction in muscle mass will occur within about 2 weeks after complete denervation.[51] Disuse atrophy such as occurs after tenotomy is characterized by an absence of fibrillation activity.

Fibrillation potentials are monophasic (negative) or biphasic (usually positive-negative in non–end plate regions and negative-positive in end plate regions) but rarely triphasic in waveform (Fig. 5–31 B' and C'). Amplitude is usually 100 to 300 μV but may be less than 50 μV or greater than 600 μV. Duration ranges from 0.5 to 5 msec. The rhythm is random and sustained as long as viable muscle tissue is present, although amplitude and duration decrease with cicatrization. Distinguishing fibrillation potentials from small motor unit potentials can be accomplished by noting that the former are not associated with reflex or volitional movements, whereas the latter are. The sound associated with fibrillation potential activity is described in Table 5–3. A marked reduction in fibrillation potential activity signals onset of successful motor nerve reinnervation.[10, 20]

Fibrillation potential activity may be modified by physiologic and pharmacologic factors. Heat enhances fibrillation activity, and a heat lamp should be used to warm muscles to be examined in animals with subnormal body temperatures. Repeated passive stretching of a denervated muscle enhances fibrillation activity also. Neostigmine increases fibrillation activity, but a preanesthetic dose of atropine has no effect.

Positive sharp waves (PSW) are commonly noted in activity recorded from denervated muscles (Fig. 5–31 B' and C'). Although sometimes referred to as positive potentials of denervation, their presence alone is not diagnostic of denervation as is true for fibrillation potentials. Moreover, a relative increase in number of positive sharp waves is not a signal of onset of reinnervation.[10] The positive sharp wave is characterized by a rapidly rising positive phase followed by a slow decay to the baseline (Fig. 5–31C'). Amplitude of the positive sharp waves ranges from 100 μV to 20 mV. The mechanism of their production is unknown, but they may represent a nonpropagated depolarization in a region of muscle fibers adjacent to the tip of the active electrode.

Complex repetitive discharges or bizarre high frequency discharges (BHFD) consist of low voltage–short duration potentials with fairly stable frequencies of 20 to 40 Hz. They often have abrupt onset and cessation. Bizarre high frequency discharges are noted in a variety of neuropathic and myopathic conditions.

Myotonic discharges are noted for their variation in amplitude and frequency, which results in sounds often simulating a diving airplane or revving motorcycle (see Table 5–3). Frequencies may range up to 1000 Hz. These discharges can be triggered mechanically or electrically or by needle insertion or movement and may be associated with myotonic diseases[22, 53] or with iatrogenic hyperadrenocorticism[21] or Cushing's disease. In the latter conditions the activity might also be termed bizarre high frequency discharges. The myotonic discharges are unaffected by neuromuscular blockade produced by curare, indicating that they reflect activity of myogenic origin.

Fasciculation potentials represent spontaneous, random discharges of motor units. Often only one or a small number of motor units are involved. This response is believed to be associated with an irritative lesion at the level of the motor neuron cell body.

Activity Associated with Voluntarily or Reflexively Induced Muscle Contractions. Potentials recorded from a normal muscle during a voluntary or reflex contraction represent the summation of the electric activity of the individual muscle fibers composing a motor unit. These potentials are termed motor unit potentials (Fig. 5–31 C and D). The contraction itself does not produce electric activity, but it may displace the electrode, causing fluctuations in the electromyogram similar to those associated with insertion activity. Motor unit potentials are characterized by their amplitude, duration, number of phases, and firing rate. The first three characteristics are determined in the same manner as those for an evoked potential (Fig. 5–33). The firing rate or frequency is the number of times a specific motor unit potential recurs each second (Fig. 5–31D). Increasing strength of muscle contraction can be produced by recruiting more motor units or by increasing firing rate of the active group of motor units. Firing rates are usually less than 60 Hz.

Amplitude of motor unit potentials is markedly influenced by electrode position. Shifting the electrode tip by 0.5 mm from the position of maximal amplitude of a motor unit potential may cause as much as a tenfold or greater reduction in the recorded potential. Thus, maximal amplitude and also shortest duration of a

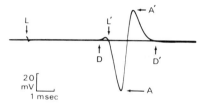

Figure 5–33. An evoked potential of a canine plantar interosseous muscle that has been superimposed on a tracing of the baseline or zero potential line. The stimulus artifact is the small deflection beneath L. Latency is the interval between L and L'; duration is the interval between D and D'; and amplitude is the difference between maximal negative (A) and maximal positive (A') deflections. The potential has three phases. The stimulus was applied to the tibial nerve at a point slightly above the tuber calcis.

particular motor unit potential are recorded from a small region. The potentials that arise in close proximity to the electrode tip produce a sharp cracking sound, whereas those arising a short distance away from the tip produce soft thumping sounds because of their lower amplitude and longer duration. Sound is helpful in correctly positioning the tip of the active electrode. Configuration will vary according to whether the electrode is in the end plate or non–end plate region of the muscle (Fig. 5–31C).

The motor unit potentials associated with the repetitive discharge of a single motor unit are remarkably similar in configuration (Fig. 5–31D) and are relatively easy to identify among the activity of two or three other motor units. Ideally, motor unit potential activity should be evaluated at various levels of tonic muscle contraction. In normally innervated muscle, the smallest potentials appear with minimal contractile tension. As the force of contraction is increased by recruitment of additional motor units, the size of the potentials increases and the firing rate of individual potentials increases. At maximal contraction, the number of motor units that are firing is so great that normally it is impossible to define the configuration of a single motor unit potential. Thus, this activity pattern is termed a full recruitment or complete interference pattern (Fig. 5–31E). In persons, clinical electromyographic examinations include evaluation of the effort pattern associated with graded voluntary contractions. A similar approach in animal electromyography is desirable but is usually precluded by lack of subject cooperation. Therefore, activity associated with minimal contractions and that associated with maximal or near maximal contractions is evaluated in animal electromyography.

Methods for inducing an effort pattern in limb muscles in animals include use of flexor (pedal) reflexes for flexor muscles and increasing weight bearing for antigravity muscles. The latter is accomplished by placing the animal on an inclined plane or by lifting one to three of the limbs not being evaluated electromyographically. Antigravity motor unit potential activity is readily recorded from gastrocnemius muscles. Stretching the pectineus muscle by abduction of the stifle will reflexively induce motor unit potentials in the muscle in a lightly anesthetized dog.[7] Recruitment of motor unit potentials is proportional to magnitude of the stretch of the muscle. The mean firing rate for many motor units is about 10 to 15 per second, and the maximum firing rates are between 30 and 50 Hz.[13] Characteristics of motor unit potentials of muscles of dogs are summarized in Table 5–4. In five different muscles in 3 month old pigs the mean amplitude and range of motor unit potentials were 300 µV and 220 to 410 µV, respectively, and the mean duration and its range were 3.2 msec and 2.8 to 3.6 msec, respectively.[54]

The smaller the number of fibers in a motor unit, the smaller the motor unit potential that can be recorded from that motor unit. Muscles with highly refined movements have small motor units and thus small motor unit potentials. Small animals have motor unit potentials with lower amplitude and shorter duration than large animals.[20] Aged animals may have potentials with larger amplitude and longer duration than those recorded from animals of intermediate ages. Growth is associated primarily with an increase in duration of motor unit potentials.

Fasciculation potentials have the characteristics of motor unit potentials but differ in that they occur spontaneously and sporadically rather than with voluntary effort. They are not usually considered a significant abnormality when present alone. When fasciculation occurs in a large number of motor units, the resultant involuntary muscle contraction is called a spasm and may be either tonic or clonic in nature. Clonic spasms are relatively common in pectineus muscles of dogs.[7]

In chronic neuronopathies, nearby functional nerve fibers develop branches that innervate some of the denervated muscle fibers, thereby creating large motor units. The potentials of these motor units may be ten times the amplitude usually associated with motor units in a particular muscle and are commonly termed giant motor unit potentials. Because the new nerve branches have a slowed conduction ve-

Table 5–4. CHARACTERISTICS OF EVOKED POTENTIALS AND MOTOR UNIT POTENTIALS OF CANINE MUSCLE MOTOR POINTS*

Stimulation Sites	Recording Site (Muscle)	Potential*	Latency (msec)†	Amplitude (mV)†	Duration (msec)†	Phases†
—	Supraspinatus	MUP‡	—	1.37 (0.14–4.82)	2.73 (1.40–4.78)	2.1 (1.0–2.6)
—	Deltoideus	MUP	—	1.03 (0.20–2.54)	2.95 (1.90–4.51)	2.3 (1.4–3.2)
—	Biceps	MUP	—	1.01 (0.33–2.04)	2.79 (2.08–4.05)	2.4 (2.0–3.5)
—	Triceps	MUP	—	0.93 (0.36–2.47)	2.72 (1.95–3.43)	2.4 (1.9–4.1)
Radial nerve where it crosses humerus	Extensor carpi radialis	EP‡	2.2 (1.4–4.8)	54 (28–92)	12 (8.0–20)	3 (2–5)
—	Extensor carpi radialis	MUP	—	0.85 (0.17–2.22)	2.62 (1.60–4.38)	2.3 (1.4–3.2)
Radial nerve	Extensor digitorum communis	EP	2.4 (1.4–3.1)	55 (29–106)	10 (4.0–16)	3 (2–5)
Radial nerve	Extensor digitorum lateralis	EP	2.0 (1.6–2.8)	78 (28–180)	9.3 (4.4–17)	3 (2–5)
Radial nerve	Extensor carpi ulnaris	EP	2.1 (1.4–2.6)	61 (14–154)	7.8 (5.0–13)	3 (2–4)
Ulnar nerve above medial epicondyle of humerus	Flexor carpi ulnaris	EP	2.2 (1.0–3.6)	92 (38–165)	10 (3.5–16)	4 (2–6)
—	Flexor carpi ulnaris	MUP	—	1.86 (0.75–4.47)	3.17 (1.76–4.68)	2.6 (2.0–3.3)
Ulnar nerve above accessory carpal bone	Interosseus	EP	2.6 (1.8–3.4)	54 (28–152)	5.0 (3.4–12)	2 (2–4)
Median nerve craniodorsal to median epicondyle of humerus	Pronator teres	EP	2.1 (1.3–2.8)	53 (20–154)	9.0 (3.0–16)	1 (2–6)
Median nerve	Flexor carpi radialis	EP	1.8 (1.0–2.8)	60 (30–94)	8.4 (3.8–16)	3 (2–5)
—	Flexor carpi radialis	MUP	—	1.72 (0.27–5.27)	3.19 (1.69–4.45)	2.4 (1.0–2.9)
Median nerve	Flexor digitorum profundus	EP	2.0 (1.0–3.0)	67 (18–106)	8.5 (2.8–16)	3 (2–6)
—	Middle gluteal	MUP	—	0.89 (0.41–2.10)	2.31 (1.38–3.19)	2.1 (1.0–2.8)
—	Biceps femoris	MUP	—	0.75 (0.26–1.52)	2.69 (1.90–4.56)	2.2 (1.9–3.2)
—	Semitendinosus	MUP	—	0.63 (0.26–1.34)	2.74 (1.74–3.96)	2.3 (1.8–4.4)
—	Vastus lateralis	MUP	—	0.72 (0.35–1.63)	2.73 (1.94–3.86)	2.1 (1.5–2.6)
—	Gracilis	MUP	—	0.77 (0.32–1.78)	2.60 (1.77–4.24)	2.3 (2.0–3.0)
—	Pectineus	MUP	—	1.68 (0.54–4.73)	3.17 (1.46–4.53)	2.2 (1.5–3.1)
Peroneal nerve caudal to patella	Tibialis cranialis	EP	2.3 (1.4–4.0)	54 (29–90)	14 (8.0–22)	3 (2–5)
—	Tibialis cranialis	MUP	—	0.79 (0.26–1.88)	2.70 (1.51–4.06)	2.2 (1.4–3.0)
Tibial nerve caudal to distal end of femur	Gastrocnemius (lateral head)	EP	2.1 (1.2–3.2)	93 (40–140)	11 (7.0–18)	4 (2–5)
—	Gastrocnemius (lateral head)	MUP	—	1.88 (0.56–4.11)	3.36 (2.59–3.93)	2.7 (2.1–3.1)
Tibial nerve	Gastrocnemius (medial head)	EP	1.7 (1.0–3.0)	96 (30–160)	12 (6.0–17)	3 (2–5)
Tibial nerve at tuber calcis	Interosseus	EP	4.0 (3.4–4.8)	56 (22–112)	4.6 (2.8–8.0)	2 (2–4)

*Evoked potential results from Bowen JM: Electromyographic analysis of evoked potentials of canine muscle motor points. JAVMA 164:509, 1974. Motor unit potential results from Bowen JM: Unpublished data.
†Average (range).
‡MUP = motor unit potential; EP = evoked potential.

locity, increased asynchrony of onset of muscle fiber action potentials results in giant motor unit potentials being polyphasic. During recovery from neuropathies, giant motor unit potentials may be present, but the more common type of potential has a subnormal amplitude and frequently an increased number of phases; it resembles a myopathic motor unit potential (Fig. 5–31F′).

A reduction in amplitude and duration of motor unit potentials is a characteristic of primary muscle disease and reflects a decrease in the number of active muscle fibers in the motor unit. These potentials are termed myopathic motor unit potentials (Fig. 5–31F′). In human electromyography, it has been reported that the mean amplitude of 30 randomly recorded motor unit potentials should deviate by more than 40% from the normal mean value to be considered abnormal.[13] Small motor unit potentials in myopathies have the appearance of fibrillation potentials but may be distinguished from the latter by their regular rhythm and association with voluntary contractions.

Activity Induced by Electrical Stimulation of Motor Nerves. Because most peripheral nerves contain both sensory and motor fibers, suprathreshold electric stimulation of mixed nerves activates both types of fibers. The presence of a sensory response to stimulation provides important electrodiagnostic information. The potentials recorded from a muscle following stimulation of the nerve innervating the muscle are termed M, F, or H waves, depending on the pathway involved in evoking the potential. A major advantage of these potentials is that they can be evaluated without cooperation of the animal.

The M wave is the most frequently examined potential and represents an evoked potential arising from the summation of individual motor unit potentials initiated by orthodromically conducted nerve impulses. The actual number of motor unit potentials contributing to the M wave is a function of stimulus intensity. Usually a supramaximal stimulus intensity is used to enable evaluation of maximal size of the evoked potential of a particular region of a muscle.

F waves represent a long latency response to antidromic motor neuron activation. This may occur simultaneously with orthodromic conduction of a nerve impulse, which produces an M wave. When the antidromically conducted nerve impulse reaches the cell body, it initiates an orthodromically conducted nerve impulse that produces an evoked potential (F wave) with a latency of several milliseconds longer than the M wave. Transection of the ventral roots terminates the F wave response, whereas transection of the dorsal root does not. Latency may be accounted for by the antidromic and orthodromic conduction times for the nerve impulse. Stimulus strength should be supramaximal and frequency of stimulation should be about 1 Hz. Maximal amplitude of the F wave in the dog is about 3% of the associated M wave response.[39] Mean amplitudes of F waves are between 200 and 300 μV. The shapes of a series of F waves can be quite variable. F waves are noted after approximately 20% of stimuli producing M waves.[39] The F wave is believed to provide a means of assessing motor neuron excitability. F wave changes in proximal neuropathies are often noted before most other EMG changes. Organophosphate compounds appear to reduce F wave activity.[24] F waves have been recorded in young chickens.[34]

The H wave has longer latency than the M wave. It is believed to be the result of activation of a monosynaptic reflex (H reflex); in persons, it reaches maximal amplitude at submaximal stimulus strength for the M wave because the afferent fibers are larger and more responsive to the stimuli. Changing position of stimulating electrodes has opposite effects on latencies of the M and H waves.

Long latency, reflex evoked muscle potentials (REMP) have been recorded from interosseous muscles of anesthetized dogs[32, 47, 50] (Fig. 5–34). The reflex evoked muscle potentials have similarities to H waves recorded from persons, except that the response is less likely to be canceled by supramaximal stimulation. The amplitude of the reflex evoked muscle potential is about 8% of that of the direct evoked muscle potential (DEMP or M wave).[50] Latency is about three times that of the M wave. Reflex evoked muscle potentials have been recorded from adult as well as 1 to 12 week old dogs.[50]

Using paired stimulus pulses separated by intervals of 2 to 1000 msec, Sims[47] demonstrated that the recovery cycle of the reflex evoked muscle potential in dogs is similar to that for the H reflex in persons. The reflex evoked muscle potential was absent for pulse intervals of 20 to 80 msec as expected for involvement of a monosynaptic reflex arc. A stimulus rate of 1 per 5 sec provided the best recording interval.

Use of reflex evoked muscle potential for examination of neurologic problems has received limited evaluation in veterinary medicine.[32] It may prove to be especially valuable for early evaluation of brachial plexus injuries. In human proximal neuropathies, the H reflex

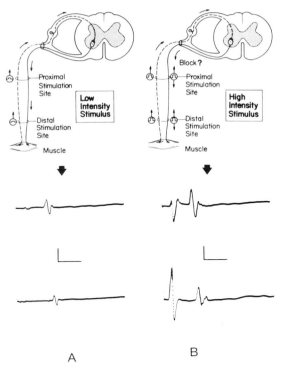

A   B

Figure 5–34. A, Low intensity stimuli applied to the ulnar nerve of a dog produces a long latency reflex evoked muscle potential (REMP) in interosseous muscle recordings. The response reflects reflex activation of motor neurons and not their direct activation because of the higher threshold of motor nerves to electric stimulation. B, When high intensity stimuli are applied to the ulnar nerve both motor and sensory fibers are activated, producing responses reflecting both direct activation and reflex activation of motor neurons. The longer latency of the reflex response arises from the longer conduction distance through the reflex arc. Note that the shift from proximal to distal stimulation sites decreases latency of the direct response and increases latency of the reflex response. (From Sims MH and Selcer RR: Occurrence and evaluation of a reflex-evoked muscle potential (H reflex) in the normal dog. Am J Vet Res 42:975, 1981.)

may be detected as being abnormally prolonged before sensory and motor examinations reveal abnormalities.

An approximation of sensory nerve conduction velocity can be derived from the reflex evoked muscle potentials resulting from stimulation at two points along the course of a mixed nerve. Because stimulus intensities are submaximal, the population of nerve fibers activated may be different at the two points of stimulation. This can lead to errors in determination of conduction velocities. Therefore, direct measurement of sensory nerve conduction velocity is preferable to use of the reflex evoked muscle potential.

The important characteristics of evoked po-

tentials (M waves) include latency, amplitude, duration, and number of phases (see Fig. 5–33). Mean values for the characteristics of evoked potentials are presented in Table 5–4. These values will vary with the type of exploring electrode and positioning of the electrode tip. Latency represents the time for nerve impulse conduction from the stimulation site to the nerve terminal, neuromuscular delay (about 0.5 msec), and time for conduction from the end plate region to the tip of the active electrode. It is best measured when the stimulating electrodes are applied to the nerve near the muscle and the exploring electrode is positioned in the end plate region. Under these conditions, latency may be termed the terminal conduction time. Some electromyographers consider single latency determinations to be a satisfactory substitute for nerve conduction velocity determinations.[15] Because nerve fiber compression prolongs latency, latency can be used to determine the level of compression along a peripheral nerve.

The amplitude of an evoked potential provides an approximate indication of the number of muscle fibers activated by nerve stimulation. Values for amplitude range from a few millivolts to over 100 mV (Table 5–4). Careful positioning of the exploring electrode at a site within the muscle at which the potential has no or minimal prodromal positivity will provide the maximal amplitude. This site is within the end plate region. During reinnervation the evoked potential amplitude increases but may never attain the control value if reinnervation is incomplete. The reduction in muscle fiber size associated with disuse atrophy also leads to a reduction in size of the evoked potential, but latency and number of phases are unaffected. Duration and number of phases of the evoked potential are a measure of the synchrony of discharge of the individual motor unit potentials and of the number of these units discharging. When synchrony decreases, the duration and number of phases increase. When the number of units responding decreases, the number of phases often increases and the duration may decrease. Normally the number of phases is less than five (Table 5–4). Demyelinating diseases affecting peripheral nerves frequently cause an increase in the number of phases (see Fig. 5–31 H').

When a motor nerve is severed, the distal segment undergoes wallerian degeneration. The degeneration begins at the site of severance and migrates peripherally. Thus, immediately after severance, the entire distal segment responds well to electric stimulation, but no response occurs when the proximal segment is stimulated. Over a period of several days the distal segment remains responsive to stimulation but only if the electrode is moved closer to the muscle each day. The evoked potential decreases in amplitude and latency increases, and, depending on length of the distal segment, conduction ceases abruptly after about 5 to 8 days.[23]

In a normal muscle the evoked potentials can be superimposed on the oscilloscope display during stimulation at a frequency of 30 per second with little evidence of fatigue being noted during a 5 second period of stimulation as long as the electrode tip is not displaced by the muscle contraction (Fig. 5–31F). In contrast, myasthenia gravis is characterized by a rapid decrease in evoked potential amplitude during stimulation at frequencies of 4 to 50 Hz[42] (Fig. 5–31G'). This response may be noted also during reinnervation and occasionally in ventral horn cell disease and syringomyelia. In contrast, repetitive stimulation has been noted to increase electromyographic response in botulism and "shaker foal" syndrome.[43, 56]

Recording Artifacts

Electric activity derived from sources other than those of electromyographic interest is considered artifact and can hinder evaluation of electromyograms. Included among recording artifacts are electric activity of cardiac muscle (a biphasic wave of long duration) and brain (temporal muscle records), electrode movement, and electric devices such as electric cautery, diathermy, electric motors, and fluorescent lighting. The source of interference should be identified and appropriate steps taken to exclude it from the electromyograms. Incorrect electrode positioning, poor electrode-tissue contact, and proximity of the electronic interference generator are common causes of interference. Use of telemetry and high quality differential amplifiers can aid in reducing electric interference. Fine wire electrodes reduce movement artifacts.[2]

NERVE CONDUCTION VELOCITY

Passage of a nerve impulse along a nerve fiber requires a finite time that is characteristic of a particular diameter of a motor or sensory nerve fiber. Demyelinating neuropathies are associated with a slowing of the conduction velocity of a nerve impulse.[41] Usually sensory nerve conduction velocities (NCV) are affected before motor NCV. Slowing of conduction velocity is rare in neuronopathies and does not occur at all in myopathies. Following severance of a motor nerve, the nerve conduction velocity of the distal segment remains normal until conduction failure occurs.[23, 48] This occurs in about 5 to 8 days in the dog and after a longer period in larger animals.

Nerve conduction velocities of certain long peripheral nerves can be measured clinically in an anesthetized animal with the aid of an electromyograph, electronic stimulator, and recording and stimulating electrodes. Sensory conduction velocity measurements require use of a signal averager because the nerve potentials must be measured directly and have small amplitude compared with amplitude of muscle potentials associated with motor nerve stimulation.

Procedure

Motor nerve conduction velocity is determined by inserting the active electrode into a muscle supplied by the nerve being evaluated and stimulating that nerve (Fig. 5–35). Single supramaximal stimuli are applied successively, preferably at two points along the course of the nerve, and the evoked potentials are photographed or displayed on a storage oscilloscope. Three evoked potentials for each site of stimulation should be superimposed to ensure that the response is stable. Latency of evoked potentials for each site of stimulation should be measured to the nearest 0.1 msec. The difference represents the conduction time for impulses in the fastest conducting fibers of the nerve segment between the proximal and distal stimulation sites. When the length of the nerve segment (measured to the nearest millimeter) is divided by the latency difference or conduction time, the conduction velocity is given in meters per second (Fig. 5–35). This procedure is termed the onset latency method for determining nerve conduction velocity.

Normal values for conduction velocities for several nerves are given in Table 5–6. Application of these values necessitates duplication of the recording and stimulating electrode position noted in the reference supplying these values. Impulse conduction to muscles in the proximal part of an extremity is faster than that to muscles in the distal part of the extremity. For radial and median nerves of the horse the

Table 5–5. CHARACTERISTIC ELECTROMYOGRAPHIC FINDINGS IN DISEASES AFFECTING THE NERVOUS SYSTEM OR STRIATED MUSCLE

Lesion or Disease	Insertion Activity	Fibrillation Potentials and Positive Sharp Waves	High Frequency Discharges	Motor Unit Potentials			Evoked Potential Amplitude	Nerve Conduction Velocity
				Amplitude	Phases	Effort Pattern		
Upper motor neuron lesion (cord compression)	Increased	Absent or few	Absent	Normal	Normal	Reduced	Reduced (disuse atrophy)	Normal
Neuropathy (spinal muscular atrophy)	Increased	Present	Bizarre	Sub- to supranormal	Increased	Reduced	Reduced	Normal
Mononeuropathy (trigeminal nerve)	Increased	Present	Bizarre	Near normal if present	Near normal if present	Reduced if present	Absent or reduced	Decreased if measurable
Traumatic polyneuropathy (brachial plexus)	Increased	Present	Bizarre	Near normal to supranormal if present	Near normal if present	Reduced if present	Absent or reduced	Normal if measurable
Hereditary polyneuropathy (neuronal abiotrophy)	Increased	Present	Bizarre	—*	—	—	Absent or reduced	Decreased
Allergic polyneuropathy	Increased	Present	Bizarre	Reduced	Increased	Reduced	Reduced	Decreased
Metabolic polyneuropathy (diabetes mellitus)	Increased	Present	Absent	Reduced	Increased	Reduced	Reduced	Decreased
Toxic polyneuropathy (acrylamide; hexacarbon solvent)	Increased	Present	Absent	Reduced	Increased	Reduced	Reduced	Decreased
Delayed neuropathy (organophosphates)	—	—	—	Reduced	—	—	Reduced	Normal
Botulism (botulin toxin)	Increased	Absent or few	Absent	Reduced	Normal to increased	Reduced	Reduced but increased by 20 Hz stimulation	Normal
Tick paralysis (tick toxin)	Normal	Absent	Absent	Reduced	Normal	Reduced	Reduced but may increase with repetitive stimulation	Normal to decreased
Myasthenia gravis	Normal	Absent or few	Absent	Reduced	Normal to increased	Normal to reduced	Reduced by 4–30 Hz stimulation	Normal
Polymyositis	Increased	Present	Bizarre	Reduced	Increased	Increased	Reduced	Normal
Nutritional myopathy	Increased	Absent or few	Bizarre	—	—	—	—	Normal
Hereditary myopathy	Increased	Absent	Myotonic-like	—	—	—	—	Normal
Endocrine myopathy (Cushing's disease)	Increased	Absent	Myotonic-like	Reduced	Increased	Increased	Reduced	Normal
Myotonic (muscular) dystrophy	Increased	Absent or few	Myotonic	—	—	—	—	Normal

*Response in affected dogs or cats has not been investigated.

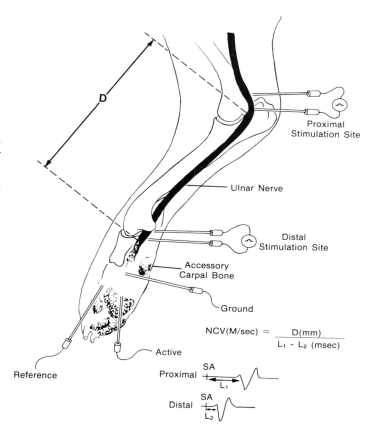

Figure 5–35. Schematic diagram of the latency technique for determination of ulnar motor nerve conduction velocity. Latency (L_2) of the evoked potential induced by stimulation at the level of the accessory carpal bone is subtracted from the latency (L_1) of the evoked potential induced by stimulation at the level of the olecranon. The difference represents the conduction time for impulses in the fastest conducting fibers of the nerve segment (D) between the stimulating electrodes. Conduction velocity is calculated with the formula given in the diagram. The active electrode tip was in an interosseous muscle.

difference is about 15%.[25] The limiting factor in determination of conduction velocity is the length of nerve accessible to stimulation at two sites. These sites should be separated by at least 100 mm. Thus, the accessible courses of the femoral, median, radial, and obturator nerves may be too short, particularly in small animals, for accurate determination of conduction velocities.

Experimental errors arise primarily from inaccuracies associated with reading the two latencies and estimating the conduction distance. These errors are influenced by the magnitudes of the conduction distance, time, and velocity.[40] Serial evaluations of the same nerve may normally be expected to vary by 4 to 6 m/sec. However, repeated bilateral measurements in normal dogs provide similar mean values.[35]

Some electromyographers consider latency a satisfactory substitute for nerve conduction velocities in clinical evaluations.[15] Because of size variations among animals within a species, latency rate has been recommended for use in place of latency.[52, 64] Latency rate is determined

by dividing the distance between the stimulating electrode and the active electrode by the latency. The latency rate is expressed in meters per second. It is especially useful when the accessible nerve segment length is less than 100 mm.

A linear relationship exists between nerve conduction velocity and temperature of tissues adjacent to the nerve down to 20°C.[36] For each degree centigrade below normal tissue temperature, a correction of 1.8 m/sec should be added to nerve conduction velocity measurements in dogs. In young chickens the correction factor is 1.1 m/sec per degree C.[34] Alternatively, a heating pad or heat lamp can be used to restore the temperature of the tissue to a normal range. Young (less than 8 weeks) and old (more than 12 years) animals have reduced nerve conduction velocity in comparison with those of animals in the intermediate age range.[55] Protein malnutrition has been reported to reduce conduction velocity reversibly in rhesus monkeys.[46]

Direct measurement of nerve conduction velocities can be accomplished by placing the tip

Table 5–6. MOTOR AND SENSORY NERVE CONDUCTION VELOCITIES*

Species	Nerve Function	Nerve Conduction Velocity (m/sec)					Reference
		Radial	*Median*	*Ulnar*	*Tibial*	*Peroneal*	
Dog	Motor	72	66	59	68	80	Walker et al, 1979
Dog	Motor	—	—	60	60	75	Lee & Brown, 1970
Cat	Motor	—	—	77	79	75	Bowen†
Chicken‡	Motor	—	—	—	35	—	Kornegay et al, 1983
Horse	Motor	79	73	71	90	90	Sprinkle, 1977
Dog	Sensory	62	—	68	—	—	Holliday et al, 1977
Dog	Sensory	65	—	69	63	64	Redding et al, 1982
Cat	Sensory	84	—	89	80	85	Redding and Ingram, 1984
Pony	Sensory	—	79	71	—	—	Blythe et al, 1983

*The reference should be examined to determine the nerve segment associated with the reported conduction velocity.
†Unpublished data. Electrode positions were similar to those used in dogs.[35]
‡Two to 4 weeks of age.

of a monopolar, insulated needle electrode adjacent to a nerve and then applying a supramaximal stimulus to the nerve either proximal or distal to the recording site. Conduction time is the interval between the stimulus artifact and the evoked nerve potential. This procedure is used for determination of sensory nerve conduction velocity. Because the nerve action potentials are of low amplitude (<50 µV), a signal averager must be used to enhance the signal-to-noise ratio. The number of responses averaged by various investigators has ranged from 64 to 1600.[26, 45] Responses are evoked at a stimulation rate of 10 Hz. The averaged evoked response amplitude is 5 to 250 µV.[26] A stimulus pulse duration of 0.1 msec is satisfactory. Threshold stimulation intensity produces a triphasic potential but is submaximal as further increase in intensity causes an increase in amplitude of evoked response. However, as stimulus intensity is increased, conduction velocity also increases. This is believed to be due to spread of the electric field and initiation of the impulse at a point closer to the recording electrodes. Therefore, a stimulus intensity of twice threshold has been recommended as being optimal for minimizing spread of the stimulus while maximizing number of fibers stimulated.[5] Errors as noted for motor nerve conduction velocity also occur in sensory nerve measurements.

Sensory nerve conduction velocity may be a more sensitive measure of presence of a neuropathy than motor nerve conduction velocity. In animals such as the horse, sensory nerves may be more accessible to evaluation than motor nerves. To avoid interference from muscle contraction when attempting measurement of sensory nerves, values should be determined for purely sensory nerves, or stimuli should be applied to a region that has a high density of sensory fibers and a low density of motor fibers, e.g., the digits. Values for conduction velocities of sensory nerves decrease at a rate of 0.1 to 0.2 m/sec/year from values for young adults.[63] In diabetic animals, sensory nerve conduction velocities are decreased.[54] Combined measurement of sensory nerve potentials and somatosensory cerebral evoked potentials is helpful in localizing a lesion affecting sensory function. In neuropathies, records of sensory nerve potentials may be difficult to obtain.

Interpretation of Results

Diagnosis of diseases affecting nerves, muscles, or the neuromuscular junction is greatly aided by information derived from an electromyographic examination. When possible and if indicated, results of histologic and histochemical evaluations of muscle biopsies and serum muscle enzyme determinations should be integrated with electromyographic and neurologic information. The distinction between neuropathies and myopathies is not easy to establish in animals, although difficulties are also encountered in this area in humans.[65] Electromyographic findings in specific neuropathies and myopathies are summarized in Table 5–5.

KINESIOLOGY

Kinesiology utilizes EMG to define the role of a specific muscle or group of muscles in posture and in simple and complex body or limb movements. Extensive kinesiologic studies on dogs during walking, trotting, and galloping have been conducted.[60]

REFERENCES

1. Allam MW, Nulsen FE, and Lewey FH: Electrical intraneural bipolar stimulation of peripheral nerves in the dog. JAVMA 114:87, 1949.
2. Basmajian JV, Stecko G: A new bipolar electrode for electromyography. J Appl Physiol 17:849, 1962.
3. Basmajian JV, Clifford HC, McLeod WD, and Nunnally HN: Computers in Electromyography. Butterworths & Co, Reading, MA, 1975.
4. Beckett SD, Walker DF, Hudson RS, et al: Corpus spongiosum penis pressure and penile muscle activity in the stallion during coitus. Am J Vet Res 36:433, 1975.
5. Blythe LL, Kitchell RL, Holliday TA and Johnson RD: Sensory nerve conduction velocities in forelimb of ponies. Am J Vet Res 44:1419, 1983.
6. Botelho SY, Steinberg SA, McGrath JT, and Zislis J: Electromyography in dogs with congenital spinal cord lesions. Am J Vet Res 28:205, 1967.
7. Bowen JM: Electromyographic analysis of reflex and spastic activities of canine pectineus muscles in the presence and absence of hip dysplasia. Am J Vet Res 35:661, 1974.
8. Bowen JM: Electromyography. In Klemm WR (ed): Applied Electronics for Veterinary Medicine and Animal Physiology. Springfield, IL, Charles C Thomas, 1976.
9. Bowen JM: Electronic evaluation of motor function and dysfunction. In Klemm WR (ed): Applied Electronics for Veterinary Medicine and Animal Physiology. Springfield, IL, Charles C Thomas, 1976.
10. Bowen JM: Denervation in the canine pectineus muscle: Quantitative electromyographic analysis of its time course. Arch Phys Med Rehabil 58:339, 1977.
11. Bowen JM: Peripheral nerve electrodiagnostics, electromyography, and nerve conduction velocity. In Hoerlein BF, Canine Neurology, 3rd ed. Philadelphia, WB Saunders Co, 1978.
12. Bryant SH, Lipicky RJ, and Herzog WH: Variability of myotonic signs in myotonic goats. Am J Vet Res 29:2371, 1968.
13. Buchthal F and Rosenfalck P: Electrophysiological aspects of myopathy with particular reference to progressive muscular dystrophy. In Bourne GH (ed). Muscular Dystrophy in Man and Animals. New York, Hafner Publishing Co, 1963.
14. Chrisman CL, Burt JK, Wood PK, and Johnson EW: Electromyography in small animal clinical neurology. JAVMA 160:311, 1972.
15. Christie BGB and Coomes EN: Normal variation of nerve conduction in three peripheral nerves. Ann Phys Med 5:303, 1960.
16. Cohen HL and Brumlik J: A Manual of Electroneuromyography. New York, Harper and Row, 1968.
17. Desmedt JE (ed): New Developments in Electromyography and Clinical Neurophysiology, vols 1–3, Basel, Switzerland, S Karger, 1973.
18. DiBartola SP and Tasker JB: Elevated serum creatine phosphokinase. J Am Anim Hosp Assoc 13:744, 1977.
19. Engel WK: Focal myopathic changes produced by electromyographic and hypodermic needles ("needle myopathy"). Arch Neurol 16:509, 1967.
20. Feinstein B, Pattle RE, and Weddell G: Metabolic factors affecting fibrillation in denervated muscle. J Neurol Neurosurg Psychiat 8:1, 1945.
21. Greene CE, Lorenz MD, Munnell JF, et al: Myopathy associated with hyperadrenocorticism in the dog. JAVMA 174:1310, 1979.

22. Griffiths IR and Duncan ID: Myotonia in the dog: A report of four cases. Vet Rec 93:184, 1973.
23. Griffiths IR and Duncan ID: Some studies of the clinical neurophysiology of denervation in the dog. Res Vet Sci 17:377, 1974.
24. Hazelwood JC, Stefan GE, and Bowen JM: Motor unit irritability in beagles before and after exposure to cholinesterase inhibitors. Am J Vet Res 40:852, 1979.
25. Henry RW and Diesem CD: Proximal equine radial and median motor nerve conduction velocity. Am J Vet Res 42:1819, 1981.
26. Holliday TA, Ealand BG, and Weldon NE: Sensory nerve conduction velocity: Technical requirements and normal values for branches of the radial and ulnar nerves of the dog. Am J Vet Res 38:1543, 1977.
27. Howard FM: Electromyography and conduction studies in peripheral nerve injuries. Surg Clin North Am 52:1343, 1972.
28. Hussain S and Pettit GD: Tendon transplantation to compensate for radial nerve paralysis in the dog. Am J Vet Res 28:335, 1967.
29. Inada S, Sugano S and Ibaraki T: Electromyographic study on denervated muscles in the dog. Jap J Vet Sci 25:327, 1963.
30. Jarcho LW, Berman B, Dowben RM and Lilienthal JL: Site of origin and velocity of conduction of fibrillary potentials in denervated skeletal muscle. Am J Physiol 178:128, 1954.
31. Johnson EW, Fallon TJ and Wolfe CV: Errors in EMG reporting. Arch Phys Med Rehabil 57:30, 1976.
32. Knecht CD and Redding RW: Monosynaptic reflex (H wave) in clinically normal and abnormal dogs. Am J Vet Res 42:1586, 1981.
33. Knecht CD and St Clair LE: The radial-brachial paralysis syndrome in the dog. JAVMA 154:653, 1969.
34. Kornegay JN, Gorgacz EJ, Parker MA and Schierman LW: Motor nerve conduction velocity in normal chickens. Am J Vet Res 44:1537, 1983.
35. Lee AF and Bowen JM: Evaluation of motor nerve conduction velocity in the dog. Am J Vet Res 31:1361, 1970.
36. Lee AF and Bowen JM: Effect of tissue temperature on ulnar nerve conduction velocity in the dog. Am J Vet Res 36:1305, 1975.
37. Liu CT: Effect of aspirin on strength-duration curve of the traumatized muscle in cats. J Trauma 10:68, 1970.
38. Luco JV and Eyzaguirre C: Fibrillation and hypersensitivity to ACh in denervated muscle: Effect of length of degenerating nerve fibers. J Neurophysiol 18:65, 1955.
39. Machida M, Sato K, Asai T, and Okada A: An experimental study of the F-wave in the dog: Effects of spasticity and central muscle relaxant. Electromyogr Clin Neurophysiol 23:353, 1983.
40. Maynard FM and Stolov WC: Experimental error in determination of nerve conduction velocity. Arch Phys Med Rehab 53:362, 1972.
41. McDonald WI: The effects of experimental demyelination on conduction in peripheral nerve: A histological and electrophysiological study. II. Electrophysiological observations. Brain 86:501, 1963.
42. Miller LA, Lennon VA, Lambert EH, et al: Congenital myasthenia gravis in 13 smooth fox terriers. JAVMA 182:694, 1983.
43. Prickett ME: The "barker," "wanderer" and "shaker foal" syndrome. Proc AAEP Convention, 309, 1969.
44. Redding RW and Ingram JT: Sensory nerve conduction velocity of cutaneous afferents of the radial, ulnar, peroneal, and tibial nerves of the cat: Reference values. Am J Vet Res 45:1042, 1984.

45. Redding RW, Ingram JT and Colter SB: Sensory nerve conduction velocity of cutaneous afferents of the radial, ulnar, peroneal, and tibial nerves of the dog: Reference values. Am J Vet Res 43:517, 1982.
46. Roy S, Singh N, Deo MG, and Ramalingaswami V: Ultrastructure of skeletal muscle and peripheral nerve in experimental protein deficiency and its correlation with nerve conduction studies. J Neurol Sci 17:399, 1972.
47. Sims MH: Recovery cycle of the reflex-evoked muscle potential (H reflex): Excitability of spinal motor neurons in the healthy dog. Am J Vet Res 43:89, 1982.
48. Sims MH and Redding RW: Failure of neuromuscular transmission after complete nerve section in the dog. Am J Vet Res 40:931, 1979.
49. Sims MH and Redding RW: Maturation of nerve conduction velocity and the evoked muscle potential in the dog. Am J Vet Res 41:1247, 1980.
50. Sims MH and Selcer RR: Occurrence and evaluation of a reflex-evoked muscle potential (H reflex) in the normal dog. Am J Vet Res 42:975, 1981.
51. Solandt DY and Magladery JW: The relation of atrophy to fibrillation in denervated muscle. Brain 63:255, 1940.
52. Sprinkle FP: Nerve Conduction Velocities in the Horse. Thesis. Auburn University, Auburn, AL, 1977.
53. Steinberg S and Botelho S: Myotonia in a horse. Science 137:979, 1962.
54. Steiss JE, Bowen JM, and Williams CH: Electromyographic evaluation of malignant hyperthermia-susceptible pigs. Am J Vet Res 42:1173, 1981.
55. Swallow JS and Griffiths IR: Age related changes in the motor nerve conduction velocity in dogs. Res Vet Sci 23:29, 1977.
56. Swift TR: Disorders of neuromuscular transmission other than myasthenia gravis. Muscle Nerve 4:334, 1981.
57. Tanzi F, Taglietti V, Zucca G, et al: Computerized EMG analysis. Electromyogr Clin Neurophysiol 19:495, 1979.
58. Thiele B and Bohle A: Number of single fibre action potentials contributing to the motor unit potential. Electroenceph Clin Neurophysiol 41:668, 1976.
59. Thomson FK and Bowen JM: Electrodiagnostic testing: Mapping and clinical use of motor points in the dog. JAVMA 159:1763, 1971.
60. Tokuriki M: Electromyographic and joint-mechanical studies in quadrupedal locomotion. III. Gallop. Jap J Vet Sci 36:121, 1974.
61. Tradati F: L'esame elettrodiagnostico nella patologia neuromuscolare del cane. Clinica Vet (Milano) 86:347, 1963.
62. Tursky B: Integrators as measuring devices of bioelectric output. Clin Pharm Therap 5:887, 1964.
63. Vandendriessche G, Vanhecke J, and Rosselle N: Normal sensory conduction in the distal segment of the median and radial nerve: Relation to age. Electromyogr Clin Neurophysiol 21:511, 1981.
64. Walker TL, Redding RW and Braund KG: Motor nerve conduction velocity and latency in the dog. Am J Vet Res 40:1433, 1979.
65. Warmolts JR and Engel WK: A critique of the "myopathic" electromyogram. Trans Am Neurol Assoc 95:173, 1970.
66. Warmolts JR and Engel WK: Open biopsy electromyography. I. Correlation of motor unit behavior with histochemical muscle fiber type in human limb muscle. Arch Neurol 27:512, 1972.
67. Wiederholt WC: "End-plate noise" in electromyography. Neurology 20:214, 1970.

Section 3

RW Redding, DVM, PhD
LJ Myers II, DVM, PhD

EVOKED RESPONSE

An evoked response is a graphic recording of the electric events occurring in a particular part of the nervous system as a result of stimuli given by the investigator or clinician to receptors or afferent nerve fibers. In most cases, the recordings are made using electrodes placed at a considerable distance from the generators (source) and therefore have been called far field recordings. Recordings made under these conditions are volume conducted potentials and obey the laws of unit charge through a conducting medium, in this case through body fluids. Although the latency of the response is for all practical purposes instantaneous and not affected by the electrode distance, the farther removed the electrodes are from the source, the smaller the recorded response. Clinically used evoked responses are usually in the nanovolt to microvolt range.

Because these electrochemical events (evoked potentials) are small in comparison with the background activity such as electroencephalographic (EEG) activity, it is necessary to use equipment designed to "average out" random background activity and at the same time "average in" the desired signal. Such signal averaging devices are available and are used clinically to evaluate the auditory, visual, somatosensory, olfactory, and gustatory systems.

In addition, evoked responses of greater magnitude are recorded from skeletal muscle and nerve trunks (see Nerve Conduction Velocity and Electromyography above).

RECORDING EQUIPMENT

The hardware needed to record evoked potentials is shown in the simplified block diagram (Fig. 5–36).

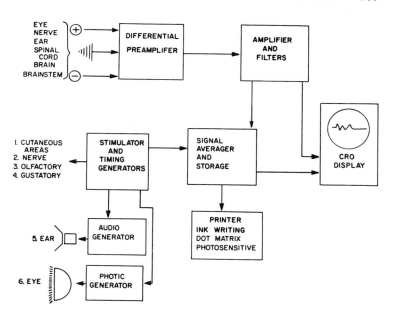

Figure 5–36. Block diagram of evoked response system.

Preamplifier

One of the most important units of the system is the preamplifier. The quality of the first stage of the amplification must be high for good signal acquisition. The preamplifier should be of the differential type with a high input impedance and have a good common mode rejection capacity. A good signal-to-noise ratio is also essential, as the major source of system noise will occur in the preamplifier section. Input impedance is an important consideration in veterinary evoked potential recordings because needle electrodes are used much more frequently than in recordings from human subjects. The effective source impedance is frequently 5 to 35 KΩ in needle type recordings. Equipment for surface disk electrodes may be designed for lower input impedances, from 1 to 5 KΩ. Such equipment will not record input from high impedance needles accurately.

The postamplifier must be of high quality and should contain high and low bandpass filters. Appropriate filtering of the amplified signal can shorten the averaging process, but inappropriate filtering can distort waveform amplitudes and latencies. The frequency content of the recorded potentials is such that a bandpass of 50 to 1000 cycles is adequate. However, a 3000 Hz bandwidth is frequently used.

The Signal Averager

Signal averagers are designed to extract low amplitude evoked responses from ongoing higher amplitude background activity (Fig. 5–37). Most modern signal averagers use analog (continuous signals) to digital (discrete signal) converters and digital memory for storing numeric data. The memories used for signal averaging are storage bins that correspond one to one with the number of discrete measures within a single sweep. The numeric value of each sample is added to the specific storage bin corresponding to its order in a sweep. This is repeated for each sweep for the desired number of sweeps (usually 64 or more). The signal averager (or summing computer) extracts the desired signal from unwanted noise because the signal averager is "time locked" to the stimulus, and, therefore, the evoked response is averaged

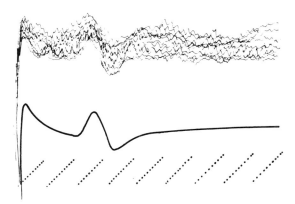

Figure 5–37. A signal averaged, sensory nerve compound action potential (lower) compared with the raw data (upper). Thirty-two epochs were averaged. Time base in staircase, each staircase is 1 msec, each dot represents 0.1 msec. Amplitude of standardization signal is 10 μV. Negative is upward.

at an exact point in time in the averager and is summed at this point in time. This provides a powerful method of extracting the time locked signal from the random background noise in which the signal is buried. The noise comes from ongoing myogenic, electroencephalographic, and electrocardiographic activities, which are random and therefore canceled by the repeating averager, whereas the neuronal activities that have been specifically evoked by the stimulus are progressively enhanced.

Automatic Artifact Rejection

Automatic artifact rejection must be part of a signal averaging system. If a signal entering the averager exceeds a preset voltage threshold, that sweep is rejected as containing artifact. This is especially useful when recording from animals, because movement is frequently encountered. It should be realized, however, that there are limitations to artifact rejection. Excessive rejection results in a poor tracing, and other methods such as reduction of gain of the amplifier and quieting of the animal result in a better recording.

Data Manipulation

A signal averaging system must be able to store data from an averaging run and display those data for observation before printing a permanent record. The stored data can then be manipulated for more accurate measurement if necessary. The amplitude of the storage signal can be increased or decreased by manipulation of the controls. In addition, the time base may be increased to visualize early potentials if so desired. Any changes made must be noted on the record so that measurements are accurate.

Electrodes

In human medicine, electrodes used for evoked potentials recording are usually surface disk or cup type secured by tape or collodion after proper skin preparation. In veterinary evoked potential recordings, needle electrodes are more commonly used and require high impedance input preamplifiers as described above.

Graphics

For research, comparative, and legal reasons, records of evoked potentials must be made. Although time and amplitude measurements may be made with the cursors (electronic point marking devices) on the stored display screen, it is necessary to confirm or measure other aspects of the evoked potentials. Two types of permanent recordings are usually used. A graphic plot of the data (x and y coordinates) is printed on an 8 × 11 inch paper by a write-out unit using pen or dot matrix type recording. Some averaging systems use a fiberoptic scope, which prints on linographic photosensitive paper. Alternatively, a photograph of the display screen may be made.

Measurements

Various methods of measurements are used in evaluation of evoked potentials. Unfortunately, different authors use different polarity input and various points of measurement. Onset latencies or peak latencies of the positive and negative peaks are used. Onset latencies are measured from the onset of stimulation to the onset of the first deflection from baseline indicating the arrival of the first action potentials of a series. This type of measurement is usually used in calculation of maximum conduction velocity of sensory nerves and spinal cord potentials. Peak latencies are measured from onset of stimulus to the peak of either a negative (N) or positive (P) wave. Peak points are labeled sequentially P or N1, etc., or one may use the time in milliseconds from stimulus to the peak, i.e., N_4, N_{43}, N_{125}. This type of measurement is used in auditory and visual evoked potential evaluation.

An evoked response provides information relating to the sensory, integrative, and output systems involved. Most or all of the anatomic structures involved in the neural processing resulting from a stimulus and corresponding response can be evaluated. Although an evoked response may be performed with the intent of evaluating either the sensory or the output system, assessment of systems and the integration between the two is required. In the past, for example, the brain stem auditory evoked response (BAER) was used to evaluate the sense of hearing; however, recently its use has been expanded to evaluate lesions of the central nervous system, particularly of the brain stem.

Prior to the early 1960s, recording of evoked responses of the brain, brain stem, and spinal cord was difficult. While evoked muscle potentials and electroretinograms were frequently recorded, brain stem auditory, somatosensory, and visual evoked responses were recorded only with great difficulty using the technique of superimposition of sequential evoked responses. Detection of the waveforms of the evoked responses was sometimes impossible. The advent of the signal averaging computer made the technique of recording these responses comparatively simple; with the signal averager, the clinical use of evoked responses increased dramatically.

EVOKED POTENTIALS RECORDING

Some of the parameters used in recording evoked potentials are summarized in Table 5–7.

Auditory Potentials

Brain Stem Auditory Evoked Response

The brain stem auditory evoked response (BAER) is the time locked brain stem activity associated with an auditory stimulus usually within 10 msec of the stimulus.[33] It is highly constant in latency of waveforms, consisting of seven waves, the first five of which are used clinically. Although anatomic correlates for each wave are not proved with certainty, it is thought that the first is associated with the vestibulo-cochlear nerve, the second associated to an extent with the cochlear nucleus function, the third with the nucleus of the trapezoid body, and the fourth and fifth with the lemniscal nuclei and caudal colliculus (Fig. 5–38).

The brain stem auditory evoked response has been used in dogs,[20] horses,[23] cattle,[14] and cats[10] in localizing and lateralizing brain stem lesions, such as infarcts; in evaluating inner ear injury,[23] in evaluating certain drug effects, such as ototoxicity of neomycin;[24] and in definitively determining brain death. Several cases have occurred in which wave peak and/or interpeak latencies have been lengthened, and subsequent necropsy has shown brain stem lesions diagnosed by the BAER in the dog. Current research indicates a high proportion of dogs with vestibular signs or recurrent seizures exhibit abnormal BAER.

Middle and Long-Latency Potentials

A set of evoked potentials associated with auditory stimuli can be recorded at times later than the brain stem auditory evoked response. These are commonly termed middle and long

latency auditory evoked potentials, although terminology is not always consistent. Middle latency auditory evoked potentials (MLAEP) occur between 10 and 50 msec following an auditory stimulus, whereas long latency auditory evoked potentials (LLAEP) occur between 50 and 600 msec following an auditory stimulus (Fig. 5–38). These potentials have been evaluated in the dog[34] and cat,[15, 36] and anatomic and clinical correlation of these responses is currently being studied.

Somatosensory Potentials

Spinal Evoked Potentials

Spinal evoked potentials (SEP) are elicited by electric stimulation of a peripheral nerve and recorded with electrodes placed near the spinal cord at selected spinal segments[7, 18] (Fig. 5–39).

Spinal evoked potentials have been used in veterinary medicine to determine both spinal cord function and, indirectly, peripheral nerve conduction.[17, 26] Only a few publications[17, 18, 21, 26, 29] dealing with the dog and the cat are currently available. The spinal evoked response can be used to localize a spinal cord lesion by analysis of latencies, spinal conduction velocities, and wave forms of the response.[6, 8]

Somatosensory Cortical Evoked Potentials

The somatosensory cortical evoked potentials (SSEP) in the dog and cat have been described by several authors.[21, 29, 30] These potentials are a group of waveforms with highly reliable latencies (Fig. 5–40); they generally must be obtained from animals anesthetized with sodium pentobarbital owing to the depression of these waveforms by most other anesthetics.[12] As in the case of the spinal evoked potential, electric stimulation of a peripheral nerve is used to elicit the potential, but the recording electrodes are placed near the contralateral somatosensory cortex, the ipsilateral somatosensory cortex, or the cisterna magna.[26]

Peripheral Sensory Nerve Potentials (see Section 2, Electromyography)

Visual Potentials

The Electroretinogram

The electroretinogram (ERG) is the recorded electrical activity of the retina evoked by a photic stimulus and is composed of three waves:

Table 5–7. PARAMETERS OF EVOKED POTENTIALS

| Evoked Potential | Stimulus Values | | | Analysis Duration | Amplifier Sensitivity | Number of Responses Averaged |
	Amplitude	Duration	Frequency			
Electroencephalographic audiometry	70 dB	1.0 sec	400–40,000 Hz	5–10 sec	50 μV/cm	1
Brain stem auditory evoked response	50–70 dB (90 dB if necessary)	0.1 msec	10–20 Hz	10 msec	5–10 μV/cm*	64–256
Spinal evoked potential	3–10 V	0.1 msec	5–10 Hz	10–20 msec	5–10 μV/cm*	64–256
Somatosensory cortical evoked potential	3–10 V	0.1 msec	5–10 Hz	20 msec	5–10 μV/cm*	128–512
Nerve conduction velocity (sensory)	3–10 V	0.1 msec	10 Hz	10–20 msec	5–10 μV/cm*	64–256
Electroretinogram	Photic	0.01 msec	2 Hz	10 msec	50–100 μV	4–16 (if averaged)
Visual evoked potential	Photic	0.01 msec	2 Hz	200–300 sec	50–100 μV*	128–512
Electroencephalographic olfactometry	10–15M benzaldehyde	10 sec	—	10–20 sec	50 μV/cm	1
Electroolfactogram	Odor saturated	500 msec	0.2 Hz	3 sec	100 μV/cm	1–16

*Electronic amplification of stored evoked potential may be necessary.

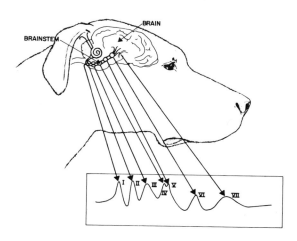

Figure 5–38. Brain stem auditory evoked response. Idealized diagram of waveforms recorded by signal averaging. Neural elements that are believed to sequentially generate the auditory waves: Wave I—cochlea, spiral ganglia, and CN VIII; wave II—cochlear nuclei; wave III—nucleus of the trapezoid body; waves IV and V—lateral lemniscus and lemniscal nuclei and caudal colliculus, respectively (these two waves are frequently combined to form one wave); wave VI—medial geniculate body; wave VII—auditory radiations. Positive is upward.

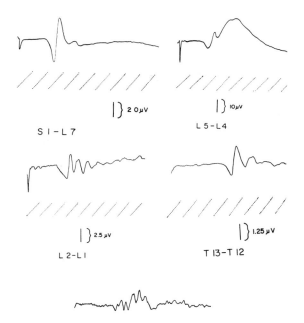

Figure 5–39. Spinal evoked potentials from a cat at different levels of the spinal cord. The tibial nerve was stimulated by rectangular 0.1 msec pulses at 10 Hz. Active recording needle at junction of vertebral bodies indicated. Negative is upward.

Figure 5–40. Short latency somatosensory signal averaged potentials recorded from cisterna magna (CM), ipsilateral sensory cortical area (ISC), and contralateral sensory cortical area (CSC). Active recording needle electrode is subcutaneous in scalp in CSC and ISC and on dura in CM. Numbers indicated are onset of potentials, viz, P–1 is onset of positive developing potential and N–1 is onset of negative developing potential. Negative is upward.

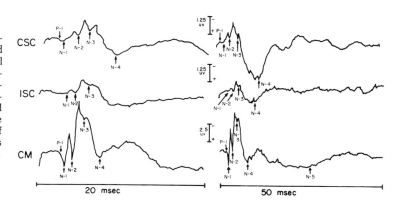

the A wave corresponding primarily to the activation of visual pigment and photoreceptors; the B wave, corresponding primarily to the bipolar cells of the retina; and the C wave, which probably originates in the pigment epithelium and which does not have a known clinical significance[1] (Fig. 5–41). Only the A and B waves are normally used to clinically evaluate retinal function in veterinary medicine.[32]

The electroretinogram is relatively easy to evoke and record, and there are reports of recordings from sheep,[35] swine,[37] cats, dogs,[29] and horses. An averaging computer is not usually required. A storage oscilloscope, polygraph, or electroencephalograph is adequate to measure the ERG. A recording electrode is placed anterior to or on the cornea of the eye of interest, a reference electrode is placed posterior to the orbit, and a stimulus of flashing light is directed into the eye. This light may be white, blue or red filtered.

A characteristic of the ERG in clinical use is the relationship between ERGs recorded under scotopic and photopic conditions. A scotopic ERG exhibits a higher amplitude than an ERG recorded under photopic conditions (Fig. 5–41). A scotopic ERG is recorded after an animal has been dark adapted for a period required to completely restore rod function. Ideally, this is approximately 20 to 30 minutes; but, practically, over 60% of the increase in amplitude of the scotopic ERG is seen within 3 to 5 minutes. The reason for the higher amplitude of the scotopic ERG is the addition of rod function to the cone function seen in photopic conditions. Thus, both photopic and scotopic ERGs are advisable in retinal evaluation.

A number of diseases in domestic animals have been described in which the ERG is altered. Progressive retinal atrophy seen in the poodle,[4] the rod dysplasia of the Norwegian elkhound,[2, 3] and the rod-cone dysplasia of the Irish setter[5] breeds are best known. In these syndromes, the ERG provides the earliest diagnosis currently available.[28] In the Irish setter and Norwegian elkhound the earliest finding clinically is night blindness (nyctalopia). Developing nyctalopia may be diagnosed as early as 6 weeks of age by the reduction of amplitude in the scotopic ERG, whereas clinical signs of the disease may not be apparent for 1 to 2 years. Advanced degeneration of the retina is made obvious by reduction or absence of the photopic ERG. Progressive retinal atrophy in the poodle is detected as early as 9 weeks of age by observation of prolonged duration and decreased amplitude of all waves of the ERG.[4] Retinal degeneration also occurs in cats, but no diagnosis based on the ERG is yet reported. Nyctalopia in which the scotopic ERG is not significantly larger in amplitude than the photopic has also been described in appaloosa horses. A retinopathy caused by vitamin E deficiency has also been described in dogs.[31]

The ERG is also used to evaluate the degree of retinal degeneration in animals with cataracts and, therefore, determine the advisability of surgical removal of the cataracts.

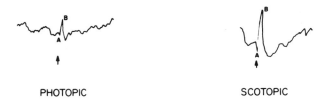

PHOTOPIC SCOTOPIC

Figure 5–41. Electroretinographic recordings from a normal dog under photopic (light adapted), scotopic (dark adapted), flicker stimuli up to 40 Hz. Positive is upward.

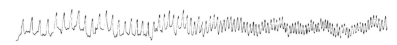

40 Hz

FLICKER

50 μV

200 ms

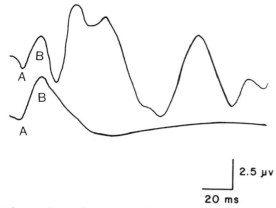

Figure 5–42. Signal averaged, short latency visual evoked response (VER) from a normal dog (upper). Simultaneously recorded electroretinogram (ERG) (lower). Note that the first waves of the VER are volume conducted ERG. A and B waves of the ERG are indicated. Positive is upward.

The Visual Evoked Response

The visual evoked response (VER) has been recorded in dogs.[19, 22] horses, swine,[37] and cats.[13] It is the time locked EEG activity evoked by light flash stimuli, although the VER has also been performed using certain light patterns. The response consists of a variable number of waves in the cat with reported high variability of waveforms.[13] Amplitude of these waves is extremely low, ranging from 0.5 to 2.0 μV (Fig. 5–42).

Clinically, the VER has not been used extensively in veterinary medicine but has been reported to be useful in the diagnosis of amaurosis (blindness not originating from the eye) in the syndrome of arsanilic acid poisoning in swine.[37] In this disease the ERG appears to be normal, but the waveforms of the VER are absent. It has also been used to evaluate visual acuity in the dog[9] and cat.[16] The VER has use in human medicine to diagnose forebrain and brain stem lesions, particularly in cases of multiple sclerosis, but this application in veterinary medicine has not yet been reported.

Olfactory Potentials

Electroencephalographic Olfactometry

Electroencephalographic olfactometry has been developed recently to evaluate the sense of smell in the dog. It involves recording of the standard EEG and the EMG of the neck musculature in response to a controlled olfactory stimulus. The EEG component of the recording is extremely difficult to evaluate owing to extensive EMG artifact, and the EMG of the neck and head musculature increases in amplitude with increasing concentrations of odoriferous substances. It is a useful technique to approximate the threshold stimuli for olfactory sensation in the dog (Fig. 5–43) and has been used to demonstrate olfactory deficits in cases of canine parainfluenza and canine distemper.

Electroolfactogram

The electroolfactogram (EOG) is the electric response of the olfactory mucosa recorded with a flexible catheter electrode in response to a 500 msec saturated vapor olfactory stimulus (ethyl butyrate) applied to the mucosa.[25] The electroolfactogram evoked by this technique is a biphasic, long latency response with average onset of 214 msec and average amplitude of 144 μV in mesaticephalic dogs. This evoked response is yet in the experimental stage but

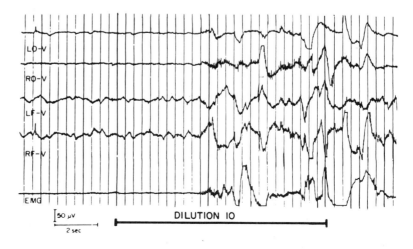

Figure 5–43. Electroencephalographic olfactometry. EEG and EMG recorded before, during, and after olfactory stimulation (horizontal line below EMG). Stimulus was 10^{-10} M benzaldehyde. Note that EMG and EEG and artifact response occurred approximately 2 seconds after onset of stimuli.

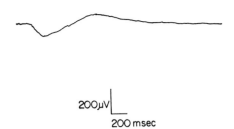

$200\mu V$
200 msec

Figure 5–44. Electroolfactogram from a normal dog. Active recording electrode placed on olfactory mucosa. Negative is upward.

shows promise in the diagnosis of anosmia, and perhaps hyposmia, in the dog (Fig. 5–44).

Olfactory Evoked Cortical Response

The olfactory evoked cortical response (OFR) is the time locked EEG activity associated with an olfactory stimulus. It has been used clinically in human medicine but has yet to be so employed in veterinary medicine. It is an experimental diagnostic technique that may eventually be used in diagnosis of anosmia and hyposmia, and further study may show it to be beneficial in a manner similar to the brain stem auditory evoked response in diagnosis of brain lesions.

Gustatory Potentials

Gustatory Evoked Response

The gustatory evoked response (GER) is an experimental technique with potential for diagnosis of ageusia (inability to taste) and hypogeusia (reduced ability to taste). Much developmental work remains to be done on this potential prior to its clinical use.

REFERENCES

1. Adrian ED: The electric response of the human eye. J Physiol 104:84, 1945.
2. Aguirre, GD and Rubin LF: Progressive retinal atrophy (rod dysplasia) in the Norwegian elkhound. JAVMA 158:208, 1971.
3. Aguirre, GD and Rubin LF: The early diagnosis of rod dysplasia in the Norwegian elkhound. JAVMA 159:429, 1971.
4. Aguirre, GD and Rubin LF: Progressive retinal atrophy in the miniature poodle: An electrophysiologic study. JAVMA 160:191, 1972.
5. Aguirre GD and Rubin LF: Rod-cone dysplasia (progressive retinal atrophy) in Irish setters. JAVMA 166:157, 1975.
6. Bennett MH: Effects of compression and ischemia on spinal cord evoked potentials. Exp Neurol 80:508, 1983.
7. Bernhard CG: The spinal cord potentials in leads from the cord dorsum in relation to peripheral source of afferent stimulation. Acta Physiol Scand 29 (Suppl) 106:1, 1953.
8. Bernhard CG and Widen L: On the origin of the negative and positive spinal cord potential evoked by stimulation of low threshold cutaneous fibers. Acta Physiol Scand 20 (Suppl) 106:42, 1953.
9. Bromberg N and Dawson W: Preliminary measures of canine visual spatial resolutions with electrophysiological techniques. Trans 11th Ann Scientific Program of the College of Veterinary Ophthalmologists, Chicago, November 2 and 3, 1980.
10. Buchwald JS and Huang C-M: Far field acoustic response: Origins in the cat. Science 189:392, 1975.
11. Buchwald JS, Hinman C, Norman RJ, et al: Middle and long latency auditory evoked responses recorded from the vertex of normal and chronically lesioned cats. Brain Res 205:91, 1981.
12. Coles, JG, Wilson, GJ, Sima AF, et al: Intraoperative detection of spinal cord ischemia using somatosensory cortical evoked potentials during thoracic aortic occlusion. Ann Thorac Surg 34:299, 1982.
13. Creel, D, Dustman RE, and Beck EC. Intensity of flash illumination and the visually evoked potential of rats, guinea pigs and cats. Vision Res 14:725, 1974.
14. Crowell WA, Divers TJ, Byers TD, et al: Neomycin toxicosis in calves. Am J Vet Res 42:29, 1981.
15. Farley GR and Starr A: Middle and long latency auditory evoked potentials in cat. I. Component definition and dependence on behavioral factors. Hearing Res 10:117, 1983.
16. Harris LR: Contrast sensitivity and acuity of a conscious cat by the occipital evoked potential. Vision Res 18:175, 1978.
17. Hoerlein BF, Redding RW, Hoff EJ, and McGuire DA: Evaluation of dexamethasone, DMSO, mannitol and solcoseryl in acute spinal cord trauma. J Anim Hosp Assoc 19:216, 1983.
18. Holliday TA, Weldon, NE, and Ealand BG: Percutaneous recording of evoked spinal cord potentials of the dog. Am J Vet Res 40:326, 1979.
19. Howard DR and Breazile JE: Normal visual cortical-evoked response in the dog. Am J Vet Res 33(11):2155, 1972.
20. Kay R, Palmer AC, and Taylor PM: Hearing in the dog as assessed by auditory brainstem evoked potentials. Vet Rec 114:81, 1984.
21. Kornegay JN, Marshall AE, Purinton PT, and Oliver JE: Somatosensory evoked potentials in clinically normal dogs. Am J Vet Res 42:70, 1981.
22. Malnati GA, Marshall AE, and Coulter DB: Electroretinographic components of the canine visual evoked response. Am J Vet Res 42(1):159, 1981.
23. Marshall AE, Byars TD, Whitlock RH, and George LW: Brainstem auditory evoked response in the diagnosis of inner ear injury in the horse. JAVMA 178:282, 1981.
24. Morgan JL, Coulter DB, Marshall AE, and Goetsch DD: Effects of neomycin on the waveform of auditory-evoked brain stem potentials in dogs. Am J Vet Res 41:1077, 1980.
25. Myers LJ, Nash R, and Elledge HS: Electroolfactography: A technique with potential for diagnosis of anosmia in the dog. Am J Vet Res 45:2296, 1984.
26. Nash R: Reference Values for the Feline Somtosensory Evoked Response. Thesis (MS). Auburn University, Auburn, AL, 1984.
27. Parry HB, Tansley K, and Thompson LC: The electroretinogram of the dog. J Physiol 120:28, 1953.

28. Parry HB, Tansley K, and Thompson LC: Electroretin-ogram during development of hereditary retinal degen-eration in the dog. Br J Ophthalmol 39:349, 1955.

29. Purinton PT, Oliver JE, and Bradley WE: Difference in routing of pelvic visceral afferent fibers in the dog and cat. Exp Neurol 73:725, 1981.

30. Purinton PT, Oliver JE, Kornegay JN, and Bradley WE: Cortical averaged evoked potentials produced by pudendal nerve stimulation in dogs. Am J Vet Res 44:446, 1983.

31. Riis RC, Sheffy BE, Loew E, et al: Vitamin E deficiency retinopathy in dogs. Am J Vet Res 42:74, 1981.

32. Rubin LF: Clinical retinography in dogs. JAVMA 151:1456, 1967.

33. Sims MH and Moore RE: Auditory-evoked response in the clinically normal dog: Early latency components. Am J Vet Res 45:2019, 1984.

34. Sims MH and Moore RE: Auditory-evoked response in the clinically normal dog: Middle latency components. Am J Vet Res 45:2028, 1984.

35. Smith EL, Witzel DA, and Pitts DG: The waveform and scotopic CFF of the sheep electroretinogram. Vision Res 16:1241, 1976.

36. Starr A and Farley GR: Middle and long latency auditory evoked potentials in cat. II. Component dis-tributions and dependence on stimulus factors. Hearing Res 10:139, 1983.

37. Witzell DA, Smith EL, Beerwinkle KR, and Johnson JH: Arsanilic acid-induced blindness in swine: Electro-retinographic and visually evoked responses. Am J Vet Res 37:521, 1976.

38. Young W and Flamm ES: Effect of high-dose cortico-steroid therapy on blood flow evoked potentials, and extra cellular calcium in experimental spinal injury. J Neurosurg 51:667, 1982.

Section 4   *DB Coulter, DVM, PhD*

TYMPANOMETRY AND ACOUSTIC REFLEX

OBJECTIVES

Tympanometry uses impedance audiometry to evaluate the mobility and patency of the tympanic membrane, the functional condition of the middle ear, and the ventilation capability of the auditory (eustachian) tube. The acoustic reflex, middle ear muscle contraction after a loud noise, can also be evaluated by impedance audiometry.

INSTRUMENTATION AND TECHNIQUE

Most commercially available electroacoustic impedance bridges contain instrumentation for monitoring acoustic impedance at the plane of the tympanic membrane, changing air pressure in the external ear canal, eliciting the acoustic reflex, and recording the impedance (compli-ance) changes.[5]

Figure 5–45 is a diagram of the basic nonre-cording instrument components needed for tympanometry and testing of the acoustic reflex. A low frequency, relatively intense, continuous pure tone signal delivered by the probe sealed in the external ear canal is reflected back to the microphone (Fig. 5–45) and is measured as a sound pressure level. The sound pressure level varies with the acoustic impedance (compliance) of the middle ear system. The low frequency selected by manufacturers can affect the ap-pearance of tympanograms.

Tympanometry

For tympanometry, the ear probe is sealed in the external ear canal while the instrument delivers a continuous low frequency sound and the air pressure is varied in the closed ear canal. The external ear canal pressure (relative to atmospheric pressure) is varied from about $+300$ mm H_2O to -300 mm H_2O over a 3 to 5 second period. A plot of the sound pressure level (impedance) is recorded. Various tympan-ograms are shown in Figure 5–46.

Acoustic Reflex

For testing the acoustic reflex, a loud sound is introduced in addition to the low frequency sound. The external ear canal pressure is set at a point of maximal tympanic membrane com-pliance as determined by tympanometry. The stimulus (loud sound) results in a small change in the impedance (compliance) of the middle ear system. Because the acoustic reflex is bilat-eral (like the pupillary light reflex) even with unilateral stimulation, both ipsilateral and con-tralateral acoustic reflexes can be elicited and recorded. The ipsilateral reflex is both elicited and recorded in the same ear. The contralateral reflex is elicited in one ear by a loud sound and recorded from the other ear.

INTERPRETATION

Tympanometry

Most of the abnormalities that cause changes in middle ear impedance (compliance) are

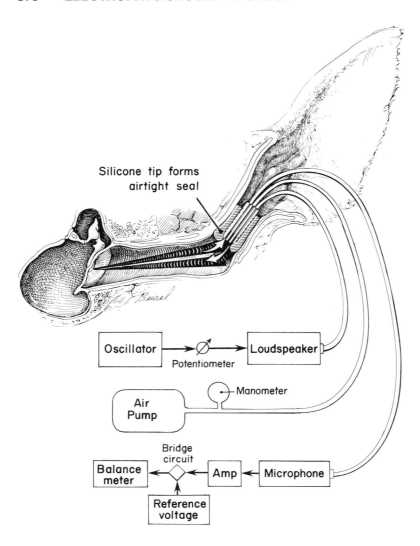

Silicone tip forms
airtight seal

Figure 5–45. A schematic representation of the basic instrumental components of an impedance audiometer with the probe (tip) placed in the external ear canal. The recording components are not shown. (From Penrod JP and Coulter DB: The diagnostic uses of impedance audiometry in the dog. J Am Anim Hosp Assoc 16:941, 1980.)

shown in Figure 5–46. Normal tympanograms of animals vary with breed, age, and sex, but these variations are not well documented. The physical volume test, which is used to determine the size of the external ear canal in cubic centimeters, is, therefore, quite variable in animals. If the external ear canal is blocked with wax or debris, the trace and/or reading of the impedance audiometer will be quite small (near 0.2 ml), or if the probe is pressed against the ear canal wall, the physical volume will be low (near 0.2 ml). If the pressure in the middle ear approximates atmospheric pressure, maximum compliance will be near zero ($\pm$ 100 mm H_2O). Amplitude of a normal tympanogram reflects skeletal muscle tone. The amplitude of a tympanogram from a conscious dog will be lower than that from a tranquilized or anesthe-

tized dog.[6] Tympanograms can be normal in appearance in the presence of neural deafness.

Loss of compliance (high impedance) of the tympanic membrane (Fig. 5–46 b and c) is associated with age and otitis media with effusion. Injury can decrease membrane compliance. However, large surgical incisions in the membrane of cats that left visual scars could not be detected tympanometrically 1 month after surgery.[7]

A perforated tympanic membrane may permit the low frequency probe tone to reflect back from the external ear canal and the middle ear, resulting in a large volume measure and no deflection as the pressure changes (Fig. 5–46d). With a perforated membrane, it may be difficult to raise the pressure in the external ear canal as the air escapes out of the auditory tube.

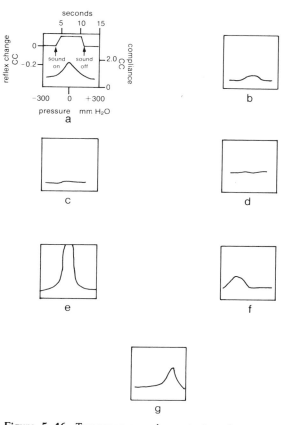

Figure 5–46. Tympanograms demonstrating changes in middle ear impedance (compliance). a, Tympanogram of a normal middle ear. Note that maximal compliance of the tympanic membrane occurs near zero pressure, i.e., middle ear pressure equals atmospheric pressure. At the top of scheme a normal acoustic reflex is shown. The tracing deflects when the loud sound is turned on and returns to baseline when the sound is turned off. The deflection can be either up or down and be normal. b, Tympanogram from an ear with an intact but stiff (reduced compliance) tympanic membrane. Loss of compliance often occurs with middle ear effusion. c, Tympanogram from an ear with a noncompliant tympanic membrane. The membrane is so stiff that no discernable point of maximal compliance is evident. d, Tympanogram from an ear with a perforated tympanic membrane. The elevated trace is the result of the low frequency sound being reflected from a larger (in cubic centimeters) cavity. e, Tympanogram from an ear with a tympanic membrane with excessively high compliance, eg, with disarticulated bony ossicles. f, Tympanogram from an ear with a nonpatent auditory tube. g, Tympanogram from an ear of an animal that is anesthetized with a gas anesthetic. Certain gases will accumulate in the middle ear during anesthesia when the animal is not opening the auditory tube by yawning or swallowing. The greater amplitude is due to an increase in tympanic membrane compliance as a result of relaxation of the skeletal muscles in the middle ear.

A flaccid tympanic membrane or discontinuity of the middle ear ossicular chain results in excessively high compliance (Fig. 5–46e).

The normal auditory tube pumps fluid from the middle ear into the pharynx and periodically

opens during yawning and swallowing to maintain the middle ear at atmospheric pressure.[4, 8] If the tube is blocked owing to inflammation or mucus and the ingress of air is prevented, the trapped oxygen and nitrogen are absorbed by the middle ear mucosal surface, creating a negative pressure. Because tympanic membrane compliance is maximal when external ear canal pressure equals middle ear pressure, a blocked auditory tube results in a tympanogram similar to the one shown in Figure 5–46f. Such a tympanogram may be an early sign of serous otitis media.[9] Serial tympanometry improves diagnostic capabilities in screening for serous otitis media. After gas anesthesia, significant negative pressures in the middle ear may even cause rupture of a tympanic membrane, especially if the membrane has been weakened prior to or during surgery.[11]

Certain gas anesthetics will accumulate in the middle ear during anesthesia when the animal is not opening the auditory tube by yawning, gulping, or swallowing. When this occurs, the tympanogram resembles that shown in Figure 5–46g. The increased amplitude is due to an increase in tympanic membrane compliance as a result of relaxation of the skeletal muscles in the middle ear.

Acoustic Reflex

When a loud sound is introduced by an instrument into the external ear canal, the impedance bridge (Fig. 5–45) picks up the small change in impedance of the middle ear, which is recorded as a deflection (Fig. 5–46a). Because the reflex contraction of the middle ear muscles is bilateral with unilateral stimulation, both ipsilateral and contralateral acoustic reflexes can be recorded. In some birds, the reflex cannot be elicited by a loud sound, although the stapedius muscle does contract during vocalization.[2] The reflex is variable in mammals.[1] The tensor tympani muscle does not contract during the reflex in humans and monkeys. In domestic animals the tensor tympani muscle contracts but not to the extent of the smaller stapedius muscle. There are a few otherwise normal animals that do not show the reflex at any sound level. On the other hand, the reflex can sometimes be recorded even when the tympanic membrane is perforated or other middle ear injury has occurred. The reflex can be elicited from an anesthetized animal. The effects of anesthesia have not been well documented in domestic animals.

The acoustic reflex is more useful when combined with tympanometry. A combination of a negative middle ear pressure and a loss of acoustic reflex is highly suggestive of middle ear effusion.

The reflex decay test is conducted by presenting the loud sound for about 10 seconds. The recorded deflection of the trace is monitored during the stimulus period. In many, but not all, normal ears the deflection will be maintained during the loud sound. With eighth cranial nerve disorders, the deflection often decays (is not maintained).[3] This test has not been well documented in domestic animals.

Facial paralysis (the seventh cranial nerve innervates the stapedius muscle) or middle ear disorders of one ear (unilateral) may be manifested by a loss of the reflex when the recording probe is in the affected ear. Reflex loss is found with both ipsilateral and contralateral stimulation.

In severe cochlear hearing loss or an eighth nerve disorder, the reflex (both ipsilateral and contralateral) cannot be elicited from the affected ear, but the reflex can be elicited in the affected ear by stimulating the normal contralateral ear.[3]

Intraaxial brain stem disorders may result in an absence of contralateral reflexes but the presence of ipsilateral reflexes. If all acoustic reflexes are present and normal in an animal with brain stem signs, it is probable that the disorder is anterior to the acoustic reflex arc.

Acoustic impedance measurements are not tests of hearing, but coupled with brain stem auditory evoked responses, do aid in differentiating conductive malfunction from neural lesions.[10]

REFERENCES

1. Borg E: Excitability of the acoustic m. stapedius and m. tensor tympani reflexes in the nonanesthetized rabbit. Acta Physiol Scand 85:374, 1972.
2. Counter SA and Borg E: Physiological activation of the stapedius muscle in Gallus gallus. Acta Otolaryngol 403:13, 1979.
3. Hayes D and Jerger J: Impedance audiometry in otologic diagnosis. Otolaryngol Clin North Am 11:759, 1978.
4. Honjo I, Okazaki N, Nozoe T, et al: Experimental study of the pumping function of the Eustachian tube. Acta Otolaryngol 92:311, 1970.
5. Jerger J: Clinical experience with impedance audiometry. Arch Otolaryngol 92:311, 1970.
6. Kitzman JV, Chambers JN, and Coulter DB: The effects of halothane-and-oxygen anesthesia, and of halothane-nitrous oxide-and-oxygen anesthesia on tympanograms in the dog. J Aud Res 22:87, 1982.
7. Margolis RH, Osguthorpe JD, and Popelka GR: The effects of experimentally-produced middle ear lesions on tympanometry in cats. Acta Otolaryngol 86:428, 1978.
8. Murphy D: Negative pressure in the middle ear by ciliary propulsion of mucus through the Eustachian tube. Laryngoscope 89:954, 1979.
9. Orchik DJ, Morff R, and Dunn JW: Impedance audiometry in serous otitis media. Arch Otolaryngol 104:409, 1978.
10. Penrod JP and Coulter DB: The diagnostic uses of impedance audiometry in the dog. J Am Anim Hosp Assoc 16:941, 1980.
11. Perreault L, Normandin N, Plamondon L, et al: Tympanic membrane rupture after anesthesia with nitrous oxide. Anesthesisology 57:325, 1982.

Section 5   *JE Oliver, Jr, DVM, MS, PhD*

URODYNAMIC ASSESSMENT

A variety of pressure, flow, and electrophysiologic measurement techniques have been developed to assess the function of the lower urinary tract[2, 3, 5] Most of these are available at a few referral centers. Cost of equipment, frequency of use, and value derived will probably restrict use in veterinary practice. Integration of the data derived from each of these tests into the final diagnosis is discussed in Chapter 13. The tests described have been used on dogs and cats; there is little information available on their use in other domestic animals.[1] Table 5–8 summarizes the data provided by each test.

CYSTOMETRY

Cystometry, the recording of the cystometrogram (CMG), consists of inflating the bladder with a fluid or gas while concurrently recording intravesical pressure.[11, 12] Cystometry is principally a test of detrusor muscle function. The presence or absence of a detrusor reflex can be documented objectively. In addition, the CMG provides data on the threshold volume and pressure, the capacity of the bladder, the ability of the bladder to fill at a normal pressure, and

Table 5–8. INFORMATION PROVIDED BY URODYNAMIC TESTS

	Detrusor Reflex	Detrusor Tone	Urethral Reflex	Urethral Tone	Urethral Obstruction	Pelvic Nerve	Pudendal Nerve	Sacral Spinal Cord	Spinal Cord and Brain
Cystometrogram	+	+				+		+	+
Urethral electromyogram			+				+	+	
Urethral closure pressure profile				+	+				
Uroflowmetry	+			+	+				
Spinal evoked response—bladder						+		+	
Spinal evoked response—urethra							+	+	
Anal evoked response—urethra							+	+	
Cortical evoked response—urethra							+	+	+

+, The test provides information on this function or structure.

the presence of uninhibited bladder contractions.[5, 9]

Techniques and Equipment

Simple open manometer measurement systems using a bottle of sterile water, drip chamber, and manometer have been replaced with automatic recording systems using pressure transducers. These can be purchased commercially* or derived from common laboratory equipment. Gas cystometry is preferred in the author's laboratory, because it is faster, cleaner, and reliable. Some believe that water cystometry is more physiologic. Carbon dioxide (CO_2) is the preferred gas to avoid the possibility of air embolism. A CO_2 tank with a flow meter is required. Water may be delivered by

*For example, Browne Medical, Santa Barbara, CA 93101.

a syringe pump or other laboratory pump. Peristaltic pumps are less desirable because of artifact production. The CO_2 or liquid source is connected in parallel to a pressure transducer and to a catheter in the patient (Fig. 5–47). The pressure transducer is connected to a suitable amplifier and strip chart recorder. Commercial systems are self-contained and have simplified controls.

To perform a cystometrogram, the patient is sedated with xylazine (2 mg/kg subcutaneously).[12] Other drugs have been tested and are less satisfactory. Less than 50% of the animals will tolerate the procedure without sedation.[11] A catheter is placed in the bladder and the bladder emptied. Foley catheter is used in female dogs and the largest size possible regular cather in male dogs and cats. The Foley cather is advantageous in preventing leakage of the gas. After calibration of the machine, the tubing is connected to the catheter and flow of CO_2 started. After a small initial rise in pressure as

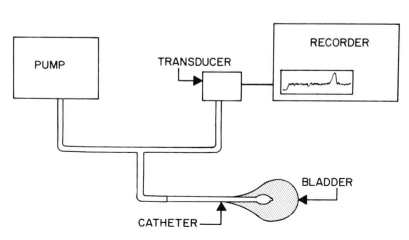

Figure 5–47. Equipment for recording the cystometrogram. (From Oliver JE Jr and Young WO: Evaluation of pharmacologic agents for restraint in cystometry in the dog and cat. Am J Vet Res 34:665, 1973.)

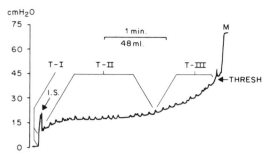

Figure 5–48. Cystometrogram of a dog showing segments of the tonus limb. T–I, Resting pressure; T–II, bladder filling pressure change (smooth muscle elasticity); T–III, bladder filling pressure change after capacity is reached. Scale indicates time and volume. Thresh, threshold of detrusor reflex; M, maximal contraction; I.S., initial spike, an artifact.

$$T-II = \frac{\text{pressure at inflection} - \text{resting pressure} \times 100}{\text{volume}}$$

(From Oliver JE Jr and Young WO: Air cystometry in dogs under xylazine-induced restraint. Am J Vet Res 34:1433, 1973).

the catheter is cleared of fluid, the pressure should remain relatively constant until capacity is reached (Fig. 5–48). As the bladder reaches its capacity, the pressure will gradually start increasing, or a detrusor contraction will occur, causing a sharp rise in pressure. After allowing 1 to 2 seconds to see that the pressure rise is sustained, the catheter must be disconnected from the tubing. Sustained increase in pressure can cause damage to the bladder. If there is no detrusor reflex when the pressure reaches 50 cm H_2O, the test should be stopped to avoid damaging the bladder.

Interpretation

Normal values for the CMG of dogs are given in Table 5–9. The presence or absence of the detrusor reflex is the most important information obtained. More than 90% of normal dogs will have a detrusor reflex using this method.

The resting pressure is rarely of significance. The tonus limb II (T-II) measurement indicates elasticity of the bladder wall. Low values are not significant. High values indicate a loss of elasticity usually caused by inflammation or collagen deposition in the bladder wall. Threshold volume correlates to body size, but it is quite variable. Threshold pressure is relatively consistent but has not shown any correlation to clinical problems. Maximal contraction pressure may be decreased in dogs with voiding problems, but care must be taken in interpretation

because leakage around the catheter will lower this value.

A subjective assessment of bladder sensation may be obtained if the animal becomes apprehensive or restless as the bladder reaches capacity.

URETHRAL CLOSURE PRESSURE PROFILE

The urethral closure pressure profile (UCPP) measures the intraluminal pressure of the urethra throughout its length.[5, 14] Ideally, bladder pressure is measured simultaneously. The parameters calculated from a UCPP are illustrated in Figure 5–49.

Technique and Equipment

The same equipment used for cystometry may be used for the urethral closure pressure profile, with the addition of a device to withdraw the catheter at a constant rate. Commercial equipment is available or a simple device can be constructed.[14] Catheters with side holes must be used. The number and position of holes or catheter size does not seem to matter.[5] Withdrawal rate and recorder speed should be coordinated. The author usually records at twice the speed of withdrawal. Fluid or gas perfusion may be used, but all of the data in animals are based on fluid perfusion. Sterile saline is perfused with a syringe pump at the rate of 2

Table 5–9. NORMAL VALUES FOR CYSTOMETROGRAMS (CMG) OF DOGS, USING XYLAZINE FOR RESTRAINT

Measurement	Mean ± SD Values (N = 41)*
Tonus limb I	9.7 ± 4.3
Tonus limb II	12.6 ± 12.2
Threshold pressure	24.4 ± 10.0
Threshold pressure minus tonus limb I	14.4 ± 8.7
Threshold volume	206.6 ± 184.4
Maximal contraction pressure	77.6 ± 33.8

*N, Number of CMG. All values are given in centimeters of water, except for threshold volume, which is given in milliliters of air (see Fig. 5–48).

From Oliver JE Jr and Young WO: Air cystometry in dogs under xylazine-induced restraint. Am J Vet Res 34:1433, 1973. Used by permission.

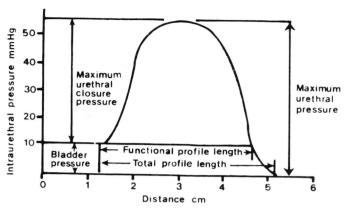

Figure 5–49. Schematic representation of the urethral closure pressure profile. (From Rosin A, Rosin E, and Oliver JE Jr: Canine urethral pressure profile. Am J Vet Res 41:1113, 1980.)

ml/min. Other devices for perfusion may be used, but a peristaltic pump is not satisfactory.[14]

Maximum urethral closure pressure (MUCP) and functional profile length (FPL) are the two most important parameters. MUCP is the maximum urethral pressure minus intravesical pressure. FPL is the length of the urethra where urethral pressure exceeds bladder pressure. Low MUCP or short FPL is associated with incontinence. The point of maximum urethral pressure is usually at the level of the striated sphincter. Stricture may cause a pressure rise at other locations.[13] Normal values are given in Table 5–10.

Multiple channel catheters are being used in humans to record bladder and urethral pressure simultaneously. Limitations on length and diameter have precluded their use in most animals. Such a recording system provides much more information about the physiologic interaction of bladder and urethra.

ELECTROMYOGRAPHY

Electromyography (EMG) of the urethral and anal sphincter and other muscles innervated by the pudendal nerve provides useful information about the status of the motor unit and sacral spinal cord segments.[5, 9, 10] Techniques are described in Section 2, Electromyography, above.

EMG is also useful when recorded with the cystometrogram. Many of the commercial units have provision for recording a channel of electric activity along with the pressure channel. Urethral EMG is more important than anal EMG. The recording can be done with either needle electrodes or a catheter electrode. Urethral EMG can also be recorded during urethral pressure profilometry.

UROFLOWMETRY

The measurement of urine flow during voiding has been called uroflowmetry. A number of methods of measuring flow have been reported in humans.[2, 3, 5] Only one method of uroflowmetry has been reported in veterinary medicine. Moreau et al[6–8] used an electromagnetic flow transducer to record the flow of urine collected in a funnel. They simultaneously recorded intravesical pressure (cystometrogram). The infusion of the bladder and intravesical pressure were accomplished by placement of two catheters into the bladder through the abdominal wall. A urethral EMG could be recorded also.

Uroflowmetry and cystometry recorded simultaneously provide a more complete dynamic picture of micturition. The major disadvantage of this technique is the necessity to place two catheters through the abdominal wall. Moreau et al[6] found minimal deleterious effects of this procedure in a study on 12 dogs. Hematuria and pyuria were noted in a few animals. Leakage from the punctures was not found. Bacter-

Table 5–10. NORMAL VALUES FOR URETHRAL PRESSURE PROFILES OF DOGS, USING XYLAZINE FOR RESTRAINT*

	Maximal Urethral Pressure (mm Hg)	Maximal Urethral Closure Pressure (mm Hg)	Functional Profile Length (cm)
Female dogs	27.1 ± 12.5	23.9 ± 11.8	7.2 ± 1.9
Male dogs	32.7 ± 4.1	28.3 ± 4.0	28.3 ± 3.9

*All values are mean ± standard deviation (see Fig. 5–49).

Modified from Rosin A, Rosin E, and Oliver JE Jr: Canine urethral pressure profile. Am J Vet Res 41:1113, 1980.

iuria was induced in 4 of the 12 dogs. However, this procedure has the potential for leakage. Leakage has occurred in animals following cystocentesis using a 22 gauge needle. These have been animals with some form of neurogenic bladder. Using two 3.5 Fr catheters could increase the risk significantly. The author prefers not to do a cystocentesis if bladder function is abnormal.

OTHER ELECTROPHYSIOLOGIC TESTS

Signal averaging has added several potentially useful tests in the evaluation of neurogenic bladder disorders.[2, 5] The bulbocavernosus reflex and other pudendal reflexes can be measured directly.[4] Stimulation of the urethra or dorsal nerve of penis evokes a reflex contraction of the anal sphincter muscle that can be recorded by a needle or anal plug electrode. This provides objective evaluation of the sensory and motor components of the pudendal nerve.

Spinal evoked response can be recorded from stimulation of the pudendal nerve with a needle electrode.

Combinations of the various tests described can provide information about many of the components of the nervous system involved in micturition. A good, safe, reliable method of evaluating the physiologic process of micturition, including the detrusor reflex and urethral activity, has not been developed for use in animals.

REFERENCES

1. Attenburrow DP and James ED: Urinary incontinence in a pony mare. Equine Vet J 13:206, 1981.
2. Barrett DM and Wein AJ: Controversies in Neurourology. New York, Churchill Livingston, 1984.
3. Bors E and Comarr AE: Neurological Urology. Baltimore, University Park Press, 1971.
4. Bradley WE, Timm GW, Rockswold GL, and Scott FB: Detrusor and urethral electromyelography. J Urol 114:891, 1975.
5. Hald L and Bradley WE: The Urinary Bladder, Neurology and Dynamics. Baltimore, Williams & Wilkins, 1982.
6. Moreau PM, Lees GE, and Gross DR: Simultaneous cystometry and uroflowmetry (micturition study) for evaluation of the caudal part of urinary tract in dogs: Studies of the technique. Am J Vet Res 44:1765, 1983.
7. Moreau PM, Lees GE, and Gross DR: Simultaneous cystometry and uroflowmetry (micturition study) for the evaluation of the caudal part of the urinary tract in dogs: Reference values for healthy animals sedated with xylazine. Am J Vet Res 44:1174, 1983.
8. Moreau PM, Lees GE, and Hobson HP: Simultaneous cystometry and uroflowmetry for evaluation of micturition in two dogs. JAVMA 183:1084, 1983.
9. Oliver JE JR: Disorders of micturition. In Hoerlein BF: Canine Neurology, 3rd ed. Philadelphia, WB Saunders Co, 1978.
10. Oliver JE Jr and Lorenz MD: Handbook of Veterinary Neurologic Diagnosis. Philadelphia, WB Saunders Co, 1983.
11. Oliver JE Jr and Young WO: Evaluation of pharmacologic agents for restraint in cystometry in the dog and cat. Am J Vet Res 34:665, 1973.
12. Oliver JE JR and Young SO: Air cystometry in dogs under xylazine-induced restraint. Am J Vet Res 34:1433, 1973.
13. Rosin AE and Barsanti JA: Diagnosis of urinary incontinence in dogs: Role of the urethral pressure profile. JAVMA 178:814, 1981.
14. Rosin A, Rosin E, and Oliver J: Canine urethral pressure profile. Am J Vet Res 41:113, 1980.

II Diseases of the Nervous System

Chapter 6   KG Braund, DVM, PhD

Degenerative and Developmental Diseases

METABOLIC STORAGE DISEASES

Metabolic storage diseases are rare inherited diseases of humans and animals. As a result of partial or complete deficiency of a single lysosomal enzyme, there is an accumulation or "storage" of that enzyme's substrate and substrate by-products within lysosomes (organelles responsible for the intracellular digestion of polymeric material such as protein, polysaccharides, mucopolysaccharides, and complex lipids)[23, 172, 173] (Fig. 6–1). Although lysosomal storage diseases are often widespread throughout the body, clinically, the majority affect the central nervous system (Table 6–1, Fig. 6–2).

Certain generalizations can be made about this group of diseases:[22]

1. These diseases are rare and occur mainly in dogs and cats.

2. Animals are usually normal at birth.

3. Affected animals fail to grow as rapidly as their littermates.

4. As these conditions usually have a recessive mode of inheritance, only part of a litter is likely to be affected.

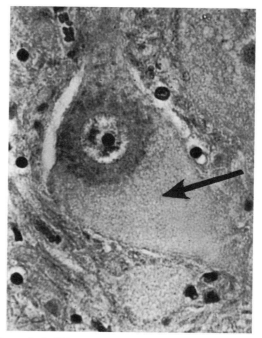

Figure 6–1. GM$_1$ gangliosidosis in a Siamese cat. A neuron contains a large amount of storage material (arrow). Hematoxylin and eosin, high power.

Table 6–1. STORAGE DISEASES IN DOMESTIC ANIMALS

Disease	Enzyme Deficit (Storage Product)	Signalment	Clinical Signs	Human Disease	Reference
Gangliosidosis GM$_1$ Type 1	β-Galactosidase (ganglioside)	Beagle-cross dogs (3 mo); domestic cats (2–3 mo); Friesian cattle (CNS—1 mo)	Tremors, incoordination, spastic paraplegia, impaired vision	Norman-Landing disease	21, 79, 80, 267
Type 2	β-Galactosidase (ganglioside)	Siamese, Korat, and domestic cats (2–3 mo)	As above	Derry's disease	6–10
Gangliosidosis GM$_2$ Type 1	Hexosaminidase A (ganglioside)	German short haired pointer dogs (6–9 mo)	Ataxia, incoordination, impaired vision, dementia	Tay-Sachs disease	181, 182, 222
Type 2	Hexosaminidase A & B (ganglioside)	Domestic cats (2 mo)	Same as cats with GM$_1$ gangliosidosis	Sandhoff's disease	56, 57
Type 3	Hexosaminidase A (ganglioside)	Yorkshire swine (CNS—3 mo)	Ataxia, incoordination, hypermetria	Bernheimer-Seitelberger disease	263, 268
Glucocerebrosidosis	β-Glucosidase (glucocerebroside)	Sydney silky dog (6–8 mo)	Ataxia, incoordination, tremors, hypermetria	Gaucher's disease	137, 309
Sphingomyelinosis	Sphingomyelinase (sphingomyelin)	Siamese, domestic cats (2–4 mo); poodle dogs (2–4 mo)	Ataxia, incoordination, tremors, hypermetria	Niemann-Pick disease	33, 61, 262, 291, 315
Globoid cell leukodystrophy	β-Galactosidase (galactocerebrosidase)	Cairn terrier, West Highland (2–5 mo); beagle, blue-tick (4 mo); mixed, poodle (2 yr); basset hound (1½–2 yr); Pomeranian (1½ yr); domestic cat (5–6 wk), Polled Dorset sheep (4–18 mo)	Ataxia, incoordination, tremors, progressive paraparesis, hypermetria, impaired vision	Krabbe's disease	27, 96, 101, 166, 168, 208, 223, 264, 296, 333
Metachromatic leukodystrophy	Arylsulfatase (sulfatide)	Domestic cat (2 wk)	Progressive motor dysfunction, seizures, opisthotonos		6
Mucopolysaccharidosis	Arylsulfatase B (mucopolysaccharide)	Siamese, domestic cat (4–7 mo)	Progressive paraparesis	Maroteaux-Lamy disease	60, 143, 196
	α-L-Iduronidase (mucopolysaccharide)	Domestic cat (10 mo)	Progressive paraparesis	Hurler's syndrome	144
Glycoproteinosis	(?Glycoprotein)	Beagle, basset hound, poodle dogs (5 mo–9 yr)	Depression, progressive seizures	Lafora's disease	88, 148, 155, 209, 300
Mannosidosis	α-Mannosidase (mannoside)	Domestic cat (7 mo); Angus, Murray gray cattle	Ataxia, incoordination, tremors and aggression (calves)	Mannosidosis	34, 145, 170, 176, 310, 318
	β-Mannosidase (mannoside)	Nubian goats (birth–1 yr)	Ataxia, recumbency	β-Mannosidosis	146
Glycogenesis	α-Glucosidase	Lapland dogs (1½ yr); domestic cat; Corriedale sheep (6 mo); Shorthorn & Brahma cattle (3–9 mo)	Incoordination, exercise intolerance	Pompe's disease	211, 224, 235, 273, 281
Fucosidosis	α-L-Fucosidase	Springer spaniel dogs (2 yrs)	Incoordination, behavioral changes, dysphonia, dysphagia, seizures		138, 185, 203
Ceroid lipofuscinosis	Unknown abnormality	English setter (1 yr); dachshund (3½–7 yr); cocker spaniel (1½ yr); Chihuahua, Saluki dogs (2 yr); Siamese, domestic cats (2–7 yr); South Hampshire sheep (6–18 mo)	Personality change, visual impairment, ataxia, incoordination, jaw champing, seizures	Batten's disease, Ceroid lipofuscinosis	2, 62, 129, 192, 193, 196, 238, 259, 266, 269, 284, 307

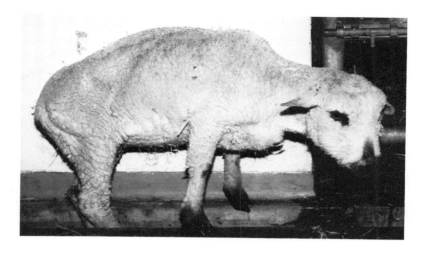

Figure 6–2. Ovine ceroid lipofuscinosis (OCL). This two year old South Hampshire ewe is in the terminal stages. The ewe is totally blind, with some residual pupillary constrictor responses to bright light; has profound dementia; and tends to wander and become stuck in fences, gates, or drains (as shown). Seizure activity is evident as intermittent episodes of jaw chomping, head nodding, and face, neck, and occasionally thoracic limb muscle spasms. The ewe has severe cerebral atrophy (brain weight approximately half of normal) with widespread astrogliosis, neuronal loss, and cellular lipofuscin accumulation. (Courtesy of RD Jolly, Massey University, New Zealand.)

5. Specific diseases are known to be present in certain breeds.

6. There is often a history of inbreeding.

7. Many manifest as neurologic disorders in young animals, usually at a few months of age.

8. The disease is always progressive and has a fatal outcome.

9. The age of onset and speed of progression are usually directly related.

10. More than one system may be involved.

There are a number of plant intoxications of ruminants and horses that clinically and pathologically mimic inherited storage diseases.[174]

Diagnosis of metabolic storage diseases can be made by determining lysosomal enzyme activities from brain, viscera, or a preparation of white blood cells. The activity of the deficient enzyme will be low, whereas the activity of other lysosomal enzymes tends to be increased. Specialized laboratories are usually necessary to confirm a diagnosis.

The outlook for specific therapy is not encouraging.

An unclassified lysosomal storage disease has been reported in Abyssinian cats.[196, 302] Several unclassified leukodystrophies have been reported in cats,[97, 149] and a hereditary "cavitating" leukodystrophy has been described in Dalmatian dogs.[17] A suspected neurologic storage disease has been reported in cattle.[142]

NEURONAL ABIOTROPHIES AND DEGENERATIONS

There are many degenerative disorders affecting the nervous system of domestic animals. The majority are hereditary, or suspected of being hereditary in nature, and are characterized by premature aging and degeneration and death of various neuronal cell populations. The cause and pathogenesis are not known. The mechanism of premature degeneration of cells is termed abiotrophy, implying an inherent lack of trophic or nutritive factor. Degenerative diseases tend to be breed related. Clinical signs frequently occur in young animals, usually within a few months after birth. An exception to this rule is degenerative myelopathy in German shepherd dogs, which is observed most often in dogs over 5 years of age. Progressive signs of neurologic deficits generally are present with degenerative disorders.

Antemortem diagnosis is based on clinical signs, age, and breed and on ruling out acquired diseases. Examination of biopsy material from selected sites, such as the cerebellum, may confirm a diagnosis in some instances. In general, electrodiagnostic aids, clinical biochemistry, and radiology are of limited value in the diagnosis of degenerative disease. Prognosis is guarded to poor. There is no treatment.

Inherited Cerebellar Degeneration in the Kerry Blue Terrier

This is an autosomal recessive disease that affects Kerry blue terriers. Degenerative lesions are initially observed in the Purkinje cell (+/- granule cell) layers, followed by symmetric, bilateral neuronal degeneration in the olivary nuclei after 3 to 4 months of clinical signs. Several months later, neurons of the substantia nigra and caudate nuclei degenerate in a symmetric fashion.[69]

Clinical signs of stiffness of pelvic limbs and head tremors reflect cerebellar disease and are seen between 8 and 16 weeks of age. Subsequent signs include dysmetria-hypermetria and often inability to stand by 1 year of age.

Inherited Degeneration in the Rough Coated Collie

This is an autosomal recessive disease reported in rough coated collie dogs in Australia in which there is early and rapid degeneration of Purkinje cells and granule cells of the cerebellum.[136] Other changes include neuron depletion in cerebellar roof nuclei, lateral vestibular nuclei, inferior olivary nuclei, and ventral horns of spinal cord.

Pelvic limb incoordination occurs between 1 and 2 months of age. Subsequently, animals develop a broad based stance, hypermetria, and head tremors, and occasionally a bunny hopping gait.

A similar disorder has been reported recently in the border collie working sheepdog in New Zealand.[121]

Inherited Cerebellar Degeneration in the Gordon Setter

This is an autosomal recessive, late onset cerebellar disease affecting mature Gordon setters between 6 and 30 months of age.[58, 65–67, 71] Lesions are restricted to the cerebellum and characterized by profound loss of Purkinje cells throughout most of the cerebellar cortex. The molecular layer is moderately thinned and the granule cell layer varies in thickness. Dogs appear normal during the first 6 months of life, but between 9 and 18 months they may develop a mild thoracic limb stiffness, hypermetria, broad based stance, and occasional stumbling. Nystagmus occurs late. These signs progress slowly or remain static after a short period of progression.

Cerebellar Degeneration in Arabian Horses

Arabian horses demonstrate Purkinje cell loss, often with a paucity of granule neurons, for which a hereditary basis is presumed.[86, 103, 248] Onset of signs is from birth to a few months of age. Clinical signs are characterized by symmetric spasticity of all limbs, dysmetria-hypermetria, and intention tremor. Signs may progress rapidly, then remain stabilized or slowly progress. Prognosis is guarded. There is no treatment.

A similar clinical and pathologic syndrome is reported in Gotland ponies, with onset of signs from birth to 6 months. An autosomal recessive inheritance has been documented for this disease.[19]

Cerebellar Degeneration in Other Breeds/Species

Cerebellar degenerations, usually involving Purkinje cells, have been reported in families of Samoyeds (with swollen axons of Purkinje neurons in the granule cell layer), Airedale terriers, Finnish harriers, and Bern running dogs. A genetic basis has been suggested. A similar disorder has been observed in single litters of Labrador retrievers, golden retrievers, beagles, cocker spaniels, Cairn terriers, and Great Danes.[65–67, 71] Cerebellar cortical atrophy characterized by selective degeneration of Purkinje cells of the cerebellum has been described in lambs (daft lamb disease), Yorkshire piglets, and several breeds of calves.[13, 68, 157, 161, 317] In lambs the disease is inherited as a single autosomal recessive trait. The hereditary nature of the disorder in calves and piglets remains to be clarified.

Hereditary Ataxia in Smooth Haired Fox Terriers

Hereditary ataxia is an autosomal recessive disorder in smooth haired fox terriers that has been reported as a clinical entity in Sweden since 1941.[18, 20] A similar condition has been described in Britain in Jack Russell terriers, a type of short legged, smooth haired terrier developed within the smooth haired fox terrier breed. Pathologically, a focal, wallerian degeneration is found in the dorsolateral and ventromedial white matter of cervical and thoracic spinal cord. In the Jack Russell terriers, degenerative changes are found in central auditory pathways and peripheral nerves.

Clinical signs in both breeds occur between 2 and 6 months of age, when weakness and pelvic limb incoordination are observed.[18, 140] The incoordination progresses to involve all limbs, and a prancing or dancing type of gait is observed. Animals appear to be unable to gauge the extent of a movement, which is unpredictable in direction.[246]

Hereditary Neuroaxonal Dystrophy

Domestic tricolor cats have been found to have an autosomal recessive condition that is characterized pathologically by gross atrophy of the cerebellar vermis and microscopically by marked ballooning of cell processes (spheroids) in nuclear groups extending from the medulla to the thalamus and cerebellar vermis.[324] These changes are accompanied by loss of neurons, including Purkinje and granule cells of the cerebellar vermis. Inner ear lesions have been reported.

Clinical signs occur in kittens at approximately 5 to 6 weeks of age, at which time head tremors and head shaking are observed. Signs progress to marked incoordination of gait and hypermetria. Affected kittens have an abnormal coat color.

Similar clinical and neuropathologic findings are reported in Suffolk sheep[50] and in Rottweiler and collie sheep dogs.[44, 45, 59] The genetic pattern in the dog is suggestive of an autosomal recessive trait. The clinical manifestations of canine neuroaxonal dystrophy are chiefly those of a slowly progressive cerebellar ataxia with incoordination, hypermetria, and wide based stance beginning in the first year of life. The signs progress slowly. Some Rottweilers have been observed up to 6 years of age. The cerebellar ataxia persisted, but there was no loss of strength or mentation. Results of cerebrospinal fluid, electroencephalographic, and electromyographic examinations were normal.[44]

Hereditary Quadriplegia and Amblyopia in the Irish Setter

This is an autosomal recessive, lethal disease of Irish setters. Animals are affected at birth. Although they make coordinated walking or paddling movements, they are unable to stand or walk unaided, and propel themselves on their bellies with a swimming type of action.[251] Signs progress to visual impairment, amblyopic nystagmus, head tremor, and seizures. No convincing neuropathologic changes have been found to account for the clinical signs.[246, 251]

Hereditary Neuronal Abiotrophy in Swedish Lapland Dogs

This is an autosomal recessive disease that has been reported in Swedish Lapland dogs.[278, 279] Degeneration of Purkinje cells and spinal ganglion cells occurs, together with diffuse axonal degeneration in the medullary rays of the cerebellum and projections of the dorsal roots and cranial nerves II, V, and VII and in the dorsal funiculus of the spinal cord and spinocerebellar tracts. Neuronal degeneration and loss are observed in the ventral gray matter in cervical and lumbar intumescences.[278, 279]

Only the spinal cord lesions are detected clinically. Signs appear in affected puppies at 5 to 7 weeks of age. The onset is marked by thoracic or pelvic limb weakness that progresses rapidly to tetraparesis. Subsequent muscle wasting and deformity are most pronounced in distal portions of the limbs. Spinal reflexes are reduced or absent, and electromyographic examination reveals denervation potentials.

Hereditary Canine Spinal Muscular Atrophy

Hereditary canine spinal muscular atrophy is a dominantly inherited lower motor neuron disease in Brittany spaniels. The motor neurons of selected brain stem nuclei and ventral horn of the spinal cord are characterized by chromatolysis, neuronal depletion, and neurofibrillary abnormalities in perikarya, dendrites, and proximal axons.[53–55] Three phenotypic variants have been recognized: (1) Early onset: Pups become weak by 1 month of age and are tetraparetic by 3 to 4 months; (2) Intermediate onset: Clinical signs develop between 4 and 6 months of age, pups are tetraparetic by 2 to 3 years; (3) Late onset: This is characterized by slowly progressive disease with dogs surviving well into adult life.

In all three phenotypes muscle weakness first appears in proximal muscles of limb girdles and trunk. Animals walk in a waddling fashion. Progressive atrophy ensues in proximal muscles of pelvic limbs and lumbar paraspinal muscles. In some dogs, cranial nerve abnormalities are observed and include weakness and atrophy of facial muscles (causing wrinkling of facial skin and wide palpebral fissures), depressed gag reflex, and decreased muscle tone in the tongue. Severely affected animals remain in lateral recumbency and are unable to raise their heads.[206]

Electromyography reveals sporadic fibrillations, fasciculations, and occasional polyphasic potentials. Nerve conduction studies are normal. Degenerative changes in peripheral nerves result in neurogenic atrophy in more proximal skeletal muscles.

Hereditary Progressive Neurogenic Muscular Atrophy in Pointer Dogs

A hereditary disorder has been described in pointer dogs.[160] Clinical signs of weakness, dysphonia, and diminished tendon reflexes are observed in affected dogs at about 5 months of age. Progressive muscular atrophy occurs in all limbs and trunk, particularly in the shoulder region. Muscle fasciculations are present. Animals eventually become tetraplegic. On EMG examination, fibrillation potentials and positive sharp waves are noted.

Axonal degeneration is found in peripheral

nerves.[163] Numerous accumulated lipidlike granules occur in ventral horn cells of the spinal cord and in hypoglossal and spinal accessory nuclei of the brain stem.

Stockard's Spinal Muscular Atrophy of Dogs

This degenerative condition was produced in 1936 by crossbreeding Great Danes with bloodhounds and St Bernards. Pathologic changes observed are degeneration and depletion of motor and preganglionic sympathetic neurons in ventral and intermediolateral horns of lumbar spinal cord.[294] The disease is transmitted through an inheritable factor involving at least three dominant genes.

Clinical signs occur at 3 months of age and are characterized by sudden onset of paresis and posterior paralysis and atrophy of pelvic limb appendicular muscles. Prognosis is poor. There is no treatment.

Lower Motor Neuron Disease

A hereditary basis has not been established for several diseases occurring in young animals in which pathologic changes are restricted to lower motor neurons in spinal cord and brain stem. A neurologic syndrome has been reported in New Zealand involving nine dogs, seven of which were sheepdogs of the collie type.[135] Seven of the dogs were from 3 to 9 months of age, one was 1 year old and one 2 years old. In the central nervous system, lesions were restricted to the spinal cord and were characterized by depletion of large motor neurons at various levels, accompanied by degeneration of ventral spinal roots and neurogenic atrophy of appendicular muscle.

Clinical signs included a sudden onset of posterior paresis with rapid progression (2 to 4 weeks) to flaccid paralysis and/or tetraplegia.

Degeneration of lower motor neurons and white matter in ventral columns has been reported in three Siamese kittens from two different litters. Body tremors and dysmetria were noted at 10 days of age.[105]

A similar disorder has been reported in a kitten.[308] Neuronal degeneration and depletion were observed in the large motor neurons of the lateral parts of the ventral horns in cervical and lumbar intumescences, wallerian degeneration of ventral roots, and neurogenic atrophy of appendicular muscle. The degeneration of nerve cells was characterized by abnormal accumulation of neurofilaments. The cat was the only one affected in a litter of four. At 3 to 4 weeks of age weakness was noted in all limbs. This progressed to complete tetraplegia within 2 to 3 weeks. Lower motor neuron signs associated with neurofibrillary accumulation have also been reported in enzootic ataxia of sheep[34] and goats,[49] a puppy,[72] a zebra,[152] and piglets.[150] The condition in sheep and goats is a slowly progressive degenerative disorder of specific populations of neurons that is related to copper deficiency in the dam and offspring. Affected Yorkshire piglets showed progressive ataxia and marked weakness associated with diffuse wallerian-type degeneration in the spinal cord white matter and ventral peripheral nerve roots. There was neurofilamentous accumulation in motor neurons of the brain stem and spinal cord, although no association with low copper intake could be found.[150]

A newly recognized, heritable, neurodegenerative disorder of newborn, horned Hereford calves has been reported from Canada.[275] Generalized tremor, difficulty in standing, and stiff ataxic movements were noted. There was neurofibrillary accumulation in neurons of the central, peripheral, and autonomic nervous systems, with concomitant axonal degeneration in spinal cord white matter and in ventral nerve roots.

Pelvic limb spasticity occurred in all 61 Landrace piglets from eight litters in South Africa. At 2 weeks, affected piglets became paraplegic. Neuronal degeneration was described in the red nucleus, cerebellar nuclei, and lumbar spinal cord, with no etiology being determined.[237]

Demyelination in Miniature Poodles

A suspected hereditary disorder in miniature poodles has been reported.[81, 219, 293] Pathologically, diffuse demyelination was found throughout all columns of the spinal cord. Focal areas of malacia were also observed in cerebellar peduncles and tegmentum. Clinical signs first appeared between 2 and 4 months of age. Initial signs of pelvic limb paresis progressed to spastic paraplegia and tetraplegia. Prognosis is poor. There is no treatment.

Cerebrospinal Dysmyelinogenesis

Abnormal myelination of the nervous system has been reported in a variety of animal species.[77, 95, 102, 162] The hereditary nature of this disorder has been established in the pig.[134, 261]

Table 6–2. CONGENITAL TREMOR OF PIGS—DIAGNOSTIC TAXONOMY

Cause	AI (Virus, Hog Cholera)	AII (Virus Unknown)	AIII (Genetic Sex-Linked Recessive)	AIV (Genetic, Autosomal Recessive)	AV (Chemical Trichlorfon)	B (Unknown)
Field Observations						
Proportion of litters affected	High	High	Low	Low	High	Variable
Proportion of pigs affected within litter (approx.)	≥ 40%	≥ 80%	25%	25%	≥ 90%	Variable
Mortality among affected pigs	Medium–high	Low	High	High	High	Variable
Sex of affected pigs	Both	Both	Male	Both	Both	Any
Breed of dam (pure or crossbred)	Any	Any	Landrace	Saddleback	Any	Any
Recurrence in successive litters of same parents	No	No	Yes	Yes	Yes	?
Duration of outbreak	≤ 4 mo	≤ 4 mo	Indefinite	Indefinite	≤ 1 mo	?
Laboratory Observations						
Macroscopic						
Cerebellum:whole brain ratio (≤ 8% = abnormal)	↓	?	?	?	↓	↓?
Spinal cord size (weight)	↓	?	↓	↓	↓	?
Microscopic (CNS)						
Myelin deficiency	+	+	+	+	+	?
Myelin aplasia (partial)	−	−	+	−	−	?
Oligodendrocytes swollen	+	+	−	−	−	?
Oligodendrocytes reduced in number	?	?	+	?	?	?
Neurochemistry (spinal cord)						
Total DNA	↓	?	↓	↓	↓	?
Whole lipid/g	↓	↓	↓	↓	↓	?
Cerebrosides/g	↓	↓	↓	↓	↓	?
Lipid hexose:phosphorus ratio	↓	↓	↓	↓	~	?
Cholesterol esters characteristic of demyelination	+	+	−	+	−	−
Serology						
Maternal antibodies to hog cholera	+	−	−	−	−	−

+, Present; −, absent; ~, not significantly changed; ↓ decreased.

*Type A, A form of congenital tremor with defined pathologic characters and known etiology; type B, a form of congenital tremor as yet inadequately characterized and/or of unknown etiology.

From Done JT and Bradley R: Nervous and muscular system. Reprinted by permission from Diseases of the Swine, Sixth Edition, edited by AD Leman © 1985 by The Iowa State University Press, Ames, Iowa 50010.

Affected Landrace and saddleback pigs are affected with congenital tremor types AIII (sex linked) and AIV (recessive), respectively. Other causes of congenital tremor ("dancing pig disease," "myoclonic congenita," "trembles") are recognized, and the differential characteristics of these diseases are given in Table 6–2.[76]

Dysmyelination of the CNS in chow chow dogs is believed to be hereditary.[305, 306] In these dogs, a severe myelin deficiency is found throughout the central nervous system, especially in subcortical white matter and foliated white matter of the cerebellum. Axons have thin or uncompacted myelin sheaths, separated from each other by massive astrocytosis, and bizarre myelin formations. Peripheral nerves are normally myelinated. The myelin deficiency in absence of degenerative changes indicates a disorder of myelin formation rather than breakdown. Retarded myelination may be due to a dysfunction of delay in glial maturation. Animals show clinical signs at 2 to 4 weeks of age. Clinical signs are characterized by wide based stance, hypermetria, head and body intention tremors, and often a bunny hopping gait. Clinical signs plateau from 6 to 12 months, followed by gradual improvement. A similar myelin disorder has been reported in male springer spaniels that is suggestive of an intrinsic defect of oligodendrocyte metabolism. A sex linked, recessive inheritance has been proposed for this condition.[131]

Cerebrospinal hypomyelinogenesis has been observed in a 5 week old Dalmatian puppy.[125] On pathologic examination, myelin was not found anywhere in the CNS. There was no evidence of active white matter degeneration. The peripheral nervous system was normally myelinated. Generalized body tremors were present at birth. The puppy could not walk voluntarily, and horizontal pendular nystagmus was observed.

Another degenerative myelin disorder has been recognized in Charolais cattle in the United Kingdom, France, and Canada.[24, 247] The etiology and pathogenesis of this chronic progressive neurologic disorder are unknown; however, the nature of the pathologic process suggests a basic derangement of the myelin bearing cell. Lesions are restricted to the white matter of the central nervous system and are characterized by plaques composed of axons surrounded by masses of small processes and disorganized myelin sheaths. Oligodendrocytic processes are hypertrophied and hyperplastic. Lesions are most marked in the internal capsule, cerebellar white matter, and spinal cord.

Clinical signs are first recognized at 8 to 24 months of age and progress from slight ataxia to recumbency over a period of 1 to 2 years.

Hereditary hypomyelinogenesis has been reported in Jersey, Hereford, Shorthorn, and Angus-Shorthorn breeds of cattle.[157, 283, 331]

Fibrinoid Leukodystrophy of Labrador Retrievers

A fibrinoid leukodystrophy characterized by symmetric dysmyelination and perivascular gliosis of cerebral and cerebellar hemispheres has been observed in Labrador retriever dogs.[221, 290] Clinical signs noted at about 6 months of age included pelvic limb paresis, progressive ataxia, and generalized weakness.

Hereditary Myelopathy of Afghan Hounds

This disease in Afghan hounds has an autosomal recessive mode of inheritance.[4] Histologic lesions are limited to the spinal cord from caudal cervical regions to midlumbar segments and to dorsal nucleus of the trapezoid body. Cavitation and necrosis occur in white matter, especially in midthoracic cord segments. Funicular axons remain intact. Gray matter involvement is confined to the dorsal nucleus of the trapezoid body and to the periphery of the spinal ventral gray columns. The cause of these lesions has not been determined.[4, 63]

Clinical signs occur between 3 and 8 months of age. Pelvic limb paresis and ataxia are the first signs observed. Within 1 to 3 weeks, these signs progress to paraplegia, thoracic limb paresis, and truncal ataxia. Pelvic limbs and caudal thorax may be analgesic.[4, 47, 63]

Leukoencephalomyelopathy of Rottweiler Dogs

A demyelinating disorder of the spinal cord and brain has been reported in two rottweiler dogs.[113] A 3 year old female and a 4 year old male had a slowly progressive course for 7 to 9 months. There was a common grandsire on their sire's side. Clinical signs included ataxia, tetraparesis, dysmetria, delayed proprioceptive positioning, and exaggerated spinal reflexes. All diagnostic studies including CSF analysis, EMG, and myelography were normal. One dog was treated with corticosteroids for 2 months without improvement. Demyelinating lesions were found in the brain stem, deep cerebellar white matter, and spinal cord. The cause is unknown.

Degenerative Myelopathy in Dogs

This degenerative disease may have an inherited basis. It is most often observed in German shepherd dogs over 5 years of age. A similar condition has been reported in other breeds of large dogs.[130] The pathogenesis of this disease is unknown. It is unrelated to intervertebral disk degeneration, spondylosis deformans, or osseous metaplasia of dura mater. Vitamin deficiency, trauma, and vascular disease have been suggested as possible causes.[3] Morphometric data[31] do not support the hypothesis that this disease represents a "dying back" neuropathy.[130] More recent suggestions that immunologic factors (suppressor cells) may play a role[311, 312] need further clarification. The significance of reportedly abnormal activities of brush border and lysosomal enzymes in the intestines of dogs with degenerative myelopathy is unknown.[320] Pathologically, the most severe lesions are found in the thoracic spinal cord and are characterized by degeneration of white matter, especially in dorsolateral and ventromedial funiculi. Dorsal root involvement and loss of neurons in dorsal gray horns of spinal cord have been observed in some German shepherd dogs.[3, 130] The onset of the disease is insidious. Initial signs include pelvic limb ataxia and paresis. The signs progress slowly to truncal ataxia and severe pelvic limb paresis. Knuckling of paws of pelvic limbs is commonly observed. Some dogs have a depressed patellar reflex. Sphincter function remains normal. The disease is usually slowly progressive.

Diagnosis is based on clinical syndrome, breed, and age. Results of radiography and myelography are normal, which distinguishes degenerative myelopathy from disk protrusion and neoplasia. There is no satisfactory treatment currently available. A similar disorder has been reported in cats.[218] The cause is unknown and treatment is ineffective.

Hound Ataxia

A degenerative myelopathy has been recognized in Britain in adult foxhounds, harriers, and beagles.[246, 250] Histologically, severe wallerian degeneration is found in the spinal cord, involving all tracts except dorsal columns. Changes are most severe in the midthoracic region of the cord, frequently associated with neuronal degeneration in gray matter. The etiology of this condition remains unknown, although a dietary factor may be involved.

Age of onset varies from 2 to 7 years. Initial signs are pelvic limb ataxia and exaggerated elevation of these limbs when retracted at a gallop. Occasionally the pelvic limbs are dragged. The panniculus reflex is usually absent at levels caudal to the thirteenth thoracic to the second lumbar segments. Muscle atrophy is not observed. Affected animals usually become unworkable owing to increasing pelvic limb incoordination within 6 to 18 months from the onset of symptoms.

Degenerative Myeloencephalopathies in Large Animals

Equine degenerative myeloencephalopathy (EDM) has been described in horses of several breeds and in zebras.[215, 229] Progressive ataxia and tetraparesis began at a few months of age. There was associated neuronal fiber degeneration, particularly in the dorsolateral and ventromedial funiculi in the spinal cord, and neuroaxonal dystrophy, neuronal dropout, gliosis, and pigment accumulation in spinal cord and caudal medullary, sensory relay nuclear areas. The diagnosis could only be made by ruling out other causes of progressive tetraparesis and confirmed at necropsy. Familial, nutritional, toxic, and metabolic etiologic factors were considered.

A similar syndrome affecting Morgan horses has been described,[15] wherein the neuroaxonal dystrophy is emphasized. In addition, a myelopathy affecting captive Przewalskii wild horses has recently been described.[204] The clinical syndrome was similar to EDM, although neuroaxonal dystrophy was not reported to be prominent and a mild degenerative, spinal ganglionopathy was described. This latter disease was associated with low plasma α-tocopherol values. The role of vitamin E in the pathogenesis of these equine myelopathies needs to be confirmed by controlled trials.

Ataxia and weakness associated with spinal cord degenerative lesions are reported in llamas, wildebeests, and camels,[249] and in sheep affected with Murrurundi disease and Coonabarabran disease.[139]

Spongiform Degeneration of the Central Nervous System

Variable spongiform degenerative conditions have been recognized in Egyptian Mau kittens,[184] Hereford calves,[51, 171] silky terrier puppy,[274] and Samoyed puppy.[213]

A suspected genetic disorder occurs in the Egyptian Mau breed of cat (a small breed derived from the Siamese cat). There is widespread vacuolation of white and gray matter of brain and spinal cord. There is no evidence of myelin breakdown. Clinical signs are first noticed in kittens at 7 weeks of age and are characterized by pelvic limb ataxia and hypermetria. Subsequent signs include intermittent periods of severe depression and reduced activity, with frequent flicking movements of distal pelvic limbs when at full flexion. The condition appears to improve with age.

There is some similarity of this disorder to congenital brain edema of horned Hereford calves[171] and to hereditary neuraxial edema of polled Hereford calves.[25, 51] Calves are alert but unable to stand at birth and lie in lateral recumbency. In the syndrome in polled calves, auditory and tactile stimulation (especially on the tip of the nose) induces extensor rigidity of the limbs. Affected horned Hereford calves can stand if assisted and move with an ataxic gait. In addition, there are prominent tonic muscle spasms. Prognosis is hopeless, as there is no treatment. Both these bovine diseases, particularly the latter, are characterized pathologically by status spongiosus. Reduced myelin formation and myelin breakdown are also present in congenital brain edema.

Spongiform degeneration has also been described in the dog. In a Samoyed puppy, a generalized vacuolation of white matter throughout brain and spinal cord has been reported, with most severe changes being found in the cerebellum. Pelvic limb tremor was observed at 12 days of age, progressing to generalized tremors over the next 5 days. A similar spongiform change is described in the cerebral and cerebellar white matter, but not in spinal cord, of silky terrier puppies.[274] A large number of Alzheimer type II protoplasmic astrocytes are found in severely affected areas. Clinical signs are noted at birth and consist of uncontrolled intermittent contractures of the paravertebral muscles, especially of the thoracolumbar region, at intervals of approximately two per second. Occasionally the pelvic limbs are lifted off the ground during these contractures. The episodes are intensified with excitement. Low intensity contractions continue during sleep. Signs do not appear to be progressive.

CONGENITAL MALFORMATIONS

Congenital malformations constitute structural abnormalities of prenatal origin that are present at birth and that seriously interfere

Table 6–3. CONGENITAL MALFORMATIONS OF NERVOUS TISSUE

Induction Disorders
Anencephaly[42, 99]
Meningoencephaloceles/cranium bifidum[254]
Meningomyeloceles/spina bifida
Arnold-Chiari malformations[38, 301]
Vertebral anomalies

Neuronal Migration and Proliferative Disorders
Cerebral abnormalities
  Congenital hydrocephalus
  Hydranencephaly
  Porencephaly
  Aplasia[28]
Convolutional abnormalities
  Lissencephaly
  Polymicrogyria
Commissural abnormalities
  Agenesis of corpus callosum[37]
Cerebellar abnormalities
  Aplasia/hypoplasia

Maturational Disorders
Malformations of cytoarchitecture
  Heteropias[162]
Defects of myelin metabolism
  Dysmyelinogenesis

with viability or physical well-being. Diverse and dissimilar, genetic and environmental insults may produce similar morphologic defects if they occur at the same time during nervous system development[179, 180] (Table 6–3). Normal ontogeny, a process of predetermined events occurring in proper sequence to ensure normal development of the CNS, may be divided into three developmental phases with characteristic disorders:[158] (1) Embryogenesis, characterized by induction to form neural plate, groove, and tube, followed by segmentation. Induction and segmentation failures during this period will produce a variety of dysraphic states, including anencephaly,[42, 99] cranium bifidum and spina bifida,[254] meningoencephaloceles, and meningomyeloceles. (2) Neuronal migration-proliferation. Disorders occurring during this phase include various malformations affecting the cerebral hemispheres (congenital hydrocephalus, hydranencephaly, porencephaly), convolutions (lissencephaly), commissures (agenesis of corpus callosum),[37] cerebellum (aplasia-hypoplasia), and brain stem (agenesis of cranial nerve nuclei) tissue. (3) Maturation of cellular organization, synaptic development, and myelin formation. Major developmental processes occurring at this time include (a) attainment of proper alignment, orientation, and layering of cortical neurons; (b) elaboration of axonal and dendritic ramifications; (c) establishment of synaptic contacts; (d) proliferation and differentiation of glia; and (e) myelin production. Disorders are characterized by malformations of cytoarchitecture (heterotopias), neurotransmission disorders, and defects of myelin metabolism (eg, globoid leukodystrophy). Most of these disorders are generally considered heredofamilial, metabolic, or neurodegenerative processes. Diagnosis of these malformations is difficult and requires enzymic and pathologic confirmation. These disorders are discussed above; see Metabolic Storage Diseases and Neuronal Abiotrophies and Degenerations.

Congenital Malformations of the Cerebrum

Congenital Hydrocephalus

Congenital hydrocephalus has been reported in most species of domestic animals and is one of the most common congenital malformations of the canine nervous system.[219] It has multiple causes and usually is divided into communicating (nonobstructive) and noncommunicating (obstructive) forms. The latter type results from a block within the ventricular system and represents the most common cause of hydrocephalus.[286] Congenital stenosis, forking, gliosis, and septum formation of mesencephalic aqueduct have been described in animals and persons.[12, 94, 158, 277] In communicating hydrocephalus, cerebrospinal fluid passes through the ventricular system into the subarachnoid space where absorption is impaired.

In a recent epizootiologic study of canine hydrocephalus, small, "toy," and brachycephalic breeds (e.g., Maltese, Yorkshire terrier, English bulldog, Chihuahua, Lhasa apso, pomeranian, toy poodle) were identified as being at high risk, thus supporting previous studies.[95, 162, 286, 246] The smaller the adult dog (whether dwarf or miniature in size, or brachycephalic), the higher the risk of hydrocephalus. In this study 53% of 564 hydrocephalic dogs manifested clinical signs by 1 year of age.

A distinction between congenital and acquired forms of hydrocephalus may be difficult from a clinical viewpoint, especially because infectious agents are believed to cause hydrocephalus postnatally in young puppies.[151] Furthermore, the confusion in terminology is reflected in the results of a recent epizootiologic study from 14 veterinary schools in the United States in which 30% of 564 dogs classified as having "hydrocephalus due to congenital origin" were over 2 years of age.[286]

The pathophysiology of hydrocephalus remains unclear. Autoradiographic studies in dogs[164] demonstrated transependymal flow of albumin and fluid. A reversal of CSF flow has been documented in experimental communicating hydrocephalus in the dog.[295] Cranial trauma, infectious agents causing encephalitis and meningitis, and neoplasia have all been incriminated in acquired hydrocephalus in animals.[162] In Siamese cats, hereditary hydrocephalus is transmitted as an autosomal recessive trait.[289] In obstructive hydrocephalus, pressure from ventricular enlargement may result in disruption of pellucid septum and atrophy of associated structures including subcortical white matter, optic radiation, internal capsule, and auditory radiation. In severe cases the cerebral hemispheres contain extremely large fluid filled lateral ventricles, with the cerebral cortex often being reduced to 3 to 4 mm in thickness (Fig. 6–3). On gross inspection the brain may be enlarged with loss of gyral pattern and decreased depth of sulci. Owing to in-

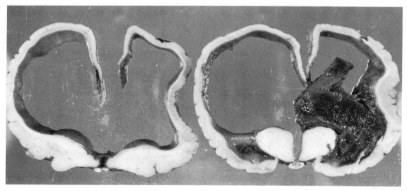

Figure 6–3. Severe hydrocephalus in a Chihuahua. Notice the thinning of the cerebral cortex. There is an intraventricular hematoma. (From Oliver JE Jr and Lorenz MD: Handbook of Veterinary Neurologic Diagnosis. Philadelphia, WB Saunders Co, 1983.)

creased intracranial pressure, herniated portions of the cerebellum and terminal medulla oblongata may be found.[219] The entire ventricular system may be dilated in communicating hydrocephalus. The mesencephalic aqueduct is often stenotic in obstructive hydrocephalus. The ependymal lining is frequently disrupted and false diverticula may be observed. A pronounced subependymal edema is usually present.

Clinical examination of newborn and immature hydrocephalic animals will often indicate an enlarged, dome-shaped cranium and open sutures and/or fontanelles in an animal that continuously cries out, has visual and auditory impairment, and exhibits altered mental status (ranging from hyperexcitability to severe depression). Gait is often incoordinated and clumsy, and affected animals may circle and press their heads into objects. Pupils may be dilated and fixed. Ventrolateral strabismus may be evident.[70] The strabismus is frequently caused by the encroachment on the orbit from the expanding frontal bones, in which case eye movements are normal.

Diagnosis of hydrocephalus is based on clinical signs and is confirmed by radiographic demonstration of enlarged lateral ventricles by ventriculography (Fig. 6–4). Plain radiography will often reveal a ground glass appearance throughout the cranial vault. Cranial sutures and/or open fontanelles may be evident after the normal age for closure and skull ossification.

Electroencephalographic traces usually have a characteristic pattern of high amplitude (25–200 µV), slow wave (1–5 Hz) activity, often with a superimposed fast frequency of 10 to 12 Hz (see Fig. 5–15). Electroencephalography has proved useful in substantiating a clinical diagnosis of occult hydrocephalus in absence of radiographic abnormalities.[265]

Prognosis is poor. Treatment of animals with severe congenital hydrocephalus is futile because of the large amount of tissue destruction and atrophy. Indeed, the efficacy of glucocorticosteroids and surgical shunt procedures in animals with "acquired" hydrocephalus remains uncertain owing to the lack of well-controlled clinical trials and to incomplete knowledge of the underlying pathogenesis. Successful shunting procedures have been reported in "acquired" hydrocephalus in older dogs.[98, 110, 154]

Dexamethasone, administered orally (1 mg divided 4 times daily for 3–5 lb dogs), has been used empirically. This dose is gradually reduced over a 2 to 3 week course of therapy. Some animals may be maintained on alternate day dosage schedules. Glucocorticosteroids are believed to primarily affect brain bulk and CSF production, not CSF absorption.[167]

Hydrocephalus occurs widely in cattle and has been reported in virtually all major beef and dairy herds.[122, 127] Several inherited hydrocephalus syndromes have been described in Hereford and Shorthorn breed cattle,[127, 128] with additional features including cerebellar hypo-

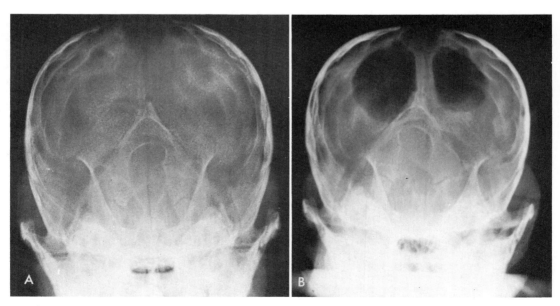

Figure 6–4. A, Anteroposterior radiograph of a dog with hydrocephalus. B, Pneumoventriculogram demonstrating the enlarged ventricles.

plasia, microphthalmia, myopathy, and retinal dysplasia.

Porencephaly

This congenital disorder represents a circumscribed cerebral defect that communicates with the ventricular system. It is a rare disorder thought to be secondary to fetal vascular maldevelopment. There is no treatment.

Hydranencephaly

This malformation is characterized by virtual absence of the cerebral hemispheres and basal ganglia with remnants of mesencephalic structures. The cerebral hemispheres are replaced by CSF filled sacs lined by leptomeninges, a glial membrane, and ependymal remnants. The pathogenesis of this anomaly is not always certain. A fetal cerebrovascular accident may result in massive necrosis and reabsorption of tissue.[158] In utero viral infections with destruction of large portions of CNS tissue occur with blue tongue virus[210, 243, 244] and Akabane virus,[141, 190, 191] resulting in hydranencephaly in newborn lambs and calves. Hydranencephaly believed to be associated with feline panleukopenia virus has been reported in a cat.[123] Affected animals may have dummylike characteristics; they are blind, ataxic, unable to suckle, and indifferent to their environment. Unilateral hydranencephaly has been observed in an 8 month old miniature poodle whose only clinical sign was a visual defect.[68] Congenital hydranencephaly and cerebellar hypoplasia has been reported in calves, for which an environmental rather than inherited cause was postulated.[126]

Lissencephaly

This rare defect is characterized by a small, smooth appearing brain with few or no gyri present and derangement of cells of the cerebral cortex. It results from disturbance of neuronal migration and proliferation during development. This anomaly has been reported in Lhasa apso dogs,[124, 332] wire haired fox terriers, Irish setters,[66] and a cat with cerebellar hypoplasia.[105]

Clinical signs are usually detected in the first year of life and are characterized by erratic behavior patterns (episodes of aggressiveness, growling at imaginary objects, confusion, hyperactivity), visual deficits, and seizures. Apart from abnormal wave tracings detected electroencephalographically, results of routine ancillary diagnostic tests are normal.

Prognosis is guarded. Treatment is symptomatic. Seizures may be controlled with anticonvulsant therapy.

Other, rare malformations of the prosencephalon are recorded in various species.[68]

Congenital Malformations of the Cerebellum

As with most other congenital anomalies, malformations of the cerebellum in domestic animals usually result from unknown causes. Various forms of agenesis (absence of the whole or parts), aplasia (faulty development with no tissue differentiation), and hypoplasia (faulty development with some tissue differentiation)[219] have been reported in dogs[52, 82, 105, 183, 219] and in other domestic species.[43, 66, 67, 87, 89, 126, 162, 194]

In utero infection with feline panleukopenia virus results in destruction of actively dividing granule neurons and hypoplasia of the granule cell layer[169] (Fig. 6–5). Purkinje cells may also be destroyed.[169]

Cerebellar hypoplasia and degeneration occur in utero in cattle infected with bovine virus diarrhea.[32, 178] The degree of cerebellar lesion observed at term ranged from slight gross deformity to almost complete absence of any cerebellar tissue.

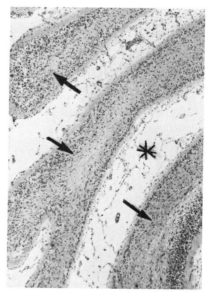

Figure 6–5. Cerebellar hypoplasia due to panleukopenia infection in a 5 day old kitten. There is a marked distention of the arachnoidal space (asterisk) due to atrophy of the cerebellar folia. Note the absence of an external granular cell layer and the extreme hypocellularity of the internal granular cell layer (arrows). Hematoxylin and eosin, low power.

Blue tongue virus[243, 244] and Akabane virus[141] may destroy fetal cerebellar tissue in a nonselective fashion in cattle and sheep. Similarly, hog cholera virus administered to pregnant sows will result in cerebellar lesions.[89]

In animals born with congenital malformations clinical signs will be present at birth or, in the case of dogs and cats, when they first begin to ambulate. The signs of cerebellar disease are generally nonprogressive, are symmetric, and vary from dysmetric-hypermetric gait, head tremor, and wide based stance to opisthotonos and extensor rigidity of the limbs (e.g., in calves). Abnormal nystagmus may be seen. Diagnosis is usually based on age, breed and species, history (e.g., of viral infection), and clinical signs. There is no treatment.

Malformation of Foramen Magnum

An abnormally large foramen magnum, which has been termed occipital dysplasia, resulting from a defect in development of the occipital bone, has been described in small dogs.[11, 153, 234, 256] The abnormality consists of a dorsal midline extension of the foramen magnum into the occipital bone.

Clinical signs of cervical pain, personality changes, and seizures as described in the initial report[11] have not been substantiated by others.[256] Varying degrees of enlargement of the foramen magnum occur normally in small and toy breed dogs. Frontal radiographs of the skull readily reveal the enlargement. Clinical evidence of neurologic disease in such dogs (e.g., Yorkshire terrier, Pomeranian, Maltese, miniature and toy poodles, Chihuahuas) most likely reflects some other intracranial disease such as hydrocephalus.[256] The Arnold-Chiari malformation consisting of caudal extension of cerebellar and pontomedullary tissue has been reported in calves, lambs, and a dog.[38, 301]

Congenital Malformations of the Cranial Nerves

Optic Nerve Hypoplasia

A malformation of parts of the eyeball occurs as a hereditary disease in collie dogs.[282, 330] Abnormal development of optic nerve (and retina) may produce blindness. Pathologically, there is no stenosis of the optic canal, but there is a reduction in size of the optic nerve and atrophy and reduced number of optic nerve fibers. Vacuolation and paucity of neurons were observed in ganglion cells of retina.[162] Bilateral hypoplasia of the optic nerve of unknown etiology has been reported in the cat,[14] dog,[92, 117, 186, 314] and horse.[118] According to several reports, optic nerve foramina may be reduced in diameter.[92, 186]

Diagnosis is suggested by a history of visual impairment from birth. There is usually a menace deficit and reduced or absent pupillary reflexes in affected eyes.

In vitamin A deficient calves, acquired optic neuropathy resulting from progressive osseous constriction within the optic canal must be distinguished from optic nerve hypoplasia. Prognosis is poor. There is no treatment.

Congenital Deafness

Deafness as a result of disease in the receptor organ or a lesion of the auditory pathways is known as nerve deafness. Congenital deafness in animals is usually associated with degeneration, hypoplasia, or aplasia of the spiral organ.[1, 159, 207] Congenital deafness is frequently associated with pigmentation disorders such as a white coat color and blue eyes.[1, 16, 26, 270, 323] In cats, the disorder is associated with a dominant autosomal gene.[16] A hereditary pattern has been suggested for Old English sheepdogs, cocker spaniels, Dalmatians, and bull terriers.[162]

Pathologic changes consist of total or partial agenesis of the organ of Corti, the spiral ganglion, and the cochlear nuclei.[162] Additionally, in congenitally deaf collie and Dalmatian puppies, partial collapse of the saccule, atrophy of the saccular nerve, and obliteration of the cochlear duct have been described.[156, 207] Neonatal and young immature animals are presented for hearing deficits. The deficit is usually present from birth, or within a few weeks postnatally,[26, 270] and is permanent. Some animals are affected unilaterally.

Definitive diagnosis of deafness is aided by brain stem auditory evoked response testing (see Chapter 5).

Congenital Vestibular Disease

There are several reports of peripheral vestibular abnormality in young dogs and cats. It has been seen in cocker spaniels, German shepherd dogs, Doberman pinschers, Akita dogs, and Siamese and Burmese cats.[68] Clinical signs, which usually begin at 3 to 12 weeks of age, include head tilt, circling, ataxia, and, in some cases, deafness. Nystagmus is not a feature of this disorder, but there is a deficit in normal eye movements.

The few animals that have been examined histologically had no detectable lesions.

The signs are generally not progressive, and improvement is usually seen over a period of weeks. This is probably due to compensation rather than resolution of the problem. There is no treatment.

Genetic studies have not been done, but there have been multiple cases observed in the breeds listed.

Congenital Malformations of the Vertebral Column and Spinal Cord

Myelodysplasia

Myelodysplasia is a congenital malformation resulting from defective development of any part of the spinal cord before complete differentiation of gray and white matter. Myelodysplastic conditions in animals include spina bifida, sacrococcygeal dysgenesis, and spinal dysplasia.

Spina Bifida

This anomaly results from failure of fusion of the halves of the dorsal spinous processes with or without protrusion of the spinal cord or its membranes (or both) (Fig. 6–6). Spina bifida manifesta, cystica, and operta are synonymous subclassification indicating presence of meningocele, myelocele, or meningomyelocele, respectively.[322] Spina bifida occulta is characterized by a bony defect without visible protrusion of enclosed vertebral canal structures.[219] Myelodysplasia, consisting of gliosis, hydromyelia (dilation of the central canal), syringomyelia (cavitations within the spinal cord), or abnormal position of the central gray matter and anomalies of dorsal and ventral horns may also occur with spina bifida.[219, 322]

The embryonic pathogenesis of this anomaly is controversial. One theory is that there is overgrowth of cells of the dorsal neural tube that interferes with fusion of the neural tube and vertebral arches.[260] Another theory suggests that vertebral arches fail to fuse as a result of a neuroschistic bleb.[245]

Spina bifida has been reported in most domestic species.[36, 40, 46, 95, 107, 108, 153, 162, 177, 198, 201, 219, 253] There is a high incidence of spina bifida in young English bulldogs.[153, 322] The conditions may occur anywhere along the vertebral column but is most common in the lumbar region. The malformation usually does not interfere with gray matter to the extent that lower motor neuron signs become evident. Clinical signs are often noticed when affected animals begin to ambulate and may include pelvic limb ataxia and paresis, fecal and urinary incontinence, perineal analgesia, and flaccid anal sphincters. The site of the bony defect may be marked by dimpling of the overlying skin, streaming of hair coat, and palpable cavitation in the dorsal spinous process.[219, 322]

Diagnosis is based on age, clinical signs, breed, and radiography. Plain radiographs will demonstrate abnormalities ranging from nonfusion of dorsal laminae to a cleft spinous process. However, myelography may demonstrate protrusion of spinal cord, meninges, or both (Fig. 6–7).

Prognosis is guarded to poor. Treatment is usually not attempted.

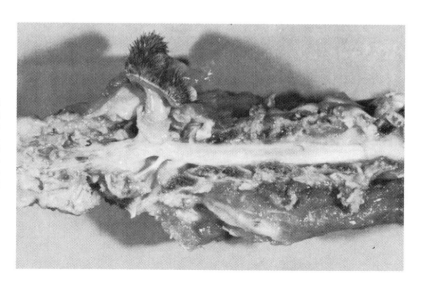

Figure 6–6. Myelomeningocele in an English bulldog puppy with spina bifida. Myeloschisis, a cleft in the dorsal part of the spinal cord, is also present. (From Oliver JE Jr and Lorenz MD: Handbook of Veterinary Neurologic Diagnosis. Philadelphia, WB Saunders Co, 1983.)

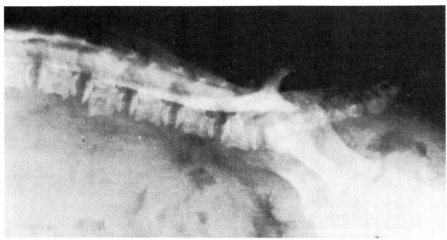

Figure 6–7. Myelogram demonstrating a myelomeningocele in an English bulldog puppy (same patient as in Figure 6–6). (From Oliver JE Jr and Lorenz MD: Handbook of Veterinary Neurologic Diagnosis. Philadelphia, WB Saunders Co, 1983.)

Caudal Dysgenesis

Congenital malformations of the sacrocaudal spinal cord and vertebrae have been well described in tailless Manx cats, in which the disease is transmitted as an autosomal dominant trait.[202, 205, 299] Neurologic signs, including plantigrade posture, hopping gait, pelvic limb paresis-paraplegia, fecal and urinary incontinence, and perianal sensory loss, are associated with agenesis or dysgenesis of caudal vertebrae and, in some cats, severe sacral dysgenesis and spina bifida. Pathologically, subcutaneous cyst formation, meningocele, myelomeningocele, syringomyelia, dystematomyelia, shortening of the spinal cord and absence of cauda equina, and anomalies of the dorsal horn have been described in affected animals.[64, 165, 188, 202, 212] Affected animals may steadily deteriorate after birth and become paraplegic, or a partial disability may remain stationary.[165]

Diagnosis is based on breed, age, clinical signs, and lumbrosacral radiography (Fig. 6–8). Prognosis is guarded. There is no treatment. Mildly affected animals may attain longevity if fecal and urinary incontinence are managed.

A similar disorder has been reported in a Maltese kitten.[106]

Spinal Dysplasia

This congenital myelodysplasia most commonly occurs in Weimeraner dogs and is considered to be an inherited condition transmitted by a codominant gene with reduced penetrance and variable expressivity.[288] The disorder has also been reported in other breeds of dogs,[68, 120, 220, 236, 288, 304] in Charolais cattle,[200] and in a Thoroughbred foal.[41] Prenatal studies have shown that dysraphic changes, resulting from abnormal migration of mantle cells, are evident in embryos (24–28 days of gestation) obtained by mating severely dysraphic Weimeraner dogs.[90, 91]

Pathologically, the malformation includes hydromyelia, duplication of central canal or an absent central canal, syringomyelia (usually in dorsal columns), chromatolysis and loss of nerve cell bodies in gray matter, aberrations in the dorsal median septum and ventral median fissure, and gray matter ectopias (Fig. 6–9).[48, 220]

Clinical signs usually appear by 4 to 6 weeks of age; however, abnormal spinal reflexes reportedly are observed in newborn dysraphic pups.[83] Affected animals have a symmetric, bunny hopping pelvic limb gait, wide based stance, and overextension of pelvic limbs with depressed proprioception. Less constant signs include scoliosis, abnormal hair streams in the dorsal neck region, and koilosternia (gutterlike depression of the chest).[220] Clinical signs neither progress nor retrogress. Animals can lead a normal life. There is no treatment.

Occipitoatlantoaxial Malformations

An occipitoatlantoaxial malformation has been reported in Arabian foals of both sexes. The condition is believed to be inherited in an autosomal recessive manner.[199, 217] In most animals there is no discernible atlantooccipital joint, with complete fusion of the atlas with the occipital bone. The axis may be displaced, and the dens may be hypoplastic. The foramen of the atlas may be markedly reduced in size.

Clinical signs may be present at birth or within the first few weeks or months. Affected animals may be unable to stand or may manifest severe ataxia and paresis. Clinical signs are progressive. Affected horses extend their necks more often than normal, and a clicking sound may be heard when the animal's head moves. The malformation can be palpated in the living animal.

Diagnosis is based on historical, signalment, clinical, and radiographic data. Other malformations in this region of the skeleton of horses have been discussed.[217] A similar disorder has been described in Holstein cattle.[316] Odontoid process angulation, probably of congenital origin and causing cord compression, has been reported in dogs.[257, 297]

Atlantoaxial Subluxation

This is a condition of instability of the atlantoaxial articulation that produces excessive flexion of the joint and may result in severe, acute neurologic deficit. The disorder results from separation, absence, or malformation of the dens.[115, 116, 195, 255] The pathogenesis of this developmental malformation is unknown. Although hereditary factors may be involved in some lines of miniature and toy breeds of dogs in which this congenital anomaly is most common, fracture and insufficient ligamentous support of the dens may occur in any breed. Congenital atlantoaxial subluxation occurs most commonly in dogs less than 1 year of age; however, older animals exposed to various stresses may also be affected.

Congenital absence of the dens or lack of fusion between dens and axis[195] results in decreased stability between the atlas and axis, thus causing the cranial aspect of the axis to rotate dorsally into the vertebral canal with subsequent spinal cord compression.[109]

Clinical signs vary according to the degree of luxation. They may range from cervical rigidity and pain to spastic paraparesis and sometimes tetraplegia. The signs may develop slowly over several months, or they may occur acutely.

When atlantoaxial luxation is suspected, survey radiographs should be made without anesthesia before manipulating the animal exces-

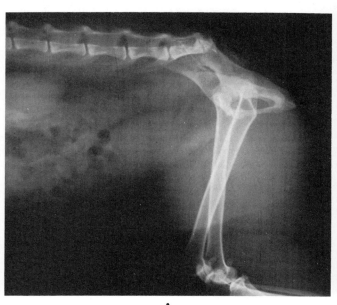

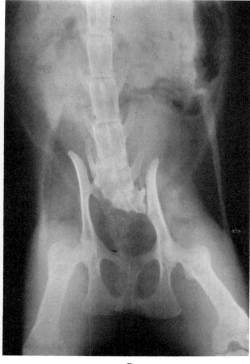

A   B

Figure 6–8. Radiographs of a manx cat with sacrococcygeal dysgenesis. A, Lateral view. B, Ventrodorsal view. There is complete agenesis of the caudal vertebrae and segmental fusion defect with malformation of the sacral vertebrae. A sacroiliac luxation is present on the right side.

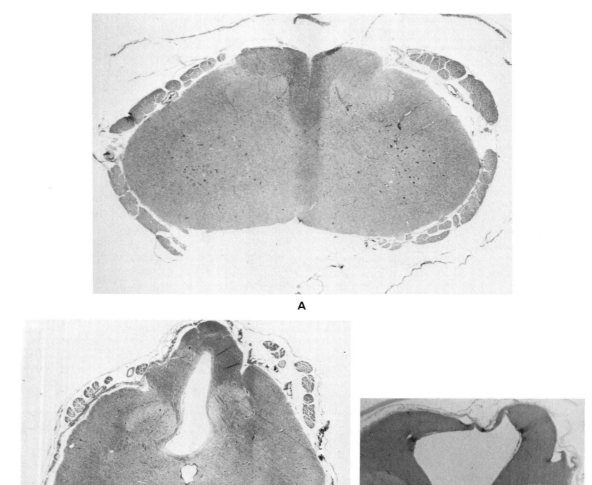

Figure 6–9. A, Spinal cord dysplasia in a Weimeraner, lumbar spinal cord. Note the complete lack of the central canal. B, Syringomyelia in a Labrador retriever puppy. Note the fluid cavity in the dorsal midline of the spinal cord. C, Bovine spinal cord malformation. Section of spinal cord at L4 from a 1 month old, female Holstein calf with myelodysplasia. There is absence of the central canal and of the ventral median septum with a large syrinx dorsally. There is poor differentiation of the fused ventral horns, and asymmetric remnants of the dorsal funiculi remain. The calf had a moderate, hypometric, ataxic, bunny-hopping paraparesis with bilaterally active reflexes (flexor, patellar, and toe extension/Babinski). Hematoxylin and eosin, low power.

sively. Lateral view radiographs will reveal widening of the space between the arch of the atlas and spinous process of the axis, angulation of the axis relative to the atlas, and the rounded end of the axis indicating the absence of the dens (Fig. 6–10). Oblique views may be useful

in determining the presence or absence of the dens. Open mouth frontal[234] and flexed lateral views are not necessary in most cases and are likely to cause severe compression of the spinal cord.[239]

The prognosis is guarded. Treatment of spinal

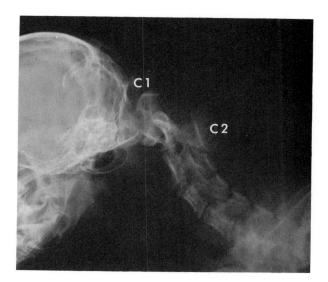

Figure 6–10. An atlantoaxial luxation with absence of the dens.

cord trauma using glucocorticoid and/or mannitol may be indicated. Stabilization of the luxation is mandatory[109, 111, 112] (see Chapter 17).

Miscellaneous Congenital Vertebral Anomalies

A wide variety of congenital abnormalities of the vertebral column can occur in animals, but the majority, at least in dogs, are minor and cause no clinical signs.[232]

Vertebral anomalies often result from disruption of normal development and regression of the embryonic notochord, abnormal segmentation of mesoderm into somites, or altered vascularization and ossification of the vertebrae.[5] Some of these vertebral anomalies have been classified in the horse.[217]

Block vertebrae result from disturbed somite segmentation. This anomaly may involve incomplete separation of vertebral bodies, arches, or the entire vertebra (Fig. 6–11b). Block vertebrae are generally stable and rarely clinically significant.[232]

The *butterfly vertebra* is an anomaly that results from persistence of the notochord or sagittal cleavage of notochord producing a sagittal cleft of the vertebral body (Fig. 6–11a). Butterfly vertebrae are most often detected in brachycephalic, screw tailed breeds (French and English bulldogs, pugs, Boston terriers, and Pekingese). This anomaly is rarely clinically significant.

Hemivertebra is a malformation that may be caused by hemimetameric displacement of so-

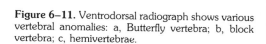

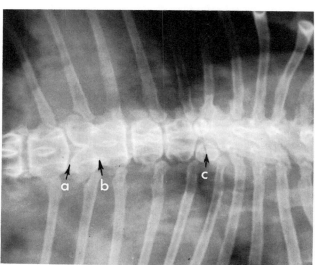

Figure 6–11. Ventrodorsal radiograph shows various vertebral anomalies: a, Butterfly vertebra; b, block vertebra; c, hemivertebrae.

mites, resulting in right and left hemivertebrae and scoliosis, or it may be produced by altered vascularization and ossification of vertebrae[285] (Fig. 6–11c).

Although the majority of cases do not produce any obvious clinical signs,[232] hemivertebra is more often associated with neurologic deficits than any other congenital vertebral anomaly. Affected animals are usually less than 1 year of age.[77, 78] Neurologic signs may result from progressive kyphosis, ultimately producing cord compression, or may follow vertebral luxation or fracture at the site of hemivertebra following a sudden jump, fall, or trauma. This condition is seen quite frequently in dogs and is reported in a quarterhorse filly[189] and a Saanen-cross kid goat.[276] The breeds of dogs that have been reported to be most commonly affected are the screw tailed breeds (the English bulldog, French bulldog, and Boston terrier).[77, 84] (The kinked tail is due to hemivertebrae in the coccygeal region.[77]) Vertebrae most commonly affected are in the region T7 to T9. Clinical signs include varying degrees of pelvic limb paresis and paralysis, muscular atrophy, pain on palpation of the vertebral column, and often fecal and urinary incontinence. In addition, abnormal spinal conformation, including scoliosis and kyphosis, may be present. Radiographs show an obvious abnormality of the vertebral column affecting a single or, in some cases, several vertebrae (Fig. 6–11). There is usually a marked dorsal deviation of the thoracic vertebral column with one or more wedge-shaped vertebral bodies. Disk spaces are usually well preserved. The vertebral end plates are smooth and of normal thickness. Myelography will often outline compression of the subarachnoid space over one or more of the anomalous vertebrae.

A relationship between abnormal congenital vertebral development and neonatal mortality has been suggested in English bulldogs.[84]

Diagnosis of clinically significant hemivertebrae is based on age, breed, clinical history, clinical signs, and radiography. Dogs may be treated with surgical decompression and stabilization.

DEGENERATIVE DISEASES OF THE VERTEBRAL COLUMN AND MENINGES

Cervical Malformation-Malarticulation

This disease is considered to represent a developmental malformation and malarticulation of cervical vertebrae in dogs and horses. This disorder has been termed wobbler syndrome, equine sensory ataxia, vertebral instability, vertebral subluxation, cervical spondylolisthesis, cervical stenosis, and cervical spondylopathy.[68, 74, 85, 104, 111, 216, 258, 271, 287, 319, 327] It occurs most frequently in Thoroughbred horses and Great Dane and Doberman pinscher dogs. The cause of this disorder is unknown but is probably multifactorial. Rapid growth rates and nutrition,[147, 216] mechanical factors,[327] and genetic factors[214, 287] have all been suggested as playing a role. One study refuted a pure hereditary basis in horses.[93] The age of onset of clinical signs varies from 3 months to 9 years. In general, Great Danes are affected at less than 2 years of age, Doberman pinschers more frequently manifest signs when 2 years of age or older,[68, 73, 214, 327] and horses are more frequently affected at midcervical sites at 6 months to 2 years of age and at caudal cervical sites in older animals.[272] There is no sex predisposition in dogs, although more male than female horses are affected.[271, 319]

The underlying deformity is a narrowing of the diameter of the vertebral canal that may be apparent only on flexion and/or extension of the neck[216, 241, 327, 328] (see Figs. 4–20 and 4–21). One or more of the caudal cervical vertebrae may be unstable and malarticulated so that the craniodorsal aspect of the vertebral body is displaced dorsally into the vertebral canal,[68] or the cranial border of the vertebral orifice protrudes into the canal[68, 216] (see Fig. 4–5). If the displacement appears on both flexed and extended radiographic views, it is considered to be stable. As a result of abnormal stresses on vertebrae associated with malarticulation, the cervical vertebrae may become malformed. In dogs there may be deformity and exostoses of the cranioventral region of the ventral bodies, and degenerative changes have been observed in associated intervertebral disks, sometimes with encroachment of articular processes into the vertebral canal.[29, 327] Interarcuate ligaments and dorsal longitudinal ligaments may become hypertrophic.[287] Dural and synovial cysts may form in the exuberant periarticular tissues and become a soft tissue component to compression of the spinal cord.[100, 119, 319]

In the spinal cord, degenerative changes characterized by white and gray matter necrosis are seen at the site of spinal cord compression. Wallerian-like neuronal fiber degeneration of white matter is seen above and below the compressive lesion.

Clinical signs are related to the severity of spinal cord compression and are therefore var-

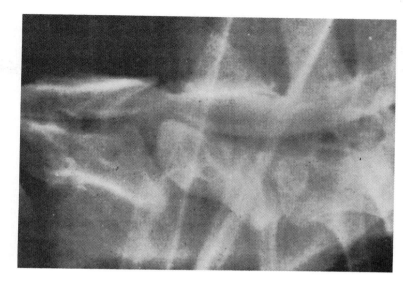

Figure 6–12. Myelogram of a 4 year old Doberman pinscher with cervical spondylopathy. Note the subluxation of C6 and the stenosis of the vertebral canal at this level. (From Oliver JE Jr and Lorenz MD: Handbook of Veterinary Neurologic Diagnosis. Philadelphia, WB Saunders Co, 1983.)

iable in nature and degree. The most common sign is pelvic limb ataxia and paresis, with or without thoracic limb involvement. Clinical signs usually are first noticed in pelvic limbs. Affected animals can have difficulty rising from lateral recumbency or from a sitting position and frequently have a hypermetric gait in thoracic limbs. The digits may knuckle when the animal walks, and nails or hoofs are often worn excessively as a result of scuffing and dragging. Most dogs have a conscious proprioceptive deficit, and dogs and horses usually demonstrate a wide based stance. Sometimes pain may be elicited upon neck manipulation, especially extension. Clinical signs tend to be slowly progressive but can be abrupt in onset when external trauma is suspected as playing a major precipitating role.

Diagnosis is based on historical, signalment, clinical, and radiographic data. In older dogs similar signs are frequently caused by a type II disk protrusion. Many animals have more than one site of compression, which may not be apparent on survey radiography. Therefore, myelography is essential to establish an accurate diagnosis and prognosis, especially if surgery is to be considered (Fig. 6–12; see also Fig. 4–12).

Prognosis for spontaneous recovery is poor;[68, 73, 216] however, marked improvement has been reported following decompressive and stabilizing surgery (see Chapter 17).

There have been isolated reports of a similar cervical malformation-malarticulation in other canine breeds, including Rhodesian ridgeback, Old English sheepdog, Irish setter, fox terrier, boxer, chow chow, Weimeraner, golden retriever, and Pyrenean mountain dog. A possible hereditary malformation of C2–C3 vertebrae occurs in basset hounds less than 6 months of age.[252] Spinal cord compression has been successfully relieved by surgery.[246]

Spondylosis Deformans

This is a degenerative disorder of the vertebral column characterized by the presence of vertebral osteophytes at intervertebral spaces, resulting in the formation of spurs or complete bony bridges.[133, 230, 231, 329] Although the condition is believed to be associated with degenerative changes in the anulus fibrosus of the intervertebral disks, it is rarely observed in chondrodystrophoid breeds that are frequently affected with disk disease.[231]

Spondylosis deformans has been reported in dogs, cats, male cattle, and pigs.[75, 234, 313] The incidence increases with age. In dogs, vertebral sites most often affected are T9–T10 and L7–S1. The distribution at areas of maximal spinal mobility in dogs[30, 133] suggests that mechanical factors may play a role in the pathogenesis.

Osteophytes tend to develop on ventral, lateral, and dorsolateral aspects of vertebral margins. Osteophytic projections into the vertebral canal with compression of the spinal cord are rare (Fig. 6–13; see also Fig. 4–8).

Spondylosis deformans in dogs tends to be a subclinical disorder. Localized pain or lameness may occur in association with fracture of bony spurs or bridges. Diagnosis is based on radiographic findings. Osteophytes have a smooth ventral border and a curved beaklike appearance. Treatment is symptomatic. Prognosis is good.

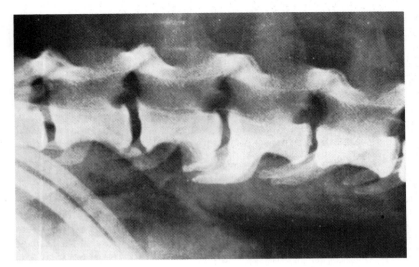

Figure 6–13. Spondylosis of the lumbar vertebrae and dural ossification were incidental findings in this English bulldog. These changes seldom cause neurologic signs. (From Oliver JE Jr and Lorenz MD: Handbook of Veterinary Neurologic Diagnosis. Philadelphia, WB Saunders Co, 1983.)

Dural Ossification

This is a degenerative disorder of dogs characterized by deposition of bone plaques on the inner surface of the dura mater. These plaques occur in more than 60% of both large and small breeds over 2 years of age and occur most often in cervical and lumbar areas of the spine.[233, 280] The etiology of this condition (also known as osseous metaplasia of the dura mater and ossifying pachymeningitis) is unknown.

At necropsy, gross plaques of bone tissue are found. In extreme cases, the dura may be transformed into a solid bony tube.[219, 303] The plaques often contain marrow cavities. In general, dural ossification rarely causes clinical disease, but spinal cord compression with secondary degenerative changes in white and gray matter has been reported in dogs with dural ossification.[219, 321] Degenerative changes may also occur in nerve roots closely associated with plaques.[219] Affected animals may have a history of chronic (months) paresis, often with atrophy of limb musculature.[219, 321] It is detected radiographically, usually as an incidental finding, and is characterized by thin radiopaque linear shadows in cervical and lumbar areas, especially at the site of intervertebral foramina (Fig. 6–13; see also Fig. 4–9).

If a definitive diagnosis is made in a dog with neurologic signs, decompressive surgery may be attempted. More common disorders should be given priority in the differential diagnosis of chronic spinal cord compression.

Lumbosacral Stenosis

Stenosis or narrowing of the vertebral canal, intervertebral foramina, or both in the lumbosacral area is an entity recently reported in dogs.[240, 298] Acquired or degenerative stenosis may develop in association with tumors or infectious processes, intervertebral disk prolapse, degenerative spondylosis deformans, or vertebral luxation.[240] Thickened lamina, pedicles, articular surfaces, and ligaments often accompany acquired lumbar stenosis. A form of congenital ("idiopathic") stenosis in dogs has been reported and is characterized by shortening of the pedicles, thickened and sclerotic apposition of the lamina and articular processes, infolding and hypertrophy of the flaval ligament, and sclerotic and bulbous articular processes that bulge into the dorsal half of the canal.[298]

Large breed dogs, the German shepherd in particular, were most commonly affected in one study of dogs with acquired stenosis.[240] Smaller breed dogs were more often affected with the congenital form.[298]

Irrespective of etiology, dogs with lumbosacral vertebral stenosis usually manifest a syndrome complex that reflects varying degrees of cauda equina involvement, depending on the level and extent of the lesion. Commonly reported clinical signs include pain on palpation of the lumbosacral area, difficulty in rising, slight pelvic limb paresis or lameness in one pelvic limb, tail paresis, hypotonia of anal sphincter with fecal incontinence, paresthesia of perineal area, tail, or pelvic limbs, and urinary incontinence.[240, 298]

Diagnosis is based on clinical signs, radiographic evidence of stenosis of lumbosacral canal using plain films or contrast study (such as epidurography), interosseous vertebral venography,[225] and electromyographic changes in muscles innervated by nerves forming the cauda equina,[240] namely, femoral, sciatic, obturator, pudendal, and pelvic nerves (see Fig. 4–16).

Prognosis is usually favorable if the stenosis is treated by surgical decompression using dorsal laminectomy, facetectomy, and foraminotomy.[240, 298] Medical treatment has usually been ineffective.[240]

UNCLASSIFIED FAMILIAL AND DEVELOPMENTAL ANOMALIES OF UNKNOWN CAUSE

Scotty Cramp

Scotty cramp is an inherited paroxysmal neurologic disorder with a recessive mode of transmission in Scottish terrier dogs.[226–228] The condition is also variously described as muscular hypertonicity, muscular cramping, and hyperkinesis. Although there are no structural changes observed in the central or peripheral nervous systems or in muscle, physiologic studies have demonstrated that the defect appears to be in those neuronal systems that control or moderate muscle contraction. Pharmacologic studies suggest that the disorder may be associated with serotonic transmitters, because antiserotonin agents markedly increase the severity of clinical signs.

Clinical signs may be elicited by exercise, excitement, stress, and poor health. The condition may occur in animals at any age; however, signs tend to be more prevalent in young dogs. Affected dogs appear normal when at rest or on initial exercise. As the exercise continues, clinical signs are usually observed; these progressively increase in severity during the episode. Initial signs may be abduction of the thoracic limbs or arching of the lumbar spine, followed by pelvic limb stiffening, occasional catapulting of the pelvic limbs into the air, and falling and curling into a ball, with the tail and pelvic limbs tightly flexed against the body. Respiration may momentarily cease, and facial muscles may be contracted. Animals do not lose consciousness. Signs usually remit within 10 minutes. Multiple episodes may occur over a 24 hour period. The disorder is usually nonprogressive.

Diagnosis is based on the clinical signs, because results of all laboratory tests are within normal limits. Historical information may reveal a family history of hyperkinesis. Signs can be induced using methylsergide, a serotonin antagonist. The drug is administered orally at a dosage of 0.3 mg/kg, and the animal is exercised 2 hours later.

Treatment consists of daily oral dosing of acepromazine maleate (0.1 to 0.75 mg/kg every 12 hours) or diazepam (0.5 mg/kg every 8 hours). Vitamin E (125 IU/kg/day) may also be effective. Sometimes, behavioral modification or environmental change may be sufficient.

A similar condition has been reported in young Dalmatian dogs.[326]

Spastic Paresis (Bovine Spastic Paralysis, Elso Heel)

This disease occurs quite frequently in young dairy and beef calves, particularly those nursing with their dams at pasture. Progressive, continual spasm of the gastrocnemius and digital flexor muscles occurs from 1 to 8 months of age. Calves show an upright posture and one side is usually worse than the other, with the worst limb held caudally. The limb is advanced as a pendulum, and ultimately the calf has great difficulty moving.[39]

There appear to be overactive stretch reflexes operative and some suggestion that it is an extrapyramidal dopaminergic central disorder present, with no lesions visible in the CNS.

Achilles tenotomy, tibial neurectomy, and selective tibial neurectomy each help to resolve the clinical spasms and are salvage procedures to be considered. There is evidence that the disorder is not inherited, but it is probably best not to breed affected animals. Similar disorders have been recorded in adult cattle.[132, 292]

Spastic Syndrome (Periodic Spasticity, Barn Cramps, Standings Disease, Stretches)

This syndrome occurs in older cattle, especially bulls at artificial insemination studs.[39, 132, 246] There are extensor muscle spasms of the back and hindquarters with caudal extension of the pelvic limbs and difficulty in moving, especially immediately on rising. Signs progress until there is muscle atrophy and great difficulty in getting up. There are no consistent lesions present and no treatment for the syndrome.

Uncommon Muscle Spasms and Paretic Disorders of Calves

Several other rare paralytic diseases, and diseases characterized by muscle spasms, for which there are no neuropathologic lesions demonstrated and no known cause or treatment, are reported as isolated events.[39, 246]

Skeletal Deformities in Calves

A high frequency of paraparesis was seen in young calves in a herd of Angus cattle in Canada.[242] There were focal, premature synostoses of vertebral growth plates associated with stenosis of the thoracolumbar vertebral canal and resulting spinal cord compression. This syndrome may be related to known toxic and nutritional disorders affecting the bovine skeleton.

Calcium Phosphate Deposition Disease in Great Danes

This possibly familial disorder was seen clinically as progressive ataxia and paraplegia in 1 to 2 month old puppies.[325] Periarticular calcium phosphate mineralization occurred, along with deformity of bones in the axial and appendicular skeleton and mineralization of soft tissues. Caudal cervical vertebral canal stenosis caused compression of the spinal cord. The exact pathogenesis of the changes was not determined.

Multiple Cartilaginous Exostoses

Multiple cartilaginous exostoses (MCE) is a benign proliferative disease of cartilage and bone.[114] Any bone that is formed by enchondral ossification may be affected; however, vertebrae, ribs, and long bones are the most frequent location of exostoses. The condition has been reported in dogs, cats, and horses. There is no apparent sex or breed predisposition, although a familial tendency is probable. The condition is related to abnormal differentiation of cartilage cells that give rise to exostoses.

Neurologic signs in animals relate to spinal cord compression secondary to vertebral exostoses, which are most common in thoracic and lumbar regions. Signs progress from pelvic limb paresis to paraplegia. Onset of neurologic signs occurs prior to 1 year of age. Diagnosis is based on radiography, myelography, and microscopic examination of a biopsy specimen. Surgical excision is necessary in animals with evidence of progressive spinal cord compression. Prognosis is guarded.

REFERENCES

1. Adams EW: Hereditary deafness in a family of foxhounds. JAVMA 128:302, 1956.
2. Appleby EC, Longstaffe JA, and Bell FR: Ceroid-lipofuscinosis in two Saluki dogs. J Comp Pathol 92:375, 1982.
3. Averill DR: Degenerative myelopathy in the aging German Shepherd dog: Clinical and pathologic findings. JAVMA 162:1045, 1973.
4. Averill DR and Bronson RT: Inherited necrotizing myelopathy of Afghan hounds. J Neuropathol Exp Neurol 36:734, 1977.
5. Bailey CS: An embryological approach to the clinical significance of congenital vertebral and spinal cord abnormalities. J Am Anim Hosp Assoc 11:426, 1975.
6. Baker HJ: Inherited metabolic disorders of the nervous system in dogs and cats. In Kirk RW (ed): Current Veterinary Therapy V. Philadelphia, WB Saunders Co, 1974, p 700.
7. Baker HJ and Lindsey JR: Animal model of human disease: Human GM1 gangliosidosis. Animal model: Feline GM1 gangliosidosis. Am J Pathol 74:649, 1974.
8. Baker HJ, Lindsey JR, McKann GM, and Farrell DF: Neuronal GM1 gangliosidosis in a Siamese cat with β-galactosidase deficiency. Science 174:838, 1971.
9. Baker HJ, Mole JA, Lindsey JR, and Creel RM: Animal models of human ganglioside storage diseases. Fed Proc 35:1193, 1976.
10. Baker HJ, Reynolds GD, Walkley SU, et al: The gangliosidoses: Comparative features and research applications. Vet Pathol 16:635, 1979.
11. Bardens JW: Congenital malformations of the foramen magnum in dogs. Southwest Vet 18:295, 1965.
12. Barlow RM and Donald LG: Hydrocephalus in calves associated with unusual lesions in the mesencephalon. J Comp Pathol 73:410, 1963.
13. Barlow RM, Linklater KA, and Young GB: Familial convulsions and ataxia in Angus calves. Vet Rec 83:60, 1968.
14. Barnett KC and Grimes TD: Bilateral aplasia of the optic nerve in a cat. Br J Ophthalmol 58:663, 1974.
15. Beech J: Neuroaxonal dystrophy of the accessory cuneate nucleus in horses. Vet Pathol 21:384, 1984.
16. Bergsma DR and Brown KS: White fur, blue eyes, and deafness in the domestic cat. J Hered 62:171, 1971.
17. Bjerkas I: Hereditary "cavitating" leukodystrophy in Dalmatian dogs. Acta Neuropathol 40:163, 1977.
18. Bjorck G, Dyrendahl S, and Olsson SE: Hereditary ataxia in Smooth-haired Fox Terriers. Vet Rec 69:87, 1957.
19. Bjorck G, Everz KE, Hansen HJ, and Henrickson B: Congenital cerebellar ataxia in the Gotland pony breed. Zentralbl Veterinarmed (A) 20:341, 1973.
20. Bjorck G, Mair W, Olsson SE, and Sourander P: Hereditary ataxia in Fox Terriers. Acta Neuropathol (Suppl) 1:45, 1962.
21. Blakemore WF: GM1 Gangliosidosis in a cat. J Comp Pathol 82:179, 1972.
22. Blakemore WF: Lysosomal storage diseases. Vet Ann 15:242, 1975.
23. Blakemore WF and Palmer AC: Cerebral lipidoses and leucodystrophies in animals. Vet Ann 12:129, 1971.
24. Blakemore WF, Palmer AC, and Barlow RM: Progressive ataxia of Charolais cattle associated with disordered myelin. Acta Neuropathol 29:127, 1974.
25. Blood DC and Gay CC: Hereditary neuroaxial edema of calves. Aust Vet J 47:520, 1971.
26. Bosher SK and Hallpike CS: Observations on the histologic features, development, and pathogenesis of the inner ear degeneration of the deaf white cat. Proc R Soc Lond (Biol) 162:147, 1965.
27. Boysen BG, Tryphonas L, and Harries NW: Globoid cell leukodystrophy in the bluetick hound dog. 1. Clinical manifestations. Can Vet J 15:303, 1974.
28. Bradfield T: A Dalmatian with partial aplasia of cere-

bral hemispheres. Southwest Vet 22:323, 1969.

29. Braund KG and Mayhew IG: Unpublished data, 1979.

30. Braund KG, Taylor TKF, Ghosh P, and Sherwood AA: Spinal mobility in the dog. A study in chondrodystrophoid and non-chondrodystrophoid animals. Res Vet Sci 22:78, 1977.

31. Braund KG and Vandevelde M: German Shepherd dog myelopathy. A morphologic and morphometric study. Am J Vet Res 39:1309, 1978.

32. Brown T-T, deLahunta A, Bistner SI, et al: Pathogenetic studies of infection of the bovine fetus with bovine viral diarrhea virus. 1. Cerebellar atrophy. Vet Pathol 11:486, 1974.

33. Bundza A, Lowden JA, and Charlton KM: Niemann-Pick disease in a poodle dog. Vet Pathol 16:530, 1979.

34. Burditt LJ, Chotai K, Hirani S, et al: Biochemical studies on a case of feline mannosidosis. Biochem J 189:467, 1980.

35. Cancilla PA and Barlow RM: Structural changes of the central nervous system in swayback (enzootic ataxia) of lambs. Acta Neuropathol 6:251, 1966.

36. Chesney CJ: A case of spina bifida in a Chihuahua. Vet Rec 93:120, 1973.

37. Cho DY and Leipold HW: Agenesis of corpus callosum in calves. Cornell Vet 68:99, 1978.

38. Cho DY and Leipold HW: Arnold-Chiari malformation and associated anomalies in calves. Acta Neuropathol 39:129, 1977.

39. Cho DY and Leipold HW: Congenital defects of the bovine central nervous system. Vet Bull 47:489, 1977.

40. Cho DY and Leipold HW: Spina bifida and spinal dysraphism in calves. Zentralbl Veterinarmed (A) 24:680, 1977.

41. Cho DY and Leipold HW: Syringomyelia in a Thoroughbred foal. Equine Vet J 9:195, 1977.

42. Cho DY and Leipold HW: Anencephaly in calves. Cornell Vet 68:60, 1978.

43. Cho DY and Leipold HW: Cerebellar cortical atrophy in a Charolais calf. Vet Pathol 15:264, 1978.

44. Chrisman CL, Cork LC, and Gamble DA: Neuroaxonal dystrophy of Rottweiler dogs. JAVMA 184:464, 1984.

45. Clark RG, Hartley WJ, Burgess GS, et al: Suspected neuroaxonal dystrophy in collie sheep dogs. NZ Vet J 30:102, 1982.

46. Clarke L and Carlisle CH: Spina bifida with syringomyelia and meningocoele in a short-tailed cat. Aust Vet J 392, 1975.

47. Cockrell BY, Herigstad RR, Flo GJ, and Legendre AB: Myelomalacia in Afghan hounds. JAVMA 162:362, 1973.

48. Confer AW and Ward BC: Spinal dysraphism: A congenital myelodysplasia in the Weimaraner. JAVMA 160:1423, 1972.

49. Cordy DR and Knight HD: California goats with a disease resembling enzootic ataxia or swayback. Vet Pathol 15:179, 1978.

50. Cordy DR, Richards WPC, and Bradford GE: Systemic neuroaxonal dystrophy in Suffolk sheep. Acta Neuropathol 8:133, 1967.

51. Cordy DR, Richards WPD, and Stormont C: Hereditary neuraxial edema in Hereford calves. Pathol Vet 6:487, 1969.

52. Cordy DR and Snelbaker HA: Cerebellar hypoplasia and degeneration in a family of Airedale dogs. J Neuropathol Exp Neurol 11:324, 1952.

53. Cork LC, Griffin JW, Adams RJ, and Price DL: Hereditary canine spinal muscular atrophy. Am J Pathol 100:599, 1980.

54. Cork LC, Griffin JW, Choy C, et al: Pathology of

motor neurons in accelerated hereditary canine spinal muscular atrophy. Lab Invest 46:89, 1982.

55. Cork LC, Griffin JW, Munnell JF, et al.: Hereditary canine spinal muscular atrophy. J Neuropathol Exp Neurol 38:209, 1979.

56. Cork LC, Munnell JF, and Lorenz MD: The pathology of feline GM2 gangliosidosis. Am J Pathol 90:723, 1978.

57. Cork LC, Munnell JF, Lorenz MD, et al: GM2 ganglioside lysosomal storage disease in cats with B-hexosaminidase deficiency. Science 196:1014, 1977.

58. Cork LC, Troncoso JC, and Price DL: Canine inherited ataxia. Ann Neurol 9:492, 1981.

59. Cork LC, Troncoso JC, Price DL, et al: Canine neuroaxonal dystrophy. J Neuropathol Exp Neurol 42:286, 1983.

60. Cowell KR, Jezyk PF, Haskins ME, and Patterson DF: Mucopolysaccharidosis in a cat. JAVMA 169:334, 1976.

61. Crisp CE, Ringler DH, Abrams GD, et al: Lipid storage disease in a Siamese cat. JAVMA 156:616, 1970.

62. Cummings JF and deLahunta A: An adult case of canine neuronal ceroid-lipofuscinosis. Acta Neuropathol 39:43, 1977.

63. Cummings JF and deLahunta A: Hereditary myelopathy of Afghan hounds, a myelinolytic disease. Acta Neuropathol 42:173, 1978.

64. Deforest ME and Basrur PK: Malformations and the Manx syndrome in cats. Can Vet J 20:304, 1979.

65. deLahunta A: Comparative cerebellar disease in domestic animals. Scientific Proc, Am Coll Vet Intern Med, 1979, p 10.

66. deLahunta A: Comparative cerebellar disease in domestic animals. Comp Cont Educ 2:8, 1980.

67. deLahunta A: Diseases of the cerebellum. Vet Clin North Am 10:91, 1980.

68. deLahunta A: Veterinary Neuroanatomy and Clinical Neurology, 2nd ed. Philadelphia, WB Saunders Co, 1983.

69. deLahunta A and Averill DR: Hereditary cerebellar cortical and extrapyramidal nuclear abiotrophy in Kerry Blue Terriers. JAVMA 168:1119, 1976.

70. deLahunta A and Cummings JF: The clinical and electroencephalographic features of hydrocephalus in three dogs. JAVMA 146:954, 1965.

71. deLahunta A, Fenner WR, Indrieri RJ, et al: Hereditary cerebellar cortical abiotrophy in the Gordon setter. JAVMA 177:538, 1980.

72. deLahunta A and Shively GN: Neurofibrillary accumulation in a puppy. Cornell Vet 65:240, 1975.

73. Denny HR, Gibbs C, and Gaskell CJ: Cervical spondylopathy in the dog—a review of thirty-five cases. J Small Anim Pract 18:117, 1977.

74. Dimock WW and Errington BJ: Incoordination of equidae: Wobblers. JAVMA 95:261, 1939.

75. Doige CE: Pathological changes in the lumbar spine of pigs: Gross findings. Can J Comp Med 43:142, 1979.

76. Done JT: The congenital tremor syndrome in pigs. Vet Ann 16:90, 1975.

77. Done JT: Developmental disorders of the nervous system in animals. Adv Vet Sci Comp Med 21:69, 1977.

78. Done SH, Drew RA, Robins GM, and Lane JG: Hemivertebra in the dog: Clinical and pathological observations. Vet Rec 96:313, 1975.

79. Donnelly WJC, Hannon J, Sheahan BJ, and O'Connor PJ: Cerebrospinal lipidosis in Friesian calves. Vet Rec 91:225, 1972.

80. Donnelly WJC, Sheahan BJ, and Rogers TA: GM1 gangliosidosis in Friesian calves. J Pathol 111:173, 1973.

81. Douglas SW and Palmer AC: Idiopathic demyelination of brain-stem and cord in a miniature poodle puppy. J Pathol Bact 82:67, 1961.

82. Dow RW: Partial agenesis of the cerebellum in dogs. J Comp Neurol 72:569, 1940.

83. Draper DD, Kluge JP and Miller WJ: Neurologic, pathologic, and genetic aspects of spinal dysraphism in dogs (Abstr). Anat Histol Embryol 4:369, 1975.

84. Drew RA: Possible association between abnormal vertebral development and neonatal mortality in bulldogs. Vet Rec 94:480, 1974.

85. Dueland R, Furneaux RW, and Kaye MM: Spinal fusion and dorsal laminectomy for midcervical spondylolisthesis in a dog. JAVMA 162:366, 1973.

86. Dungworth DL and Fowler ME: Cerebellar hypoplasia and degeneration in a foal. Cornell Vet 56:17, 1966.

87. Edmonds L, Crenshaw D, and Selby LA: Micrognathia and cerebellar hypoplasia in an Aberdeen Angus herd. J Hered 64:62, 1973.

88. Edmonds HL, Hegreberg GA, van Gelder NM, et al: Spontaneous convulsions in beagle dogs. Fed Proc 38:2424, 1979.

89. Emmerson JL and Delez AL: Cerebellar hypoplasia, hypomyelinogenesis and congenital tremors of pigs associated with prenatal hog cholera vaccination of sows. JAVMA 147:47, 1965.

90. Engel HN and Draper DD: Comparative prenatal development of the spinal cord in normal and dysraphic dogs: Embryonic stage. Am J Vet Res 43:1729, 1982.

91. Engel HN and Draper DD: Comparative prenatal development of the spinal cord in normal and dysraphic dogs: Fetal stage. Am J Vet Res 43:1735, 1982.

92. Ernest JT: Bilateral optic nerve hypoplasia in a pup. JAVMA 168:125, 1976.

93. Falco MJ, Whitwell K and Palmer AC: An investigation into the genetics of "Wobbler Disease" in Thoroughbred horses in Britain. Equine Vet J 8:165, 1976.

94. Fankhauser R: Hydrocephalus studien. Schweiz Arch Tierheilkd 101:407, 1959.

95. Fankhauser R and Luginbuhl H: Pathologische Anatomie des Zentralen und Peripheren Nervensystems der Haustiere. Berlin, Paul Parey, 1968, p 208.

96. Fankhauser R, Luginbuhl H, and Hartley WJ: Leukodystrophie von Typus Krabbe beim Hund. Schweiz Arch Tierheilkd 105:198, 1965.

97. Fatzer R: Leukodystrophische eskrankungen im gehirn junger katzen. Schweiz Arch Tierheilkd 117:641, 1975.

98. Few AB: The diagnosis and surgical treatment of canine hydrocephalus. JAVMA 149:286, 1966.

99. Field B and Wanner RA: Cerebral malformation in a Manx cat. Vet Rec 96:42, 1975.

100. Fisher LF, Bowman KF, and MacHarg MA: Spinal ataxia in a horse caused by a synovial cyst. Vet Pathol 18:407, 1981.

101. Fletcher TF, Kurtz HJ, and Low DG: Globoid cell leukodystrophy (Krabbe type) in the dog. JAVMA 149:165, 1966.

102. Foulkes JA: Myelin and dysmyelination in domestic animals. Vet Bull 8:441, 1974.

103. Fraser, H: Two dissimilar types of cerebellar disorder in the horse. Vet Rec 78:608, 1966.

104. Fraser H and Palmer AC: Equine incoordination and wobbler disease of young horses. Vet Rec 80:338, 1967.

105. Frauchiger E and Frankhauser R: Vergleichende Neuropathologie des Menschen und Tiere. Berlin, Springer Verlag, 1957.

106. Frye FL: Spina bifida occulta with sacro-coccygeal agenesis in a cat. Anim Hosp 3:238, 1967.

107. Frye FL and McFarland LZ: Spina bifida with rachischisis in a kitten. JAVMA 146:481, 1965.

108. Furneaux RW, Doige CE, and Kaye MM: Syringomyelia and spina bifida occulta in a Samoyed dog. Can Vet J 14:317, 1973.

109. Gage ED: Atlanto-axial subluxation. In Bojrab MJ (ed): Current Techniques in Small Animal Surgery. Philadelphia, Lea & Febiger, 1975, p 376.

110. Gage ED and Hoerlein BF: Surgical treatment of canine hydrocephalus by ventriculoatrial shunting. JAVMA 153:1418, 1968.

111. Gage ED and Hoerlein BF: Surgical repair of cervical subluxation and spondylolisthesis in the dog. J Am Anim Hosp Assoc 9:385, 1973.

112. Gage ED and Smallwood JE: Surgical repair of atlanto-axial subluxation in a dog. Vet Med Small Anim Clin 65:583, 1970.

113. Gamble DA and Chrisman CL: A leukoencephalomyelopathy of Rottweiler dogs. Vet Pathol 21:174, 1984.

114. Gambardella PC, Osborne CA, and Stevens JB: Multiple cartilaginous exostoses in the dog. JAVMA 166:761, 1975.

115. Geary JC: Canine spinal lesions not involving disks. JAVMA 155:2038, 1969.

116. Geary JC, Oliver JE, and Hoerlein BF: Atlanto-axial subluxation in the canine. J Small Anim Pract 8:577, 1967.

117. Gelatt KN and Leipold HW: Bilateral optic nerve hypoplasia in two dogs. Can Vet J 12:91, 1971.

118. Gelatt KN, Leipold HW, and Coffman JR: Bilateral optic nerve hypoplasia in a colt. JAVMA 155:627, 1969.

119. Gerber H, Fankhauser R, Straub R, and Ueltschi G: Spinale Ataxia beim Pferd, veruusacht durch Synoviale Cysten in der Halswirbelsaul. Schweiz Arch Tierheilkd 122:95, 1980.

120. Gieb LW and Bistner SI: Spinal cord dysraphism in a dog. JAVMA 150:618, 1967.

121. Gill JM and Hewland ML: Cerebellar degeneration in the border collie. NZ Vet J 8:170, 1980.

122. Gilmore JPW: Congenital hydrocephalus in domestic animals. Cornell Vet 46:487, 1956.

123. Greene CE, Gorgacz EJ, and Martin CL: Hydranencephaly associated with feline panleukopenia. JAVMA 180:767, 1982.

124. Greene CE, Vandevelde M, and Braund KG: Lissencephaly in two Lhasa Apso dogs. JAVMA 169:405, 1976.

125. Greene CE, Vandevelde M, and Hoff EJ: Congenital cerebrospinal hypomyelinogenesis in a pup. JAVMA 171:534, 1977.

126. Greene HJ: Congenital hydranencephaly and cerebellar hypoplasia in calves. JAVMA 173:1008, 1978.

127. Greene HJ, Leipold HW, and Hibbs CM: Bovine congenital defects: Variations of internal hydrocephalus. Cornell Vet 64:596, 1974.

128. Greene HJ, Saperstein G, Schalles R, and Leipold HW: Internal hydrocephalus and retinal dysplasia in shorthorn cattle. Irish Vet J 32:65, 1978.

129. Greene PD, and Little PB: Neuronal ceroid-lipofuscin

storage in Siamese cats. Can J Comp Med 38:207, 1974.

130. Griffiths IR and Duncan ID: Chronic degenerative radiculomyelopathy in the dog. J Small Anim Pract 16:461, 1975.

131. Griffiths IR, Duncan ID, McCulloch M, and Harvey MJA: Shaking pups: A disorder of central myelination in the spaniel dog. Part 1. Clinical, genetic, and light microscopical observations. J Neurol Sci 50:423, 1981.

132. Hamilton GF: Periodic spasticity of cattle, and spastic paresis. *In* Howard JL (ed): Current Veterinary Therapy: Food Animal Practice. Philadelphia, WB Saunders Co, 1981, p 1096.

133. Hansen H-J: A pathologic-anatomical study on disk degeneration in the dog. Acta Orthop Scand (Suppl 11) 1952.

134. Harding JDJ, Done JT, Harbourne JF, and Gilbert FR: Congenital tremor type A III in pigs: An hereditary sex-linked cerebrospinal hypomyelinogenesis. Vet Rec 92:527, 1973.

135. Hartley WJ: Lower motor neuron disease in dogs. Acta Neuropathol 2:334, 1963.

136. Hartley WJ, Barker JSF, Wanner RA, and Farrow BRH: Inherited cerebellar degeneration in the Rough Coated Collie. Aust Vet Pract June:1, 1978.

137. Hartley WJ and Blakemore WF: Neurovisceral glucocerebroside storage (Gaucher's disease) in a dog. Vet Pathol 10:191, 1973.

138. Hartley WJ, Canfield PJ, and Donnelly TM: A suspected new canine storage disease. Acta Neuropathol 56:225, 1982.

139. Hartley WJ and Loomis LM: Murrurundi disease: An encephalopathy of sheep. Aust Vet J 57:399, 1981.

140. Hartley WJ and Palmer AC: Ataxia in Jack Russell Terriers. Acta Neuropathol 26:71, 1973.

141. Hartley WJ, Wanner RA, Della-Porta AJ, and Snowdon WA: Serological evidence for the association of Akabane virus with epizootic bovine congenital arthrogryposis and hydranencephaly syndromes in New South Wales. Aust Vet J 51:103, 1975.

142. Hartley WJ and Webb RF: A suspected new storage disease in cattle. Vet Pathol 19:616, 1982.

143. Haskins ME, Bingel SA, Northington JW, et al: Spinal cord compression and hindlimb paresis in cats with mucopolysaccharidosis VI. JAVMA 182:983, 1983.

144. Haskins ME, Jezyk PF, Desnick RJ, et al: Mucopolysaccharidosis in a domestic short-haired cat—a disease distinct from that seen in the Siamese cat. JAVMA 175:384, 1979.

145. Healy PJ and Cole AE: Heterozygotes for mannosidosis in Angus and Murray grey cattle. Aust Vet J 52:385, 1976.

146. Healy PJ, Seaman JT, Gardner JA, and Sewell CA: β Mannosidase deficiency in Anglo nubian goats. Aust Vet J 57:504, 1981.

147. Hedhammer A, Wu F-M, Krook L, et al: Overnutrition and skeletal disease: An experimental study in growing Great Dane dogs. Cornell Vet (Suppl 5) 64:1, 1974.

148. Hegreberg GA and Padgett GA: Inherited progressive epilepsy of the dog with comparisons to Lafora's disease of man. Fed Proc 35:1202, 1976.

149. Hegreberg GA, Thuline HC, and Francis BH: Morphologic changes in feline leukodystrophy. Fed Proc 30:341, 1971.

150. Higgins RJ, Rings DM, Fenner WR, and Stevenson S: Spontaneous lower motor neuron disease with neurofibrillary accumulation in young pigs. Acta Neuropathol (Berl) 59:288, 1983.

151. Higgins RJ, Vandevelde M, and Braund KG: Internal hydrocephalus and associated periventricular encephalitis in young dogs. Vet Pathol 14:236, 1977.

152. Higgins RJ, Vandevelde M, Hoff EJ, et al: Neurofibrillary accumulation in the zebra (*Equus burchelli*). Acta Neuropathol 37:1, 1977.

153. Hoerlein BF: Canine Neurology, 2nd ed. Philadelphia, WB Saunders Co, 1971, p 217.

154. Hoerlein BF: Canine Neurology, 3rd ed. Philadelphia, WB Saunders Co, 1978.

155. Holland JM, Davis WC, Prieur DJ, and Collins GH: Lafora's disease in the dog. Am J Pathol 58:509, 1970.

156. Hudson WR and Ruben RJ: Hereditary deafness in the Dalmatian dog. Arch Otolaryngol 75:213, 1962.

157. Hulland TJ: Cerebellar ataxia in calves. Can J Comp Med 21:72, 1957.

158. Icenogle DA and Kaplan AM: A review of congenital neurologic malformations. Clin Pediatr 20:565, 1981.

159. Igarashi M, Alford BR, Cohn AM, et al: Inner ear anomalies in dogs. Ann Otol Rhinol Laryngol 81:249, 1972.

160. Inada S, Sakamoto H, Haruta K, et al: A clinical study on hereditary progressive neurogenic muscular atrophy in Pointer dogs. Jap J Vet Sci 40:539, 1978.

161. Innes JRM, Rowlands WT, and Parry HB: An inherited form of cortical cerebellar atrophy in ("daft") lambs in Great Britain. Vet Rec 61:225, 1949.

162. Innes JRM and Saunders LZ: Comparative Neuropathology. New York, Academic Press, 1962.

163. Izumo S, Ikuta F, Igata A, et al: Morphological study on the hereditary neurogenic amyotrophic dogs: Accumulation of lipid compound-like structures in the lower motor neuron. Acta Neuropathol (Berl) 61:270, 1983.

164. James AV, Burns B, Flor WF, et al: Pathophysiology of chronic communicating hydrocephalus in dogs (*Canis familiaris*). J Neurol Sci 24:151, 1975.

165. James CC, Lassman LP, and Tomlinson BE: Congenital anomalies of the lower spine and spinal cord in Manx cats. J Pathol 97:269, 1968.

166. Johnson GR, Oliver JE, and Selcer R: Globoid cell leukodystrophy in a beagle. JAVMA 167:380, 1975.

167. Johnson I, Gilday DL, and Hendrick EB: Experimental effects of steroids and steroid withdrawal on cerebrospinal fluid absorption. J Neurosurg 42:690, 1975.

168. Johnson KH: Globoid leukodystrophy in the cat. JAVMA 157:2057, 1970.

169. Johnson RH, Margolis G, and Kilham L: Identity of feline ataxia virus on the feline panleukopenia virus. Nature 214:175, 1967.

170. Jolly RD: The pathology of the central nervous system in pseudolipidosis of Angus calves. J Pathol 103:113, 1971.

171. Jolly RD: Congenital brain oedema of Hereford calves. J Pathol 114:199, 1974.

172. Jolly RD: Lysosomal storage diseases. Neuropathol Appl Neurobiol 4:419, 1978.

173. Jolly RD and Blakemore WF: Inherited lysosomal storage diseases: An essay in comparative medicine. Vet Rec 92:391, 1973.

174. Jolly RD and Hartley WJ: Storage diseases of domestic animals. Aust Vet J 53:1, 1977.

175. Jolly RD, Janmaat A, West DM, and Morrison I: Ovine ceroid lipofuscinosis: A model of Batten's disease. Neuropathol Appl Neurobiol 6:195, 1980.

176. Jolly RD and Thompson KG: The pathology of bovine mannosidosis. Vet Pathol 15:141, 1978.

177. Jubb KVF and Kennedy PC: Pathology of Domestic Animals, 2nd ed. New York, Academic Press, 1970, p 344.

178. Kahrs RF, Scott FW, and deLahunta A: Congenital cerebellar hypoplasia and ocular defects in calves following bovine viral diarrhea-mucosal disease infection in pregnant cattle. JAVMA 156:1443, 1970.
179. Kalter H and Warkany J: Congenital malformations. N Engl J Med 308:424, 1983.
180. Kalter H and Warkany J: Congenital malformations. N Engl J Med 308:491, 1983.
181. Karbe E: Animal model of human disease: GM2-gangliosidosis (amaurotic idiocies) types I, II, and III. Animal model: Canine GM2-gangliosidosis. Am J Pathol 71:151, 1973.
182. Karbe E and Schiefer B: Familial amaurotic idiocy in male German shorthair pointers. Pathol Vet 4:223, 1967.
183. Kay WJ and Budzelovich GN: Cerebellar hypoplasia and agenesis in the dog. J Neuropathol Exp Neurol 29:156, 1970.
184. Kelly DF and Gaskell CJ: Spongy degeneration of the central nervous system in kittens. Acta Neuropathol 35:151, 1976.
185. Kelly WR, Clague AE, Barnes RJ, et al: Canine α-L-fucosidosis: A storage disease of Springer spaniels. Acta Neuropathol 60:9, 1983.
186. Kern TJ and Riis RC: Optic nerve hypoplasia in three miniature poodles. JAVMA 178:49, 1981.
187. Kilham L, Margolis G, and Colby ED: Congenital infections of cats and ferrets by feline panleukopenia virus manifested by cerebellar hypoplasia. Lab Invest 17:465, 1967.
188. Kitchen H, Murray RE, and Cockrell BY: Spina bifida, sacral dysgenesis and myelocele. Am J Pathol 66:203, 1972.
189. Klaasen JK and Wagner PC: Congenital vertebral abnormalities in a foal. Equine Pract 3:11, 1981.
190. Kono S, Moriwaki M, and Nakagawa M: Akabane disease in cattle: Congenital abnormalities caused by viral infection. Spontaneous disease. Vet Pathol 19:246, 1982.
191. Kono S and Nakagawa M: Akabane disease in cattle: Congenital abnormalities caused by viral infection. Experimental disease. Vet Pathol 19:267, 1982.
192. Koppang N: Neuronal ceroid-lipofuscinosis in English setters. J Small Anim Pract 10:639, 1970.
193. Koppang N: Canine ceroid-lipofuscinosis. A model for human neuronal ceroid-lipofuscinosis and aging. Mech Ageing Devel 2:421, 1973/1974.
194. Kronevi T, Ostensson K, and Lesser J: A case of partial cerebellar hypoplasia in a cat. Nord Vet Med 30:221, 1978.
195. Ladds P, Guffy M, Blauch B, and Splitter G: Congenital odontoid process separation in two dogs. J Small Anim Pract 12:463, 1970.
196. Lange AL, Van den Berg PB, and Baker MK: A suspected lysosomal storage disease in Abyssinian cats. Part II. Histopathological and ultrastructural aspects. J South Afr Vet Assoc 48:201, 1977.
197. Langweiler M, Haskins ME, and Jezyk PF: Mucopolysaccharidosis in a litter of cats. J Am Anim Hosp Assoc 14:748, 1978.
198. Leathers CW, Wagner PC, and Milleson B: Cervical spina bifida with meningocele in an Appaloosa foal. J Vet Orthop 1:55, 1979.
199. Leipold HW, Brandt GW, Guffy M, and Blauch B: Congenital atlanto-occipital fusion in a foal. Vet Med Small Anim Clin 69:1312, 1974.
200. Leipold HW, Cates WF, Radostits OM, and Howell WE: Spinal dysraphism, arthrogryposis and cleft palate in newborn Charolais calves. Can Vet J 10:268, 1969.
201. Leipold HW, Dennis SM, and Huston K: Congenital defects in cattle. Nature, cause, and effect. Adv Vet Sci Comp Med 16:103, 1972.
202. Leipold HW, Huston K, Blauch B, and Guffy MM: Congenital defects of the caudal vertebral column and spinal cord in Manx cats. JAVMA 164:520, 1974.
203. Littlewood JD, Herrtage ME, and Palmer AC: Neuronal storage disease in English Springer spaniels. Vet Rec 112:86, 1983.
204. Liu S-K, Dolensek EP, Adams CR, and Tappe JP: Myelopathy and vitamin E deficiency in six Mongolian wild horses. JAVMA 183:1266, 1983.
205. Long SE and Berepubo NA: A 37XO chromosome complement in a kitten. J Small Anim Pract 21:627, 1980.
206. Lorenz MD, Cork LC, Griffin JW, et al: Hereditary muscular atrophy in Brittany spaniels: Clinical manifestations. JAVMA 175:833, 1979.
207. Lurie MH: The membranous labyrinth in the congenitally deaf collie and dalmatian dog. Laryngoscope 58:279, 1948.
208. Luttgen PJ, Braund KG, and Storts RW: Globoid cell leukodystrophy. J Small Anim Pract 24:153, 1983.
209. Mackenzie CD and Johnson RP: Lafora's disease in a dog. Aust Vet J 52:144, 1976.
210. MacLachlan NJ and Osburn BI: Bluetongue virus-induced hydranencephaly in cattle. Vet Pathol 20:563, 1983.
211. Manktelow BW and Hartley WJ: Generalized glycogen storage disease in sheep. J Comp Pathol 85:139, 1975.
212. Martin AH: A congenital defect in the spinal cord of the Manx cat. Vet Pathol 8:232, 1971.
213. Mason RW, Hartley WJ, and Randall M: Spongiform degeneration of the white matter in a Samoyed pup. Aust Vet Pract 9:11, 1979.
214. Mason TA: Cervical vertebral instability (Wobbler syndrome) in the doberman. Aust Vet J 53:440, 1977.
215. Mayhew IG, deLahunta A, Whitlock RH, and Geary JC: Equine degenerative myeloencephalopathy. JAVMA 170:195, 1977.
216. Mayhew IG, deLahunta A, Whitlock RH, et al: Spinal cord disease in the horse. Cornell Vet (Suppl 6) 68:1, 1978.
217. Mayhew IG, Watson AG, and Heissan JA: Congenital occipitoatlantoaxial malformation in the horse. Equine Vet J 10:103, 1978.
218. Mesfin GM, Kusewitt D, and Parker A: Degenerative myelopathy in a cat. JAVMA 176:62, 1980.
219. McGrath JT: Neurologic Examination of the Dog, 2nd ed. Philadelphia, Lea & Febiger, 1960.
220. McGrath JT: Spinal dysraphism in the dog. Pathol Vet (Suppl) 2:1, 1965.
221. McGrath JT and Batt R: A leukodystrophy in the dog. J Neuropathol Exp Neurol 34:78, 1975.
222. McGrath JT, Kelly AM, and Steinberg SA: Cerebral lipidosis in the dog. J Neuropathol Exp Neurol 27:141, 1968.
223. McGrath JT, Schutta H, Yaseen A, and Steinberg S: A morphologic and biochemical study of canine globoid cell leukodystrophy. J Neuropathol Exp Neurol 28:171, 1969.
224. McHowell J, Dorling PR, Cook Rd, et al: Infantile and late onset form of generalised glycogenosis type II in cattle. J Pathol 134:266, 1981.
225. McNeel SV and Morgan JP: Intraosseous vertebral

venography: A technic for examination of the canine lumbosacral junction. J Am Vet Radiol Soc 19:168, 1978.

226. Meyers KM, Dickson WM, Lund JE, and Padgett GA: Muscular hypertonicity. Arch Neurol 25:61, 1971.

227. Meyers KM, Lund JE, Padgett G, and Dickson WM: Hyperkinetic episodes in Scottish terrier dogs. JAVMA 155:129, 1969.

228. Meyers KM and Schaub, RG: The relationship of serotonin to a motor disorder of Scottish terrier dogs. Life Sci 14:1895, 1974.

229. Montali RJ, Bush M, Sauer RM, et al: Spinal ataxia in Zebras. Vet Pathol 11:68, 1974.

230. Morgan JP: Spondylosis deformans in the dog. A morphologic study with some clinical and experimental observations. Acta Orthop Scand (Suppl 96) 1967.

231. Morgan JP: Spondylosis deformans in the dog: Its radiographic appearance. J Am Vet Radiol Soc 8:17, 1967.

232. Morgan JP: Congenital anomalies of the vertebral column of the dog: A study of the incidence and significance based on a radiographic and morphometric study. J Am Vet Radiol Soc 9:21, 1968.

233. Morgan JP: Spinal dural ossification in the dog. Incidence and distribution based on a radiographic study. J Am Vet Radiol Soc 10:43, 1969.

234. Morgan JP: Radiology in Veterinary Orthopedics. Philadelphia, Lea & Febiger, 1972.

235. Mostafa IE: A case of glycogenic cardiomegaly in a dog. Acta Vet Scand 11:197, 1970.

236. Neufeld JL and Little PB: Spinal dysraphism in a dalmatian dog. Can Vet J 15:335, 1974.

237. Newsholme SJ and Marshall LW: Unilateral hindleg spasticity: An outbreak of a specific clinical condition in suckling piglets. J South Afr Vet Assoc 51:195, 1980.

238. Nimmo Wilkie JS and Hudson EB: Neuronal and generalized ceroid-lipofuscinosis in a Cocker spaniel. Vet Pathol 19:623, 1982.

239. Oliver JE Jr and Lewis PE: Lesions of the atlas and axis in dogs. J Am Anim Hosp Assoc 9:304, 1973.

240. Oliver JE Jr, Selcer RR, and Simpson S: Cauda equina compression from lumbosacral malarticulation and malformation in the dog. JAVMA 173:207, 1978.

241. Olsson S-E, Starenborn M, and Hoppe F: Dynamic compression of the cervical spinal cord: A myelographic and pathologic investigation in Great Dane dogs. Acta Vet Scand 23:65, 1982.

242. Orr JP and McKenzie GC: Unusual skeletal deformities in calves in a Saskatchewan beef herd. Can Vet J 22:121, 1981.

243. Osburn BI, Johnson RT, Silverstein Am, et al: Experimental viral-induced congenital encephalopathies. II. The pathogenesis of bluetongue vaccine virus infection in fetal lambs. Lab Invest 25:206, 1971.

244. Osburn BI, Silverstein AM, Prendergast RA, et al: Experimental viral-induced congenital encephalopathies I. Pathology of hydranencephaly and porencephaly caused by bluetongue vaccine virus. Lab Invest 25:197, 1971.

245. Padget D: Neuroschisis and human embryonic development. J Neuropathol Exp Neurol 29:192, 1970.

246. Palmer AC: Introduction to Animal Neurology, 2nd ed. Oxford, Blackwell Scientific, 1976.

247. Palmer AC, Blakemore WF, Barlow RM, et al: Progressive ataxia of Charolais cattle associated with a myelin disorder. Vet Rec 91:592, 1972.

248. Palmer AC, Blakemore WF, Cook WR, et al: Cerebellar hypoplasia and degeneration in the young Arab

horse. Clinical and neuropathological features. Vet Rec 93:62, 1973.

249. Palmer AC, Blakemore WF, O'Sullivan B, et al: Ataxia and spinal cord degeneration in llama, wildebeeste, and camel. Vet Rec 107:10, 1980.

250. Palmer AC and Medd RK: Hound ataxia. Vet Rec 109:43, 1981.

251. Palmer AC, Payne JE, and Wallace ME: Hereditary quadriplegia and amblyopia in the Irish setter. J Small Anim Pract 14:343, 1973.

252. Palmer AC and Wallace ME: Deformation of cervical vertebrae in basset hounds. Vet Rec 80:430, 1967.

253. Parker AJ and Byerly CS: Meningomyelocoele in a dog. Vet Pathol 10:266, 1973.

254. Parker AJ and Cusick PK: Meningoencephalocele in a dog. Vet Med Small Anim Clin 69:206, 1974.

255. Parker AJ and Park RD: Atlanto-axial subluxation in small breeds of dogs. Diagnosis and pathogenesis. Vet Med Small Anim Clin 68:1133, 1973.

256. Parker AJ and Park RD: Occipital dysplasia in the dog. J Am Anim Hosp Assoc 10:520, 1974.

257. Parker AJ, Park RD, and Cusick PK: Abnormal odontoid process angulation in a dog. Vet Rec 93:559, 1973.

258. Parker AJ, Park RD, Cusick PK, and Jeffers CB: Cervical vertebral instability in the dog. JAVMA 163:71, 1973.

259. Patel V, Koppang N, Patel B, and Zeman W: p-Phenylene diamine-mediated peroxidase deficiency in English setters with neuronal ceroid-lipofuscinosis. Lab Invest 30:366, 1974.

260. Patten B: Overgrowth of the neural tube in young human embryos. Anat Rec 113:381, 1952.

261. Patterson DSP, Sweasey D, Brush PJ, and Harding JDJ: Neurochemistry of the spinal cord in British saddleback piglets affected with congenital tremor type A-IV, a second form of hereditary cerebrospinal hypomyelinogenesis. J Neurochem 21:397, 1973.

262. Percy DH and Jortner BS: Feline lipidosis. Arch Pathol 92:136, 1971.

263. Pierce KR, Kosanke SD, Bay WW, and Bridges CH: Animal model of human disease: GM2 gangliosidosis. Animal model: porcine cerebrospinal lipodystrophy (GM2 gangliosidosis). Am J Pathol 83:419, 1976.

264. Pritchard DH, Napthine DV, and Sinclair AJ: Globoid cell leucodystrophy in polled Dorset sheep. Vet Pathol 17:399, 1980.

265. Prynn RB and Redding RW: Electroencephalogram in occult canine hydrocephalus. JAVMA 152:1651, 1968.

266. Rac R and Giesecke PR: Lysosomal storage disease in Chihuahuas. Aust Vet J 51:403, 1975.

267. Read Dh, Harrington DD, Keenan TW, and Hinsman EJ: Neuronal-visceral GM1 gangliosidosis in a dog with β-galactosidase deficiency. Science 194:442, 1976.

268. Read WK and Bridges CH: Cerebrospinal lipodystrophy in swine. Pathol Vet 5:67, 1968.

269. Read WK and Bridges CH: Neuronal lipodystrophy—occurrence in an inbred strain of cattle. Pathol Vet 6:235, 1969.

270. Rebillard G, Rebillard M, Carlier E, and Pujol R: Histo-physiological relationships in the deaf white cat auditory system. Acta Otolaryngol 82:48, 1976.

271. Reed SM, Bayly WM, Traub JL, et al: Ataxia and paresis in horses. Part I. Differential diagnosis. Comp Cont Ed 3:588, 1981.

272. Reed SM, Newbry J, Bayly WM, et al: Cervical

vertebral malformation/malarticulation in the horse. Proc XII Ann Sci Progr, Am Coll Vet Intern Med 1984, p 201.

273. Richards RB, Edwards JR, Cook RD, and White RR: Bovine generalized glycogenosis. Neuropathol Appl Neurobiol 3:45, 1977.

274. Richards RB and Kakulas BA: Spongiform leukoencephalopathy associated with congenital myoclonia syndrome in the dog. J Comp Pathol 88:317, 1978.

275. Rousseau CG, Klavano GG, Johnson ES, et al: A newly recognized neurodegenerative disorder of horned Hereford calves. Can Vet J 24:296, 1983.

276. Rowe CL: Hemivertebra in a goat. Vet Med Small Anim Clin 74:211, 1979.

277. Sahar A, Hochwald GM, Kay WJ, and Ransohoff J: Spontaneous canine hydrocephalus: Cerebrospinal fluid dynamics. J Neurol Neurosurg Psychiatr 34:308, 1971.

278. Sandefeldt E, Cummings JF, deLahunta A, et al: Hereditary neuronal abiotrophy in the Swedish Lapland dog. Cornell Vet 63 (Suppl 3):1, 1973.

279. Sandefeldt E, Cummings JF, deLahunta A, et al: Hereditary neuronal abiotrophy in Swedish Lapland dogs. Am J Pathol 82:649, 1976.

280. Sandersleben J von and el Sergany MA: Ein Beitrag zur sogenannten Pachymeningitis spinalis ossificans des Hundes unter Berucksichtigung pathogenetischer und atiologischer Gesichtspunkte. Zentralbl Veterinarmed (A) 13:526, 1966.

281. Sandstrom B, Westman J, and Ockerman PA: Glycogenosis of the central nervous system in the cat. Acta Neuropathol 14:194, 1969.

282. Saunders LZ: Congenital optic nerve hypoplasia in collie dogs. Cornell Vet 42:67, 1952.

283. Saunders LZ, Sweet JD, Martin SM, et al: Hereditary congenital ataxia in Jersey calves. Cornell Vet 42:559, 1952.

284. Schmidt U: Generalisierte Lipofuscinose bei einer Katze. Berl Munch Tierarztl Wochenschr 4:70, 1974.

285. Schmorl G and Junghanns H: The Human Spine in Health and Disease, 2nd ed. New York, Grune and Stratton, 1971.

286. Selby LA, Hayes HM, and Becker SV: Epizootiologic features of canine hydrocephalus. Am J Vet Res 40:411, 1979.

287. Selcer RR and Oliver JE: Cervical spondylopathy—wobbler syndrome in dogs. J Am Anim Hosp Assoc 11:175, 1975.

288. Shelton MC: A Possible Mode of Inheritance for Spinal Dysraphism in the Dog with a More Complete Description of the Clinical Syndrome. Thesis. Iowa State University, Ames, IA, 1977.

289. Silson M and Robinson R: Hereditary hydrocephalus in the cat. Vet Rec 84:477, 1969.

290. Simpson ST: Unpublished data, 1980.

291. Snyder SP, Kingston RS, and Wenger DA: Animal model of human disease: Niemann-Pick disease. Sphingomyelinosis of Siamese cats. Am J Pathol 108:252, 1982.

292. Stashak TS and Mayhew IG: The nervous system. In Jennings PB (ed): The Practice of Large Animal Surgery. Philadelphia, WB Saunders Co, 1984, p 1032.

293. Steinberg SA: Clinico-pathologic conference. JAVMA 143:404, 1963.

294. Stockard CR: An hereditary lethal factor for localized motor and preganglionic neurons. Am J Anat 59:1, 1936.

295. Strecker E-P, Bush M, and James AV: Cerebrospinal fluid imaging as a method to evaluate communicating hydrocephaus in dogs. Am J Vet Res 34:101, 1973.

296. Suzuki Y, Austin J, Armstrong D, et al: Studies in globoid leukodystrophy: Enzymatic and lipid findings in the canine form. Exp Neurol 29:65, 1970.

297. Swaim SF and Greene CE: Odontoidectomy in a dog. J Am Anim Hosp Assoc 11:663, 1975.

298. Tarvin G and Prata RG: Lumbosacral stenosis in dogs. JAVMA 177:154, 1980.

299. Todd NB: The inheritance of taillessness in Manx cats. J Hered 52:228, 1961.

300. Tomchick TL: Familial Lafora's disease in the beagle dog. Fed Proc 32:8, 1973.

301. Van den Akker S: Arnold-Chiari malformation in animals. Acta Neuropathol (Suppl) 1:39, 1962.

302. Van den Berg PB, Baker MK, and Lange AL: A suspected lysosomal storage disease in Abyssinian cats. Part I: Genetic, clinical and clinical pathological aspects. J South Afr Vet Assoc 48:195, 1977.

303. Vandevelde M: Unpublished data, 1976.

304. Vandevelde M: Unpublished data, 1978.

305. Vandevelde M, Braund KG, Luttgen PJ, and Higgins RJ: Dysmyelination in Chow Chow dog: Further studies in older dogs. Acta Neuropathol 55:81, 1981.

306. Vandevelde M, Braund KG, Walker TL, and Kornegay JN: Dysmyelination of the central nervous system in the Chow-Chow dog. Acta Neuropathol 42:211, 1978.

307. Vandevelde M and Fatzer R: Neuronal ceroid-lipofuscinosis in older dachshunds. Vet Pathol 17:686, 1980.

308. Vandevelde M, Greene CE, and Hoff EJ: Lower motor neuron disease with accumulation of neurofilaments in a cat. Vet Pathol 13:428, 1976.

309. Van De Water NS, Jolly RD, and Farrow BRH: Canine Gaucher disease—the enzymatic defect. Aust J Exp Biol Med Sci 57:551, 1979.

310. Walkley SU, Blakemore WF, and Purpura DP: Alterations in neuron morphology in feline mannosidosis. Acta Neuropathol 53:75, 1981.

311. Waxman FJ, Clemmons RM, and Hinrichs DJ: Progressive myelopathy in older German Shepherd dogs. II. Presence of circulating suppressor cells. J Immunol 124:1216, 1980.

312. Wasman FJ, Clemmons RM, Johnson G, et al: Progressive myelopathy in older German Shepherd dogs. I. Depressed response to thymus-dependent mitogens. J Immunol 124:1209, 1980.

313. Weisbrode SE, Monke DR, Dodaro ST, and Hull BL: Osteochondrosis, degenerative joint disease and vertebral osteophytosis in middle-aged bulls. JAVMA 181:700, 1982.

314. Weisse I and Stotzer H: Hypoplasie des Nervus opticus und Kolobom der papille bei einem jungen Beagle. Berl Munch Tierarztl Wochenschr 86:1, 1973.

315. Wenger DA, Sattler M, Kudoh T, et al: Niemann-Pick disease: A genetic model in Siamese cats. Science 208:1472, 1980.

316. White ME, Pennock PW, and Seiler RJ: Atlanto-axial subluxation in five young cattle. Can Vet J 19:79, 1978.

317. White ME, Whitlock RH, and deLahunta A: A cerebellar abiotrophy of calves. Cornell Vet 65:476, 1975.

318. Whitten JH and Walker D: "Neuronopathy" and "pseudolipidosis" in Aberdeen Angus calves. J Pathol Bact 74:281, 1957.

319. Whitwell KE: Causes of ataxia in horses. In Practice. Vet Rec (Suppl) 2:17, 1980.

320. Williams DA, Sharp NJH, and Batt RM: Enteropathy associated with degenerative myelopathy in German Shepherd dogs. Sci Proc, Am Coll Vet Intern Med, 1983, p 40.

321. Wilson JW, Greene HJ, and Leipold HW: Osseous

metaplasia of the spinal dura mata in a Great Dane. JAVMA 167:75, 1975.

322. Wilson JW, Kurtz HJ, Leipold HW, and Lees GE: Spina bifida in the dog. Vet Pathol 16:165, 1979.

323. Wolff D: Three generations of deaf white cats. J Hered 33:39, 1942.

324. Woodard JC, Collins GH, and Hessler JR: Feline hereditary neuroaxonal dystrophy. Am J Pathol 74:551, 1974.

325. Woodard JC, Shields RP, Aldrich HC, and Carter RL: Calcium phosphate deposition disease in Great Danes. Vet Pathol 19:464, 1982.

326. Woods CB: Hyperkinetic episodes in two Dalmatians. J Am Anim Hosp Assoc 13:255, 1977.

327. Wright F, Rest JR, and Palmer AC: Ataxia of the Great Dane caused by stenosis of the cervical vertebral canal: Comparison with similar conditions in the Bas-sett hound, Doberman Pinscher, Ridgeback and the Thoroughbred horse. Vet Rec 92:1, 1973.

328. Wright JA: A study of the radiographic anatomy of the cervical spine in the dog. J Small Anim Pract 18:341, 1977.

329. Wright JA: Spondylosis deformans of the lumbosacral joint in dogs. J Small Anim Pract 21:45, 1980.

330. Yakely WL, Wyman M, Donovan EF, and Fechheimer NS: Genetic transmission of an ocular fundus anomaly in collies. JAVMA 152:457, 1968.

331. Young S: Hypomyelinogenesis congenita (cerebellar ataxia) in Angus-Short-Horn calves. Cornell Vet 52:84, 1962.

332. Zaki FA: Lissencephaly in Lhasa apso dogs. JAVMA 169:1165, 1976.

333. Zaki F and Kay WJ: Globoid cell leukodystrophy in a miniature poodle. JAVMA 163:248, 1973.

Chapter 7   *KG Braund, DVM, PhD*
BD Brewer, MS, DVM
IG Mayhew, BVSc, PhD

Inflammatory, Infectious, Immune, Parasitic, and Vascular Diseases

VIRAL DISEASES OF THE CENTRAL NERVOUS SYSTEM

In utero viral diseases of the CNS frequently result in congenital malformations (see Chapter 6).

Canine Distemper

Canine distemper encephalomyelitis (CDE) is caused by a paramyxovirus closely related to measles virus of humans and to rinderpest virus of cattle.[115] Even though the incidence is decreasing, canine distemper encephalomyelitis is still one of the most common central nervous system disorders in the dog. The virus initially invades and multiplies in lymphatic tissue and then spreads to epithelial and nervous tissue.[6, 8] Results of experimental studies suggest that central nervous system infection may be initiated by migrating virus infected lymphocytes.[250] This pantropic or neurotropic virus usually affects both white and gray matter.

Several clinical syndromes have been recognized in dogs:[26, 273]

Canine Distemper Encephalitis in Immature Animals. Microscopic lesions are generally found in many of the visceral organs, including the bladder, kidney, gastrointestinal tract, bronchioles, and tonsils. Lesions in the central nervous system are characterized by mononuclear perivascular cuffing, gliosis, microglial proliferation, and inflammatory cell infiltration of the pia arachnoid.[118, 181] In many cases, ependymal and subependymal edema and vacuolation are evident and are often accompanied by a proliferation of subependymal glial cells. Adventitial cell proliferation and endothelial swelling are commonly seen. Neuronal changes including nuclear pyknosis and shrunken cells, chromatolysis, and neuronophagia are found in the cerebral cortex, pontomedullary nuclei, Purkinje cells, and gray matter of the spinal cord. Intranuclear and intracytoplasmic inclusion bodies may be present in neuronal cells, astrocytes, histiocytes, meningeal cells, and ependymal cells. The distribution of inclusion bodies in distemper virus encephalitis is erratic, and their presence is not an indication of the severity of the disease process.

Changes in the white matter vary according to the duration and intensity of the infection. There is an apparent predilection for change in the central white matter of the cerebellum, the cerebellar peduncles, the optic nerves and

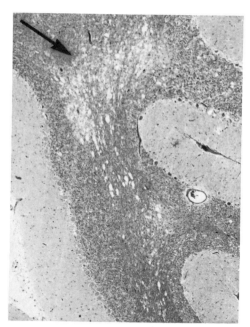

Figure 7–1. Canine distemper encephalitis produces this typical lesion in the cerebellum. Note the area of necrosis in the white matter (arrow). Hematoxylin and eosin, low power.

tracts, and the spinal cord (Fig. 7–1). Demyelinating lesions can be focal or disseminated, isolated or confluent. The demyelinating component of canine distemper encephalitis is of comparative medical interest[223, 251, 286] and has

been proposed as a model of multiple sclerosis and subacute sclerosing panencephalitis (SSPE) in humans.[137]

The mechanism of demyelination in canine distemper encephalitis is unknown. Some workers have suggested that demyelination results from direct virus activity on the oligodendrocyte.[109, 251] Others consider that immunologic mechanisms are involved.[140, 148] Results of a recent study indicate that both mechanisms may play a role: a direct viral effect in acute demyelination, and a local immune response in chronic, progressive demyelination.[275]

Nerve fibers may undergo degeneration, resulting in the formation of swollen axonal ovoids. Pronounced gliosis may be evident in association with these changes. In many severe lesions, there is evidence of tissue necrosis, edema, and macrophage infiltration. These lesions are often situated in the cerebellar peduncles or central white matter.

This is the most common form of distemper virus infection and is frequently characterized by systemic evidence of gastrointestinal and respiratory disturbances: vomiting, diarrhea, coughing, and seromucopurulent oculonasal discharges. Hyperkeratosis of the footpad may be seen. Additionally, many animals have conjunctivitis and chorioretinitis (Fig. 7–2). Neurologic signs are quite varied and usually suggest a multifocal distribution of lesions. Cortical and subcortical signs include generalized sei-

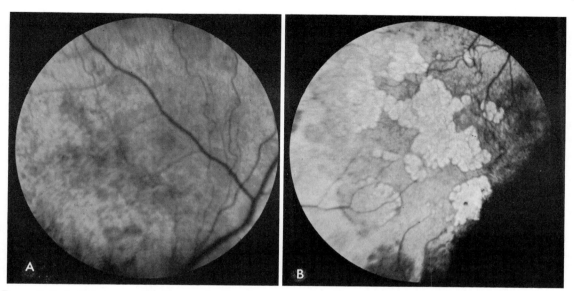

Figure 7–2. A, This is a confirmed case of active distemper retinitis. Note the irregular borders of the lesions that are characteristic of the early stages of distemper. B, Chronic chorioretinitis in a dog that had had respiratory distemper 4 months previously. The predominant clinical sign at that time was pelvic limb paresis. Note the hyperreflective lesions that have smooth and slightly pigmented borders.

zures and sometimes personality changes such as depression and disorientation. Signs of localization in the brain stem include incoordination, hypermetria, falling, head tilt, and nystagmus. Occasionally monoplegia and paraplegia are observed. A sign that is characteristic of distemper encephalitis is myoclonus or, more correctly, flexor spasm.[180] Appendicular flexor muscles, abdominal muscles, and the cervical musculature are the most frequently involved. Sometimes the masseteric, temporalis, and periorbital muscles are affected. These rhythmic contractions are not necessarily associated with limb paresis or paralysis and usually persist during sleep. The movements are temporarily abolished by intravenous injection of local anesthetic agents. The muscle contractions are caused by an abnormality in the motor neuron-interneuron pool in the spinal cord. It is not dependent on sensory nerves or descending pathways from the brain. Visual impairment is frequently reported and is generally associated with abnormal pupillary reflexes. Canine distemper virus is probably the most common cause of convulsions in dogs less than 6 months of age.

Multifocal Encephalitis Secondary to Canine Distemper Virus in Mature Animals. In mature dogs between the ages of 4 and 8 years, canine distemper virus can produce a type of encephalitis that is characterized by a chronic course.[26, 273] It is not unusual for an animal to be presented for care with a history of neurologic signs that have been present for 12 months. The incidence of this disease is relatively low and does not appear to be related to breed or sex. Animals that have received vaccinations against distemper virus may be affected. This disease is not preceded by, nor is it coincident with, the systemic signs that are seen in younger dogs. Furthermore, it is not unusual for this slowly progressive disease to remain clinically and pathologically static.

The pathologic changes that occur in mature dogs with this disease are usually restricted to the central nervous system. The lesions tend to be multifocal and necrotizing and are frequently found in the cerebellopontine angle adjacent to the fourth ventricle, in the cerebellar and cerebral peduncles, in the central cerebellar white matter, in the optic tracts, and in spinal cord white matter. Cystic lesions may be noted along with a loss of the original architecture of the tissues and strong fibrillary astrogliosis. The focal lesions may be associated with thick, perivascular, mononuclear cuffs. Small, plaquelike demyelinative lesions may be found in the capsula interna and corona radiata. Inclusion bodies are rarely found, and when present are usually located within astrocytic nuclei. Lesions generally are not found in the cerebral cortex.

The initial neurologic signs that are commonly seen in mature dogs with distemper virus encephalitis include weakness of the pelvic limbs, generalized incoordination, and occasional falling. These signs frequently progress to tetraplegia. Generalized seizures or personality changes are not features of this disease, and affected animals maintain a normal mental state. Many dogs will have unilateral or bilateral menace deficits, with normal or abnormal pupillary reflexes. Some animals have signs of facial paralysis, head tilt, and nystagmus. Although head tremors may be seen, myoclonic movements or flexor spasms are not present.

Old Dog Encephalitis. This disease, in which canine distemper virus has been incriminated as the etiologic agent, is a subacute or chronic progressive panencephalitis that occurs rarely in mature dogs. Various synonyms have been used, including disseminated encephalomyelitis in mature dogs, subacute diffuse sclerosing encephalitis, and chronic dementia distemper.

Affected animals are usually over 6 years of age; however, younger dogs may be affected. There are no related systemic signs, nor is there any apparent predisposition according to breed or sex. The most common initial neurologic sign is visual impairment. Old dog encephalitis is an invariably progressive disorder and is accompanied by the development of increasing mental depression, compulsive circling, hyperkinesia, and head pressing against objects (obstinate progression).[47] A bilateral menace deficit of a central or peripheral nature is also a common sign. An affected animal may manifest a personality change and fail to recognize its owners. Signs of involvement of the brain stem are rare.

Pathologic changes associated with the disorder are restricted to the central nervous system and are characterized by disseminated perivascular infiltration with lymphocytes and plasma cells, diffuse microglial proliferation, astrogliosis, neuronal degeneration, and neuronophagia (Fig. 7–3). The lesions have a diffuse distribution throughout all divisions of the cerebral cortex. Similar lesions are usually found throughout the basal nuclei, thalamus, hypothalamus, and midbrain. The perivascular mononuclear cuffs often extend beyond the Virchow-Robin space and infiltrate the nervous parenchyma. Diffuse demyelination is seen in

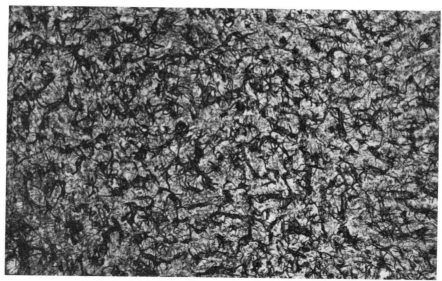

Figure 7–3. Chronic progressive distemper encephalitis. Note the diffuse fibrillary astrogliosis in the cerebral cortex. Maurer stain for astrocytes, medium power.

subcortical areas, internal capsule, and cerebral peduncles and often is observed in the pontine area and middle cerebellar peduncles. Large eosinophilic inclusion bodies are seen in the nuclei and cytoplasm of neuronal and glial cells. Necrotizing lesions may be present in the cerebral cortex, characterized by diffuse loss of neuronal cells with replacement of the parenchyma by fibrillary astrocytes.

Old dog encephalitis is clinically and pathologically different from multifocal distemper encephalitis in mature dogs. The nature of the lesions (diffuse sclerosis versus multifocal necrosis) and their topographic localization (cerebral cortex and upper brain stem versus lower brain stem and spinal cord) are quite distinct in old dog encephalitis and multifocal distemper encephalitis, respectively. In contrast to multifocal distemper encephalitis, the cerebellum is mostly spared in old dog encephalitis. Clinical differentiation between the two diseases is facilitated by the development of progressive cortical and subcortical signs (mental depression, unresponsiveness, obstinate progression) in old dog encephalitis.

The interest generated by old dog encephalitis is related to its clinical, pathologic, and immunologic similarities with subacute sclerosing panencephalitis in humans,[2, 159, 160] even though there appear to be different mechanisms operating in the maintenance of persistent infection and pathogenesis of these two chronic viral diseases.[95]

DIAGNOSIS AND TREATMENT

The diagnosis of canine distemper encephalomyelitis (in young dogs especially) is usually based on history and clinical signs. The index of suspicion is higher in affected dogs that are not vaccinated. Hematologic and biochemical data are nonspecific, and electroencephalographic traces may indicate presence of inflammatory disease only. Cerebrospinal fluid analysis may reveal a moderate pleocytosis (15 to 60 white blood cells per cubic millimeter) of mononuclear cells (lymphocytes and macrophages) and elevated gamma globulin levels.[51] Increased β-glucuronidase levels have been reported in serum and cerebrospinal fluid.[164] Specific neutralizing antibody in CSF occurs 2 to 3 weeks after onset of disease and is the most definite evidence for canine distemper. It is normally not present in the CSF of vaccinated dogs, dogs that develop circulating antibody quickly and remain asymptomatic after exposure, or dogs that die from acute canine distemper infection.[6] Results of fluorescent antibody (FA) testing for viral antigen in smears made from conjunctival or tracheal washes may be positive,[6] especially in young dogs; however, the fluorescent antibody test can be positive in recently vaccinated animals.[94]

Ophthalmoscopic examinations may detect a chorioretinitis[74] characterized by areas of hyperreflectivity and bright colored "medallion" lesions, indicative of past or latent infection.[130]

Examination of buffy coat smears may demonstrate inclusion bodies in lymphocytes, particularly in the early phase of the disease. The use of immunofluorescent techniques to detect canine distemper viral antigen in brain sections and other tissues from dogs of all ages has been described.[6, 149, 272]

Experimental transmission of distemper encephalitis from young dogs and from dogs with multifocal distemper encephalitis has been relatively easy;[140, 213] however, it is only recently that canine distemper virus has been isolated from dogs with old dog encephalitis.[116]

The suggested link between ownership of a dog with the associated possible exposure to canine distemper virus and multiple sclerosis[44, 45] has not been substantiated.[9, 19, 147, 153]

There is no treatment, and dogs with progressive neurologic signs leading to incapacitation need to be euthanatized. The prognosis is better in dogs with nonprogressive neurologic sequelae such as intermittent seizures, myoclonus, and visual impairment, although only seizures may respond to medication.

Postvaccinal Canine Distemper Encephalomyelitis

Postvaccinal canine distemper encephalomyelitis occurs in young animals, especially those less than 6 months of age. It has been recognized as a disease entity for a number of years and is believed to be associated with vaccination with live virus.

The pathogenesis of this disease is unclear. It may result from insufficient attenuation of the vaccine virus, which causes subsequent infection of the central nervous system, from the triggering of a latent paramyxovirus infection by vaccination, or from an enhanced susceptibility of the animal. This disorder has been reported after combined distemper and infectious canine hepatitis vaccination in the dog.[23, 71, 99]

Pathologic changes in the brain are characterized by multifocal neuronal degeneration, neuronophagia, axonal degeneration, perivascular cuffing, and mild to moderate gliosis. The lesions are seen at all levels but tend to be most severe in the ventral pontine area where malacia may also be seen. Purkinje cells frequently remain unaffected. Intranuclear and intracytoplasmic inclusion bodies are present in many neuronal cells. Ultrastructural examination of the inclusion bodies reveals the presence of nucleocapsids with the features of the paramyxovirus group.[23, 99]

Clinical signs are usually seen within 1 to 2 weeks after vaccination. They include anorexia, listlessness, and slight pyrexia. Neurologic signs occur 1 to 3 days after the onset of these nonspecific signs. Sudden changes in temperament, viciousness (attacking owners, other dogs, and inanimate objects), aimless wandering, howling, incoordination, and terminal convulsions may be seen in acute cases of approximately 24 hours duration. In subacute cases (a disease course of 2 to 3 days), pelvic limb incoordination, circling, depression, and visual impairment are frequently observed.

This disorder differs from spontaneous distemper infection in young dogs. The clinical differences include an absence of systemic signs and an alteration in personality to viciousness, which is similar in nature and clinical course to that seen in the furious form of rabies encephalitis. Pathologically, postvaccinal distemper encephalitis is distinguished by the virtual absence of visceral inclusions and of demyelination in the area of the cerebellopontine angle, the presence of many neuronal inclusions, diffuse pontine tegmental malacia, and large numbers of degenerating axonal ovoids.

Prognosis is guarded, and treatment is symptomatic.

Rabies

All warm blooded mammals are susceptible to rabies encephalitis; however, there is considerable interspecies susceptibility. Wildlife is the chief natural reservoir of rabies. In most northern countries such as Canada, Greenland, and the Soviet Union, foxes are the main vectors. In other parts of the world, wolves (Iran), mongooses (the Caribbean), skunks and raccoons (the United States), and bats (Latin America) play important roles in transmitting rabies.[254] In the United States, dogs play a relatively small part in current epizootics. Dog vaccination helped to decrease cases of canine rabies in the United States from 5000 in 1946 to 180 in 1973, thus eliminating the major route of rabies transmission to humans.

Rabies is caused by a rhabdovirus, which is destroyed by lipid solvents and low pH.[85] Transmission most often occurs through bite wounds from infected animals that are secreting virus in their saliva. Infection may also occur by wound or abrasion contamination from infected saliva or other infected material. Airborne transmission and infection through mucous membranes may also occur.

The incubation period is variable, ranging from 2 weeks to 1 year, depending on the amount of virus transmitted, site of inoculation, and nature of the wound.[21]

Rabies virus is highly neurotropic and reaches the central nervous system via passive centripetal movement in the axoplasmic compartment of peripheral nerves.[76, 231] Following the entry of the virus into the CNS, usually the spinal cord, its ascending course to the brain is rapid.[190, 191] In humans and animals, rabies infection is usually extremely widespread in the brain. The virus has a significantly higher tropism for neurons than for glia.[260] Negri bodies (viral antigen aggregates) are often largest in the largest neurons, such as the pyramidal cells of the hippocampus (Fig. 7–4), ganglionic neurons of pontine nuclei, and Purkinje cells of the cerebellum.[190] Centrifugal spread of virus to sites involved in bite transmission is via peripheral nerves and involves target cells exposed to body surfaces. Salivary gland mucous epithelium is the major source of virus shed into secretions in species that maintain rabies in nature. These include the dog, fox, skunk, raccoon, and bat.[190] Results of recent experimental studies indicate that dogs can excrete rabies virus in the saliva up to 13 days before clinical signs are exhibited,[73] thus necessitating a longer observation period in prospectively rabid dogs than the 10 days currently recommended.

Pathologically, rabies is characterized by a

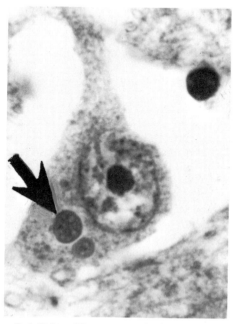

Figure 7–4. Rabies. The neuron in the hippocampus shows intracytoplasmic viral inclusions, or Negri bodies (arrow). Hematoxylin and eosin, high power.

multifocal, mild polioencephalomyelitis with mononuclear perivascular infiltrates, diffuse glial proliferation, regressive changes in neuronal cells, and glial nodules.[118] There is a predilection for localization in the brain stem, especially the substantia nigra, red nucleus, and periaqueductal gray matter of the midbrain; the pontine nuclei; the reticular formation; the floor of the fourth ventricle; and the hypothalamus. Other areas commonly affected include the gray matter of the spinal cord, hippocampus, globus pallidus, and thalamic nuclei. Intracytoplasmic Negri bodies are usually most numerous in hippocampal neurons and Purkinje cells.

Initial clinical signs tend to be nonspecific and include apprehension, restlessness, anorexia, and vomiting. A change in temperament may be noted at this stage, and excessive salivation may occur. These signs, which may be present for 2 to 5 days, are followed by either the dumb or the furious form of the disease.[118, 181] Approximately 25 to 30% of affected animals exhibit the furious form,[21] which is characterized by increased restlessness, wandering, viciousness (attack of animals, humans, or inanimate objects), howling, polypnea, drooling of saliva, and sometimes convulsions. Death usually occurs between 4 and 8 days after the onset of clinical signs. It is usually the furious form of rabies that occurs in cats.

The dumb or paralytic form of rabies encephalomyelitis is more common and is characterized by progressive ascending spinal paresis or paralysis, paralysis of the lower jaw, pharyngeal and hypoglossal paralysis (resulting in difficulty in eating and drinking, and drooling of saliva), and facial paralysis. In dogs, a noticeable change in the character of the bark occurs as a result of the pharyngeal paralysis. Death as a result of respiratory failure occurs between 3 and 6 days after the onset of clinical signs.

Recently, dogs infected with rabies experimentally have developed clinical signs and recovered. Previously rabies was considered invariably fatal in the dog. These findings place an increased responsibility on the veterinarian in managing animals with encephalitis.

It should be noted that clinical signs associated with rabies in dogs are often so variable that a distinction between the furious and dumb forms may be unjustified.[127] As a result, the diagnosis of rabies must be based on laboratory confirmation; histopathologic examinations of brain sections or smears for presence of an acute meningoencephalitis and identification of Negri bodies; and fluorescent antibody test on tactile facial hair follicles obtained from skin biopsy or on brain samples and mouse inoculation. Mouse inoculation has the disadvantage of a 3 week observation period to establish a negative diagnosis. The rabies fluorescent antibody test is widely used, for it is an extremely accurate and rapid technique.

There is no treatment. Animals exposed to rabies that have not been immunized should be euthanatized. If the animal has had adequate rabies vaccination and has been exposed (and the owners do not want euthanasia), the animal should be revaccinated and closely confined under observation for at least 30 days.

There is little benefit to be derived from classifying rabies (paralytic versus dumb forms) in large animals. In the horse, the presenting signs have included colic, suspected stifle injury, radial paralysis, difficult urination, hyperesthesia, and personality changes.[129] The signs have progressed, usually within several days, to obvious, severe neurologic disease with the clinical course ranging from 1 to 7 days. The CSF has been normal, been mildly abnormal, or evidenced moderate elevations in mononuclear cell numbers and protein levels. Rabies must be discussed in the differential diagnosis of many equine neurologic cases, but when severe unusual signs of gray matter lesions are present (ie, loss of reflexes, hypersensitivity, or loss of sensation) rabies should be strongly considered.

Signs of rabies in food animals are equally variable and have been documented in cattle, pigs, sheep, and goats. Of 97 rabid cattle, 52 were heard bellowing and 37 experienced excessive salivation.[232] Twenty appeared choked, 21 had pelvic limb paralysis, 31 were ataxic, 12 were hyperesthetic, and 8 had muscle spasms or generalized convulsions.

In one outbreak in 16 pigs, all exhibited nose twitching, rapid chewing movements, excessive salivation, and convulsions, and died between 12 and 48 hours following onset of clinical signs.[189]

Postvaccinal Rabies Encephalomyelitis

A paralytic syndrome occasionally occurs in dogs and cats as a result of infection of the central nervous system by rabies modified live vaccine virus derived from chick embryos. Clinical signs appear within 7 to 21 days after vaccination.[15, 210]

Pathologic findings are inconclusive. Acute nonsuppurative meningoencephalomyelitis has been reported.[267] The lower motor neuron signs seen neurologically suggest that the tissue lesions are associated with polioencephalomyelitis. Negri bodies may not be found in the brain, and virus may not be detected in saliva. High levels of rabies virus antibody in serum and cerebrospinal fluid have been reported in dogs with the postvaccinal syndrome.[72, 210] At present, there is no evidence to suggest that the vaccine virus reverts to its original virulence. Rabies virus has been isolated from brain, and rabies antigen has been demonstrated by fluorescent antibody techniques.[210]

Clinicopathologic correlations are not definitive, but ascending lower motor neuron paralysis, beginning in the pelvic limbs following vaccination in the thigh, appears to be the most prominent neurologic derangement. In this regard, the syndrome is similar to the dumb form of rabies. Paralysis of the cranial nerves, as well as attendant changes such as the character of the bark and excessive salivary drooling, have been observed,[72] and mental status may be depressed. Clinical recovery has been reported in dogs within 1 to 2 months.[72, 210]

The clinical differentiation between postvaccinal syndrome and the naturally acquired form of rabies infection may be difficult and is therefore dependent on a history of possible natural exposure to rabies. Appropriate public health precautions need to be taken.

Postvaccinal, progressive encephalomyelitis has occurred in horses vaccinated in the neck musculature with a modified, live, ERA strain rabies vaccine.[172] Some horses recovered completely. The exact etiopathogenesis of this syndrome is not defined.

Canine Herpesvirus Infection

Sporadic outbreaks of neonatal death in puppies caused by an infection with a herpesvirus have been reported.[39] Transmission occurs in utero, by direct contact with diseased littermates, or by inhalation or ingestion of infected material. The virus is believed to spread to the CNS via the hematogenous route, after initial replication in the oronasopharynx.[211] The high susceptibility of newborn puppies to disseminated canine herpesvirus (CHV) infection is related to their relatively low body temperature.[38] Older puppies appear to be resistant to the virus[292] and can serve as asymptomatic carriers.

In the CNS, an acute encephalitis is a feature of this disease. The main lesions are focal or laminar areas of necrosis involving mainly the Purkinje cell and granular layers of the gray matter of the cerebellum. Focal gliosis and perivascular cuffing by lymphocytes and macrophages are often seen in cerebrum, thalamus, and pons. Intracellular inclusions may be observed occasionally in neurons and glial cells adjacent to the malacic areas. Meningitis with necrosis of capillary walls may be found. Perivascular edema and hemorrhages occur in many visceral organs.[292]

The syndrome is characterized by acute onset of signs including crying, diarrhea, dyspnea, and abdominal tenderness.[39] Terminal depression and death usually occur 1 to 3 days after the onset of clinical signs. Findings at necropsy include ecchymoses and foci of necrosis in lung, liver, and kidney; diffuse pulmonary congestion; and splenomegaly.[212]

Diagnosis is based on age, clinical signs, and pathologic findings. There is no treatment.

Equine Herpesvirus Type 1 Infection

Equine herpesvirus type 1 (EHV-1) is rarely associated with neurologic disease in horses. Most often the respiratory form of EHV-1 or abortion occurs in animals in contact with the neurologically affected animal. Occasionally, the respiratory form or abortion may precede, or abortion may follow, the onset of neurologic signs in the same horse. However, the neurologic syndrome may be seen independent of other forms of equine herpesvirus type 1 infection. All ages of animals may be affected,[89] but mares between 3 and 9 months pregnant seem particularly susceptible.[119] Several horses are likely to be affected at the same time, and occasionally large numbers of animals may be simultaneously affected.[89] Vaccination is not necessarily protective. There is now evidence for the existence of a separate neurotropic subtype of equine herpesvirus 1, but the pathogenic mechanism is unclear.[177]

Histopathologic lesions may be scattered diffusely throughout the brain and spinal cord and consist of a vasculitis with resultant foci of ischemic or hemorrhagic infarction involving white matter and, less frequently, gray matter. Clinical signs vary, but the typical horse has a sudden onset of symmetric or mildly asymmetric pelvic limb ataxia that does not progress after the first few days. Bladder paralysis is common, as is a hypotonic tail and anus. Rapid, fulminating progression to complete paralysis has occurred. Hemiparesis, focal brain stem signs, and even diffuse cerebral disease have also been reported.

The CSF is usually xanthochromic with an elevated protein content but normal white blood cell count. However, the CSF rarely may be within normal limits, and certainly may be normal within 2 weeks of the onset of signs.

Diagnosis is by clinical signs (especially disturbances in bladder function associated with pelvic limb ataxia), association with respiratory disease or abortion on the farm, lack of significant progression, and typical CSF changes. Complement fixation and serum neutralization tests on paired sera will aid in the diagnosis. The absence of increased equine herpesvirus type 1 antibody concentration does not rule out the disease, nor does an increased concentration prove that the neurologic signs are due to equine herpesvirus type 1. Virus isolation from buffy coat, aborted fetuses, or respiratory tract of affected and contact animals is strong evidence of the cause of an outbreak. Viral isolation is possible from CNS tissue[222, 258] but cannot always be accomplished.

There is no proven therapy for this condition, other than supportive care, although antiinflammatory therapy is indicated. The prognosis is fair to good for full recovery in animals that are not recumbent. However, some animals have residual damage.[222] Recumbent animals have been reported to recover, but this is rare.[89]

A particularly severe form of myeloencephalitis has occasionally occurred following the intramuscular use of a modified live rhinopneumonitis vaccine, which has since been removed from the market.[162]

Aujeszky's Disease

This disease, also known as pseudorabies, mad itch, and infectious bulbar paralysis, affects most species of wild and domestic animals except horses.[118] Swine are the natural host of the causative virus (herpesvirus suis), and survivors may serve as inapparent carriers of infection. Aujeszky's disease in species other than swine, namely cattle, dogs, cats, and wildlife, is usually fatal. The virus is believed to reach the central nervous system by traveling centripetally in the peripheral nerves, probably in the axoplasm.[93, 166] The mode of transmission to dogs and cats is usually the consumption of virus contaminated tissues of swine, cattle, rats, and mice.[92] The virus may also gain entrance to the body via scratches or abrasions from contaminated objects and via the respiratory system in cattle.[50]

The virus is highly neurotropic, and the most extensive brain changes in the dog and cat occur in the medulla, followed by the pons, thalamus, cerebellum, and cerebral cortex. Microscopically, a moderate meningoencephalitis is observed, with perivascular mononuclear infiltrations, proliferation of neuroglia and accompanying neutrophil leukocytes, as well as Cowdry type A intranuclear inclusions in glia, ganglia, and neurons.[67, 118, 135]

The incubation period in the dog and cat ranges from 2 to 10 days. Death usually occurs within 24 to 48 hours after onset of clinical signs.[113] Classically, the most characteristic clinical manifestations are intense localized pruritus of the face or limbs, with scratching or chewing to the point of self-mutilation. However, recent reports suggest that pruritus may not always be a constant feature.[87, 93, 280] Early in the course of the disease, fever, restlessness, emesis, excessive salivation, and dyspnea may be noted, followed by incoordination, vocalization, anisocoria, ptosis, and facial tremors. Convulsions, coma, and death quickly ensue.[92, 113] Treatment does not alter the course of the disease.

Clinical distinction from rabies can be made by noting the presence of intense pruritus and/or observing that affected animals are not aggressive to animate and inanimate objects. Diagnosis may be suggested by clinical and histologic data, substantiated by neuropathologic findings, and confirmed by fluorescent antibody test of brain tissue or by laboratory animal (usually rabbit) inoculation with tissue extracts.

The clinical appearance, morbidity, and mortality of pseudorabies in the pig vary with the ages of the group affected and have been recently reviewed.[50] Neurologic signs include dullness, muscular tremors, weakness, ataxia, disorientation, convulsions, and death. Blindness with a head tilt has been reported in feeder pigs. Pruritus and aggressive behavior are not as common as in other affected species.

Cattle, sheep, and goats may experience sudden death or, more commonly, intense pruritus, excitement, and aggressiveness. Pruritus is not always present, however. The disease is usually fatal in these species and should be particularly considered in the differential diagnosis of a rapidly progressing neurologic disease in animals exposed to swine.

Infectious Canine Hepatitis

Infectious canine hepatitis is caused by an adenovirus (CAV-1) and is a highly contagious systemic disease of younger dogs and foxes. The virus is transmitted by direct contact with infected animals (via saliva, respiratory secretions, urine, or feces) or by contact with contaminated objects. The virus spreads to local lymph nodes via the oropharynx and is disseminated throughout the body by the hematogenous route.[7] It has special predilection for vascular endothelium and liver, kidney, and lymph nodes.[291] Signs of encephalitis related to damage of vascular endothelium are rare in the dog but may include rapidly progressive tetraparesis, coma, seizures, and death. These signs may be accompanied by vomiting, abdominal pain, fever, and jaundice.

Diagnosis is suggested by clinical signs and clinical pathologic data, substantiated by demonstration of the virus in blood or biopsy material, and confirmed by histologic examination of tissues. Large intranuclear inclusion bodies are found in hepatic cells.

Treatment is usually futile.

Feline Coronavirus Disease

This disease, also known as feline infectious peritonitis, is caused by a coronavirus.[197] Two forms have been reported: an effusive ("wet") form resulting from diffuse fibrinous peritonitis accompanied by excessive abdominal fluid,[287, 288] and a noneffusive ("dry") form characterized by perivascular granulomas around small blood vessels in various sites, especially meninges, brain, and uvea.[242]

Coronavirus infection is common in cats; however, the majority of infections are subclinical. Approximately 50% of cats with clinical coronavirus disease also test positive for feline leukemia virus.[209] The prevalence of coronavirus infection is highest in cats 1 to 2 years of age. There is no breed or sex predisposition. The route of infection and incubation period are uncertain. The CNS lesions may result from an immune complex–mediated vasculitis.

Central nervous system pathology is more often observed in the noneffusive form of feline coronavirus disease[151, 208, 242] than in the effusive form.[287, 288] However, cats without neurologic deficits may still have microscopic CNS involvement.[142] The pathologic lesions typical of feline coronavirus disease in the CNS include a pyogranulomatous inflammatory cell infiltration of leptomeninges, choroid plexus, ependyma, and brain parenchyma. Perivascular cuffing is prominent. Subependymal periventricular necrosis is commonly observed, as is the infiltration of macrophages, lymphocytes, neutrophils, and plasma cells. Inflammatory vascular changes are sometimes present, and many animals have associated panophthalmitis.[70, 142, 151, 157, 242]

The clinical neurologic vagaries of feline coronavirus disease were recognized in earlier reports[142, 151, 157, 242] and include pelvic limb paresis, nystagmus, anisocoria, seizure, tetraparesis, and intention tremors. Multifocal or diffuse CNS involvement is typical of feline coronavirus disease.

Premortem diagnosis is often difficult. It is suggested by clinical signs, including ocular changes, laboratory evidence of increased levels in CSF protein and neutrophils, and plasma hypergammaglobulinemia. Serial determinations of the virus antibody level may substantiate the diagnosis. Confirmation generally is made by neuropathologic examination.

The prognosis for affected cats is poor; most animals die within a few weeks or months. There is no satisfactory treatment.

Canine Parvovirus–Induced Encephalitis

There has been a recent report of a generalized form of canine parvovirus infection causing necrotizing vasculitis and leukomalacia, especially in the cerebrum, in a 7.5 week old Dalmatian puppy.[125] Neurologic signs were characterized by sudden onset of circling and blindness. The pathogenesis may be similar to that of feline panleukopenia virus in cats.

Equine Viral Encephalomyelitides

The equine viral encephalomyelitides constitute a group of clinically similar neurologic diseases with generally high mortality rates. Eastern (EEE), western (WEE), and Venezuelan (VEE) equine encephalitis are of consequence to the Americas. Eastern equine encephalitis is found in all of the states along the eastern seaboard and Gulf Coast and also in Michigan, Wisconsin, and Alberta. Western equine encephalitis occurs primarily in the western and midwestern United States and has caused regular epizootics in western Canada and Central and South America. It has also been found in isolated cases in many of the eastern states. Venezuelan equine encephalitis has been a problem in South and Central America and Texas, and an endemic form exists in the Florida Everglades but is unassociated with equine disease.[177]

The histologic lesion in all cases is that of a meningoencephalomyelitis with a predominance of gray matter involvement including neuronal degeneration, gliosis, and perivascular cuffing. The clinical signs usually appear as those of diffuse cerebral disease—depression, somnolence, dementia, head pressing, circling, blindness with normal pupillary response, and convulsions. Cranial nerve signs and even signs of spinal cord disease may be evident and can even be the presenting complaint, with cerebral signs following. A fever may or may not be noted at the time of examination. The CSF may be normal but usually will exhibit an elevated cell count, an elevated protein level, or both. The cell type varies for unknown reasons and may include a preponderance of neutrophils, monocytes, or lymphocytes. Large numbers of eosinophils may also be seen.

Diagnosis is by history (usually, but not always, a lack of appropriate vaccination), clinical signs, and abnormal CSF. Neutralizing, HI, or CF antibodies are usually present at the time of the most severe neurologic signs and can be compared with antibody levels for the other encephalitides if there is a history of vaccination. A lack of antibodies does not rule out the disease. The virus is readily isolated from fresh or frozen brain tissue, and the histopathology is quite typical.

There is no specific treatment for viral encephalitis, and the prognosis varies with the type of virus: 75 to 90% of eastern equine encephalitis cases are fatal, with the prognosis for survival significantly better with western or Venezuelan equine encephalitis. Antiinflammatory drugs, control of seizures, and intensive nursing care are indicated. Surviving horses may have residual CNS damage, however. The use of killed vaccines is beneficial in preventing the disease. Vaccination should begin before the mosquito season and often needs to be given twice per year.[177]

Several other togaviruses can cause encephalitis in horses.[177] Main drain virus has been reported as a potential cause of equine viral encephalomyelitis in a horse in California.[62] Eastern and western equine encephalitis have been associated with naturally occurring and experimentally induced neurologic disease in calves,[220] and eastern equine encephalitis has been associated with clinical and experimental disease in dogs and pigs.[221]

Equine Infectious Anemia

Equine infectious anemia (EIA) results in a variety of clinical disease syndromes, the least common of which appears to be neurologic disease. At necropsy of neurologically affected horses, typical lesions in lymph nodes, spleen, liver, and kidney are seen.[108] Neuropathologic findings include nonsuppurative granulomatous ependymitis, meningitis and encephalomyelitis, and plasmacytic, lymphocytic infiltration of the brain and spinal cord.[179]

The reported clinical signs most frequently involve pelvic limb ataxia, often with evidence of a multifocal or diffuse disease process. The animals may or may not have serum or CSF antibodies, as detected by the agar gel immunodiffusion (AGID) test. Neurologic signs may begin acutely or insidiously, and affected horses may be otherwise completely normal on physical examination or may have weight loss, anemia, and ventral edema. The CSF analysis has been within normal limits or grossly abnormal and suggestive of a nonsuppurative leptomeningitis.[106, 179, 182]

Diagnosis is by clinical signs, positive agar gel immunodiffusion test, or necropsy. Because of the potentially contagious nature of the disease and the progressive course of the neurologic signs and histopathologic lesions,[179] affected horses should be euthanatized.

Scrapie

Scrapie is a fatal, progressive, slow-viral disease of sheep and goats of Europe, India, Africa, Asia, and North and South America.[245] It is seen in all breeds of sheep, but in the United States the Suffolk breed seems to have the highest incidence. It occurs mainly in sheep between 2 and 5 years old, although it has been seen in slightly younger sheep. Transmission is both horizontal (animal to animal) and vertical (maternal to offspring), with a genetic factor thought to determine which infected animal manifests clinical signs. Signs include inappropriate apprehension and excitement followed by ataxia and fine head and neck tremor. Later signs include weight loss, impaired vision, and abortion. Pruritus is manifested by incessant scratching, biting, and wool loss in the absence of dermatitis. Repeated pricking of the skin of the back with a pin appears to be misinterpreted, with the affected sheep moving toward the noxious stimulus.[201]

Diagnosis is based on signs and typical histopathologic lesions, particularly neuronal degeneration and vacuolization. There is no known treatment or preventative. Federal reg-

ulations usually require slaughter of all in-contact sheep and goats.

A chronic wasting disease associated with spongiform encephalopathy occurs in captive deer in the United States.[283] Behavioral aberrations, weight loss, and death in 2 weeks to 8 months occur. There is no treatment.

Maedi and Visna

Maedi is a slowly progressive interstitial pneumonia of adult sheep; visna is a slowly progressive encephalomyelitis most likely caused by the same retrovirus. This disease has spread throughout much of the world, having been diagnosed in the Netherlands, France, England, United States, Germany, South Africa, Africa, Asia, and other locations. The disease appears in sheep 2 years of age or older. Both conditions may occur in the same sheep, but more often they occur separately. Transmission may be through the milk or via the respiratory tract.

Clinical signs of visna typically begin with ataxia, followed later by torticollis, circling, and lip tremors. All clinically affected sheep die within several months. Antemortem diagnosis is based on clinical signs, mononuclear pleocytosis in CSF, and the detection of circulating antibodies. This virus can persist in the presence of antibody; thus, antibodies signal that the sheep is infected with, and is possibly excreting, the virus, rather than convalescing from the disease. Typical lesions can be seen at necropsy. Prevention is by eradication.

Caprine Arthritis-Encephalitis

Caprine arthritis-encephalitis (CAE) is a disease with almost worldwide distribution, which is prevalent in the United States. It is caused by a retrovirus and usually manifests itself as an ascending paresis in young goats and an insidious arthritis in adults. The virus is antigenically similar to the retrovirus that causes visna and maedi in sheep, but it has not been possible to infect any other species with this particular virus.

The arthritic form of caprine arthritis-encephalitis is the most common. The encephalitic form occurs in younger goats, frequently between 2 and 4 months of age, although adults are infrequently affected. Initially, pelvic limb weakness and ataxia are seen, often asymmetrically. Affected kids are bright, alert, and responsive. Some are febrile. The disease often progresses to hemiplegia or tetraplegia and will become static. A few kids will develop a concurrent clinical interstitial pneumonia. Spinal reflexes are frequently intact (in contrast with swayback), indicative of upper motor neuron disease. However, mild to severe multifocal lower motor neuron signs may be present. Kids with this disease have also been found to be blind and to have a head tilt and facial nerve paresis, in addition to ataxia.[198] Because of the nature of the disease, the CSF will usually exhibit a pleocytosis, usually with mononuclear cells prevailing.

The diagnosis of caprine arthritis-encephalitis is based on clinical signs, typical postmortem lesions of leptomeningeal and focal parenchymal necrosis with perivascular infiltration of lymphocytes and histiocytes, and, in chronic cases, the demonstration of significant antibody levels to caprine arthritis-encephalitis virus by an agar gel immunodiffusion test. Unfortunately, there is no treatment. Prevention and control have recently been discussed.[134]

Porcine Hemagglutinating Encephalomyelitis

This neurotropic porcine coronavirus (hemagglutinating encephalomyelitis virus [HEV]) appears in two forms: a peracute to acute neurologic form, and a subacute to chronic form characterized by vomiting and emaciation known as vomiting and wasting disease (VWD).[185] Infection with HEV is common, but clinical disease is rare and usually seen in pigs early in life. CNS infection is by extension through the peripheral nerves, and microscopic evidence of nonsuppurative encephalomyelitis is often extensive.

Clinical signs of the neurologic form include hyperesthesia, muscle tremors, ataxia, paddling, and coma. Morbidity and mortality vary but may approach 100%. Definitive diagnosis depends on viral isolation from the CNS or demonstration of infected neurons by immunofluorescence.

Porcine Enteroviral Encephalomyelitis

Enteroviral encephalomyelitis (EE) of pigs has been given a variety of names including Teschen disease, Talfan disease, porcine polio-myelitis, and benign enzootic paresis, which most likely represent various manifestations of one virus. Morbidity and mortality vary tremendously in different outbreaks, piglets being more susceptible to the disease. The disease variability seems to be related to the strain of the virus, host susceptibility, environment, and geographic location of the disease outbreak.[34]

The pathologic lesions seen are those of a nonsuppurative inflammation involving primarily the gray matter, typical of many viral CNS diseases—neuronal degeneration, glial cell proliferation, and vascular congestion and cuffing. Clinical signs include ascending, progressive pelvic limb ataxia and weakness with generalized muscle tremors. In severe cases nystagmus, convulsions, opisthotonos, and coma may appear.

There is no treatment for enteroviral encephalomyelitis, but some animals will survive with variable recovery periods, some having permanent neurologic signs and some remaining as carriers of the virus. Diagnosis is based on postmortem examination and viral isolation.

Infectious Bovine Rhinotracheitis Virus Meningoencephalomyelitis

The herpesvirus (bovine herpesvirus type 1) of cattle causing infectious bovine rhinotracheitis (IBR) is known to cause several disease syndromes in cows and calves: respiratory problems, keratoconjunctivitis, genital infections, generalized neonatal infection, abortion, and less commonly CNS disease. The CNS form may be seen as a distinct entity in a particular herd or may occur in conjunction with one of the other forms of the disease in the same animal or in contact animals. Histopathologic lesions of the CNS include areas of malacia and hemorrhage, variable presence of inclusion bodies in the neurons of the brain and spinal cord, and perivascular cuffing with mononuclear cells and neutrophils. Gliosis and chromatolysis may be seen.[20] Typical signs include depression with intermittent periods of excitement, ataxia, blindness, intermittent generalized tremor, opisthotonos, convulsions, and death. Occasionally only ataxia and paralysis of the pelvic limbs may be seen.[14, 20, 82, 184] Fever may or may not be present.

Diagnosis is confirmed by isolation of the virus from the CSF, brain, nasal mucosa, or other body tissues.[14, 17] Paired serum neutralization titers may indicate a recent infection.

The prognosis is poor for all but the mildly affected animals, and no treatment has been suggested to be efficacious.

Malignant Catarrhal Fever

Malignant catarrhal fever is a viral disease of cattle, thought to be transmitted through contact with sheep or deer. It is characterized by a wide variety of clinical signs, including panophthalmitis, purulent nasal and ocular discharges, exudative dermatitis, lymphadenopathy, high fever, diarrhea, hyperemia of mucous membranes, and occasionally encephalitis with depression, circling, ataxia, and convulsions terminally.

Histologically, the CNS lesion is one of vasculitis and diffuse meningitis and encephalomyelitis. The CSF may exhibit an elevated total protein content and a mononuclear pleocytosis.[213] Definitive diagnosis requires a combination of history, clinical signs, gross pathology, and histopathology.

Borna Disease

Borna disease is an encephalomyelitis caused by an unclassified slow virus that mainly affects horses but may infect sheep, goats, cattle, and rabbits.[124] Geographically, the disease is limited to Central Europe, Syria, Lebanon, and Egypt. The virus is thought to be transmitted via a tick or through ingestion or inhalation.

Neurologic signs include depression, blindness, teeth grinding, ataxia, hyperexcitability, and convulsions.

Louping-Ill

Louping-ill is a flavoviral encephalomyelitis that is tick-borne and occurs in Scotland, England, and Ireland.[124] In addition to sheep, the disease occurs occasionally in people, cattle, horses, dogs, and swine. Clinical signs are similar to those described for Borna disease.

Allergic Encephalomyelitis

A disseminated, demyelinating encephalomyelitis has been reported as a complication of rabies vaccination using phenolized brain tissue vaccines.[121] This disorder is now of mainly historical interest because this vaccine has been replaced by chick embryo or tissue culture–modified live virus vaccines. The demyelination is believed to result from immunologic reaction to myelin in brain origin vaccines. An ascending paralysis was observed in affected animals.

INFLAMMATORY DISORDERS OF UNKNOWN ETIOLOGY

Granulomatous Meningoencephalomyelitis

This is a nonsuppurative inflammatory disorder of dogs that is characterized by disseminated perivascular cuffs composed of reticuloendothelial elements and lymphoplasmic infiltrates. This pathologic description also fits so-called reticulosis.[66, 138, 141] According to Fankhauser et al,[66] reticulosis is a proliferative reaction of reticulohistiocytic cells originating from adventitia of vessels within the CNS. Controversy concerning the origin of the macrophages[48] awaits further clarification.[271] When the cells in the granulomatous lesions are predominantly reticulohistiocytic with a high mitotic index, the lesion has been called neoplastic reticulosis. When many inflammatory cells (lymphocytes, plasma cells) are present and the mitotic index is low, the lesion has been termed inflammatory reticulosis.[66, 141, 266]

In an attempt to simplify the confusion in terminology, the term granulomatous meningoencephalitis (GME) will be used in lieu of reticulosis. Three forms of this disease are considered to occur:[54] focal (formerly known as primary or neoplastic reticulosis),[66, 141, 266] disseminated (formerly termed inflammatory reticulosis),[141, 266] and ocular (formerly classified as ocular reticulosis).[266]

Focal granulomatous meningoencephalitis is characterized by massive perivascular sheets of reticulohistiocytic cells that merge to form solid tumor-like nodules, often surrounded by reticulin fibers. The mitotic index is usually high. The most pronounced lesions are found in the white matter of the cerebral hemispheres and in the brain stem.[66, 229, 271]

The disseminated form consists of massive perivascular cuffs with lymphocytes, plasma cells, and histiocytic elements, often in clusters and scattered throughout the CNS, especially in white matter.[26, 48, 229]

The ocular form is characterized by diffuse infiltration of posterior segments of the eyes, optic nerves, chiasma, or tracts by reticulohistiocytic and lymphoplasmic cells.[75, 228] Disseminated or focal lesions in other areas of the CNS may accompany the ocular form.[83, 229, 243]

The cause of granulomatous meningoencephalitis is unknown. A possible viral etiology has been speculated[66] and, although distemper and rabies-like inclusion bodies have been reported in focal and disseminated granulomatous meningoencephalomyelitis,[37, 270, 274] definitive evidence by viral isolation and transmission studies is lacking. Toxoplasma-like organisms have been reported in one dog.[4]

Granulomatous meningoencephalitis appears most commonly in young and middle aged dogs, with an age range between 1 and 10 years.[30, 48, 229] Poodles may be more susceptible than other breeds.

Onset of clinical signs may be acute or chronic, usually with a progressive course over a 2 to 8 week period. Clinical signs are variable and reflect lesion localization. The ocular form is characterized by acute onset of visual impairment and dilated unresponsive pupils as a result of unilateral or bilateral optic neuritis. Ophthalmoscopic examination may reveal a hyperemic and edematous optic disc.[75, 83, 243] Focal disease may produce signs suggestive of a space occupying lesion, whereas with the disseminated disorder, there may be evidence of a diffuse disease process involving several areas of the neuraxis. Common clinical signs may include incoordination, ataxia and falling, cervical pain, head tilt, nystagmus, facial and/or trigeminal nerve paralysis, circling, seizures, and decreased awareness or depression.[30, 48, 229]

Examination of cerebrospinal fluid usually reveals pleocytosis (50–400 white blood cells per cubic millimeter) with a predominant population of mononuclear cells (lymphocytes, monocytes, and macrophages). The protein content of CSF may be slightly elevated. Electroencephalographic tracings are abnormal, with slow wave–high voltage activity.[30]

A tentative diagnosis may be based on clinical and laboratory data; however, confirmation requires microscopic evaluation of the CNS. Prognosis is poor. Long-term treatment is unsatisfactory, although temporary remission is often achieved with glucocorticoid administration.[75, 83, 229, 243]

Feline Polioencephalomyelitis

This is a chronic, slowly progressive neurologic disease recently described in immature and mature cats.[267] In this report five of six cats were female and of different breeds. The cause of feline polioencephalomyelitis is unknown; however, the pathologic changes suggest a viral infection. A similar disease has been reported in lions and tigers.[77] A viral cause was suspected, but viral isolation attempts were unsuccessful.

Pathologic changes consist of severe neuronal degeneration and loss, especially in segments of the thoracic spinal cord and, to a lesser extent, in the cerebral cortex, basal and diencephalic nuclei, midbrain, periaqueductal gray matter, and oculomotor and pontomedullary nuclei. Diffuse degeneration of white matter (demyelination and axonal necrosis) is usually present in ventral and lateral columns of the spinal cord.

Clinical signs include incoordination, paresis, and hypermetria. Intention tremors may be seen involving the head. The mental status is invariably one of alertness. Function of the cranial nerves tends to be normal, except for depressed direct and consensual pupillary reflexes in some animals. Postural reactions and segmental spinal reflexes may be noticeably depressed in affected limbs. Occasionally, a localized area of apparent hyperesthesia is evident. In some cases, a psychomotor-like pattern of seizures has been reported in sleeping animals that is characterized by hallucinations, wild stares, clawing, and hissing and biting at imaginary objects.

Results of laboratory procedures are nonspecific. Prognosis is guarded. Data on treatment are lacking.

Chronic Encephalitis of Pug Dogs

This is a chronic progressive neurologic disease recognized in pug dogs 9 months to 4 years of age.[54] The course of the disease varies from 1 to 6 months. The etiology is unknown. Pathologically, a granulomatous encephalitis is observed affecting white and gray matter, primarily in the cerebrum. The most common clinical signs are seizures (generalized and partial). Circling, visual deficits, and intermittent screaming have also been observed in some affected dogs. Death is often preceded by coma or status epilepticus.

Cerebrospinal fluid has moderate pleocytosis (mononuclear), and protein levels may be slightly increased. Diagnosis is based on signalment, historical, clinical, and pathologic data. Prognosis is poor, and treatment is unrewarding.

BACTERIAL DISEASES OF THE CENTRAL NERVOUS SYSTEM

Bacterial Meningitis

In contrast with domestic large animals, meningitis is not a common disease of the dog and cat. Bacterial invasion of the CNS usually results in both encephalomyelitis and meningitis. Bacterial infections of the CNS occur via hematogenous spread from distant foci within the body; by direct extension from sinuses, ears, and eyes; as a result of trauma (eg, bite wound); or from contaminated surgical instruments (eg, spinal needle). In neonatal herbivores, failure of passive transfer of neonatal immunoglobulins via colostrum is the single most important factor in neonatal sepsis and bacterial meningoencephalomyelitis.

Basilar empyema can occur secondary to otitis interna or as a sequela to the rupture of a pyogenic mass that formed in the basilar venous sinus after dehorning or rhinitis. Organisms usually disseminate via CSF pathways and produce cerebrospinal meningitis with microabscess formation. One important source of bacterial infection of meninges and CNS parenchyma in dogs is bacterial endocarditis.

Bacteria are probably the most common causes of purulent meningitis. Organisms that have been cultured from dogs with bacterial meningitis include *Pasteurella* sp, *Pasteurella multocida*, *Staphylococcus aureus*, *Staphylococcus epidermidis*, *Staphylococcus albus*, *Actinomyces* sp, and *Nocardia* sp.

Pathologic changes that are characteristic of bacterial meningitis include diffuse infiltration of inflammatory cells into the leptomeninges by both polymorphonuclear and mononuclear cells. Frequently, inflammation is found throughout the entire subarachnoid space of the brain and spinal cord. Vasculitis is often pronounced.

Bacterial invasion of CNS parenchyma is characterized by mononuclear and polymorphonuclear inflammatory infiltration and large perivascular cuffing. Necrosis of gray and white matter may be observed with infiltrations of macrophages, neutrophils, and plasma cells. Irrespective of the etiologic agent, bacterial meningitis usually is acute in onset and tends to be characterized by a group of clinical signs that include hyperesthesia, pyrexia, and cervical rigidity. Pyrexia is believed to be secondary to bacterial invasion of the blood stream and cerebrospinal fluid, accompanied by the release of leukocytic pyrogen and hypothalamic stimulation. In humans, inflammation of the subarachnoid space activates protective reflexes resulting in nuchal rigidity and hyperextension of the neck and vertebral column. A similar mechanism probably exists in the dog and serves as an explanation of the signs of cervical rigidity and the occasionally seen opisthotonos with thoracic limb hyperextension. In addition, emesis, anorexia, and seizures may be observed.[26, 36, 112, 145, 196]

Cattle with basilar epidural empyema (also called pituitary abscess) may have a stargazing attitude, bradycardia, blindness, dilated pupils, a dropped jaw, and facial, tongue, and pharyngeal paralysis.

All large animals may be victims of bacterial meningitis. Signs of bacterial meningitis in large animals include hyperesthesia of the head and neck, depression, somnolence, convulsions, blindness, and ataxia. Fever, omphalophlebitis, polyarthritis, and ophthalmitis may accompany meningitis.

The clinical diagnosis of bacterial meningitis is supported by the finding of highly pleocytic cerebrospinal fluid (500 to 1000 or more white blood cells per cubic millimeter) with a high proportion of polymorphonuclear cells. The protein content of the cerebrospinal fluid is usually increased as well (100–200 mg/dl). Low CSF glucose values relative to plasma glucose are typical. Affected neonatal herbivores will most often have low circulating immunoglobulin levels. Electroencephalographic traces may demonstrate high voltage–fast or slow wave activity. Definitive diagnosis is made by bacterial culture of CSF. Blood cultures may incriminate a pathogenic organism when CSF cultures are negative.

Rickettsial infections (Rocky Mountain spotted fever or *Ehrlichia*) should be considered in dogs with evidence of meningitis and negative culture results. In addition, parasitic migration through the CNS can result in aseptic, suppurative meningitis.[173, 174]

Prognosis is guarded. Appropriate use of antibiotics, according to the culture results, is basic to successful therapy of bacterial meningitis (encephalomyelitis). Correction of the immunodeficiency is mandatory in neonatal large animals. Chloramphenicol has the highest penetrability of the central nervous system, followed by sulfonamides and trimethoprim. Ampicillin and penicillin enter the nervous system only with meningeal irritation. Aminoglycosides do not penetrate the CNS, even when inflammation exists[32] (see Chapter 15). Intrathecal administration of antibiotics should only be considered in refractory cases. Glucocorticoids, in general, are contraindicated in the treatment of bacterial or fungal meningitis; however, a suppurative meningitis of unknown etiology has been observed in some dogs with clinical and laboratory evidence of bacterial meningitis (encephalomyelitis), in which abatement of signs occurred only following glucocorticoid therapy.[54] An immunologic pathogenesis is suspected.

Neuraxial Abscessation

Intracranial or intraspinal abscessation may result from bacterial meningitis (encephalomyelitis), or from vertebral osteomyelitis.[22, 105, 178, 226, 246, 249] Clinical signs usually will reflect a space occupying lesion. Diagnostic and therapeutic procedures are the same as those for bacterial meningitis (encephalomyelitis). Prognosis is guarded, especially if the mass lesion is large and encapsulated, making it refractory to antibiotic therapy.

Cerebral abscesses are probably more common in sheep, goats, and calves. These abscesses may be silent, associated with overt meningitis, or cause signs of a space occupying lesion. In the latter case, one can expect contralateral impaired vision, menace deficit and decreased facial sensation, circling or turning the head toward the side of the lesion, and contralateral deficits in postural reactions. When sufficient size is obtained or with associated severe cerebral edema, signs of brain stem compression may also be seen, including asymmetric pupil size, ataxia, and weakness (Fig. 7–5). CSF changes depend on the degree of meningeal or ependymal involvement. Typical offending bacteria include *Staphylococcus aureus*, *Fusobacterium necrophorum*, or *Corynebacterium pyogenes* in food animals and *Streptococcus equi* or *Actinobacillus mallei* in horses. Therapy is based on prolonged use of appropriate antibiotics, although surgical drainage has been discussed.[246]

Diskospondylitis and Vertebral Osteomyelitis

Diskospondylitis is intervertebral disk infection with concurrent osteomyelitis occurring in contiguous vertebral bodies. This disorder occurs in young to middle aged adult dogs, usually of the larger breeds. Male dogs are affected twice as often as females. Juvenile large animals are more often affected than adults.

Diskospondylitis may occur following 'iatrogenic trauma of the vertebral column (eg, disk curettage), foreign body migration, paravertebral injection, or, more commonly, blood-borne septic emboli.[107, 126, 143, 144, 155] *Staphylococcus aureus* was the most common organism identified by cultures of blood, urine and bone in one study involving dogs.[143] Other organisms identified include *Brucella canis*, *Nocardia*, *Streptococcus canis*, and *Corynebacterium diphtheroides*. Fungi have also been cultured from vertebrae.[206, 289] A cause and effect relationship between urinary tract infection and diskospondylitis remains to be established. Bacteria often involved include *Corynebacterium pyogenes* in cattle; *Corynebacterium pseudotuberculosis* in sheep and goats; *Salmonella* sp, *Actinobacillus equuli*, and *Corynebacterium equi* in foals; and

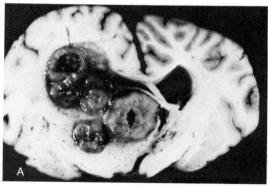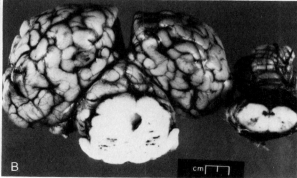

Figure 7–5. Equine brain abscess. This 4 year old pony mare showed progressive, intermittent depression, circling, and seizures over a 2 month period. Cerebrospinal fluid contained 27,000 white cells, mostly neutrophils. The mare became depressed, exhibited asymmetric cranial nerve function, and finally became comatose. A, A large, multiloculated abscess was found in the region of the left lateral ventricle. Chains of gram positive organisms were seen in the abscess. B, The asymmetric caudal herniation of both occipital lobes and the tonsil of the cerebellum compressed the midbrain pons (left) and the caudal medulla oblongata (right), respectively.

Mycobacterium tuberculosis and *Brucella abortus* in adult horses.

Clinical signs are variable, ranging from subtle spinal hyperesthesia to severe paresis or paralysis.[107, 114, 143] Affected animals may manifest depression, anorexia, and pyrexia.[143] The clinical neurologic signs reflect the degree of bone proliferation and compression of spinal cord.

Radiographic abnormalities include a concentric area of lysis of adjacent vertebral end plates early in the disease process. More chronic lesions are characterized by varying degrees of bone lysis and proliferation, vertebral sclerosis, shortening of vertebral bodies, and narrowed intervertebral disk spaces (Fig. 7–6 and see Fig. 4–7).

Diagnosis is based on clinical, laboratory, and radiographic data. The hemogram may or may not reflect the presence of an infection. Blood and urine cultures should be obtained before starting antibiotic therapy. Percutaneous aspiration of the infected vertebrae using fluoroscopic control is a technique with promise. Brucella determinations should be checked because of the public health significance.

Prognosis is usually favorable with aggressive long-term antibiotic therapy if the vertebrae are stable. Until culture results are available, the organism should be assumed to be a staphylococcus. The cephalosporins have been effective in the majority of small animal cases. In large animals the bone damage is often so extensive before the case is presented that the outlook is much worse for full resolution. Vertebral curettage may expedite clinical resolution. In severe spinal cord compression, decompression and vertebral immobilization may be indicated.[81, 246]

Tetanus

Tetanus is a bacterial disease caused by *Clostridium tetani* that can affect all domestic animals and humans.[181] Disease occurs as a result of localization of tetanus spores in an anaerobic environment, such as a necrotic wound, and conversion to a vegetative, toxin producing form. The organisms produce an exotoxin within 4 to 8 hours, which travels via peripheral nerves to the central nervous system.[217] A transsynaptic migration of tetanus toxin occurs in spinal cord motor neurons.[233] Toxin binds the release of inhibitory neurotransmitter from interneurons, resulting in release of motor neurons (especially alpha) from inhibition, with subsequent hyperexcitability.

Considerable species differences exist in susceptibility to tetanus. The dog is much less susceptible than the horse. In horses tetanus is most frequently seen in neonatal foals, in postpartum mares, and after surgery or injury. In the food animal species it is particularly associated with shearing, tail docking, ear tagging, castration, dog bite wounds, parturition, and metritis. Clinical signs usually are observed within 5 to 10 days of infection[63, 133, 181, 298] and include stiffness of gait with extensor rigidity in all limbs, dyspnea, and spasms of the masticatory and pharyngeal muscles, resulting in trismus and dysphagia. The tail may be elevated, facial muscles contracted to give a sneering expression (risus sardonicus) with wrinkling of the forehead, and the third eyelid protruded (Fig. 7–7). In severe disease, the animal may be recumbent and opisthotonic. Death results from respiratory failure. Affected animals are hypersensitive to external stimuli.

Diagnosis of the severe form of tetanus is largely based on characteristic clinical data. Mild forms of the disease may be difficult to diagnose because there are no specific ancillary aids available. There is a lack of the usually observed electric silence following needle insertion in electromyographic studies. Results of conduction studies are normal.

Prognosis is usually favorable with treatment in animals still able to stand. Therapy consists

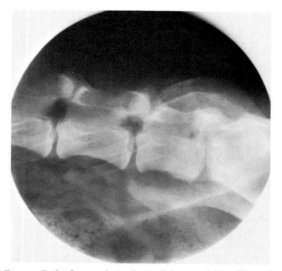

Figure 7–6. Canine brucellosis diskospondylitis. There is lysis and proliferation of bone at L7–S1 involving both vertebrae, which is characteristic of inflammatory lesions. *Brucella canis* was isolated in pure culture from the spinal lesion taken at surgery and from the testicle. The agglutination titer was 1:200.

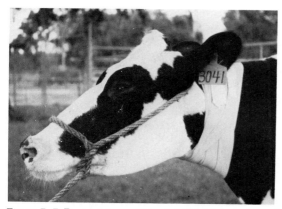

Figure 7–7. Bovine tetanus. This adult Holstein cow showed a stiff gait, elevated tail—head, bloat, and extended head posture (as shown), with rigid facial expression, flared nostrils, and immobile eyelids and ears. In addition, there was trismus and spasm of retractor muscles of the eyeball with resulting protrusion of the nictitating membrane when the head was manipulated. These classic signs of tetanus occurred a few weeks after calving. The cow survived with feeding and hydration via a rumen fistula, sedation, systemic administration of procaine penicillin, uterine lavage, vaccination for *Clostridium tetani*, and tetanus antitoxin administered intravenously and in the lumbosacral subarachnoid space.

of wound débridement, administration of crystalline penicillin (20,000–50,000 IU/kg four times daily in dogs), and immediate administration of tetanus antitoxin (TAT) (100–500 IU/kg intravenously). A test dose (eg, 0.1 ml) of antitoxin can be given subcutaneously 20 minutes prior to the intravenous dosage and the animal observed for any allergic reaction. Large animals should probably receive 2000 to 10,000 IU of homologous antitoxin or much higher doses if nonhomologous antitoxin is used. Early in the course of the disease, intrathecally administered antitoxin (up to 30,000 IU per adult large animal) is probably quite beneficial in shortening the clinical course.[177] In addition, performing this procedure allows CSF analysis and exclusion of bacterial meningitis from the diagnosis. Muscle spasms can be controlled using diazepam, xylazine, glycerylguiacol, or barbiturates, and sedation can be attained using chlorpromazine, barbiturates, or chloral hydrate. Long-term (3–4 weeks) supportive care may be needed; toxin remains bound for some time. Ventilatory assistance and insertion of a nasogastric or pharyngostomy tube may be required for animals with respiratory distress or severe trismus and pharyngeal spasms, respectively. Affected animals should be placed in a quiet environment and cotton wool placed in their ears. The problem of bloat must be dealt with in the ruminant as it frequently accompanies

signs of tetanus. Once adult horses or cattle become recumbent, the prognosis for recovery from tetanus is poor.

Horses should be vaccinated 3 times as juveniles and at least every 5 years as adults.[177] All large animals should receive active (toxoid) or passive protection prior to surgical procedures or susceptible periods such as calving.

Canine Idiopathic Pyogranulomatous Meningoencephalomyelitis

Pyogranulomatous meningoencephalomyelitis is an acute, rapidly progressive disease of 2 to 3 weeks duration that, to date, has been recognized only in mature pointers.[26, 265]

The cause of the meningoencephalomyelitis is unknown. Results of special histologic stains for microorganisms, cultures of blood and cerebrospinal fluid, and studies of animal inoculations have all been negative. Clinical and pathologic data suggest a bacterial etiology.

Pathologic changes are found throughout the brain and spinal cord but are most severe in the cranial segments of the cervical spinal cord and in the caudal brain stem. These changes are characterized by extensive mononuclear (plasma, lymphocytic cells) and polymorphonuclear inflammatory infiltrations in the leptomeninges and parenchyma. Large perivascular cuffs are seen. In some cases, central necrosis of gray matter and edema are found in segments of the cervical cord along with infiltration of macrophages, monocytes, neutrophils, and plasma cells. These changes are probably secondary to impaired spinal circulation from the meningeal reaction. An increased population of reticuloendothelial cells is occasionally observed among the perivascular cells. Focal ependymitis may be present along ventricular pathways.

Clinical signs include cervical rigidity, kyphosis, nose held close to the ground, reluctance to move, and an incoordinated gait. Occasionally, brachycardia, vomiting, and atrophy of the cervical muscles are seen. Signs of parenchymal involvement include paralysis of the trigeminal and facial nerves and Horner's syndrome.

Marked, predominantly neutrophilic pleocytosis (500–1000 white blood cells per cubic millimeter) and an increased concentration of protein (sometimes over 700 mg/dl) are found on examination of the cerebrospinal fluid of affected animals.

Diagnosis is based on signalment, clinical, and pathologic data.

In the small series of cases so far observed, prognosis has been poor. Temporary remission of signs has resulted following antibiotic therapy.

Thromboembolic Meningoencephalitis

Thromboembolic meningoencephalitis (TEME), a bacterial disease of cattle caused by the gram negative bacillus *Hemophilus somnus*, is a disease typically seen in 8 to 12 month old feedlot cattle during the winter. It has also been observed in pastured and dairy cattle.[54, 247]

The gross CNS lesions are multifocal areas of hemorrhagic necrosis with histologic evidence of severe vasculitis with thrombosis, necrosis of vessel walls, and intense neutrophil accumulation perivascularly. Fibrinopurulent polyarthritis, laryngeal necrosis, myositis, chorioretinitis, pleuritis, or pneumonia may be seen also.

Affected animals are usually febrile. Neurologic signs include partial paralysis of multiple cranial nerves, blindness (rarely unilateral), depression, ataxia, paresis, seizures, and death. Sudden death in a few animals is sometimes the first suggestion of a herd problem, but this may have been preceded by herd respiratory problems. CSF analysis reveals an elevated protein level and neutrophilic pleocytosis.

Treatment with tetracyclines, sulfonamides, or penicillin-streptomycin may be useful in the early stages of the disease. A vaccine is currently available that reportedly is somewhat effective in preventing the neurologic form of thromboembolic meningoencephalitis in the feedlot but not as useful for the respiratory or reproductive forms of the disease.[247]

Listeriosis

Listeriosis is an acute, infectious but noncontagious disease of a wide variety of mammalian and avian species, which is worldwide in distribution but more prevalent in temperate and colder climates. The etiologic agent is a gram positive, β-hemolytic bacillus, *Listeria monocytogenes*, which resides in soil and silage and is resistant to environmental hazards.[94]

This disease is characterized by three different syndromes: (1) placentitis with abortion in the last trimester; (2) septicemia with miliary abscessation; and (3) suppurative meningoencephalitis with multiple microscopic abscesses in the brain stem.[156] This discussion will be limited to the neurologic form of the disease.

In the case of encephalitic listeriosis, the organisms probably gain entry through abrasions of the mouth, eyelids, nose, or muzzle.[40] Although some outbreaks in sheep and goats have been associated with silage feeding, often this is not part of the history. Generally, a single animal is affected, and in the case of cattle, it is usually a cow of at least 1 year of age.[225] Swine are rarely affected clinically but may exhibit the CNS or, more commonly, the septicemic form of the disease, which is usually fatal.[156] Horses rarely may be affected, with no evidence of exposure to ruminants or silage.[177] The bacteria enter branches of the cranial nerves (especially CN V, VII, IX, X, and XII) and ascend to the brain stem.[40] Clinical signs vary with the cranial nerves and brain stem areas involved and include depression, upper motor neuron signs to the ipsilateral limbs (knuckling, paresis, rigidity), and localizing lower motor neuron cranial nerve signs, most often asymmetric. These include facial paralysis, dysphagia, head tilt, nystagmus, and circling. The animals are anorectic and often febrile, and an endophthalmitis may be present. Diagnosis can usually be made on physical and neurologic examination when multiple cranial nerves are involved. Examination of the CSF is useful as almost all affected animals will have an increased number of white blood cells and usually an elevated protein content. The white blood cells often are predominantly mononuclear but may be mixed. Hematology is not useful, except to suggest a stress leukogram.

Treatment can be successful if the animals can swallow, are not recumbent, and are not too far along in the course of the disease. Although tetracycline has been recommended for cattle, the authors have had reasonable success in goats using high levels of penicillin (40,000 IU/kg intravenously, four times daily) until improvement is noted, followed by at least a 7 day course of intramuscular penicillin (20,000–40,000 IU/kg twice daily). Supportive therapy may be necessary.

Postmortem diagnosis is based on histology and culturing and identifying *L. monocytogenes* because significant gross lesions are not always seen. Isolation may require prior storage of culture specimens at 4°C for several days.

Enterotoxemia

Clostridium perfringens type D produces an epsilon toxin that is thought to increase vascular permeability, resulting in hemorrhage and edema. Ultimately, liquefactive necrosis is produced in the brain and spinal cord tissue. The microscopic lesion is also known as focal symmetric encephalomalacia. The disease is most commonly seen in well-nourished suckling kids and lambs, goats experiencing sudden feed changes, feedlot lambs 2 to 3 weeks after fattening begins, and feedlot cattle. It may also be seen in adult animals. Sudden death is typical, but neurologic signs include ataxia, trembling, rigid limb extension, opisthotonos, convulsions, coma, and death.[124, 201]

Lambs,[124] and particularly feeder pigs,[194] afflicted with the enterotoxemic form of colibacillosis can experience neurologic signs associated with the neuropathologic lesions similar to those discussed above.

Hemophilus Polyserositis of Pigs (Glasser's Disease)

Glasser's disease is caused by the gram negative, pleomorphic rod *Hemophilus parasuis*. It is characterized pathologically by a fibrinous pleuritis, pericarditis, peritonitis, meningoencephalitis, and arthritis in any combination, with meningitis being observed most frequently.[94]

Clinical signs may include fever, depression, lameness (usually involving multiple joints), and coughing or dyspnea. Neurologic signs most often manifested are muscle tremors, ataxia, and recumbency. Diagnosis is by history of stress, clinical signs, necropsy findings, and, ultimately, bacterial culture.

Glanders and Botryomycosis

These disorders, associated with *Pseudomonas mallei* and *Staphylococcus* sp, respectively, have been reported to involve the brains of horses.[118]

Meningoencephalitis Following Hot Iron Disbudding of Goat Kids

Death of goat kids occurs hours to several weeks following overzealous application of a hot iron to horn buds.[290] Sudden death may occur without neurologic signs, or there may be anorexia, pyrexia, somnolence, blindness, and recumbency. There are degrees of focal, cerebral necrosis with inflammation and edema of the frontal cortices underlying areas of the frontal bone necrosis. Bacteria may be cultured from the meninges and brain, and these may be involved in the pathogenesis of sudden death.

PROTOZOAL DISEASES OF THE CENTRAL NERVOUS SYSTEM

Toxoplasmosis

Toxoplasmosis is an infectious condition caused by the protozoan parasite *Toxoplasma gondii* and occurs in acquired and congenital forms in humans and animals.[61, 238] Cats are the definitive host for this parasite. The three known infective stages of *Toxoplasma* are bradyzoites, tachyzoites, and sporozoites. The three modes of transmission are carnivorism, fecal contamination, and transplacental or congenital infection. These modes of transmission involve the different infective stages as follows: carnivorous ingestion of bradyzoites, tachyzoites, or both; contamination with feline feces containing sporozoites of sporulated oocysts; and transplacental infection of the fetus with tachyzoites after ingestion of encysted bradyzoites or sporulated oocysts by the mother.[128] Toxoplasma oocysts are shed in feline feces unsporulated and are not infective until sporulated (1–5 days). Sporulated oocysts can survive in soil for several months. Land snails, earthworms, flies, and cockroaches may serve as transport hosts for oocysts. Most mammals become intermediate hosts through ingestion of oocysts.

Toxoplasma gondii is highly adapted to transmission by encysted bradyzoites via carnivorism. This applies particularly to cats. Humans, sheep, pigs, dogs, and (rarely) cats are known to transmit *T. gondii* transplacentally. In humans, congenital infection occurs only when a woman becomes infected during pregnancy.[55] Congenitally infected children may have signs of retinochoroiditis, hydrocephalus, seizures, and cerebral calcification.

The incidence of clinical toxoplasmosis is low in dogs and cats. Toxoplasmosis is a systemic infection affecting most organs and the CNS in particular.[65, 110, 139] Pathologically, perivascular cuffing and diffuse and focal infiltration by lymphocytes, plasma cells, and histiocytes, hemorrhage, edema, necrosis, and neuronal degeneration have been described throughout the CNS. In some instances, a granulomatous reaction may be observed. *Toxoplasma* organisms may be found extracellularly and/or in cysts. In skeletal muscle, pathologic changes are most often characterized by pronounced focal or disseminated myonecrosis. It has been hypothesized that immaturity and concurrent distemper infection contribute to an increased susceptibility of dogs to toxoplasmosis.[101, 188]

Clinical neurologic signs associated with toxoplasmosis are variable and may reflect a focal or multifocal disease process. In dogs signs include hyperexcitability, depression, tremor, intention tremor, paresis, paralysis, and seizures.[11, 139] In dogs less than 3 to 4 months of age, a clinical syndrome may be observed that is characterized by rigid hyperextension and gross atrophy of the pelvic limbs. This syndrome is associated with pronounced myonecrosis of pelvic limb musculature and presence of either cyst forms or proliferating free forms of Toxoplasma gondii.[59]

Clinically apparent encephalomyelitis is uncommon in cats. Pneumonia is the most important clinical manifestation of feline toxoplasmosis.[154, 279] Ocular toxoplasmosis has also been reported[262] (Fig. 7–8).

Encephalitis is quite frequently seen in aborted ruminant fetuses,[61, 238] although clinically neurologic disease is rare. The equine species appears to be resistant to developing clinical toxoplasmosis.[3]

Cerebrospinal fluid is usually abnormal, with elevated protein content and a mixed monocytic-polymorphonuclear pleocytosis. Xanthochromia will be present if hemorrhage has occurred.

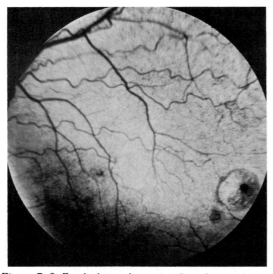

Figure 7–8. Fundic lesion from a confirmed case of toxoplasmosis. Note the hyperreflective area with a pigmented border and a dark center at the 4 o'clock position.

Several serologic procedures are available for detection of antibodies of T. gondii. The most specific, and most expensive, is the cytoplasm modifying or dye test of Sabin and Feldman. Other tests include the indirect fluorescent antibody, indirect hemagglutination, agglutination, and complement fixation.

Diagnosis may be confirmed by serologic and histopathologic studies.

Prognosis is guarded once animals manifest neurologic signs. Sulfonamides and pyrimethamine are two drugs widely used for therapy of systemic toxoplasmosis.

Sporozoan Encephalomyelitis

Toxoplasma gondii is thought to have been identified as a cause of ovine encephalitis, but nontoxoplasma organisms have also been identified.[100] Sarcocystis cysts are occasionally seen in the ovine brain, but no inflammatory reaction surrounding them or clinical signs have been associated. Reported signs associated with toxoplasmosis have ranged from ataxia, blindness, and head jerking to flaccid paraparesis only. Antemortem diagnosis might be aided by complement fixation or the Sabin-Feldman dye test. Sarcocysts, and probably other coccidian parasites, can produce nonsuppurative meningoencephalomyelitis in various domestic animals.[60, 127]

Equine Protozoal Myeloencephalitis

Equine protozoal myeloencephalitis (EPM) is a common disease of horses in the United States that live or travel east of the Rocky Mountains.[54] It has also been reported in Canada.[43] and, recently, three cases have been reported in California that apparently never left that state.[58] To date, a definitive diagnosis only can be made postmortem with histologic observation of the putative agent (an unidentified protozoan) best resembling Sarcocystis sp.[239] Occasionally, only typical lesions consisting of necrotizing nonsuppurative encephalomyelitis with a proliferative inflammation involving gray and white matter will be seen with no organisms present.[54] This is particularly so if the animal has been treated with combinations of trimethoprim-sulfadiazine or other sulfonamides and pyrimethamine.

There does not appear to be any particular age, breed, or sex predilection. However, the disease most frequently affects young adult Thoroughbred and Standardbred horses. It does

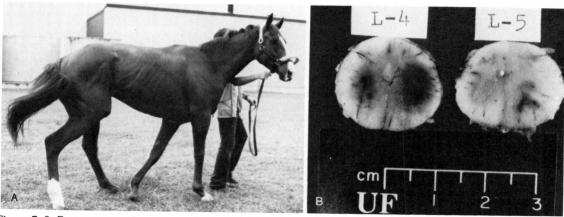

Figure 7–9. Equine protozoal myeloencephalitis (EPM). A, This young Thoroughbred gelding had an acute onset of right pelvic limb "lameness" that rapidly progressed to asymmetric paraparesis, with profound extensor weakness in the right pelvic limb and atrophy of the quadriceps muscles. B, At necropsy examination there was a brownish, soft lesion in the L4–L5 spinal cord segments, which was worse on the right side and involved white and gray matter. Protozoal organisms were associated with the nonsuppurative, necrotic myelitis.

not appear to be contagious, but a common environmental source of contamination may exist. The organism is able to infect any area of the brain and spinal cord, white or gray matter (Fig. 7–9). Thus, clinical signs vary greatly and often initially may appear as a lameness. Without therapy the disease usually will progress, occasionally rapidly.

Early signs may include symmetric ataxia and weakness, but with progression the signs often become asymmetric (Fig. 7–9). Evidence of multifocal gray matter involvement, such as various cranial nerve deficits, muscle atrophy, sensory loss, focal, patchy sweating, loss of reflexes, or monoplegia, are frequently seen.

The CSF is, unfortunately, often normal in these patients but may exhibit xanthochromia, slight to moderate increase in protein level, and a slight mononuclear pleocytosis. Numerous, small structures resembling sporozoan zoites were observed in the CSF of a mare suspected of having equine protozoal myoencephalitis. The mare was recumbent for 13 days but was discharged after 41 hospital days. Thus a definitive diagnosis was not obtained.[31]

Treatment is aimed at stopping the progression of the disease. Improvement must depend on resolution of edema and hemorrhage, remyelination of intact axons, and compensation by other areas of the CNS.[54] Therapy that appears to halt progression of the disease is trimethoprim-sulfadiazine (15 mg/kg orally, twice daily) and pyrimethamine (0.25 mg/kg orally, once a day) for up to 2 months. If the disease is recognized as being fulminant, di-methylsulfoxide (DMSO) (1–2 g/kg diluted to a 20% concentration in 5% dextrose) may be given intravenously once or twice daily for several days.

Animals that appear to respond to therapy may be treated with the same drugs if they are to be stressed considerably, as recurrence of signs is not uncommon.

Babesiosis

Babesiosis is caused by species of the protozoan parasite *Babesia*. Dogs may be infected with *B. canis*, *B. gibsoni*, and *B. vogeli*, whereas *B. felis* causes the disease in cats. Under natural conditions all babesias are transmitted by ticks. CNS involvement is rare. Piriform organisms have been observed to fill the lumen of small capillaries and small arterioles of the hippocampus and cerebrum.[219] The clinical signs may be mistaken for those of rabies. Sudden death has been reported.[195]

Encephalitozoonosis

Encephalitozoonosis is caused by the obligate intracellular protozoan parasite *Encephalitozoon caniculi*. This protozoal disease has been reported in many mammals including humans, dogs, cats, foxes, and laboratory animals. It has been reported in Africa, England, and the United States.[18, 25, 214, 215, 236, 237, 248, 263, 276, 277]

The pathogenesis of canine encephalitozoonosis is uncertain. Most probably it is transmitted transplacentally or neonatally. It is shed in urine of affected animals. Young dogs more often are affected. Vasculitis is considered to be the basic lesion in canine encephalitozoonosis.[263] Pathologically, a severe necrotizing nonsuppurative to granulomatous meningoencephalitis and nephritis have been seen in affected puppies.[214] Vasculitis and fibrinoid necrosis of small to medium arteries are present in brain and viscera.[236, 263]

Clinical signs of disease in young dogs with *Encephalitozoon* infection vary considerably and range from none to severe CNS disturbance, coma, and death. Poor growth, ataxia, tremor, blindness, and seizures are characteristic features of the disease in acute and subacute forms.[263] The clinical signs may be identical to those seen with distemper encephalitis in young dogs.

Diagnosis of this rare disease may be based on routine histopathology or culturing and electron microscopy.[25] Prognosis is poor. Insufficient data are available concerning treatment.

Canine Trypanosomiasis

These are protozoal diseases of domestic animals caused by *Trypanosoma* sp that are exotic to North America. Clinical signs vary with the host and species of parasite but include lethargy, anemia, depression, sudden death, genital infections, edema, hemorrhage, icterus, and emaciation.[94, 136] Hepatomegaly, cirrhosis, visceral lymphadenopathy, and splenomegaly are also observable.[284] Canine trypanosomiasis usually affects young male, rural dogs and produces multifocal to diffuse necrotizing granulomatous myocarditis. Trypanosomiasis may occasionally involve the central nervous system, producing a severe chronic meningoencephalitis in dogs[42] and paralysis or sleeping sickness in horses.[136]

Diagnosis is based on demonstration of organisms in blood smears. Prognosis is guarded. Treatment using lithium antimony thiomalate may be effective.

MYCOTIC DISEASES OF THE CENTRAL NERVOUS SYSTEM

Small Animals

Mycotic agents sporadically produce a granulomatous meningoencephalomyelitis in dogs and cats. The more common mycotic infections of the CNS are caused by *Cryptococcus neoformans*, *Blastomyces dermatitidis*, *Histoplasma capsulatum*, and *Coccidioides immitis*.[46, 122, 152, 203, 218, 252, 278] Each agent has a particular geographic distribution in the United States (Table 7–1). The pathogenesis is similar for blastomycosis, histoplasmosis, and coccidioidomycosis. The organism is present in the soil, producing mycelia and airborne spores. The coccidia of spores are probably inhaled, deposited in the alveoli, phagocytized, and converted into the spheric parasitic, budding yeast form. This form is disseminated via lymphatics, causing local hilar lymphadenopathy. There is hematogenous spread to other organs. The fate of the infected host is believed to depend on time and ability to develop cellular immunity to fungal antigens.

Unlike other mycotic agents, *Cryptococcus neoformans* exists only in the yeast form and has a worldwide distribution. Endemic areas have not been identified. Cryptococcosis frequently causes disease in dogs and cats that are immunodepressed.[234] Cats contract the disease more frequently than dogs.[282] The natural route of infection is generally believed to be the respiratory tract, with subsequent hematogenous and lymphogenous dissemination to other areas of the body.

As with bacteria, mycotic infections also may reach brain and spinal cord by direct spread from an adjacent infection, eg, from the nasal chambers, tooth alveolus and sinuses, outer ear, eustachian tube, middle or inner ear, petrous temporal bone, and basilar bone.

Although the incidence of CNS involvement by mycotic diseases is low, *Cryptococcus neoformans* may be more likely to be incriminated than the other organisms. Typcal clinical manifestations of mycotic diseases are summarized in Table 7–1. Neurologic signs will vary according to the location and severity. The signs may reflect either a focal mass lesion or a diffuse disease process (Fig. 7–10).

Diagnosis of mycotic infection is based on demonstration of the organisms in tissue sections or in material taken from aspirates or impression smears, culture, and serology. *Histoplasma* organisms may be found in neutrophils or monocytes of buffy coat or bone marrow smears. Organisms may be observed in CSF, which usually will be pleocytic (mononuclear and polymorphonuclear) and will have elevated protein levels. Eosinophils may be present with cryptococcosis.

Prognosis of mycotic infection is always

Table 7–1. MYCOTIC DISEASES OF THE CNS OF DOGS AND CATS

Disease	Etiology	Regional Distribution*	CNS Involvement	Predilection Sites	Clinical Signs
Cryptococcosis	*Cryptococcus neoformans*	Reported throughout US	Fairly common	Respiratory tract	Mucopurulent, watery to hemorrhagic, chronic nasal discharge; firm swelling over bridge of nose. Peripheral (cranial) lymphadenopathy, multiple skin lesions of head (ulcerated/draining). Depression, circling, ataxia, paraparesis, anisocoria, seizures, blindness, and apparent loss of smell
Blastomycosis	*Blastomyces dermatitidis*	Eastern seaboard of US	Uncommon	Lungs, lymph nodes, eyes, skin, bone, brain	Weight loss, emaciation, dyspnea, harsh bronchial sounds, fever; lymphadenopathy; ulcerated to draining skin lesions, epiphora, ocular redness and pain, corneal/lenticular opacification; blindness, lameness. Variable neurologic signs (see cryptococcosis)
Histoplasmosis	*Histoplasma capsulatum*	Eastern seaboard of US	Uncommon	Reticuloendothelial cells in liver, spleen, bone marrow, and lymph nodes	Coughing, dyspnea, hepatomegaly, splenomegaly, anemia; ocular lesions, skin nodules (ulcerated to draining). Variable neurologic signs (see cryptococcosis)
Coccidioidomycosis	*Coccidioides immitis*	Southwestern US	Uncommon	Lungs, lymph nodes, bone	Fever, cough, malaise, depression, peripheral lymphadenopathy to abscessation, lameness. Variable neurologic signs (see cryptococcosis)

*Within the USA.

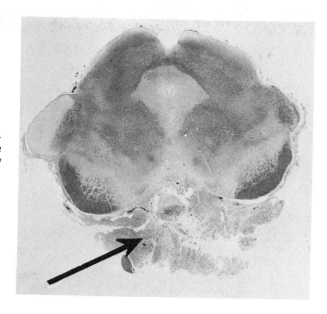

Figure 7–10. Blastomycosis in a dog, showing an extensive meningeal granuloma (arrow) on the base of the midbrain. Luxol fast blue–cresylecht violet stain, low power.

guarded, especially in the disseminated form. Most of the organisms are sensitive to treatment with amphotericin B. The treatment of choice for cryptococcosis is amphotericin B and flucytosine.[216] For the management of coccidioidal meningitis, intrathecal administration of amphotericin is recommended.

Other mycotic agents have been reported to sporadically produce CNS infection. These include *Cladosporidium trichoides*—brain abscessation;[120, 193] *Paecilomyces*—brain abscess, diskospondylitis;[206, 264] *Flavobacterium meningosepticum*—meningitis;[240] *Geotrichum candidum*—cerebral granulomas, choriomeningitis.[158]

Large Animals

Of the systemic fungal diseases of large animals, only cryptococcosis involves the CNS with any frequency. A review of this disease describes focal brain stem involvement with *Cryptococcus neoformans* producing a vestibular syndrome in a mare.[257]

Phycomycosis has involved the CNS in a horse[10] and a calf.[131]

PROTOTHECAL DISEASES OF THE CENTRAL NERVOUS SYSTEM

Prototheccosis

Protothecosis is caused by an acholoric genus of algae. Two species, *Prototheca wickerhamii* and *Prototheca zopfii,* have been shown to produce systemic disease in animals. Central nervous system involvement has been reported in dogs with both *Prototheca* sp.[117, 261]

The pathogenesis of protothecosis is uncertain. An alimentary route of exposure has been suggested. Failure of the host's immune competence may predispose to infection with this ubiquitous organism. It appears that *Prototheca* has a definite affinity for the eye in dogs. Organisms and pyogranulomatous lesions have been described in eyes, brain, spinal cord, kidneys, heart, liver, spleen, and lungs. The cellular response in dogs is frequently minimal. Clinical neurologic signs are variable, reflecting a multifocal disease process. They include visual impairment, paresis, tetraplegia, deafness, head tilt, facial hypalgesia, anosmia, and dementia. An eosinophilic pleocytosis in CSF has been reported in one affected dog.[261]

RICKETTSIAL DISEASES OF THE CENTRAL NERVOUS SYSTEM

Rickettsial diseases sporadically may involve the nervous system; however, clinical neurologic signs often are nonspecific but occasionally are suggestive of meningitis. Rickettsial organisms include *Ehrlichia canis* (canine ehrlichosis), *Neorickettsia helmintheca* (salmon poisoning), and *Rickettsia rickettsii* (Rocky Mountain spotted fever). The reason for the ataxia that is frequently seen in cases of *Ehrlichia equi* infection in horses is not understood.[90] These organisms are responsive to tetracyclines.

CHLAMYDIAL DISEASES OF THE CENTRAL NERVOUS SYSTEM

Sporadic Bovine Encephalomyelitis

Sporadic bovine encephalomyelitis (SBE), also known as Buss disease, is an infrequently occurring CNS disease that is more severe in cattle under 1 year of age. The etiologic agent appears to be a *Chlamydia*,[13, 97] although another report suggests that a paramyxovirus may cause a similar disease.[12] The disease has been documented in several countries, including the United States and Canada. Morbidity and mortality appear to vary with the age of the exposed and affected animals, with an average morbidity of 12% and mortality ranging from 30 to 40%.

Gross pathologic lesions usually include serofibrinous peritonitis, pleuritis, pericarditis, and occasionally arthritis, however, fibrous adhesions may well be lacking in animals that die acutely or are well into their convalescence. Hepatization of the lung lobes is reported. Histopathologic study of the brain reveals a leptomeningitis with severe perivascular mononuclear cuffing in areas of malacia and gliosis.

Clinical signs include stiffness, incoordination, knuckling, depression, muscle spasms, and later opisthotonos, convulsions, coma, and death. Frequently, signs of respiratory disease are concomitant, and lameness has been reported. The CSF exhibits a moderate mononuclear pleocytosis with an elevated protein level.

Diagnosis is by typical postmortem findings or a complement fixation test for antibodies, best done on acute and convalescent serum. Treatment with oxytetracycline or tylosin may be useful.

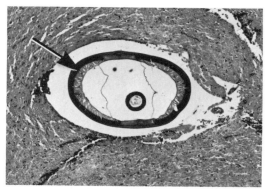

Figure 7–11. Demonstration of heartworm invasion in a dog's brain. Note the cross section of adult *Dirofilaria immitis* (arrow) in malacic brain tissue. Hematoxylin and eosin, low power.

FLY AND HELMINTH LARVAL DISEASES OF THE CENTRAL NERVOUS SYSTEM

In contrast to large domestic animals, myiasis and helminthiasis involving the CNS are rarely encountered clinically in dogs and cats. Aberrant migration and growth of parasites can result in extensive damage to neural parenchyma, including vascular rupture, necrosis, degeneration, atrophy, and proliferative (granulomatous) changes. In general, little is known of the route of migration of parasites that invade the brain, with the exception of bloodborne *Dirofilaria immitis* (Fig. 7–11). Apart from dirofilariasis, which occurs in mature dogs and cats, CNS parasitic invasion usually takes place in immature animals. Clinical signs are extremely variable, depending on the location and nature of the lesion. The signs may reflect either a mass lesion or a multifocal disease process. Diagnosis may be suggested by presence of an eosinophilic pleocytosis (together with neutrophilic and mononuclear cells) in cerebrospinal fluid. Definitive diagnosis requires isolation and/or pathologic demonstration of the parasite within the CNS.

The clinical course may be rapid or chronic, is usually progressive, and follows an acute or insidious onset of signs. Prognosis is poor and treatment ineffective.

Clinical and pathologic data for several fly and helminth larval diseases of the CNS of dogs and cats are tabulated (Table 7–2).

Table 7–2. HELMINTH AND FLY LARVAL DISEASES OF THE CNS OF DOGS AND CATS

Disease	Etiology	Species	Pathologic Changes	Clinical Signs	Reference
Cerebrospinal nematodiasis	1. *Dirofilaria immitis* (usually adults)	Dog, cat	Focal, multifocal infarction of CNS, especially brain; parenchymal compression if worms in CSF pathway	Seizures, visual impairment, depression, incoordination, paraparesis to paralysis (cord lesions)	57, 146, 162, 169, 207, 235
	2. *Toxocara canis* larvae	Dog	Focal, multifocal granulomas	As for dirofilariasis; diabetes insipidus	16, 227
	3. *Angiostrongylus cantonensis*	Dog	Multifocal granulomas throughout spinal cord and lower brain stem	Paraparesis to paraplegia; urinary and fecal incontinence; paralysis of tail; pain	170
	4. *Ancylostoma caninum*	Dog	Hemorrhagic myelomalacia	Loss of balance, torticollis, paraparesis, neck pain, tetraplegia	35
Cuterebriasis	*Cuterebra* sp larva	Dog, cat	Focal, hemorrhagic encephalomalacia	Seizures, visual impairment, depression, circling, head pressing, hysteria	102, 167, 183
Cerebral coenurosis	*Coenurus* sp	Cat	Brain swelling, cerebellar coning, tentorial herniation, cyst formation, within parenchyma	Head tilt, circling, nystagmus, falling, personality change, tetraplegia	84, 103
Cysticercosis	*Cysticercus cellulosae*	Dog	Multiple small cysts	Not provided	123

Ear Mite Infestation

Infestation with *Psoroptes cuniculi* or *Raillietina* sp appears to be common in goats[79] and is also seen in other large animals. Only rarely are noticeable scabs present in the ear, although head shaking may suggest the presence of mites. The mites live deep in the ear canal and are difficult to locate even with appropriate ear swabbing procedures. Should rupture of the tympanic membrane occur, signs of facial nerve paralysis and severe vestibular disease may become evident.[285] This condition is difficult to distinguish from an ear infection because it is often impossible to find the mites on an ear swab.

Coenurus cerebralis Infestation

Coenurosis, gid, or sturdy is the name given to the CNS disease produced by the presence of larval cysts (*Coenurus cerebralis*) of the dog tapeworm (*Taenia multiceps*), in the brain and spinal cord of sheep, goats, and, less frequently, cattle.[259] Geographically, gid has been reported in Europe, South Africa, Asia, New Zealand, Chile, and the United States. The adult tapeworm infests dogs and other Canidae, and goats and sheep are infected by the ingestion of the proglottids excreted in the feces. Mature *Coenurus* cysts, usually no more than two or three, are ultimately produced in the CNS, and the typical location appears to be the cerebrum, although the cerebellum or spinal cord can be affected. Clinical signs usually are those of a focal cerebral lesion.[201, 246],

An affected sheep might show fever and hyperesthesia during the migratory phase, and in 2 to 7 months display signs of cerebral disease, ie, impaired vision, circling, head pressing, ataxia, convulsions, and death.

The diagnosis is usually made at necropsy. Empiric treatment with albendazole or fenbendazole might be attempted, but because the cysts are antigenically completely different from the adult worm, it might well be to no avail. Hydatid cysts were suspected of causing CNS disease in a horse.[186] A successful outcome has recently been reported in 31 of 55 cases (56%) of coenurosis in which craniotomy and removal of a cyst was attempted.[241]

Oestrus ovis Infestation

Oestrus ovis is the nose bot fly of sheep and goats. The female fly deposits larvae around the nostrils of these animals, and larvae crawl up into the nasal cavity and sinuses, where they feed on the secretions of irritated mucous membranes. Rarely may they migrate to the frontal sinuses, and from there very occasionally via the ethmoid bones to the brain, or result in a frontal abscess that invades the brain. Organophosphates might be effective.[124, 163]

Parelaphostrongylus tenuis Infestation

Parelaphostrongylus tenuis is the meningeal worm of white tailed deer, which lives uneventfully in the subarachnoid space and cranial venous sinuses of its host. The larvae are ultimately shed in the feces and penetrate the footpads of certain mollusks. When these mollusks are ingested by goats, sheep, cattle, and wildlife ruminants, the larvae may migrate through the gastrointestinal wall via the peritoneal cavity and spinal nerves to the spinal cord where they randomly wander, and evoke an inflammatory response in the CNS of these aberrant hosts.

The physical examination of affected domestic animals is generally unremarkable, but abdominal cramping and hypopyon have been reported in both sheep and goats with this condition. Neurologic signs relate to the past and present location of the worm and have been reported to include tetraparesis, hemiparesis, tetraplegia, spastic gait, scoliosis, vestibular strabismus, circling, blindness, and death.[174] Although encephalitic signs have been occasionally documented in many naturally occurring cases, the complaint of lameness and/or pelvic limb paresis usually accompanies these signs. A history of possible exposure to pastures inhabited by white tailed deer seems mandatory.

Examination of the CSF is often contributory to the diagnosis. Large numbers of erythrocytes, elevated protein levels and high white blood cell counts, predominantly mononuclear cells and eosinophils, usually are present. The absence of eosinophils does not preclude the diagnosis.

The efficacy of therapy for this particular parasite has not been documented. Diethylcarbamazine, levamisole, thiabendazole, fenbendazole, or ivermectins might be reasonable drugs to try. If bacterial problems are not considered likely, glucocorticoids should probably be used concurrently in an attempt to reduce the inflammatory response. Spontaneous and possibly drug related cures have been reported.[174]

Necropsy may or may not reveal gross lesions. Histologic lesions include degenerated or intact larvae with an infiltration of mononuclear cells and eosinophils surrounding them, as well as inflammatory and malacic changes along the tracts where larvae have wandered.

Setaria digitata Disease

Setaria digitata is a filarial worm, the natural host of which is cattle. The worm lives without consequence in the peritoneal cavity of cows. Microfilaria produced by the female invade the blood stream and are transmitted by mosquitos to other animals, including sheep, goats, and horses. The worms wander at leisure and, in fact, often wander into and out of the CNS, making a definitive pathologic diagnosis difficult, but leaving malacic tracts behind.

Oftentimes, groups of animals are affected at once as reported in the Middle and Far East, and the disease generally appears during or shortly following the mosquito season.[118] Antemortem as well as postmortem diagnosis is difficult. The CSF is often normal. Clinical signs may appear acutely or insidiously, may be mild and regress completely or be severe. Most often the thoracolumbar area is involved, evidencing asymmetric signs, but cervical or brain stem lesions have been reported.[78] Treatment with diethylcarbamazine (50 mg/kg orally, once daily for 2 days) may be effective early in the disease course, and simultaneous glucocorticoid therapy should be considered.

Hypodermiasis

Hypoderma bovis, the cattle grub, is known to cause neurologic disease in both cattle and horses. *Hypoderma lineatum* has also caused neurologic problems in the horse.[177, 192] The clinical picture differs between cattle and horses, with pelvic limb paralysis following organophosphate treatment seen in cattle and encephalitis signs being seen most frequently in horses. No known relationship exists between organophosphate use and intracranial myiasis in horses.

Previously, it was thought that an interaction between a *Hypoderma* toxin and the organophosphate may have been responsible for the posterior paresis seen in cattle. Recent research disputes this idea, however.[64] Occasionally, the larvae produce liquefactive necrosis of the spinal cord, hemorrhage, or epidural lesions only, or no lesions whatever in cows with neurologic signs following organophosphate treatment. The CNS lesions of horses are produced by the extensive wandering of the parasite.

Antemortem diagnosis is difficult, as in all parasitic neurologic problems, although CSF analysis would be expected to be quite abnormal. No treatment is known to be effective. Systemic organophosphate and phenylbutazone[64] therapy could be tried.

Strongylus vulgaris Infestation

Strongylus vulgaris is known to cause encephalitis or spinal cord disease in the horse either through embolic showering from disintegration of a verminous thrombus or from damage due to the migrating worm itself. Consequently, head signs are usually those of diffuse forebrain disease, but spinal cord signs can be representative of a single focal lesion or progressive neurologic disease as the worm migrates along the spinal cord.[173]

Histopathologic changes reflect the type of disease process (infarction versus migrating tracts), and the worm is often difficult to locate owing to its propensity to migrate out of the CNS. CSF examination may reveal a massive or a mild neutrophilic pleocytosis, or it may be within normal limits.[161] Antemortem diagnosis is difficult, and this disease usually cannot be distinguished clinically from equine protozoal myeloencephalitis. No treatment has been proven to be effective, but larvicidal doses of benzimidazole anthelmintics or treatment with ivermectin, along with antiinflammatory drugs, might be of value.

Micronema deletrix Infestation

Micronema deletrix is a microscopic rhabditid nematode that is one of the more frequently reported parasites of the CNS of horses in North America. Its means of entry into the CNS is unknown, but it tends to cause diffuse forebrain signs, perhaps following earlier signs of ataxia.[5, 228] Systemic illness, sometimes relating to renal disease, can be evident.

Postmortem examination of affected animals is diagnostic, with numerous parasites surrounded by a granulomatous reaction easily located in the brain. Larvae may be expected to be present in CSF.

Other Central Nervous System Parasites

Stephanurus dentatus and *Ascaris suum* have been found in the brains and spinal cords of pigs suffering from neurologic disease.[244] Posterior paralysis is the most commonly reported clinical sign.

Draschia megastoma and *Habronema muscae* have caused brain stem and cerebral disease in horses.[176]

VASCULAR DISEASES IN THE CENTRAL NERVOUS SYSTEM

Pathologic studies over the past two decades have shown that vascular diseases in animals are no longer the rare entities they were once considered. Nevertheless, the incidence of vascular diseases is still low in comparison with other disease categories.

In general, clinical signs of vascular disease result from hemorrhage or anoxia-ischemia.

Hemorrhage

Naturally occurring intracerebral and intrameningeal hemorrhages are rare in animals. In contrast to the high incidence in humans, massive intracerebral hemorrhage resulting from spontaneous rupture of vessels and/or saccular aneurysms rarely occurs in animals.[52] Intracranial and intraspinal hemorrhage has been reported in dogs in association with arteriovenous vascular malformations, such as telangiectatic hamartomas and angiomas.[49, 68, 69, 293] Hemorrhage into primary and secondary brain tumors is frequently observed in dogs, especially oligodendrogliomas, glioblastomas, ependymomas, and hemangioendotheliomas.

Hemorrhage is often present in the CNS of animals with (1) migrating parasitic disorders, eg, cuterebriasis in dogs and *Hypoderma bovis* infestation in cattle; (2) protozoal infections, eg, toxoplasmosis in dogs and equine protozoal myeloencephalitis in horses; (3) bacterial meningoencephalitis, eg, meningitis in dogs, *E. coli* disease in calves, diplococcus infection in calves and pigs; (4) viral diseases, eg, eastern equine encephalomyelitis, malignant catarrhal fever, and infectious canine hepatitis; (5) degenerative disorders, eg, thiamine deficiency in cats, vitamin A deficiency in pigs; (6) toxins, eg, warfarin poisoning; (7) systemic metabolic disorders, eg, disseminated intravascular coagulopathies, platelet dysfunction (thrombocytopenia), and coagulation factor deficiencies; (8) cranial or spinal trauma.

Anoxia and Ischemia

In many animals lesions of the CNS may be seen that differ in regard to localization and etiology but have certain common pathologic features. The pathogenesis of these lesions is believed to be associated with hypoxia due to reduced blood and/or oxygen supply. These lesions are characterized by malacia and necrosis.

Malacias may be observed in many diverse conditions.[24, 28, 29, 150, 199, 202, 204, 224, 299] These include nigropallidal malacia in horses due to yellow star thistle poisoning; midbrain malacia of sheep associated with ingestion of *Phalaris tuberosa*; moldy corn poisoning in horses; *Clostridium perfringens* type D toxicoinfection in sheep and goats; thiamine responsive polioencephalomalacia in cattle, sheep, and goats; thiamine deficiency in dogs and cats; intoxications with lead and cyanide in dogs; hypoglycemia in dogs; cardiac arrest and vasospasm; cranial trauma; idiopathic polioencephalomalacia of dogs; x-irradiation; and decompression sickness in goats.

When the circulation to an area within the CNS is obstructed, the malacia or necrosis that ensues is called infarction. In dogs and cats, occlusive arterial disease may result from a degenerative or inflammatory process of the vessel wall, thromboembolism, severe polycythemia, or hypercoagulable state of the blood.

Generalized atherosclerosis is rare in the dog;[69] however, localized plaques have been reported in the cerebral vessels that resulted in massive infarction.[28] In aged animals of most species, varying degrees of fibrosis of intima, media, or adventitia of blood vessels are observed; however, cerebral infarction secondary to cerebral arteriosclerosis is rare[56, 69, 253] (Figs. 7–12 and 7–13).

In domestic animals, cerebrospinal infarction most often results from thrombosis or thromboembolism. Thrombosis occurs when a blood clot occludes a vessel. Thromboembolism is a term given to vascular occlusion by thrombus or other plug formed elsewhere in the body and carried to the site of obstruction. Apart from blood clots, emboli may include parasites (eg, *Dirofilaria immitis* and *Strongylus vulgaris*), tissue particles, metastatic neoplasia (eg, adenocarcinoma of mammary gland in dogs and cats), air, fat droplets, and foreign bodies. In dogs and cats thromboemboli often occur in association with bacterial endocarditis and cardiomyopathy, respectively.

Development of infarction as a result of thromboembolism of cerebrospinal vessels may depend on several factors: (1) caliber of vessel involved; (2) proportion of lumen obstructed; (3) rate of development of thrombus (time for a functional collateral circulation to develop); (4)

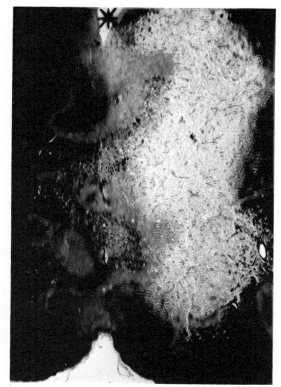

Figure 7–12. A large infarct is located in the midbrain on the right side of an 8 year old Labrador retriever. The asterisk indicates the mesencephalic aqueduct. Hematoxylin and eosin, low power.

type of artery involved, eg, functional end artery; (5) blood pressure of animal; and (6) particular vulnerability of area involved to oxygen and nutrient deprivation. Experimentally, disruption of neuronal energy metabolism following cerebral hypoxia and ischemia results in a selective vulnerability of cells in a specific topographic distribution.[27, 28, 33] The most sensitive areas include neocortex, basal nuclei, parts of the hippocampus, dorsal thalamic nuclei, and cerebellum.

The tissue reaction is uniform with pallor, disappearance of ectodermal elements, necrosis accompanied by production of gitter (macrophage) cells, and proliferation of mesenchymal elements, especially capillaries. Total necrosis of all tissue elements results in formation of cystic lesions.

Clinical signs of thromboembolism will vary depending on acuteness of vascular occlusion, location of structures supplied, and collateral arterial supply. Diagnosis may be suggested by acute or hyperacute onset of neurologic dysfunction, especially in dogs and cats with cardiac disease. Laboratory findings are nonspecific.

Tests for microfilariae should be run in areas with endemic dirofilariasis. Diagnosis is confirmed by pathologic studies.

Specific Vascular Disorders

A few specific neurologic syndromes involving blood supply to nervous tissue have been recognized in domestic animals and these will be discussed separately.

Progressive Hemorrhagic Myelomalacia

In dogs, the most undesirable sequel to spinal trauma is progressive hemorrhagic myelomalacia.[91, 268] This condition may occur within a few hours to 1 day after the initiating injury, such as acute external injury or, most commonly, acute intervertebral disk prolapse. The lesion is a combination of ischemic and hemorrhagic infarction of all parenchyma of the spinal cord. The underlying mechanism for the proposed occlusive vascular disorder is unknown. Necrosis of microvasculature and hemorrhage is believed to occur within the areas of the infarction. The condition results in complete malacia of cord segments. Clinical signs reflect the nature and level of the lesion. Initially, with T3-L3 spinal cord injury, an animal will have signs of acute onset: complete paraplegia with exaggerated pelvic limb reflexes. If the cord malacia descends to involve the lumbosacral segments,

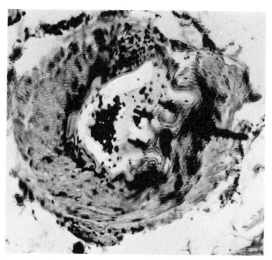

Figure 7–13. Same case as in Figure 7–12. A branch of the arteria media shows deposits of atheromatous material (dark staining material at large arrow) in the vessel wall. The irregular bulging of the intima (small arrows) produces a narrowing of the vascular lumen. Gomori's trichrome stain, medium power.

clinical signs of flaccid paraplegia with pelvic limb atonia and total areflexia will develop within 2 to 3 days. The tail will be flaccid and the anus dilated and unresponsive to stimuli. Pain perception is absent in all these areas. As the disorder progresses craniad, the thoracic limbs may become flaccid and analgesic; bilateral Horner's syndrome may occur. If the spinal cord malacia ascends to the lower to mid cervical level, respiratory paralysis will occur, resulting in death 7 to 10 days from the onset of signs.

Spinal cord damage is permanent. There is no treatment. It should be noted that this condition may develop following immediate surgical decompression of acute disk prolapse prior to any signs of progressive hemorrhagic myelomalacia.

Spinal Cord Infarction Secondary to Fibrocartilaginous Emboli

This is an ischemic necrosis of spinal cord parenchyma that has been associated with fibrocartilaginous emboli in arteries and veins.[88, 91, 104, 295, 296] Any level of the spinal cord may be involved. The disorder has been reported mainly in dogs, immature and adult, of small and large breeds, but also in a cat,[297] horse,[255, 281] three pigs,[205, 256] and lambs.[1]

The pathogenesis is not clear. Intervertebral disk material has been suggested as the source of the fibrocartilage; however, definitive evidence is lacking. It is enigmatic that this disorder occurs particularly in young adult nonchondrodystrophoid breeds of dogs that are not prone to intervertebral disk disease at this age. Pathologically, malacia and necrosis of gray and white matter are present. Infarcted areas are usually ischemic but may be hemorrhagic (Fig. 7–14). Neutrophils and phagocytic mononuclear cells may be seen.

Onset of clinical signs is typically hyperacute. Clinical signs will reflect location of the lesion within the spinal cord. Lesions that disrupt white matter will produce upper motor neuron signs (hypertonia, hyperreflexia) caudal to the level of the lesion. Infarction of gray matter will usually be asymptomatic unless it is in the area of brachial or lumbosacral intumescences, in which case complete lower motor neuron paralysis of limbs and/or tail, perineum, bladder, and rectum will be present (atonia, areflexia, analgesia). Affected animals do not typically show evidence of pain. Diagnosis is based on historical, clinical, laboratory, and pathologic findings. Plain radiographic findings are normal.

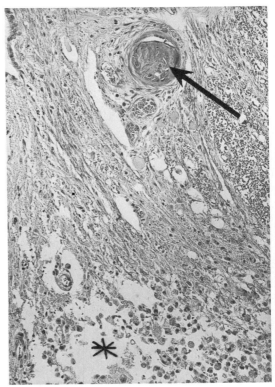

Figure 7–14. A spinal cord infarction due to a fibrocartilaginous embolus, which produces myelomalacia (asterisk). Note the small artery with embolus (arrow). Hematoxylin and eosin, medium power.

Myelography may suggest slight cord swelling. Cerebrospinal fluid analysis may reveal an elevated neutrophil count within a few hours of clinical onset. Protein levels may be elevated.

Prognosis is good to guarded and depends on the location and extent of infarction. Animals with extensive lesions of gray matter involving the brachial or lumbosacral intumescences have a poor prognosis. Any improvement should be apparent in 1 to 2 weeks. Residual effects are common. Treatment with mannitol and glucocorticosteroids has been advocated to reduce cord swelling.

Idiopathic Feline Cerebral Infarction

This is an ischemic necrosis of cerebral tissue that occurs spontaneously in adult cats of all ages and both sexes, especially in summer months.[53, 294] Lesions may be unilateral or bilateral and may involve up to 75% of one cerebral hemisphere. The major area of infarction is frequently in the distribution of the middle cerebral artery. Vascular occlusive lesions including thrombosis and vasculitis have been found only occasionally. Affected animals do not have cardiomyopathy. Clinical signs are variable but acute in onset. Signs range from depression and circling to seizures and change in attitude, often to the point of aggression. Mydriasis and visual impairment may be present. These clinical signs may be modified or disappear with time (several days to weeks). Laboratory findings are nonspecific. Abnormal brain trace pattern may be detected with electroencephalography. Diagnosis is based on historical and clinical data and substantiated by the usual clinical improvement after several days. Confirmation of diagnosis requires pathologic studies.

Prognosis is usually favorable because many of the signs seen initially will ameliorate; however, behavioral changes and uncontrollable seizures may persist.

Neonatal Maladjustment Syndrome

Neonatal maladjustment syndrome (NMS) is a well-recognized noninfectious condition of neonatal foals with a currently undefined etiology. It is characterized by gross behavioral disturbances with an initial loss of the suck reflex, followed by combinations of dementia, aimless wandering, blindness, seizures, and abnormal vocalizations occasionally resembling the barking of a dog[177, 201] (Fig. 7–15A).

Pathologic lesions described have included

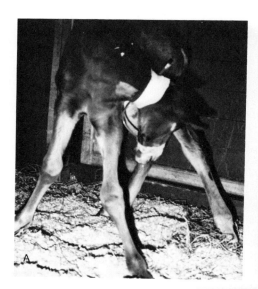
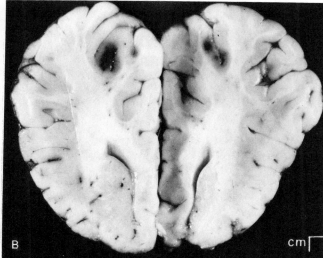

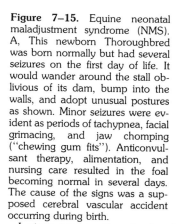
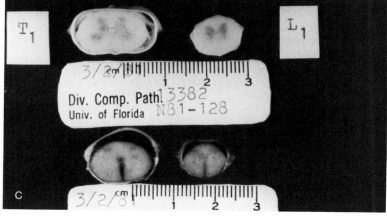

Figure 7–15. Equine neonatal maladjustment syndrome (NMS). A, This newborn Thoroughbred was born normally but had several seizures on the first day of life. It would wander around the stall oblivious of its dam, bump into the walls, and adopt unusual postures as shown. Minor seizures were evident as periods of tachypnea, facial grimacing, and jaw chomping ("chewing gum fits"). Anticonvulsant therapy, alimentation, and nursing care resulted in the foal becoming normal in several days. The cause of the signs was a supposed cerebral vascular accident occurring during birth. Lesions can sometimes be found in foals that do not survive. B, A syndrome of cerebral damage (as in A) may be associated with hemorrhagic infarcts and necrosis as seen in the frontal cortex. C, Signs of weakness or recumbency may be related to spinal cord lesions such as the prominent thoracolumbar subarachnoid hemorrhage (lower) compared with similar spinal cord segments from a foal with no subarachnoid hemorrhage (upper).

patchy areas of ischemic cerebral necrosis, cerebral edema, and parenchymal and subarachnoid hemorrhage (Fig. 7–15 B and C). Foals with neurologic signs more frequently had these types of lesions and more severe lesions than did neurologically normal foals that occasionally also had similar lesions. Further, some neurologically affected foals had no such lesions.[171]

Diagnosis is by history and clinical signs, and by ruling out disease such as trauma, meningitis, septicemia, metabolic disturbances or primary respiratory disease. Treatment consists of good nursing care, assurance of adequate colostral intake or plasma transfer, attention to acid-base balance, minimal, frequent feeding by tube if necessary, and oxygen administration by nasal tube if indicated. Convulsions can be controlled with diazepam (5–10 mg intravenously) or preferably phenobarbital (5–10 mg/kg intravenously over 30 minutes, followed by 3–6 mg/kg orally, three times daily as needed). The prognosis is moderately good for completely normal survival if good care is provided and complications such as septicemia do not occur.

Vasculitis

A severe form of meningitis and polyarteritis has been reported in beagles.[96, 132] An immunopathologic disorder has been proposed for this disorder. A similar form of necrotizing vasculitis has been observed in a 10 month old boxer dog and in a 4 month old Labrador retriever.[111]

Vascular Malformations

Vascular malformations involving the brain or spinal cord occur uncommonly in dogs,[49] horses,[86] and cattle.[41] Signs may be due to the direct, space occupying effect of the lesion or to bleeding and marginal siderosis.[175]

Acute Hematomyelia in Anesthetized Horses

Diffuse hemorrhage in the gray matter of the thoracolumbar spinal cord has resulted in permanent recumbency following general anesthesia in dorsal recumbency in horses. This appears to be a diffuse small vessel disease, but the pathogenesis is not known.[230]

Intracarotid Injection of Drugs

Occasionally, accidental intracarotid injections of various drugs occur in large animals, particularly horses, when the intrajugular site

is intended. Many times there is an immediate, acute, unilateral, cerebral ischemic episode.[80] Signs may be as mild as trotting in a circle or as profound as violent seizures or death. Water-soluble compounds are less noxious than suspensions and viscous materials. Recovery usually takes minutes to hours but may take several days, during which contralateral amaurosis and facial hypalgesia can be detected. Ischemic and hemorrhagic infarction of the forebrain may occur with vascular necrosis, edema, hemorrhage, thrombosis, and mild mononuclear cellular infiltration.

Mild syndromes usually end with complete recovery and do not warrant therapy. Anti-inflammatory drugs are possibly indicated in more severe cases.

REFERENCES

1. Abid HN and Holscher MA: Acute necrotizing myelopathy in lambs. Vet Med Small Anim Clin 78:1615, 1983.
2. Adams JM, Brown WJ, Snow HD, et al: Old dog encephalitis and demyelinating diseases in man. Vet Pathol 12:220, 1975.
3. Al-Khalid NW, Weisbrode SE, and Dubey JP: Pathogenicity of Toxoplasma gondii oocysts to ponies. Am J Vet Res 41:1549, 1980.
4. Alley MR, Jones BR, and Johnstone AC: Granulomatous meningoencephalomyelitis of dogs in New Zealand. NZ Vet J 31:117, 1983.
5. Alstad A and Berg I: Disseminated Micronema deletrix infection in the horse. JAVMA 174:264, 1979.
6. Appel MJG: Pathogenesis of canine distemper Am J Vet Res 30:1167, 1969.
7. Appel MJG, Bistner SI, Menegus M, et al: Pathogenicity of low virulence strains of two canine adenovirus types. Am J Vet Res 34:543, 1973.
8. Appel MJG and Gillespie JH: Canine distemper virus. Virol Monogr 11:1, 1972.
9. Appel MJ, Glickman LT, Raine CS, and Tourtellotte WW: Canine viruses and multiple sclerosis. Neurology 31:944, 1981.
10. Austin RJ: Disseminated phycomycosis in a horse. Can Vet J 17:86, 1976.
11. Averill DR and deLahunta A: Toxoplasmosis of the canine nervous system: Clinicopathologic findings in four cases. JAVMA 159:1134, 1971.
12. Bachmann R, Koprowski H, Jentsch G, et al: Sporadic bovine meningo-encephalitis—isolation of a paramyxovirus. Arch Virol 48:107, 1975.
13. Bannister GL, Brulanger P, Gray DP, et al: Sporadic bovine encephalitis in Canada. Can J Comp Med Vet Sci 26:25, 1962.
14. Barenfus M, Quadri C, McIntyre RW, and Schroeder E: Isolation of infectious bovine rhinotracheitis virus from calves with meningoencephalitis. JAVMA 143:725, 1963.
15. Barnard BJH, Geyer HJ, and deKoker WC: Neurologic symptoms in a cat following vaccination with high egg passage Flury rabies vaccine of chicken embryo origin. Onderstepoort J Vet Res 44:195, 1977.

16. Barron CN and Saunders LZ: Visceral larva migrans in the dog. Pathol Vet 3:315, 1966.

17. Bartha A, Hajdu G, Aldosy P, and Paczalay G: Occurrence of encephalitis caused by infectious bovine rhinotracheitis virus in calves. Acta Vet Hung 19:145, 1969.

18. Basson PA, McCully RM, and Warnes WEJ: Nosematosis: Report of a canine case in the Republic of South Africa. J South Afr Vet Med Assoc 37:3, 1966.

19. Bauer HF and Wikstrom J: Multiple sclerosis and house pets. Lancet 2:1029, 1977.

20. Beck BE: Infectious bovine rhinotracheitis encephalomyelitis in cattle and its differential diagnosis. Can Vet J 16:269, 1975.

21. Bedford PGC: Diagnosis of rabies in animals. Vet Rec 99:160, 1976.

22. Bestetti G, Buhlmann V, Nicolet J, and Fankhauser R: Paraplegia due to *Actinomyces viscosus* infection in a cat. Acta Neuropathol 39:231, 1977.

23. Bestetti G, Fatzer R, and Fankhauser R: Encephalitis following vaccination against distemper and infectious hepatitis in the dog. An optical and ultrastructural study. Acta Neuropathol 43:69, 1978.

24. Blakemore WF and Palmer AC: Delayed infarction of spinal cord white matter following X-radiation. J Pathol 137:273, 1982.

25. Botha WS, van Dellen AF, and Stewart CG: Canine encephalitozoonosis in South Africa. J South Afr Vet Med Assoc 50:135, 1979.

26. Braund KG: Encephalitis and meningitis. Vet Clin North Am 10:31, 1980.

27. Braund KG, Crawley RR, and Speakman C: Hippocampal necrosis associated with canine distemper virus infection. Vet Rec 109:122, 1981.

28. Braund KG and Vandevelde M: Polioencephalomalacia in the dog. Vet Pathol 16:661, 1979.

29. Braund KG, Vandevelde M, Albert RA, and Higgins RJ: Central (post-retinal) visual impairment in the dog—a clinical pathological study. J Small Anim Pract 18:395, 1977.

30. Braund KG, Vandevelde M, Walker TL, and Redding RW: Granulomatous meningoencephalomyelitis in six dogs. JAVMA 172:1195, 1978.

31. Brewer BD and Mayhew IG: Unpublished data, University of Florida, 1983.

32. Brewer NS: Antimicrobial agents—Part II. The aminoglycosides. Mayo Clin Proc 52:675, 1977.

33. Brierly LM, Meldrum BS, and Brown AW: The threshold and neuropathology of cerebral "anoxic-ischemic" cell change. Arch Neurol 29:367, 1973.

34. Brown T: Enteroviral encephalomyelitis of pigs. *In* Howard JL: Current Veterinary Therapy: Food Animal Practice. Philadelphia, WB Saunders Co, 1981.

35. Buick TD, Campbell RSF, and Hutchinson GW: Spinal nematodiasis of the dog associated with *Ancylostoma caninum*. Aust Vet J 53:602, 1977.

36. Bullmore CC and Sevedge JP: Canine meningoencephalitis. J Am Anim Hosp Assoc 14:387, 1978.

37. Cameron AM and Conroy JD: Rabies-like neuronal inclusions associated with a neoplastic reticulosis in a dog. Vet Pathol 11:29, 1974.

38. Carmichael LE, Barnes FD, and Percy DH: Temperature as a factor in resistance of young puppies to canine herpesvirus. J Infect Dis 120:669, 1970.

39. Carmichael LE, Squire RA, and Krook L: Clinical and pathological features of a fatal virus disease of new-born pups. Am J Vet Res 26:803, 1965.

40. Charlton KM and Garcia MM: Spontaneous listeric encephalitis and neuritis in sheep: Light microscopic studies. Vet Pathol 14:297, 1977.

41. Cho CY, Cook JE, and Leipold HW: Angiomatous vascular malformation in the spinal cord of a Hereford calf. Vet Pathol 16:613, 1979.

42. Chew M: Canine meningo-encephalitis due to *Trypanosoma evansi* infection. A report of two cases. Vet Rec 83:663, 1968.

43. Clark EG, Townsend HG, and McKenzie NT: Equine protozoal myeloencephalitis: A report of two cases from Western Canada. Can Vet J 22:140, 1981.

44. Cook SD and Dowling PC: A possible association between house pets and multiple sclerosis. Lancet 1:980, 1977.

45. Cook SD, Natelson BH, Levin BE, et al: Further evidence of a possible association between house dogs and multiple sclerosis. Ann Neurol 3:141, 1978.

46. Cordes DO and Royal WA: Cryptococcosis in a cat. NZ Vet J 15:117, 1967.

47. Cordy DR: Canine encephalomyelitis. Cornell Vet 32:11, 1942.

48. Cordy DR: Canine granulomatous meningoencephalomyelitis. Vet Pathol 16:325, 1979.

49. Cordy DR: Vascular malformations and hemangiomas of the canine spinal cord. Vet Pathol 16:275, 1979.

50. Crandell RA: Pseudorabies (Aujeszky's disease). Vet Clin North Am (Large Anim Pract) 4(2):321, 1982.

51. Cutler RWP and Averill DR: Cerebrospinal fluid gamma globulins in canine distemper encephalitis. Neurology 19:1111, 1969.

52. Dahme E and Schroder B: Kongophile Angiopathie, cerebrovascular Mikroaneurysmen und cerebrale Blutungen beim alten Hund. Zentralbl Veterinarmed (A)26:601, 1979.

53. deLahunta A: Feline neurology. Vet Clin North Am 6:433, 1976.

54. deLahunta A: Veterinary Neuroanatomy and Clinical Neurology, 2nd ed. Philadelphia, WB Saunders Co, 1983.

55. Desmonts G and Couvreur J: A prospective study of 378 pregnancies. N Engl J Med 290:1110, 1974.

56. Detweiler DK, Ratcliffe ML, and Luginbuhl H: The significance of naturally occurring coronary and cerebral arterial disease in animals. Ann NY Acad Sci 149:868, 1968.

57. Donahoe JMR and Holzinger EA: *Dirofilaria immitis* in the brains of a dog and a cat. JAVMA 164:518, 1974.

58. Dorr TE, Higgins RJ, Dangler CA, et al: Protozoal myeloencephalitis in horses in California. JAVMA 185:801, 1984.

59. Drake JC and Hime JM: Two syndromes in young dogs caused by *Toxoplasma gondii*. J Small Anim Pract 8:621, 1967.

60. Dubey JP: A review of Sarcocystis of domestic animals and of other coccidia of cats and dogs. JAVMA 169:1061, 1976.

61. Dubey JP: Toxoplasma, Hammondia, Besnoitia, Sarcocystis and other tissue cyst-forming coccidia of man and animals. *In* Kreier JP (ed): Parasitic Protozoa, vol III. New York, Academic Press, 1977, p 101.

62. Emmons R, Woodie J, Laub R, and Oshiro L: Main drain virus as a cause of equine encephalomyelitis. JAVMA 183:555, 1983.

63. English PB and Carlisle CH: Tetanus in the dog. Aust Vet J 37:62, 1961.

64. Eyre P, Boulard C, and Deline T: Local and systemic reactions in cattle to *Hypoderma lineatum* larval toxin: Protection by phenylbutazone. Am J Vet Res 42:25, 1981.

65. Fankhauser R: Toxoplasmose-encephalitis beim Hunde. Schweiz Arch Neurol Psychiatr 69:391, 1952.

66. Fankhauser R, Fatzer R, Luginbuhl H, and McGrath JT: Reticulosis of the central nervous system (CNS) in dogs. Adv Vet Sci Comp Med 16:35, 1972.

67. Fankhauser R, Fatzer R, Steck F, and Zendali JP: Morbus Aujeszky bei Hund und Katze in der Schweiz. Schweiz Arch Tierheilkd 117:623, 1975.

68. Fankhauser R and Luginbuhl H: Pathologische Anatomie des Zentralen und Peripheren Nervensystems der Haustiere. Berlin, Paul Parey, 1968, p 340.

69. Fankhauser R, Luginbuhl H, and McGrath JT: Cerebrovascular disease in various animal species. Ann NY Acad Sci 127:817, 1965.

70. Fatzer R: Meningitis und Chorio-Ependymitis granulomatosa bei Katzen. Schweiz Arch Tierheilkd 117:633, 1975.

71. Fatzer R and Fankhauser R: Enzephalomyelitis bei jungen Hunden nach Staupe-HCC-Impfung. Prakt Teirarztl 57:280, 1976.

72. Fekadu M and Baer GM: Recovery from clinical rabies of 2 dogs inoculated with a rabies virus strain from Ethiopia. JAVMA 41:1632, 1980.

73. Fekadu M, Shaddock JM, and Baer GM: Excretion of rabies virus in the saliva of dogs. J Infect Dis 145:715, 1982.

74. Fischer CA: Retinal and retinochoroidal lesions in early neuropathic canine distemper. JAVMA 158:740, 1971.

75. Fischer CA and Liu S-K: Neuro-ophthalmic manifestations of primary reticulosis of the central nervous system in a dog. JAVMA 158:1240, 1971.

76. Fischman HR and Schaeffer M: Pathogenesis of experimental rabies as revealed by immunofluorescence. Ann NY Acad Sci 177:78, 1971.

77. Flir K: Encephalomyelitis bei Gross Katzen. Dtsch Tierarztl Wochenschr 80:393, 1973.

78. Frauenfelder HC, Kazacos KR, and Lichtenfels JR: Cerebrospinal nematodiasis caused by a filariid in a horse. JAVMA 177:359, 1980.

79. Friel J and Greiner E: Psoroptic ear mites from domestic goats in Florida. Int Goat Sheep Res J, submitted, 1983.

80. Gabel AA and Koestner A: The effects of intracarotid artery injection of drugs in domestic animals. JAVMA 142:1397, 1963.

81. Gage ED: Treatment of diskospondylitis in the dog. JAVMA 166:1164, 1975.

82. Gardiner MR and Nairn ME: Viral meningoencephalitis of calves in western Australia. Aust Vet J 40:225, 1964.

83. Garmer NL, Naeser P, and Bergman AJ: Reticulosis of the eyes and the central nervous system in a dog. J Small Anim Pract 22:39, 1981.

84. Georgi JR, deLahunta A, and Percy DH: Cerebral coenurosis in a cat. Report of a case. Cornell Vet 59:127, 1969.

85. Gillespie JH and Timoney JF: Rabies and other rhabdoviruses. In Hagan WA and Bruner DW (ed): Infectious Diseases of Domestic Animals, 7th ed. Ithaca, Cornell University Press, 1981.

86. Gilmour JS and Fraser JA: Ataxia in a Welsh cob filly due to a venous malformation in the thoracic spinal cord. Equine Vet J 9:40, 1977.

87. Gore R, Osborne AD, Darke PGG, and Todd JN: Aujesky's disease in a pack of hounds. Vet Rec 101:93, 1977.

88. Greene CE and Higgins RJ: Fibrocartilaginous emboli as the cause of ischemic myelopathy in a dog. Cornell Vet 66:131, 1976.

89. Greenwood RE and Simson AR: Clinical report of a paralytic syndrome affecting stallions, mares, and foals on a thoroughbred stud farm. Equine Vet J 12:113, 1980.

90. Gribble DH: Ehrlichiosis. In Catcott EJ and Smithcors JF (ed): Equine Medicine and Surgery, 2nd ed. Santa Barbara, CA, American Veterinary Publishing, 1972, p 114.

91. Griffiths IR: Spinal cord infarction due to emboli arising from the intervertebral discs in the dog. J Comp Pathol 83:225, 1973.

92. Gustafson DP: Pseudorabies in dogs and cats. In Kirk RW (ed): Current Veterinary Therapy VI. Philadelphia, WB Saunders Co, 1977.

93. Hagemoser WA, Kluge JP, and Hill HT: Studies on the pathogenesis of pseudorabies in domestic cats following oral inoculation. Can J Comp Med 44:192, 1980.

94. Hagen WA, Bruner DW, and Gillespie JH: Hagen's Infectious Diseases of Domestic Animals, 6th ed. Ithaca, Cornell University Press, 1973.

95. Hall WW, Imagawa DT, and Choppin PW: Immunological evidence for the synthesis of all canine distemper virus polypeptides in chronic neurological diseases in dogs. Chronic distemper and old dog encephalitis differ from SSPE in man. Virology 98:283, 1979.

96. Harcourt RA: Polyarteritis in a colony of beagles. Vet Rec 102:519, 1978.

97. Harshfield GS: Sporadic bovine encephalomyelitis. JAVMA 156:466, 1970.

98. Hartley WJ: Polioencephalomalacia in dogs. Acta Neuropathol 2:271, 1963.

99. Hartley WH: A post-vaccinal inclusion body encephalitis in dogs. Vet Pathol 11:301, 1974.

100. Hartley WJ and Blakemore WF: An unidentified sporozoan encephalomyelitis in sheep. Vet Pathol 11:1, 1974.

101. Hartley WJ, Lindsay AB, and Mackinnon MM: Toxoplasma meningo-encephalomyelitis and myositis in a dog. NZ Vet J 6:124, 1958.

102. Hatziolos BC: Cuterebra larva in the brain of a cat. JAVMA 148:787, 1966.

103. Hayes MA and Creighton SR: A coenurus in the brain of a cat. Can Vet J 19:341, 1978.

104. Hayes MA, Creighton SR, Boysen BG, and Holfeld N: Acute necrotizing myelopathy from nucleus pulposus embolism in dogs with intervertebral disk degeneration. JAVMA 169:289, 1978.

105. Heavner JE and Pierce M: Brain abscess in a dog. Vet Med Small Anim Clin 76:785, 1976.

106. Held JP, McGavin MD, and Geiser D: Ataxia as the only clinical sign of cerebrospinal meningitis in a horse with equine infectious anemia. JAVMA 83:324, 1983.

107. Henderson RA, Hoerlein BF, Kramer TT, and Meyer ME: Discospondylitis in three dogs infected with Brucella canis. JAVMA 165:451, 1974.

108. Henson JB and McGuire TC: Immunopathology of equine infectious anemia. Am J Clin Pathol 56:306, 1971.

109. Higgins RJ, Krakowa S, Metzler AK, and Koestner A: Primary demyelination of CDV induced encephalomyelitis in gnotobiotic dogs. Acta Neuropathol 58:1, 1982.

110. Hirth RS and Nielsen SW: Pathology of feline toxoplasmosis. J Small Anim Pract 10:213, 1969.

111. Hoff EJ and Vandevelde M: Case report: Necrotizing vasculitis in the central nervous systems of two dogs. Vet Pathol 18:219, 1981.

112. Hudson MD: Bacterial meningitis. J Am Anim Hosp Assoc 12:88, 1976.

113. Hugoson G and Rockborn G: On the occurrence of

pseudorabies in Sweden. I. An outbreak in dogs caused by feeding abattoir offal. Zentralbl Veterinarmed (B) 19:641, 1972.

114. Hurov L, Troy G, and Turnwald G: Diskospondylitis in the dog: 27 cases. JAVMA 173:275, 1978.

115. Imagawa DT, Goret P, and Adams JM: Immunological relationships of measles, distemper and rinderpest viruses. Proc Natl Acad Sci 46:1119, 1959.

116. Imagawa DT, Howard EB, van Pelt LF, et al: Isolation of canine distemper virus from dogs with chronic neurological diseases. Proc Soc Exp Biol Med 164:355, 1980.

117. Imes GD, Lloyd JC, and Brightman MP: Disseminated protothecosis in a dog. Onderstepoort J Vet Res 44:1, 1977.

118. Innes JRM and Saunders LZ: Comparative Neuropathology. New York, Academic Press, 1962.

119. Jackson TA, Osburn BI, Cordy DR, and Kendrick JW: Equine herpesvirus 1 infection of horses: Studies on the experimentally induced neurologic disease. Am J Vet Res 38:709, 1977.

120. Jang SS, Biberstein EL, Rinaldi MG, et al: Feline brain abscesses due to *Cladosporium trichoides*. Sabouraudia 15:115, 1977.

121. Jarvis CA, Burkhart RL, and Koprowski H: Demyelinating encephalomyelitis in the dog associated with antirabies vaccination. Am J Hyg 50:14, 1949.

122. Jasmin AM, Carroll JM, Baucom JN, and Beusse DO: Systemic blastomycosis in Siamese cats. Vet Med Small Anim Clin 64:33, 1969.

123. Jauregui PH and Marquez-Monter H: Cysticercosis of the brain in dogs in Mexico City. Am J Vet Res 38:1641, 1977.

124. Jensen R and Swift B: Diseases of Sheep, 2nd ed. Philadelphia, Lea & Febiger, 1982.

125. Johnson BJ and Castro AE: Isolation of canine parvovirus from a dog brain with severe necrotizing vasculitis and encephalomalacia. JAVMA 184:1398, 1984.

126. Johnson DE and Summers BA: Osteomyelitis of the lumbar vertebrae in dogs caused by grass-seed foreign bodies. Aust Vet J 47:289, 1971.

127. Jolley WR, Jensen R, Hancock HA, and Swift BL: Encephalitis sarcocystosis in a newborn calf. Am J Vet Res 44:1908, 1983.

128. Jones SR: Toxoplasmosis: A review. JAVMA 163:1038, 1973.

129. Joyce JR and Russell LH: Clinical signs of rabies in horses. Comp Cont Ed 3:S56, 1981.

130. Jubb KV, Saunders LZ, and Coates HV: The intraocular lesions in canine distemper. J Comp Pathol 67:21, 1957.

131. Juck FA and Smith LL: Phycomycotic meningoencephalitis in a neonatal calf. Can Vet J 19:75, 1978.

132. Kelly DF, Grunsell CSG, and Kenyon CJ: Polyarteritis in a dog: A case report. Vet Rec 92:363, 1973.

133. Killingsworth C, Chiapella A, Veralli P, and deLahunta A: Feline tetanus. J Am Anim Hosp Assoc 13:209, 1977.

134. Knight AP and Jakinen MP: Caprine arthritis-encephalitis. Comp Cont Ed 4:263, 1982.

135. Knosel H: Zur Histopathologie der Aujeszky'schen Krankheit bei Hund und Katze. Zentralbl Veterinarmed (B) 15:592, 1968.

136. Knowles RC and Moulton WM: Exotic diseases. In Mansmann RA, MacAllister ES, and Pratt PW (eds): Equine Medicine and Surgery, 3rd ed. Santa Barbara, CA, American Veterinary Publications, 1982, p 366.

137. Koestner A: Animal model of human disease: Subacute sclerosing panencephalitis, multiple sclerosis. Animal

138. model: distemper-associated demyelinating encephalomyelitis. Am J Pathol 78:361, 1975.

138. Koestner A: Primary lymphoreticuloses of the nervous system in animals. Acta Neuropathol (Suppl)6:85, 1975.

139. Koestner A and Cole CR: Neuropathology of canine toxoplasmosis. Am J Vet Res 21:831, 1960.

140. Koestner A, McCullough B, Krakowka GS, et al: Canine distemper, a virus-induced demyelinating encephalomyelitis. In Zeman W and Lenette E (eds): Slow Virus Disease. Baltimore, Williams & Wilkins, 1974, p 86.

141. Koestner A and Zeman W: Primary reticuloses of the central nervous system in dogs. Am J Vet Res 23:381, 1962.

142. Kornegay JN: Feline infectious peritonitis: The central nervous system form. J Am Anim Hosp Assoc 14:580, 1978.

143. Kornegay JN and Barber DL: Diskospondylitis in dogs. JAVMA 177:337, 1980.

144. Kornegay JN, Barber DL, and Earley TD: Cranial thoracic diskospondylitis in two dogs. JAVMA 174:192, 1979.

145. Kornegay JN, Lorenz MD, and Zenoble RD: Bacterial meningoencephalitis in two dogs. JAVMA 173:1334, 1978.

146. Kotani T, Tomimura T, Ogura M, et al: Cerebral infarction caused by *Dirofilaria immitis* in three dogs. Nippon Juigaku Zasshi 37:379, 1975.

147. Krakowka S and Koestner A: Canine distemper virus and multiple sclerosis. Lancet 1:1127, 1978.

148. Krakowka S, McCullough B, Koestner A, and Olsen RG: Myelin-specific autoantibodies associated with central nervous system demyelination in canine distemper virus infection. Infect Immun 8:819, 1973.

149. Kristensen B and Vandevelde M: Immunofluorescence studies of canine distemper encephalitis on paraffin-embedded tissue. Am J Vet Res 39:1017, 1978.

150. Krook L and Kenney RM: Central nervous system lesions in dogs with metastasizing islet cell carcinoma. Cornell Vet 52:385, 1962.

151. Krum S, Johnson K, and Wilson J: Hydrocephalus associated with the noneffusive form of feline infectious peritonitis. JAVMA 167:746, 1975.

152. Kurtz HJ and Sharpnak S: *Blastomyces dermatitidis* meningoencephalitis in a dog. Pathol Vet 6:375, 1969.

153. Kurtzke JF and Priester WA: Dogs, distemper, and multiple sclerosis in the United States. Acta Neurol Scand 60:312, 1979.

154. Kyle RJ: Toxoplasma encephalitis in a cat. NZ Vet J 23:13, 1975.

155. La Croix JA: Vertebral body osteomyelitis: A case report. J Am Vet Radiol Soc 14:17, 1973.

156. Ladds PW, Dennis SM, and Njoku CO: Pathology of listeric infections in domestic animals. Vet Bull 44:67, 1974.

157. Legendre AM and Whitenack DL: Feline infectious peritonitis with spinal cord involvement in two cats. JAVMA 167:931, 1975.

158. Lincoln SD and Adcock JL: Disseminated geotrichosis in a dog. Pathol Vet 5:282, 1968.

159. Lincoln SD, Gorham JR, Davis WC, and Ott RL: Studies of old dog encephalitis. II. Electron microscopic and immunohistologic findings. Vet Pathol 10:124, 1973.

160. Lincoln SD, Gorham JR, Ott RL, and Hegreberg GA: Etiologic studies of old dog encephalitis. I. Demon-

stration of canine distemper viral antigen in the brain in two cases. Vet Pathol 8:1, 1971.

161. Little PB, Luin U, and Fretz P: Verminous encephalitis of horses: Experimental induction with *Strongylus vulgaris* larvae. Am J Vet Res 35:1501, 1974.

162. Liu I, and Castleman W: Equine posterior paresis associated with EHV-1 vaccination in California. J Equine Med Surg 12:397, 1977.

163. Livingston CW: Sheep bot fly *(Oestrus ovis)* infestation. *In* Howard JL (ed): Current Veterinary Therapy: Food Animal Practice. Philadelphia, WB Saunders Co, 1982, p. 1158.

164. Long JF, Jacoby RO, Olson M, and Koestner A: Beta-glucuronidase activity, and levels of protein and protein fractions in serum and cerebrospinal fluid of dogs with distemper associated demyelinating encephalopathy. Acta Neuropath 25:179, 1973.

165. Luttgen PJ and Crawley RR: Posterior paralysis caused by epidural dirofilariasis in a dog. J Am Anim Hosp Assoc 17:57, 1981.

166. MacCracken RM, McFerran JB, and Dow C: The neural spread of pseudorabies virus in calves. J Gen Virol 20:17, 1973.

167. MacDonald JM, deLahunta A, and Georgi J: Cuterebra encephalitis in a dog. Cornell Vet 66:372, 1976.

168. Macy DW: Colorado State University case records, 1980.

169. Mandelker L and Brutus RL: Feline and canine dirofilaria encephalitis. JAVMA 159:776, 1971.

170. Mason KV, Prescott CW, Kelly WR, and Waddell AH: Granulomatous encephalomyelitis of puppies due to *Angiostrongylus cantonensis*. Aust Vet J 52:295, 1976.

171. Mayhew IG: Observation on vascular accidents in the central nervous system on neonatal foals. J Reprod Fertil (Suppl) 32:569, 1982.

172. Mayhew IG and Brewer BD: Unpublished data, University of Florida, 1981.

173. Mayhew IG, Brewer B, Reinhard M, and Greiner E: Verminous *(Strongylus vulgaris)* myelitis in a donkey. Cornell Vet, 74:30, 1984.

174. Mayhew IG, deLahunta A, Georgi JR, and Aspros DG: Naturally occurring cerebrospinal parelaphostrongylosis. Cornell Vet 66:56, 1976.

175. Mayhew IG, deLahunta A, Whitlock RH, et al: Spinal cord disease in the horse. Cornell Vet 68 (Suppl 6):140, 1978.

176. Mayhew IG, Lichtenfels J, Greiner E, et al.: Migration of a spiruroid nematode through the brain of a horse. JAVMA 180:1306, 1982.

177. Mayhew IG and MacKay RJ: The nervous system. *In* Mansmann RA, McAllister ES, and Pratt PW (eds): Equine Medicine and Surgery, 3rd ed, vol II. Santa Barbara, CA, American Veterinary Publications, 1982.

178. McCandlish IAP and Ormerod EJ: Brain abscess associated with a penetrating foreign body. Vet Rec 102:380, 1978.

179. McClure J, Lindsay W, Taylor W, et al: Ataxia in four horses with equine infectious anemia. JAVMA 180:279, 1982.

180. McGovern VJ, Steel JD, Wyke BD, and Dodson ME: Canine encephalitis causing a syndrome characterized by tremor. Aust J Exp Biol Med Sci 28:433, 1950.

181. McGrath JT: Neurological Examination of the Dog, 2nd ed. Philadelphia, Lea & Febiger, 1960.

182. McIlwraith C and Kitchen DN: Neurologic signs and neuropathy associated with a case of equine infectious anemia. Cornell Vet 68:238, 1978.

183. McKenzie BE, Lyles DI, and Clinkscales JA: Intra-cerebral migration of Cuterebra larva in a kitten. JAVMA 172:173, 1978.

184. McKercher DG, Bibrack B, and Richards WP: Effects of the infectious bovine rhinotracheitis virus on the central nervous system of cattle. JAVMA 156:1460, 1970.

185. Mengeling WM: Encephalitis-vomiting and wasting disease complex of swine. *In* Howard JL: Current Veterinary Therapy: Food Animal Practice. Philadelphia, WB Saunders Co, 1981.

186. Miller WC and Poynter D: Hydatid cysts in a thoroughbred mare. Vet Rec 68:51, 1956.

187. Minor R: Rabies in the dog. Vet Rec 101:516, 1977.

188. Moller T and Neilsen SW: Toxoplasmosis in distemper-susceptible carnivora. Pathol Vet 1:189, 1964.

189. Morehouse LG, Kintner LD, and Nelson SL: Rabies in swine. JAVMA 153:57, 1968.

190. Murphy FA: Rabies pathogenesis. Brief review. Arch Virol 54:279, 1977.

191. Murphy FA, Bauer SP, Harrison AK, and Winn WC: Comparative pathogenesis of rabies and rabies-like viruses. Viral infection and transit from inoculation site to the central nervous system. Lab Invest 28:361, 1973.

192. Nelson DL: Cattle grubs. *In* Howard JL (ed): Current Veterinary Therapy: Food Animal Practice. Philadelphia, WB Saunders Co, 1982, p 1145.

193. Newsholme SJ and Tyrer MJ: Cerebral mycosis in a dog caused by *Cladosporium trichoides* Emmons 1952. Onderstepoort J Vet Res 47:47, 1980,

194. Nielson NO: Edema disease. *In* Leman A, et al (eds): Diseases of Swine, 5th ed. Ames, IA, Iowa State University Press, 1981, p 478.

195. Okoh AEJ: A case of cerebral babesiosis in the dog. Bull Anim Health Prod Afr 26:118, 1978.

196. Oliver JE and Lorenz MD: Handbook of Veterinary Neurologic Diagnosis. Philadelphia, WB Saunders Co, 1983.

197. O'Reilly KJ, Fishman B, and Hitchcock LM: Feline infectious peritonitis: Isolation of a coronavirus. Vet Rec 104:348, 1979.

198. O'Sullivan BM: Leukoencephalomyelitis of goat kids. Aust Vet J 54:479, 1978.

199. Palmer AC: The accident case. IV. The significance and estimation of damage to the central nervous system. J Small Anim Pract 5:25, 1964.

200. Palmer AC: Pathologic changes in the brain associated with fits in dogs. Vet Rec 90:167, 1972.

201. Palmer AC: Introduction to Animal Neurology, 2nd ed. London, Blackwell Scientific Publications, 1976.

202. Palmer AC, Blakemore WF, and Greenwood AG: Neuropathology of experimental decompression sickness (dysbarism) in the goat. Neuropath Appl Neurobiol 2:145, 1976.

203. Palmer AC, Herrtage ME, and Kaplan W: Cryptococcal infection of the central nervous system of a dog in the United Kingdom. J Small Anim Pract 22:579, 1981.

204. Palmer AC and Walker RG: The neuropathological effects of cardiac arrest in animals: A study of five cases. J Small Anim Pract 11:779, 1970.

205. Pass DA: Posterior paralysis in a sow due to cartilaginous emboli in the spinal cord. Aust Vet J 54:100, 1978.

206. Patnaik AK, Liu S-K, Wilkins RJ, et al: Paecilomycosis in a dog. JAVMA 161:806, 1972.

207. Patton CS and Garner FM: Cerebral infarction caused by heartworms *(Dirofilaria immitis)* in a dog. JAVMA 156:600, 1970.

208. Pedersen NC: Feline infectious peritonitis: Something old, something new. Feline Pract 6:42, 1976.

209. Pedersen NC: Serologic studies of naturally occurring feline infectious peritonitis. Am J Vet Res 37:1449, 1976.

210. Pedersen NC, Emmons RW, Selcer R, et al: Rabies vaccine virus infection in three dogs. JAVMA 172:1092, 1978.

211. Percy DH, Munnell JF, Olander HJ, and Carmichael LE: Pathogenesis of canine herpesvirus encephalitis. Am J Vet Res 31:145, 1970.

212. Percy DH, Olander HJ, and Carmichael LE: Encephalitis in the newborn pup due to a canine herpesvirus. Pathol Vet 5:135, 1968.

213. Pierson RE, Liggett HD, DeMartin JC, et al: Clinical and clinicopathologic observations in induced malignant catarrhal fever of cattle. JAVMA 173:833, 1978.

214. Plowright W: An encephalitis-nephritis syndrome in the dog probably due to congenital encephalitozoon infection. J Comp Pathol 62:83, 1952.

215. Plowright W and Yeoman G: Probable encephalitozoon infection of the dog. Vet Rec 64:381, 1952.

216. Prevost E, McKee JM, and Crawford P: Successful medical management of severe feline cryptococcosis. J Am Anim Hosp Assoc 18:111, 1982.

217. Price DL, Griffin J, Young A, et al: Tetanus toxin: Direct evidence for retrograde intraaxonal transport. Science 188:945, 1975.

218. Pryor WH, Huizenga CG, Splitter GA, and Harwell JF: Coccidioides immitis encephalitis in two dogs. JAVMA 161:1108, 1972.

219. Purchase HS: Cerebral babesiosis in dogs. Vet Rec 59:269, 1947.

220. Pursell A, Mitchell F, and Seibold H: Naturally occurring and experimentally induced eastern encephalomyelitis in calves. JAVMA 165:1101, 1976.

221. Pursell A, Peckham J, Cole A, et al: Naturally occurring and artificially induced eastern encephalomyelitis in pigs. JAVMA 161:1143, 1972.

222. Pursell AR, Sangster LT, Byars TD, et al: Neurologic disease induced by equine herpervirus 1. JAVMA 175:473, 1979.

223. Raine CS: On the development of CNS lesions in natural canine distemper encephalomyelitis. J Neurol Sci 30:13, 1976.

224. Read DH, Jolly RD, and Alley MR: Polioencephalomalacia of dogs with thiamine deficiency. Vet Pathol 14:103, 1977.

225. Rebhun W and deLahunta A: Diagnosis and treatment of bovine listeriosis. JAVMA 180:395, 1982.

226. Rhoades HE, Reynolds HA, Rahn DP, and Small E: Nocardiosis in a dog with multiple lesions of the central nervous system. JAVMA 142:278, 1963.

227. Richards MA and Sloper, JC: Hypothalamic involvement by "visceral" larva migrans in a dog suffering from diabetes insipidus. Vet Rec 76:449, 1964.

228. Rubin H and Woodard J: Equine infection with Micronema deletrix. JAVMA 165:256, 1974.

229. Russo ME: Primary reticulosis of the central nervous system in dogs. JAVMA 174:492, 1979.

230. Schatzmann U, Meister V, and Fankhauser R: Akute Hamatomyelie nach langerer Ruckenlage beim Pferd. Schweiz Arch Tierheilkd 121:149, 1979.

231. Schindler R: Studies on the pathogenesis of rabies. Bull WHO 25:119, 1961.

232. Schurrenberger PR, Martin RJ, and Meerdink G: Rabies in Illinois farm animals. JAVMA 156:1455, 1970.

233. Schwab ME and Thoenen H: Electron microscopic evidence for a transsynaptic migration of tetanus toxin in spinal cord motoneurons: An autoradiographic and morphometric study. Brain Res 105:213, 1976.

234. Scott DW: Feline dermatology. J Am Anim Hosp Assoc 16:349, 1980.

235. Segedy AK and Hayden DW: Cerebral vascular accident caused by Dirofilaria immitis in a dog. J Am Anim Hosp Assoc 14:752, 1978.

236. Shadduck JA, Bendele R, and Robinson GT: Isolation of the causative organism of canine encephalitozoonosis. Vet Pathol 15:449, 1978.

237. Shadduck JA and Pakes SP: Encephalitozoonosis (nosematosis) and toxoplasmosis. Am J Pathol 64:657, 1971.

238. Siim JC, Biering-Sorensen U, and Moller T: Toxoplasmosis in domestic animals. Adv Vet Sci 8:335, 1963.

239. Simpson CF and Mayhew IG: Evidence for Sarcocystis as the etiologic agent of equine protozoal myeloencephalitis. J Protozool 27:288, 1980.

240. Sims MA: Flavobacterium meningosepticum: A probable cause of meningitis in a cat. Vet Rec 95:567, 1974.

241. Skerritt GC and Stallbaumer MF: Diagnosis and treatment of conuriasis (gid) in sheep. Vet Rec 115:399, 1984.

242. Slausen DO and Finn JP: Meningoencephalitis and panophthalmitis in feline infectious peritonitis. JAVMA 160:729, 1972.

243. Smith JS, deLahunta A, and Riis RC: Reticulosis of the visual system in a dog. J Small Anim Pract 18:643, 1977.

244. Sprent J: Invasion of the nervous system in ascariasis. Parasitology 45:50, 1950.

245. Stamp JT: Slow virus infections of the nervous system of sheep. Vet Rec 107:529, 1980.

246. Stashak TS and Mayhew IG: The nervous system. In Jennings PB (ed): The Practice of Large Animal Surgery, vol II. Philadelphia, WB Saunders Co, 1984, p 983.

247. Stephans LR, Little PB, Wilkie BN, and Barnum DA: Infectious thromboembolic meningoencephalitis in cattle: A review. JAVMA 178:378, 1981.

248. Stewart CG, van Dellen AF, and Botha WS: Canine encephalitozoonosis in kennels and the isolation of encephalitozoon in tissue culture. J South Afr Vet Med Assoc 50:165, 1979.

249. Stowater JL, Codner EC, and McCoy JC: Actinomycosis in the spinal canal of a cat. Feline Pract 8:26, 1978.

250. Summers BA, Greisen HA, and Appel MJG: Possible initiation of viral encephalomyelitis in dogs by migrating lymphocytes infected with distemper virus. Lancet 2:187, 1978.

251. Summers BA, Greisen HA, and Appel MJG: Early events in canine distemper demyelinating encephalomyelitis. Acta Neuropathol 46:1, 1979.

252. Sutton RH: Cryptococcosis in dogs: A report on 6 cases. Aust Vet J 57:558, 1981.

253. Suzuki M, Fukuuchi Y, Shimazu K, et al: Cerebral atherosclerosis in the dog. II. Cerebral circulation. Arch Pathol 96:14, 1973.

254. Taylor D: Epizootic aspects. Vet Rec 99:157, 1976.

255. Taylor HW, Vandevelde M, and Firth EC: Ischemic myelopathy caused by fibrocartilaginous emboli in a horse. Vet Pathol 14:479, 1977.

256. Tessaro SV, Doige CE, and Rhodes CS: Posterior paralysis due to fibrocartilaginous embolism in two weaner pigs. Can J Comp Med 47:124, 1983.

257. Teuscher E, Vrins A, and Lemaire T: A vestibular syndrome associated with *Cryptococcus neoformans* in a horse. Zentralb Veterinarmed (A) 31:132, 1984.

258. Thoreson J and Little PB: Isolation of equine herpesvirus type 1 from a horse with acute paralytic disease. Can J Comp Med 39:350, 1975.

259. Todd KS and Dipietro JA: Cestodes. *In* Howard JL (ed): Current Veterinary Therapy: Food Animal Practice. Philadelphia, WB Saunders Co, 1981, p 931.

260. Tsiang H, Koulakoff A, Bizzini B, and Berwald-Netter Y: Neurotropism of rabies virus. An in vitro study. J Neuropathol Exp Neurol 42:439, 1983.

261. Tyler DE, Lorenz MD, Blue JL, et al: Disseminated prototheosis with central nervous system involvement in a dog. JAVMA 176:987, 1980.

262. Vainisi SJ and Campbell LH: Ocular toxoplasmosis in cats. JAVMA 154:141, 1969.

263. van Dellen AF, Botha WS, Boomker J, and Warnes WEJ: Light and electron microscopic studies on canine encephalitozoonosis: Cerebral vasculitis. Onderstepoort J Vet Res 45:165, 1978.

264. van den Hoven E and McKenzie RA: Suspected paecilomycosis in a dog. Aust Vet J 50:368, 1974.

265. Vandevelde M: Unpublished data, 1977.

266. Vandevelde M: Primary reticulosis of the central nervous system. Vet Clin North Am 10:57, 1980.

267. Vandevelde M and Braund KG: Polioencephalomyelitis in cats. Vet Pathol 16:420, 1979.

268. Vandevelde M and Fankhauser R: Zur Pathologie der Ruckenmarksblutungen beim Hund. Schweiz Arch Tierheilkd 114:463, 1972.

269. Vandevelde M and Fatzer R: Neurologische komplicaties bij drie honden na vaccinatie met een rabies-weefselktuurvaccin. Vlaams Diergeneeskd Tijdsch. 43:253, 1974.

270. Vandevelde M, Fatzer R, and Fankhauser R: Chronische-progressive Formen der Staupe-Enzephalitis des Hundes. Schweiz Arch Tierheilkd 116:391, 1974.

271. Vandevelde M, Fatzer R, and Fankhauser R: Immunohistologic studies in primary reticulosis of the canine brain. Vet Pathol 18:577, 1981.

272. Vandevelde M and Kristensen B: Observations on the distribution of canine distemper virus in the central nervous system of dogs with demyelinating encephalitis. Acta Neuropathol 40:233, 1977.

273. Vandevelde M, Kristensen B, Braund KG, et al: Chronic distemper virus encephalitis in mature dogs. Vet Pathol 17:17, 1980.

274. Vandevelde M, Kristensen B, and Greene CE: Primary reticulosis of the central nervous system in the dog. Vet Pathol 15:673, 1978.

275. Vandevelde M, Kristensen F, Kristensen B, et al: Immunological and pathological findings in demyelinating encephalitis associated with canine distemper virus infection. Acta Neuropathol 56:1, 1982.

276. van Rensburg IBJ and du Plessis JL: Nosematosis in a cat: A case report. J South Afr Vet Med Assoc 42:327, 1971.

277. Vavra J, Blazek K, Lavicka N, et al: Nosematosis in carnivores. J Parasitol 57:923, 1971.

278. Wagner JL, Pick JR, and Krigman MR: *Cryptococcus neoformans* infection in a dog. JAVMA 153:945, 1968.

279. Ward JM, Nelson N, Wright JF, and Berman E: Chronic nonclinical cerebral toxoplasmosis in cats. JAVMA 159:1012, 1971.

280. Whitley RD and Nelson SL: Pseudorabies (Aujeszky's disease) in the canine: Two atypical cases. J Am Anim Hosp Assoc 16:69, 1980.

281. Whitwell KE: Causes of ataxia in horses. *In* Practice, Vet Rec (suppl) 2:17, 1980.

282. Wilkinson GT: Feline cryptococcosis: A review and seven case reports. J Small Anim Pract 20:749, 1979.

283. Williams ES and Young S: Chronic wasting disease of captive mule deer: A spongiform encephalopathy. J Wild Dis 16:89, 1980.

284. Williams GD, Adams LG, Yaeger RG, et al: Naturally occurring trypanosomiasis (Chagas' disease) in dogs. JAVMA 171:171, 1977.

285. Wilson J and Brewer BD: Vestibular disease in a goat. Comp Cont Ed 6:S179, 1984.

286. Wisniewski H, Raine CS, and Kay WJ: Observations on viral demyelinating encephalomyelitis. Canine distemper. Lab Invest 26:589, 1972.

287. Wolf LG and Griesemer RA: Feline infectious peritonitis. Pathol Vet 3:255, 1966.

288. Wolf LG and Griesemer RA: Feline infectious peritonitis: Review of gross and histopathologic lesions. JAVMA 158:987, 1971.

289. Wood GL, Hirsch DC, Selcer RR, et al: Disseminated aspergillosis in a dog. JAVMA 172:704, 1978.

290. Wright HJ, Adams DS, and Trigo FJ: Meningoencephalitis after hot-iron disbudding of goat kids. Vet Med Small Anim Clin 78:599, 1983.

291. Wright NG: Recent advances in canine virus research. J Small Anim Pract 14:241, 1973.

292. Wright NG and Cornwell HJC: Experimental herpes virus infection in young puppies. Res Vet Sci 9:295, 1968.

293. Zaki FA: Vascular malformation (cavernous angioma) of the spinal cord in a dog. J Small Anim Pract 20:417, 1979.

294. Zaki FA and Nafe LA: Ischemic encephalopathy and focal granulomatous meningoencephalitis in the cat. J Small Anim Pract 21:429, 1980.

295. Zaki FA and Prata RG: Necrotizing myelopathy secondary to embolization of herniated intervertebral disk material in the dog. JAVMA 169:222, 1976.

296. Zaki FA, Prata RG, and Kay WJ: Necrotizing myelopathy in five Great Danes. JAVMA 165:1080, 1974.

297. Zaki FA, Prata RG, and Werner LL: Necrotizing myelopathy in a cat. JAVMA 169:228, 1976.

298. Zontine WJ and Uno T: Tetanus in a dog. Vet Med Small Anim Clin 63:341, 1968.

299. Zook BC: The pathologic anatomy of lead poisoning in dogs. Vet Pathol 9:310, 1972.

Chapter 8   *JN Kornegay, DVM, PhD*
IG Mayhew, BVSc, PhD

Metabolic, Toxic, and Nutritional Diseases of the Nervous System

Factors that alter neural metabolism have a profound effect on neurologic function. Blood gas dyscrasias, altered body temperature, water and electrolyte imbalances, accumulation of endogenous and exogenous toxins, and hormonal and nutrient excesses or deficiencies are the principal toxic, nutritional, and metabolic insults affecting the nervous system.

BLOOD GAS DYSCRASIAS

Hypoxia

Incidence

Cerebral hypoxia occurs when the amount of oxygen delivered to neurons is insufficient for aerobic metabolism. Causes of cerebral hypoxia include reduction of PaO_2 (hypoxic hypoxia), depletion of blood hemoglobin (anemic hypoxia), impaired tissue utilization of oxygen (histotoxic hypoxia), and reduction of the brain's blood supply (cerebral ischemia) due to either selective impairment of cerebral blood flow (oligemic hypoxia) or reduced cardiac output (stagnant hypoxia).[19]

Hypoxic Hypoxia. Fortunately, intrinsic safeguards protect the brain against most forms of cerebral hypoxia. Animals with severe respiratory disease often have markedly reduced PaO_2 values but rarely have neurologic clinical signs. That these animals do not experience hypoxic cerebral hypoxia is a function of chemical regulation inherent to cerebral blood vessels. Systemic hypoxia induces cerebral vessel dilation, leading to an increase in cerebral blood flow. Brain oxygenation is maintained until PaO_2 falls to 20 mm Hg.[98] Reduction of systemic oxygen tension below this point leads to failure of cerebral aerobic metabolism.

Anemic Hypoxia. The brain also appears to be protected against anemic hypoxia, in that hypoxic-type brain lesions have not been documented in association with blood loss, iron deficiency, or hemolytic anemia.[19] However, neurologic dysfunction often does occur when hemoglobin is bound to toxins such as carbon monoxide (carboxyhemoglobin) and nitrates (methemoglobin). Because neither of these forms of hemoglobin is capable of transporting oxygen, severe anemic cerebral hypoxia may occur in affected animals. Carbon monoxide exerts toxic effects by binding to hemoglobin about 250 times more readily than oxygen does.[19] Intoxication with carbon monoxide is rare in animals but has been reported in dogs that were exposed to fumes when transported in automobile trunks or truck beds.[144]

Nitrates are oxidants that convert the ferrous form of hemoglobin to the ferric state of methemoglobin. Ruminants are far more susceptible to intoxication than monogastrics because nitrates are reduced to more toxic nitrites in the rumen.[21] Sources of nitrates for grazing animals include heavily fertilized pasture and certain plants that accumulate toxic levels under natural conditions. This latter group includes *Sorghum* spp (Sudan grass and Johnson grass), *Zea mays* (corn), *Amaranthus* spp (pigweeds), *Datura* sp (jimsonweed), *Brassica oleracea*, and many others.[90, 121]

Other substances known to produce methemoglobin in animals include benzocaine,[71] phenazopyridine,[70] acetaminophen,[57] and red maple leaves.[42]

Histotoxic Hypoxia. The principal cause of histotoxic hypoxia in animals is cyanide intoxication.[69, 121] Cyanide blocks electron transfer from the cytochrome oxidase complex to molecular oxygen, thus compromising oxidative phosphorylation. The unused oxygen accumulates in tissue to the point where it is no longer released from hemoglobin. Therefore, the venous oxyhemoglobin level actually is increased. Animals may be exposed to cyanide through its use as a rodenticide or via ingestion of plants containing cyanogenetic glycosides such as *Sorghum* spp (Sudan grass, Johnson grass), *Suckleya suckleyana* (suckleya), *Prunus* spp (wild cherries), and many others.[90, 121] Chronic exposure to cyanogenetic glycoside–containing plants (eg, *Sorghum* spp) may result in neuronal death by direct effects of the glycosides on the cells.[152]

Stagnant Hypoxia. Cardiac arrest and subsequent stagnant cerebral hypoxia are encountered relatively commonly in animals, particularly in association with anesthesia.[127] An additional cause of stagnant cerebral hypoxia in animals is primary myocardial disease, in which syncope often is seen during exercise or excitement.

Oligemic Hypoxia. Focal oligemic cerebral hypoxia is common in human beings because of their high incidence of atherosclerosis with resultant infarction (stroke, cerebrovascular accident). Most cerebrovascular disease in animals is due to encephalitides such as thromboembolic meningoencephalitis of cattle[130] and feline infectious peritonitis.[185] Cerebral atherosclerosis has been described in pigs[59] but is rare in other domestic species. Occasional idiopathic cases of acute cerebral infarction also are seen, particularly in cats[33] (see Chapter 7).

Pathophysiology and Pathology

Effects of hypoxia are most pronounced in neurons, followed by oligodendroglia, astrocytes, microglia, and endothelial cells.[118] Neurons of certain cerebrocortical laminae, the hippocampus, and the Purkinje cell layer of the cerebellum are particularly sensitive to hypoxia.[19] This phenomenon of *selective vulnerability* of neurons has been attributed to differences in metabolic activity. However, studies have shown that complete cessation of cerebral blood flow is *less* injurious than incomplete ischemia.[77] This suggests that factors other than failure of metabolism may be involved in oligemic hypoxia. Pathologic processes that require oxygen, such as lipid peroxidation, may contribute.[39]

Regardless of pathogenesis, the neuronal lesion induced by cerebral hypoxia is referred to as ischemic cell change.[19] Affected neurons have eccentrically positioned pyknotic nuclei and deeply eosinophilic cytoplasm (Fig. 8–1). The resultant cerebrocortical lesion is called laminar cerebrocortical necrosis when a single layer of neurons is affected and pseudolaminar cerebrocortical necrosis when multiple layers are involved. Soon after these changes occur in the neuronal cell bodies, hypoxia-induced failure of the sodium pump leads to accumulation of sodium in neurons, glia, and endothelial cells. Water then moves into these cells to maintain osmotic equilibrium, resulting in cytotoxic edema. This increase in brain volume may lead to brain herniation[92] (Fig. 8–2).

The combined effects of diffuse neuronal ischemic cell change and cytotoxic brain edema

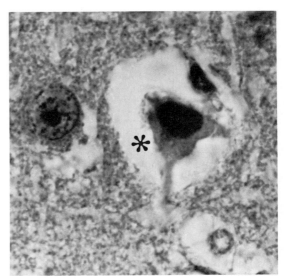

Figure 8–1. Photomicrograph of brain from horse with hypoxia. The neuron indicated by the asterisk is ischemic. Its cell body is shrunken and angulated; the nucleus is pyknotic. The neuron to its left is normal. Hematoxylin and eosin, × 250.

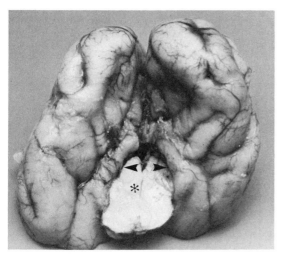

Figure 8–2. Caudal view of brain from dog that became apneic during surgery and died after several hours of artificial ventilation. The brain stem has been transected at the level of the midbrain. Portions of the parahippocampal gyri have herniated caudally through the tentorial notch, causing compression of the midbrain (arrowheads) and occlusion of the mesencephalic aqueduct (asterisk).

often result in death of the affected animal, especially when herniation occurs. If the animal survives, astrocytes and macrophages proliferate in an attempt to bridge lesions and remove necrotic debris, respectively. White matter changes usually are subtle until weeks or months later, when wallerian degeneration occurs owing to loss of cerebrocortical neurons. Severe focal oligemic hypoxia may lead to complete infarction of the involved area, with eventual cavitation.

Clinical Signs

Neurologic deficits are similar for the various forms of *diffuse* cerebral hypoxia. Clinical signs include stupor or coma, paralysis with decerebrate rigidity, seizures, blindness, and deafness. These signs may be either partially or wholly reversible after a period of days to months. Focal oligemic cerebral hypoxia usually causes less pronounced clinical signs of depression and postural reaction deficits, somatic sensory signs, and visual field deficits contralateral to the lesion.

Other clinical signs aid in differentiating the forms of cerebral hypoxia. Animals with hypoxic and stagnant hypoxia have evidence of respiratory and cardiovascular disease, respectively. A distinguishing feature of anemic hypoxia due to toxins is the coloration imparted to the mucous membranes by carboxyhemoglobin (bright red) and methemoglobin (brown). The mucous membranes are bright red in cyanide poisoning owing to the high levels of venous oxyhemoglobin. Neurologic deficits may be the only signs of oligemic hypoxia, unless there is vascular disease elsewhere in the body.

Diagnosis

A tentative diagnosis of the causes of cerebral hypoxia is based primarily on history and clinical findings. The PaO_2 is decreased except in cyanide poisoning and oligemic hypoxia. Blood concentrations of methemoglobin, carbon monoxide, and cyanide can be measured.

Treatment and Prognosis

The underlying pathogenetic mechanism should be corrected, if possible. Methylene blue (1% solution, 4–5 mg/kg orally, three times daily) has been recommended to reduce methemoglobin to hemoglobin in ruminants.[21] The dosage of methylene blue for other animals has not been well defined.[71] A single intravenous dose of 1 to 2 mg/kg has been advised in humans.[158] In treating cyanide poisoning, sodium nitrite (1% solution, 16 mg/kg intravenously) first is given to convert a tolerable fraction of hemoglobin to methemoglobin, which has a higher affinity for cyanide than does the cytochrome oxidase complex.[7] Sodium thiosulfate (20% solution, 30–40 mg/kg intravenously) then is administered so that it may serve as a substrate for the enzyme rhodenase to mediate conversion of cyanmethemoglobin to thiocyanate, which is excreted in the urine. Intracellular reductase systems convert the remaining methemoglobin to hemoglobin.

Supplemental oxygen usually also is helpful regardless of the cause of the hypoxia. Administration of 40 to 60% oxygen in an environmental unit or by nasal insufflation is indicated; 100% oxygen should be avoided as atelectasis may occur. Frequent turning of affected animals and removal of their excess oral secretions aid in preventing hypostatic congestion and aspiration pneumonia. Glucocorticoids do not have proven value in the treatment of cytotoxic edema seen with hypoxia.[4]

Acidosis

Acidosis occurs when the pH of arterial blood falls below 7.4 owing to either increased carbon dioxide (respiratory acidosis) or accumulation of acidic by-products of metabolism (metabolic acidosis). The principal causes of metabolic acidosis are shock, diabetes mellitus, and uremia; respiratory acidosis occurs when pulmonary disease impairs gas exchange. Several protective mechanisms insulate the brain against metabolic acidosis so that the pH of cerebrospinal fluid rarely is as low as that of blood.[138] Respiratory acidosis is more likely to be associated with reduction of CSF pH.[20]

The effects of acidosis on nervous tissue are poorly defined; however, the reduction in pH is presumed to alter the kinetics of many biologic enzymes, resulting in depression, delirium, or coma. These clinical effects are due in part to the accumulation of endogenous toxins in metabolic acidosis and concomitant hypoxia in respiratory acidosis.

Treatment of acidosis should include correction of the underlying disease and administration of bicarbonate-containing solutions. Bicarbonate combines with hydrogen ions to form carbonic acid, which dissociates to carbon dioxide and water. Unlike the bicarbonate ion, which is largely excluded from the brain, carbon dioxide readily crosses into the CSF, where it combines with water to form carbonic acid. The resulting transient reduction in CSF pH in the face of higher arterial pH is termed paradoxic cerebrospinal acidosis.[11] This phenomenon usually results in only mild depression and may be avoided by giving the bicarbonate slowly.

Alkalosis

Alkalosis occurs when the pH of arterial blood rises above 7.4 owing to either decreased carbon dioxide concentration (respiratory alkalosis) or loss or sequestration of body acids (metabolic alkalosis). Respiratory alkalosis results when hyperventilation is induced by either pulmonary disease or respiratory stimulants such as ammonia. Metabolic alkalosis in animals occurs most commonly when chloride is lost because of either vomiting or sequestration, as with abomasal displacement.[111]

The clinical effects of alkalosis are less pronounced than those of acidosis. The reduction of $PaCO_2$ in respiratory alkalosis constricts cerebral arterioles, reducing blood flow and causing transient confusion.[137] Metabolic alkalosis causes confusion and muscular weakness;[111, 137] compensatory hypoventilation also lowers PaO_2.[138]

Treatment of alkalosis should include correc-

tion of the underlying disease and administration of acidifying solutions. If there is concomitant hypokalemia, as is often the case with displaced abomasum, potassium should also be given.[111]

ALTERED BODY TEMPERATURE

Hyperthermia

Heat stroke occurs in animals that are confined in enclosures (automobiles, transport cages) with poor ventilation or are exercised forcibly when the ambient temperature exceeds 32.2°C (90°F).[79, 96, 149] Factors that predispose animals to heat stroke include lack of water, high humidity, obesity, dark hair-coat color, thick hair, lactation, anhidrosis, and restricted air exchange in brachycephalic animals due to upper airway malformation. The body temperature of affected animals is usually 40.6 to 43.9°C (105 to 111°F). Other signs include salivation, tachycardia, polypnea, injected mucous membranes, and sweating or panting, depending on the animal species and its principal means of dissipating heat. If the body temperature remains high, affected animals may develop cerebral edema[33] and disseminated intravascular coagulation.[146] These animals are stuporous, the mucous membranes become pale, petechiae may be present, and death ensues. Clinicopathologic abnormalities that may occur (and their causes) include respiratory alkalosis (panting), followed by metabolic acidosis (inadequate tissue perfusion, renal failure), hyperkalemia (acidosis), hypophosphatemia (alkalosis), hypocalcemia (rhabdomyolysis with calcium sequestration), and hemoconcentration (dehydration).[36, 149] The principal goal of treatment is to lower body temperature by either spraying with or submerging the animal in cold water. Rectal temperature should be monitored every 5 to 10 minutes to ensure that it does not drop below 39.5°C (103°F), as further cooling may lead to hypothermia. Animals with altered mental attitude or other neurologic defects should be given either dexamethasone (0.25–2.0 mg/kg intravenously) or mannitol (0.5–2.0 gm/kg intravenously, over a 10 minute period) to reduce cerebral edema. Those with clinical evidence of shock or disseminated intravascular coagulation may require further appropriate therapy. (Malignant hyperthermia, a paradoxic response leading to severe hyperthermia, is discussed in Chapter 14.)

Hypothermia

Animals may become hypothermic when they are exposed to severe cold and cannot seek shelter because of restraint or incapacitating disease.[44, 120, 186] Hypothermia also frequently occurs in anesthetized animals. A decrease in body temperature leads to reduction of both cerebral blood flow and brain oxygen uptake.[137] Clinical features of hypothermia include a body temperature of less than 32.2°C (90°F), altered mental attitude, and cardiac arrhythmias. Affected animals should be rewarmed using blankets and given warmed fluids and nutrients. Active rewarming of the body surface with water bottles or electric heating pads causes peripheral vasodilation. This may lead to internal cooling, with precipitation of cardiac arrhythmias.

ELECTROLYTE DISORDERS

Hypernatremia and Hyponatremia

Incidence

Hypernatremia occurs in animals that ingest or are given excessive salt or become dehydrated because of water loss or deprivation. Excessive salt ingestion (salt poisoning) and water deprivation are the most common causes of hypernatremia in pigs[156] and cattle.[126] Hypernatremia in dogs and cats usually is due to water loss subsequent to hyperventilation or diseases such as diabetes insipidus.[46] Hyponatremia results from excessive free water intake or administration of hypotonic fluids.

Pathophysiology and Pathology

Pathophysiologic effects of hypernatremia vary with the cause. When hypernatremia occurs acutely owing to excessive salt administration or ingestion, water moves rapidly from neurons into the extracellular space to maintain osmotic equilibrium. In affected human patients, the resultant brain shrinkage tears bridging veins and subdural hematomas occur.[55] Hypernatremia due to gradual fluid loss or deprivation induces neuronal production of "idiogenic osmols" to increase intracellular osmolality to the level of the extracellular fluid.[53] This reduces intracellular fluid loss; however, rapid replacement of the fluid deficit leaves neurons hypertonic with respect to the extracellular space. Neurons, therefore, imbibe water with resultant cerebral edema (water intoxication).

Pigs and cattle with either salt poisoning or water intoxication characteristically have pseudolaminar cerebrocortical necrosis.[126, 156] Brains from affected pigs also usually are infiltrated with eosinophils, possibly because the "idiogenic osmols" are chemotactic for eosinophils. Brain lesions resulting from hypernatremia in dogs and cats have not been defined.

Clinical Signs and Diagnosis

Pigs with salt poisoning may vomit and pigs and cattle may have diarrhea prior to the onset of signs of cerebrocortical disease, such as depression, ataxia, blindness, and seizures. Serum sodium levels and osmolality are increased to 180 to 190 mEq/l and 350 to 400 mOsm/kg, respectively. Chemical estimation of salt content of tissues, feed, and water is indicated in affected pigs. Hemolysis can occur in calves with excessive water intake (hyponatremia).

Therapy

The mechanism responsible for the hypernatremia must be corrected, if possible. The water deficit should be replaced with 5% dextrose over 48 to 72 hours using the following formula:[53]

$$\text{Water deficit (l)} = 0.6 \times \text{body weight (kg)}$$
$$\times \left(1 - \frac{142}{\text{serum Na (mEq/l)}}\right)$$

Serum sodium level and osmolality must be monitored closely. If neurologic function deteriorates during fluid therapy, cerebral edema probably is present and a hypertonic solution should be given. Some calves and pigs will survive with conservative therapy. When either hypernatremia or hyponatremia is possible, any specific therapy must await measurement of serum sodium concentration. The clinical signs of these conditions can be identical to those of polioencephalomalacia; consequently it may be prudent to administer thiamine.

Hypocalcemia

Incidence. Hypocalcemia (total serum calcium level <9.0 mg/dl) occurs most commonly in dairy cattle (parturient paresis, milk fever)[15] and dogs (puerperal tetany, eclampsia)[5] during lactation. Postparturient hypocalcemia also develops in sheep but is relatively rare in other species. Ruminants also may have hypocalcemia subsequent to ingestion of oxalate-containing plants (*Halogeton glomeratus*)[15] or lush green pasture (grass tetany; see Hypomagnesemia).[133] Other potential causes of hypocalcemia in dogs include hypoparathyroidism,[91, 154] renal disease,[184] ethylene glycol toxicity,[187] acute pancreatitis,[148] intestinal malabsorption,[56] hypoalbuminemia,[56] and nutritional secondary hyperparathyroidism.[117]

Pathophysiology and Pathology

The calcium ion is essential for neuromuscular transmission, muscle contraction, membrane stability, and the clotting process.[66] Failure of neuromuscular transmission and loss of membrane stability account for the signs of paresis and tetany typically caused by hypocalcemia in cattle and dogs, respectively.

Mechanisms responsible for hypocalcemia vary with each of the causative diseases. In puerperal tetany, there is excessive loss of calcium in milk. Oxalate and ethylene glycol precipitate calcium in the gut and tissues. Reduction of parathyroid hormone in hypoparathyroidism decreases renal retention, gastrointestinal absorption, and skeletal release of calcium. In kidney disease, calcium absorption in the gut is reduced owing to decreased renal hydroxylation of 25-hydroxycholecalciferol. Reduced renal clearance of phosphorus also may lead to hyperphosphatemia. Serum calcium and phosphorus levels may rise, fall, or remain unaltered with renal disease in the horse, a species that appears to metabolize calcium in an unusual manner. When the serum calcium-phosphorus product exceeds 70, calcium ion may be deposited in tissues. Calcium sequestration due to saponification of peripancreatic fatty acids is the main mechanism responsible for hypocalcemia in acute pancreatitis.

Clinical Signs

Clinical signs of hypocalcemia occur only when the level of the ionized fraction of serum calcium falls below 2.5 mg/dl.[159] Alkalosis reduces the ionized fraction of calcium, thus predisposing animals to clinical hypocalcemia. In contrast, patients with hypocalcemia due to a disproportionate reduction in protein bound calcium (as with acidosis or hypoalbuminemia) usually are clinically normal. The serum calcium concentration of hypoalbuminemic patients may be corrected using the following formula:

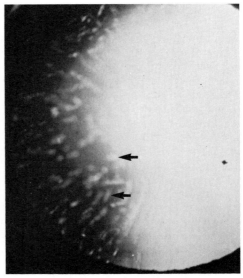

Figure 8–3. Lens, viewed in retroillumination, of dog with hypocalcemia. Note the many short linear opacities typical of hypocalcemic cataracts (arrows).

$$\text{Corrected Ca (mg/dl)} =$$
$$\text{Ca (mg/dl)} - \text{albumin (gm/dl)} + 3.5$$

Dogs with hypocalcemia usually have muscle fasciculations and convulsions; some also are depressed and may be weak with decreased spinal reflexes. Cattle also may initially have muscle tremor but usually are depressed and weak with decreased reflexes when examined. Horses may have synchronous diaphragmatic flutter ("thumps").

Prolongation of the S-T and Q-T segments has been reported on electrocardiograms of human patients with hypocalcemia[167] and was seen in an affected dog.[49] In cattle, blood pressure usually is decreased and the heart rate is increased.[15] Cataracts occur commonly in human patients with hypocalcemia[176] and also have been seen in affected dogs.[91] (Fig. 8–3).

Diagnosis

Diseases causing hypocalcemia may be subdivided based on whether there is concomitant hyperphosphatemia. Hypoparathyroidism, renal failure, and nutritional secondary hyperparathyroidism often induce hyperphosphatemia, whereas other diseases causing hypocalcemia usually have no effect on serum phosphorus levels. Further discrimination of the underlying cause of hypocalcemia is based on the characteristic clinical features of each disease.

Treatment and Prognosis

Calcium gluconate (10% solution, 0.5–1.5 ml/kg intravenously, not to exceed 10 ml) has been recommended for initial management of clinical hypocalcemia in dogs.[114] Other calcium preparations may be used, but the dose must be adjusted according to the actual calcium content of the solution. The calcium should be diluted in 5% dextrose and should then be given over 15 to 30 minutes. Calcium administration should be stopped if cardiac abnormalities are identified by auscultation or electrocardiographic monitoring.

Long-term supplementation of calcium and vitamin D may be necessary in dogs with hypocalcemia due to hypoparathyroidism and, less commonly, those with renal disease. Calcium-containing tablets or elixirs may be used to provide an approximate daily dose of 300 to 600 mg. Various vitamin D preparations have been recommended. Dihydrotachysterol acts and is metabolized more rapidly than either vitamin D_2 or D_3 and thus is probably most appropriate. A dosage of 0.01 mg/kg/day orally has been recommended,[113] but alternate day or even biweekly administration may be adequate. The serum calcium level should be closely monitored initially and should be maintained in a low normal or slightly hypocalcemic range (7.0–9.0 mg/dl). Withdrawal of the vitamin D and administration of intravenous fluids usually are adequate to correct iatrogenic hypercalcemia.

Calcium borogluconate (25% solution, 400–1000 ml) is the preferred solution for treating hypocalcemia in cattle.[15] This dose may be given intravenously with cardiac monitoring, or administered subcutaneously if the cow cannot be restrained or the heart rate is already markedly increased. Feeding a high phosphorus–low calcium ration (Ca:P of 1:3.3) during the last month of pregnancy has been advocated to stimulate parathyroid hormone production in susceptible cows.

Hypomagnesemia

Hypomagnesemia and associated muscle fasciculations and convulsions typically occur in dairy cattle and sheep grazing on lush green pasture (grass tetany, grass staggers).[133, 169] The disease is not causally related to parturition but is most common in the first 2 months after calving (lactation tetany). Clinical signs occur when serum magnesium level falls from the normal of 1.7 to 3.0 mg/dl to less than 1.0 mg/dl.

Mechanisms responsible for hypomagnesemia remain obscure; however, several factors are known to contribute.[133] Perhaps most importantly, magnesium homeostasis is not controlled nearly as closely as that of calcium. Hence, the serum magnesium level varies considerably with intake. That magnesium content of young grass is especially low is consistent with the tendency of animals to develop hypomagnesemic tetany when they graze on immature, rapidly growing pastures. Heavy fertilization of such pastures with potassium alone or with nitrogen probably also contributes, as these elements may either bind with magnesium or compete with it for absorption. The means by which hypomagnesemia causes tetany has not been explained. Impairment of cholinesterase activity at the neuromuscular end plate and reduction of the electric threshold necessary for neuromuscular transmission have been proposed.[161] Others feel that concomitant hypocalcemia is an important factor;[73] however, this is not a consistent finding in hypomagnesemic tetany.[169]

Use of solutions containing both calcium and magnesium (25% calcium borogluconate and 5% magnesium hypophosphite, 500 ml for cattle and 50 ml for sheep, intravenously) has been advocated in treating hypomagnesemic tetany.[15] Many affected animals die despite treatment. Accordingly, prevention is important. Daily feeding of magnesium oxide (60–120 gm to cattle, 7 gm to sheep) during periods of greatest susceptibility is effective.

ENDOGENOUS TOXINS

Hepatic Encephalopathy

Incidence

Hepatic encephalopathy (HE) is a syndrome in which hepatic dysfunction allows accumulation of substances that have toxic effects on the central nervous system.[23, 35, 166, 172] The three general causes are (1) acquired hepatic disease that reduces the functional detoxifying capacity of the liver,[23, 166] (2) congenital and acquired portosystemic shunts through which portal blood bypasses the liver,[35, 172] and (3) congenital deficiency of urea cycle enzymes (arginosuccinate synthetase) resulting in accumulation of ammonia.[163]

Potential causes of acquired hepatic disease[15, 23, 43, 166] include fatty liver (diabetes mellitus, pregnancy toxemia of cattle), hepatotoxicity (pyrrolizidine alkaloids, eg, *Senecio* and *Am-*

sinckia; aflatoxicosis, eg, *Aspergillus flavus*; chemicals, eg, ferrous fumarate), hepatitis (equine serum hepatitis, chronic active hepatitis), and hepatic neoplasia (bile duct carcinoma, hepatoma). In addition to reducing functional hepatic mass, these diseases also may lead to portal hypertension by impeding intrahepatic portal blood flow. This dilates existing, nonfunctional portosystemic shunts, allowing portal blood to bypass the liver.

Congenital portosystemic shunts have been described in dogs and other animals.[35, 172] The most common congenital shunt in dogs is persistence of the fetal ductus venosus; others include anomalous connection of the portal vein to either the azygous vein or the caudal vena cava and atresia of the portal vein with collateral shunts developing. When portal blood is shunted past the liver, toxins such as ammonia accumulate. In healthy animals, ammonia is converted to urea in the liver through a series of enzyme-driven reactions. A deficiency of any enzyme of this urea cycle allows accumulation of ammonia and signs of hepatic encephalopathy. Arginosuccinate synthetase deficiency has been reported in two dogs.[163]

Pathophysiology and Pathology

Ammonia level usually is increased in serum of animals with hepatic encephalopathy,[163, 166] and in serum, cerebrospinal fluid, and brain of affected human beings.[151] However, the means by which it causes encephalopathy are poorly defined. One proposed mechanism involves depletion of high energy compounds such as adenosine triphosphate (ATP).[84] Two ammonia molecules combine with α-ketoglutarate, a key intermediate in the citric acid cycle, to form glutamine. Accordingly, hyperammonemia may deplete α-ketoglutarate, thereby reducing ATP production.

The ionized and nonionized forms of ammonia are maintained in equilibrium based on the following equation:[166]

$$NH_3 + H^+ \leftrightarrows NH_4^+$$

Alkalosis shifts the equation to the left (NH_3) and acidosis shifts it to the right (NH_4^+). The nonionized form crosses cell membranes more readily. Conditions such as hypokalemia and alkalosis may exacerbate signs of hepatic encephalopathy.

The magnitude of hyperammonemia in human beings with hepatic encephalopathy does not correlate with the degree of neurologic dysfunction.[151] This has prompted studies to define other potential toxins. Mercaptans, short chain fatty acids, skatols and indoles, and biogenic amines have all been implicated in the pathogenesis of hepatic encephalopathy.[151, 188] However, the most important factor appears to be a shift in the ratio of branched chain amino acids (valine, leucine, isoleucine) to aromatic amino acids (phenylalanine, tryptophan, tyrosine).[58, 64, 164] This ratio usually is approximately 4.0 in dogs and horses but is reduced to 1.0 to 1.5 in animals with hepatic encephalopathy.[64, 164] Presumably, in hepatic disease, there is increased utilization of branched chain amino acids for energy and decreased hepatic clearance of aromatic amino acids.[58] As a result, there is decreased synthesis of norepinephrine and increased synthesis of both serotonin and "false" neurotransmitters. That this has a role in hepatic encephalopathy is supported by the correlation between the amino acid ratio and the degree of neurologic dysfunction in affected human beings[58] and dogs.[164]

The pathologic effects of HE on the brain are well defined in human beings.[41] The most characteristic lesions are hyperplasia and hypertrophy of protoplasmic astrocytes and Alzheimer type II cells. Cerebral edema and subsequent brain herniation have been identified in some human patients.[179]

Clinical Signs

Animals with hepatic encephalopathy have signs of cerebrocortical disease, including seizures, stupor or coma, altered behavior, compulsive walking, circling, head pressing, and blindness.[23, 35, 166, 172] These signs usually occur intermittently and often are exacerbated by feeding. Affected animals also may have systemic signs of hepatic disease such as polydipsia, weight loss, anorexia, and diarrhea. Those with portosystemic shunts usually have stunted growth and may have ascites.

Diagnosis

Hepatic encephalopathy should be suspected in animals with signs of cerebrocortical disease and hepatic dysfunction. There may be no hematologic abnormalities; however, affected animals often have low serum levels of albumin due to decreased hepatic synthesis and decreased serum urea nitrogen because hepatic conversion of ammonia to urea is impaired.[153, 166] A diagnosis is supported further if excretion of sulfobromophthalein (BSP) is delayed. Normally, there is less than 5% retention 30 minutes after intravenous administration of 5 mg/kg in dogs.[153] The clearance half-life of 1 gm of BSP in horses is 2.8 to 3.8 minutes.[23] Serum ammonia level usually is elevated but may be normal, in which case the ammonia tolerance test is useful.[114] This test is done in dogs and cats by giving 100 mg/kg of ammonium chloride orally and measuring serum ammonia level 30 minutes later. Whereas ammonia concentration should be normal in healthy animals, it is usually markedly increased in those with hepatic encephalopathy. Measurement of arterial ammonia may be more indicative than venous ammonia level.[147] Ammonium urate crystals also may be present in urine of affected animals. Although usually not necessary for diagnosis, the ratio of branched chain to aromatic amino acids is decreased.[164]

Once hepatic encephalopathy has been diagnosed using these tests, the cause of the hepatic dysfunction must be determined. Portosystemic shunts are identified through contrast angiography of the portal venous system[35] (Fig. 8–4). Contrast material is injected through catheters that have been placed surgically in either the splenic vein or a mesenteric vein. Animals with portosystemic shunts usually have small livers owing to hepatocyte atrophy resulting from loss of trophic intestinal substances such as insulin. Liver biopsy in these patients usually is unrewarding, as hepatocellular atrophy is the only abnormality. In contrast, liver biopsy is often the most useful test in identifying the cause of acquired hepatic encephalopathy. When serum ammonia is elevated and there is neither evidence of a portosystemic shunt nor acquired

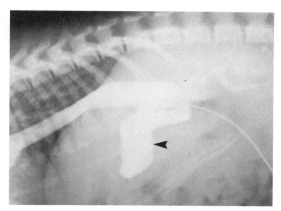

Figure 8–4. Operative mesenteric vein portogram of dog with portocaval shunt. There is an anomalous connection (arrowhead) between the portal system and systemic venous system, with no evidence of intrahepatic portal circulation.

liver disease, urea cycle enzymes may be deficient.

Treatment and Prognosis

Therapy is directed at reducing the serum levels of ammonia and other toxins through protein restriction, reduction of intestinal urea splitting bacteria, and catharsis.[23, 105, 153, 166] Animals with hepatic encephalopathy should be fed diets consisting mostly of carbohydrates with a small amount of a high quality protein source such as cottage cheese. The commercial diet K/D often is used for dogs. Antibiotics such as neomycin have been advocated in human beings to decrease ammonia-forming colonic bacteria but have had little benefit in animal patients.[166] Cathartics or enemas may be effective in reducing the contact time between nitrogenous material and the colonic mucosa. Lactulose is a nonabsorbable, synthetic disaccharide that causes an osmotic diarrhea and also reduces the pH of colonic contents, thus speeding passage of feces and increasing the amount of ionized ammonia. This drug has not been used much in animals; a dosage of 15 to 30 ml orally, four times daily, has been recommended for dogs.[153]

These therapeutic measures may alleviate signs of hepatic encephalopathy on a long-term basis and have some value in managing coma that may accompany fulminant hepatic failure. Comatose patients also should receive intravenous fluids to dilute toxins and correct hypokalemia and alkalosis. Dexamethasone and mannitol are used to reduce cerebral edema in Reye's syndrome in children[14] and may be beneficial in animals, although the potential complications of these drugs in large animals may deter their use. Amino acid mixtures prepared to restore a normal branched chain to aromatic amino acid ratio are efficacious in human patients and dogs with experimental portosystemic shunts[58] and so may have merit in treating animals with hepatic encephalopathy.

The underlying cause should be corrected if possible. This may be impossible when the liver disease is acquired and progressive, as with hepatic neoplasia and pyrrolizidine alkaloid intoxication. However, portosystemic shunts have been ligated successfully in both dogs and cats.[13, 18, 100] Before the ligature is tightened, the surgeon should be sure that the hepatic portal circulation is patent to avoid inducing severe portal hypertension. If portal hypertension already exists, subtotal ligation of the shunt may be indicated.

Uremic Encephalopathy and Neuropathy

Cerebrocortical dysfunction ranging from stupor to seizures is a common sequela of renal failure in human beings, particularly when the disease occurs acutely.[141] Peripheral neuropathy occurs even more frequently in human patients with renal disease.[142] Presumed uremic encephalopathy has been described in dogs;[184] however, uremic neuropathy has not been reported in animals.

The cerebrocortical dysfunction of uremia once was attributed wholly to dialysis (dialysis dementia), but effects of renal failure itself are now thought to contribute.[141] Factors proposed to account for uremic encephalopathy include depressed brain oxygen consumption, decreased cerebral ATPase activity, increased brain calcium and CSF phosphate levels, and accumulation of several organic acids in brain and CSF. That the signs of uremic encephalopathy are cleared rapidly by dialysis suggests that several small, water soluble molecules are responsible. Signs of peripheral neuropathy also are reversed by dialysis, again suggesting that dialyzable molecules are the cause.[142] A role for mid-sized substances has been proposed, because they cross the dialysis membrane more slowly and signs of neuropathy also are slow to reverse.

Pancreatic Encephalopathy

Confusion and behavioral changes commonly occur subsequent to acute pancreatitis in human beings.[50, 155] Although the pathogenesis of this condition remains obscure, a role for increased CSF lipase level has been proposed.[50] Although a similar syndrome has not been defined specifically in animals, pancreatic encephalopathy could contribute to the malaise frequently seen in animals with pancreatitis.

EXOGENOUS TOXINS

Exogenous toxins affecting the nervous systems of human beings are divided into those causing cerebral hypoxia (see above) and those having an affinity for specific neural structures such as myelin or myelin-forming cells, peripheral axons alone, or with central neuronal involvement, and specific brain nuclei.[119] There is considerable overlap between and within the two groups. However, the fact that neurotoxins commonly produce specific lesions allows extrapolation to pathogenesis. Examples of the general categories of neurotoxins are discussed below; others are listed in Table 8–1.

Lead Poisoning

Incidence

Lead is the principal neurotoxin among the heavy metal group. Mercury, selenium, and arsenic also have neural effects (Table 8–1). Lead poisoning (plumbism) has been reported in dogs,[93, 190] cats,[180] cattle,[31] and horses.[22] Horses usually are intoxicated by eating forage contaminated with emissions from lead smelters. Sources of lead for other species include paint, linoleum, used motor oil, and batteries.

Pathophysiology and Pathology

Plumbism causes laminar cerebrocortical necrosis and segmental demyelination of peripheral nerve fibers in animals. Neuronal necrosis has been attributed to endothelial cell proliferation and necrosis with resultant oligemic hypoxia. Segmental demyelination is presumed to result from direct effects of lead on Schwann cells and myelin itself.

Clinical Signs

Dogs, cattle, and cats with lead poisoning usually have clinical signs of cerebrocortical disease, including ataxia, seizures, blindness, and abnormal behavior.[31, 93, 180, 189] Vomiting, diarrhea, and other signs of gastrointestinal disturbance usually also occur in these species. In contrast, the principal signs of lead poisoning in horses relate to the neuropathy and include appendicular, laryngeal, and anal sphincter paresis.[22]

Diagnosis

Dogs and cattle usually have circulating nucleated red blood cells and basophilic stippling without marked anemia.[31, 150] These changes usually are absent in horses[22] and have been inconsistent in affected cats.[180] Radiopaque densities compatible with lead often are seen in the intestinal tracts of affected dogs. Some

Table 8–1. SELECTED NEUROTOXINS AFFECTING ANIMALS

Neurotoxin	Principal Species Affected	Sources	Neurologic Clinical Signs	Pathophysiology	Diagnostic Features	Neural Microscopic Lesions	Treatment
Mercury[37, 74]	Cattle, pigs	Grain treated with organomercurial fungicides	Ataxia, tremor, seizures	Inactivates mitotic spindle	Mercury levels: urine > 100 ppm; kidney > 10 ppm	Cerebrocortical (porcine) and cerebellar granular cell (bovine) necrosis; peripheral axonal degeneration and demyelination	BAL (6–7 mg/kg IM, tid until recovery)
Selenium[68, 75]	Pigs	Feed oversupplementation	Paralysis	Unknown; may bind sulfhydryl groups in plants	Selenium levels: liver 20–30 ppm	Poliomyelomalacia	Supportive
Arsenic[67, 89]	Cattle, sheep, pigs	Ingestion of herbicides & pesticides; livestock dips	Ataxia, paresis, blindness	Binds sulfhydryl groups	Arsenic levels: liver and kidney > 10 ppm	Peripheral demyelination; central white matter petechiae & perivascular demyelination	Sodium thiosulfate (100–200 ml 15% solution IV followed by 300–600 ml orally qid to horses and adult cattle; ¼ this dose to sheep)
Organophosphates, carbamates[25, 129]	Cattle, cats, sheep, pigs	Insecticides	Muscle tremors, salivation, diarrhea, miosis, seizures	Anticholinesterase	Decreased serum cholinesterase level	Peripheral axonal degeneration (chronic exposure)	Atropine (0.2 mg/kg; ¼ of dose IV, ¾ IM); 2-PAM (20 mg/kg IV or IM)
Chlorinated hydrocarbons[3, 173]	Dogs, cattle, sheep	Insecticides	Muscle tremors, increased excitability, seizures	Unknown	History of exposure, clinical signs	None	Bathing to remove dip, anesthesia
Strychnine[124]	Dogs	Pesticide	Muscle tremors, increased excitability, extensor rigidity, seizures	Blocks postsynaptic inhibition in spinal cord	History of exposure, analysis of stomach contents or tissues	None	Emetic, anesthesia, gastric lavage
Metaldehyde[171]	Dogs	Molluscicide	Muscle tremors, salivation, hyperthermia	Unknown	History of exposure, analysis of stomach contents or tissues	None	Emetic, anesthesia, gastric lavage

immature dogs also have radiopaque lines just proximal to the epiphyseal plates of long bones. These "lead lines" are due to metaphyseal sclerosis.

Blood lead concentration should not exceed 0.35 ppm (35 μg/100 ml) in healthy animals.[22, 31, 93, 180, 190] Values as high as 5.30 ppm have been reported in dogs with lead poisoning.[93] Urinary lead levels have little diagnostic value, except when measured before and after therapy with calcium ethylenediaminetetraacetate (CaEDTA). A post-treatment value of greater than 0.8 ppm is indicative of plumbism.[190] Samples of liver or kidney taken from animals with lead poisoning should contain at least 5.0 ppm of lead to be diagnostic.[125, 190]

An additional test used in diagnosing lead poisoning is measurement of urinary Δ-aminolevulinic acid (ALA).[125] This accumulates in plumbism owing to lead's inhibition of enzymes necessary for heme synthesis. Urinary ALA levels are normally less than 200 μg/100 ml in dogs and cattle but are dramatically elevated in lead poisoning.

Treatment and Prognosis

Lead in the gastrointestinal tract should be removed with enemas and emetics prior to chelation therapy. Calcium ethylenediaminetetraacetate is the most effective chelating agent; a daily dose of 100 mg/kg (not to exceed 2 gm), diluted to 10 mg/ml in 5% dextrose and given subcutaneously in four equal portions for 2 to 5 days, has been recommended for dogs.[189] Cattle and horses have been treated with a similar daily dosage divided in two equal portions and given intravenously for 1 or 2 days.[15, 22]

Hexachlorophene Toxicity

The bactericidal, fungicidal, and anthelmintic properties of hexachlorophene have led to its incorporation in soaps, antiseptic solutions, crop dusts, and anthelmintics. Hexachlorophene poisoning and associated muscle tremor have been reported in human beings,[139] cattle,[82] and dogs.[10, 178] Young animals are especially susceptible. The characteristic lesion of hexachloro-

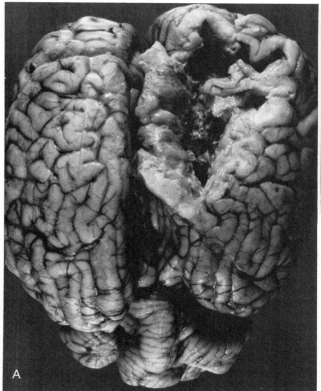

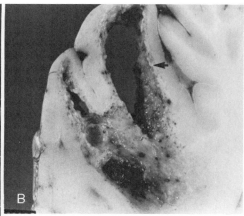

Figure 8–5. Equine leukoencephalomalacia. A, Formalin fixed brain from a miniature horse dying of a fulminant illness characterized by severe depression, recumbency, and convulsions. A large part of the right frontoparietal lobe is missing because of liquefactive necrosis of the gray matter and particularly the underlying white matter. Generalized flattening of cerebral gyri is evidence of diffuse brain swelling that resulted in herniation of the ventromedial portions of the occipital lobes (visible just rostral to the cerebellar vermis) under the tentorium cerebelli. *Fusarium* sp was present in the feedstuff and presumably the lesions were the result of a putative neurotoxin produced by the fungus. B, Transverse section of brain from horse with leukoencephalomalacia. The white matter of one gyrus (arrow) is completely cavitated, and that of an adjacent gyrus also is necrotic. Scale in lower left corner is in millimeters.

phene toxicity is vacuolation of the white matter of the central nervous system due to intramyelinic accumulation of fluid.[170] Mechanisms responsible for this lesion are poorly defined but may relate to hexachlorophene's affinity for lipids and proteins that predominate in myelin. Similar intramyelinic vacuoles result from experimental intoxication with triethyltin,[63] isoniazid,[97] and cuprizone.[168] Although there is no specific treatment for hexachlorophene toxicity, some animals recover.

Moldy Corn Poisoning

Ingestion of corn contaminated with putative neurotoxins from the fungus *Fusarium moniliforme* can be associated with a disease in horses termed leukoencephalomalacia.[6, 182] Affected horses have acute onset of signs of cerebrocortical disease, including ataxia, blindness, and circling. At the time of necropsy, the corona radiata of the cerebral cortex is necrotic and may be cavitated (Fig. 8–5). The toxin responsible for this lesion has not been identified; however, the predilection for white matter suggests that myelin may be selectively involved. There is no specific treatment.

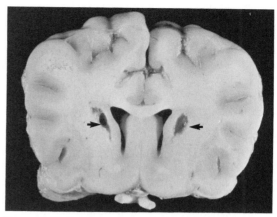

Figure 8–7. Transverse section of brain at the caudate nuclei from a dog with previous intoxication with an unknown toxin. Note the bilateral cavitating lesions in the caudate nuclei (arrows).

Yellow Star Thistle Poisoning

Chronic ingestion of yellow star thistle (*Centaurea solstitialis*) may cause bilateral necrosis of the substantia nigra and globus pallidus (nigropallidal encephalomalacia)[52, 60] (Fig. 8–6). Affected horses have difficulty eating and drinking because of dystonia of muscles of prehension, mastication, and deglutition. They may be depressed and may walk aimlessly or circle. The disease occurs most commonly in the summer and late autumn. Mechanisms responsible for this lesion are not clear. There is no specific treatment.

Focal Symmetric Encephalomalacia

Lesions of the basal nuclei, substantia nigra, and other brain stem and spinal cord regions (focal symmetric encephalomalacia) occur in lambs and kids due to *Clostridium perfringens* type D enterotoxemia.[15, 61] Similar lesions occur with *Escherichia coli* enterotoxemia (edema disease) in swine[15] (see Chapter 7). Symmetric cavitation of the caudate nuclei has been seen by the authors in a dog that ingested an unknown toxin (Fig. 8–7).

Miscellaneous Toxic Plants

Numerous plants and fungi have toxic effects on the nervous system.[15] Some are discussed in the sections on Hypoxia, Hepatic Encephalop-

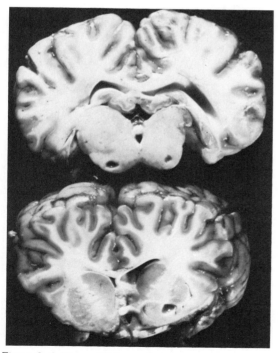

Figure 8–6. Nigropallidal encephalomalacia. The sectioned brain from a horse with yellow star thistle (*Centaurea solstitialis*) intoxication. There were signs of dystonia of the muscles of prehension and mastication and of the tongue. The liquefactive necrotic areas in both substantias nigra (top) and one (right) globus pallidus (lower) are evident as cystic cavities in the brain.

Table 8–2. EXAMPLES OF SEVERAL PLANT (AND FUNGAL) TOXICOSES OF DOMESTIC HERBIVORES THAT CAN RESULT IN SYNDROMES CHARACTERIZED BY NEUROLOGIC SIGNS

Plant	Species Affected	Neurologic Signs	Pathophysiology	Neural Lesions	Treatment*	Prognosis
Ryegrass[15,152]	Sheep, cattle, horses	Ataxia, tremor, tetany	Penitrem and fumi tremorgen mycotoxins from Penicillium sp	Secondary Purkinje cell degeneration	Diazepam	Good
Phalaris spp[15,152]	Sheep, cattle	Ataxia, tremor, weakness, seizures	Dimethyltryptamine alkaloids act as monoamine oxidase inhibitors	Neuronal pigmentation (indole melanins)	?Diazepam	Bad
Paspallum, Dallis grass[15,152]	Cattle, sheep	Ataxia, tremor	Claviceps paspalli ergot alkaloids probably neurotoxic	None	—	Good
Swainsona spp[80,152]	Sheep, cattle, horses	Weight loss, ataxia, aggressiveness	Indolizidine alkaloid (swainsonine) induces α-mannosidosis	Neuroaxonal dystrophy, neurovisceral storage products	—	Fair to very good
Locoweeds[116,152,160]	Sheep, cattle, horses	Weight loss, ataxia, aggressiveness	Indolizidine alkaloid (swainsonine) induces α-mannosidosis	Neuroaxonal dystrophy, neurovisceral storage products	Reserpine	Fair to good
Sorghum spp[1,152,174]	Horses, cattle, sheep	Ataxia, bladder paralysis	Possibly HCN or lathyrogenic toxins	Neuronal fiber degeneration, spinal cord	—	Poor to fair
Solanum esuriale[123,152]	Sheep	Exercise intolerance, weakness, arched back (humpyback)	Unknown (suspected toxin in S esuriale)	Spinal cord fiber degeneration; myopathy	—	Bad
Solanum fastigiatum,[145] S dimidiatum,[112] S kwebense[135]	Cattle	Cerebellar ataxia, "cerebellar seizures"	Suspected induction of gangliosidosis	Purkinje cell vacuolation and degeneration	—	Poor
Cycad palms[76,108,152]	Cattle, goats, horses	Ataxia, recumbency	Possibly toxic glycosides, cycasin and macrozamin	Spinal cord fiber degeneration	—	Bad
Melochia pyramidata[128]	Cattle	Ataxia, recumbency	Unknown	Spinal and nerve fiber degeneration	—	Bad
Tribulus terrestris[16]	Sheep	Asymmetric pelvic limb weakness	Possibly neuromuscular process	None	—	Bad
Karwinskia humboldtiana[27]	Goats	Hypermetria, weakness	Unknown	Peripheral neuropathy, central neuroaxonal dystrophy, myopathy	—	Bad
Nardoo fern, Marsilea drummondii[140]	Sheep	Depression, blindness, convulsions	Probably a thiaminase	Polioencephalomalacia	Thiamine	Good if early
Birdsville indigo, Indigofera linnaei[140]	Horses	Weight loss, ataxia, weakness	Arginine antagonist alkaloids: indospicine, canavanine	None	Arginine rich feeds (gelatin, lucerne)	Good
Mexican fireweed, Kochia scoparia[40]	Cattle	Blindness (nephrosis, hepatitis)	Saponins, alkaloids, oxalates; possibly thiaminase	?Polioencephalomalacia	—	Poor
Buckeye, Aesculus spp[45]	Cattle	Staggering, convulsions	Glycosides and alkaloids described	Unknown	—	Fair
Helichrysum argyrosphaerum[9]	Sheep, cattle	Peripheral blindness, nystagmus, weakness	Unknown	Patchy status spongiosus, white matter	—	Fair for life, bad for vision

*Treatment should also include removal of toxic plants and cathartics.

athy, and Thiamine Deficiency. Examples of other plant and fungal toxicoses of animals are given in Table 8–2.

ENDOCRINOPATHIES

Hypoglycemia

Incidence

Hypoglycemia occurs when there is decreased production or release of glucose or when there is increased tissue utilization of glucose or its substrates. Potential causes of decreased production in animals include inadequate glycogen stores in toy breed puppies[165] and neonatal pigs and foals,[62] hepatic insufficiency,[2] starvation,[134] glycogen storage diseases,[8, 177] and hypoadrenocorticism.[54] Increased tissue utilization may occur with lactation,[12, 95] pregnancy,[81, 106] and extreme exercise[86] or when there is excess insulin due to either iatrogenic administration or excess production by pancreatic β-cell tumors (insulinomas)[26, 29, 85, 99] or extrapancreatic neoplasms (insulin-like substances).[99, 162] Hypoglycemia also has been reported in human beings[115] and dogs[17] with sepsis, presumably due to both impaired production and increased utilization.

Pathophysiology and Pathology

Glucose is maintained at normal serum levels (45–60 mg/dl in ruminants; 70–110 mg/dl in other species) through the interaction of hepatic glycogenolytic and gluconeogenetic enzymes and hormones from the pancreas, adrenal glands, pituitary gland, intestine, and thyroid glands.[65] Insulin and glucagon, secreted by pancreatic β and α cells, respectively, are especially important in glucose homeostasis. Insulin facilitates transport of glucose and amino acids across cell membranes of some tissues, increases hepatic glycogen by activating the enzyme glycogen synthetase and inhibiting glycogenolysis, decreases hepatic gluconeogenesis, and acts together with somatotropin to stimulate growth. Glucagon directly opposes the effects of insulin by stimulating both glycogenolysis and gluconeogenesis. Epinephrine, thyroxine, and glucocorticoids also increase gluconeogenesis.

Ischemic neuronal cell change similar to that of cerebral hypoxia is the principal lesion of hypoglycemia.[19] Neurons of the cerebral cortex are affected most commonly, with either focal or laminar involvement being possible. Other pathologic changes vary with the inciting disease. β-Cell tumors usually are malignant and often metastasize to regional lymph nodes and other organs.[26, 29, 85, 99] Dogs with insulinomas also may have a polyneuropathy.[29] Glycogen storage diseases usually cause a massive accumulation of glycogen in the liver.[177]

Heavily lactating cattle and pregnant sheep that become hypoglycemic often develop fatty livers.[95, 109] In these animals, free fatty acids are oxidized as an alternate energy source. Ketone bodies formed by the oxidation normally are metabolized through the citric acid cycle. However, they accumulate in the liver and serum (ketosis) of some animals during heavy lactation or pregnancy, because a necessary intermediate of the citric acid cycle (oxaloacetate) is exhausted by the heavy demands of gluconeogenesis.[94] The fatty liver further impedes gluconeogenesis, creating a cyclic effect.

Clinical Signs

Clinical signs of hypoglycemia usually occur when the blood glucose level falls below 45 mg/dl in dogs and between 20 and 40 mg/dl in cattle. Affected animals may be euglycemic and clinically normal, except following either prolonged fasting or extreme exercise. Clinical signs of hypoglycemia are caused by either adrenergic stimulation or neuronal glucose deprivation.[99] The adrenergic signs result from activation of hypothalamic glucoreceptors and include tachycardia, tremor, and apprehension. Neuronal glucose deprivation leads to seizures, weakness, depression, and confusion. The adrenergic signs often predominate when hypoglycemia is acute in onset, whereas the neurogluconeopenic features often follow gradual declines in blood glucose concentration.

Diagnosis

Establishing hypoglycemia as the cause of neurologic dysfunction in human patients has classically been based on demonstrating Whipple's triad: fasting blood glucose of less than 40 mg/dl, exacerbation of clinical signs by fasting, and remission of these signs after intravenous glucose administration.[181] These features are not unique to any of the potential causes of hypoglycemia, so further diagnostic studies are always indicated. In fact, blood glucose level may be normal in dogs with insulinomas, even after a 24 hour fast.[29, 85] In these patients, fasting for 48 or even 72 hours is indicated, together with measurement of serum insulin levels. Patients that remain euglycemic and have normal immunoreactive serum insulin concentrations (9.8–20 µU/ml) still may be proven to have insulinomas by calculating the fasting insulin-glucose ratio.[85] The ratio usually is considerably higher in dogs with insulinomas than in those that are normal. Use of an amended insulin-glucose ratio has been advocated in dogs:[26]

$$\frac{\text{Serum insulin } (\mu U/ml) \times 100}{\text{Plasma glucose } (mg/dl) - 30}$$

The amended ratio should be less than 30 but usually is markedly elevated in dogs with insulinomas. In rare cases in which results of these tests are all normal and an insulinoma is still suspected, the glucagon tolerance test may be indicated.[85] Glucagon (0.03 mg/kg, intravenously, not to exceed 1.0 mg) is given and either glucose or insulin is measured at 0, 1, 3, 5, 15, 30, 45, 60, 90, 120, and 180 minutes. The glucagon should lead to excessive secretion of insulin in dogs with β-cell tumors. Results compatible with insulinoma include (1) a peak blood glucose concentration of less than 135 mg/dl, (2) a serum glucose concentration of less than 50 mg/dl within 120 minutes, (3) a decrease of blood glucose level after 1 to 2 minutes, (4) a serum insulin concentration of greater than 50 µU/ml within 1 minute, and (5) an insulin-glucose ratio greater than 75 after 1 minute.[85] Other insulin secretalogues (leucine, tolbutamide) have not been widely used in veterinary medicine.

Treatment

Dextrose (50% solution, 1–4 mg/kg intravenously in dogs and 500 ml intravenously in cattle) should be given to animals with clinical signs of hypoglycemia.[15, 30] Use of glycerine or propylene glycol (225 gm orally twice daily for 2 days, followed by 100 gm daily for 2 days) has been recommended in cattle to obviate the need for repeated glucose administration.[15] Dogs with suspected insulinomas should be given 10% dextrose intravenously continuously until further studies are done or the tumor is resected. This is done to avoid hypoglycemia induced by insulin secreted by the tumor in response to the 50% dextrose bolus.

Once a diagnosis of insulinoma has been established in a dog, a laparotomy should be done and all resectable primary and metastatic foci of tumor should be removed.[26] There is controversy regarding what should be done when no neoplastic tissue is found at surgery.

Because neither lobe of the pancreas has a greater incidence of tumors,[29, 85] blind biopsy probably is not indicated. Medical therapy (see below) may be helpful.

Food and water should be withheld for 3 to 5 days after surgery to reduce the likelihood of pancreatitis. Some dogs may still develop pancreatitis, so daily postoperative measurement of serum amylase and lipase levels is indicated. Dogs that become hyperglycemic after surgery may require temporary or continuous insulin supplementation. Other dogs may continue to have seizures, even though they are euglycemic, apparently because of residual neuronal injury.[29] Use of anticonvulsants is indicated in these dogs. Because most insulinomas in dogs are malignant, recurrence of neoplastic tissue and clinical hypoglycemia is common. However, dogs may remain free of clinical signs for many months following surgery and again normalize after tumor tissue is removed a second time.

Medical management of hypoglycemia due to insulinomas with diazoxide (3–12 mg/kg orally, three times daily) has been successful in some dogs.[99, 132] Diazoxide inhibits insulin secretion, enhances epinephrine-induced glycogenolysis, and directly inhibits glucose uptake by tissues. Streptozotocin, which selectively destroys pancreatic β cells, appears to have little value in dogs because of severe side effects.[81]

Diabetes Mellitus

Hyperglycemia due to diabetes mellitus may cause hyperosmolality, with resulting confusion or coma.[32] Ketoacidosis in these patients may also alter consciousness. These signs usually remit with insulin and fluid therapy. Care should be taken to avoid rapid correction of acidosis with bicarbonate, as paradoxic cerebrospinal acidosis may occur (see Acidosis above). Rapid correction of serum hyperosmolality also should be avoided because this shifts water to the brain, leading to cerebral edema.

A polyneuropathy also may occur in dogs with diabetes mellitus (see Chapter 14).

Hypothyroidism

Dogs with hypothyroidism may have atherosclerosis[106] and so could have cerebral lesions and associated neurologic dysfunction. Others may have facial nerve paralysis or a subclinical polymyopathy (see Chapter 14).

Hyperadrenocorticism

Hyperadrenocorticism may be due to either pituitary or adrenal gland adenomas. Animals with pituitary neoplasia and thalamic compression or invasion usually have neurologic dysfunction (see Chapter 9). Dogs with hyperadrenocorticism also may have a polymyopathy (see Chapter 14).

NUTRITIONAL DISEASES

Thiamine Deficiency

Incidence

The etiology, pathogenesis, and lesions of thiamine deficiency vary between monogastric animals[51, 88, 143] and ruminants.[107, 136] Thiamine is synthesized by the normal bacterial flora of the rumen and the cecum in herbivores, so dietary deficiency should not occur in these animals. However, thiamine deficiency does occur in cattle when there is a change in rumen flora so that bacteria either no longer produce thiamine or they produce thiaminase. Exclusive feeding of concentrated rations to feedlot calves and lambs predisposes to thiamine deficiency, perhaps by inducing ruminal acidosis that alters the microflora. Ingestion of thiaminase-containing plants such as bracken fern (*Peridium aquil-*

inum) and horsetail (*Equisetum arvense*) also can lead to thiamine deficiency in horses.[51] Experimental feeding of the thiamine antagonist amprolium to ruminants produces lesions identical to those of spontaneous thiamine deficiency.[102] However, efforts to identify a similar naturally occurring thiamine antagonist have thus far been inconclusive.[47] Thiamine deficiency in small animals may result from either dietary deficiency or ingestion of all-fish diets high in thiaminase.

Pathophysiology and Pathology

Thiamine deficiency causes cerebrocortical necrosis (polioencephalomalacia) in ruminants[48, 107, 136] (Fig. 8–8) and foci of symmetric necrosis in the periventricular gray matter, lateral geniculate nuclei, oculomotor nuclei, caudal colliculi, and vestibular nuclei of small animals.[88, 143] Neural lesions in horses dying of bracken fern are not well described. The exact mechanisms responsible for these lesions remain obscure. Presumably, thiamine deficiency alters neuronal metabolism in a way similar to both hypoxia and hypoglycemia, because all cause neuronal necrosis. There are thiamine dependent enzymes in both the citric acid cycle (α-ketoglutarate dehydrogenase) and the pentose phosphate shunt (transketolase).[110] The pentose phosphate pathway appears to be particularly important for glucose metabolism in rumi-

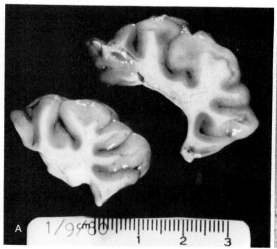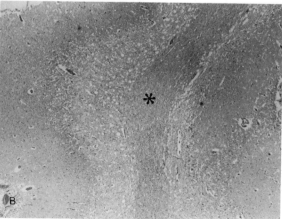

Figure 8–8. A, Ovine polioencephalomalacia. Sections of freshly cut cerebrum from a young sheep dying following signs of subacute diffuse cerebral disease and coma. Well-demarcated yellow areas, which were soft, can be seen in the cortical gray matter. These areas fluoresced under ultraviolet light, indicating that there was severe tissue destruction: laminar cortical necrosis. Flock mates similarly affected responded to large doses of thiamine and recovered. B, Photomicrograph of gyrus of cerebral cortex from cow with polioencephalomalacia due to presumed thiamine deficiency. The white matter of the gyrus is indicated by the asterisk. There are vacuoles within the deep cerebrocortical laminae on each side of the white matter. These vacuoles are due to neuronal drop out and edema. Superficial and mid laminae appear relatively normal. Hematoxylin and eosin, × 5.

nants.[87] In addition, thiamine triphosphate has a role in neuromuscular transmission.[175]

Clinical Signs and Diagnosis

Polioencephalomalacia due to thiamine deficiency in ruminants often occurs in 6 to 9 month old feedlot animals but may occur in animals 1 month of age and older.[107, 136] Clinical signs include blindness, head pressing, muscle tremor, nystagmus, and opisthotonos. Younger animals often die within 24 to 48 hours, whereas older cattle may survive for several days. Because of decreased activity of thiamine dependent enzymes, intermediate metabolites, such as pyruvate and lactate, accumulate in the blood.[48] Erythrocyte transketolase activity usually is decreased.[103]

Clinical signs of thiamine deficiency in small animals include vestibular ataxia, seizures, depression, and marked cervical ventroflexion.[88, 143] In horses there are systemic signs of weight loss and cardiac irregularities, and prominent ataxia and tremor with terminal convulsions.[51, 152]

Therapy

Thiamine hydrochloride (10 mg/kg intravenously, every 3 hours for 5 doses) often is effective in ruminants when given within a few hours of the onset of signs, and similar doses should be used in horses.[15] Ruminants treated later in the disease course usually do not recover. Depending on the suspected cause (toxic plants, ingested thiaminase, rumenal thiaminase production), purgatives and oral antibiotics may be used. If cerebral edema and herniation (evident by dilated, poorly responsive pupils) and coma are present, then intravenous mannitol (0.5 gm/kg intravenously) should be administered and repeated as necessary. The diet should be changed to consist of at least 50% roughage. Small animals should be given 50 to 100 mg of thiamine intravenously daily until there is improvement.[122] If a favorable response is not seen within a few days, another diagnosis should be considered.

Copper Deficiency

Kids and lambs nursing dams that are on copper-deficient pasture may develop a neurologic syndrome termed swayback or enzootic ataxia.[34, 101, 157] Ataxia, tremor, blindness, and death may occur at birth (congenital swayback) or progressive ataxia and weakness may develop at 1 to 6 months of age (delayed swayback) (Fig. 8–9A). Lesions of congenital swayback develop in utero and include cavitation of the cerebral white matter and hypoplasia of cerebellar granule and Purkinje cells. In delayed swayback, chromatolysis of neurons within brain stem nuclei and ventral horn cells of the spinal cord occurs after birth as a consequence of axonal injury. Failure to maintain the axon also leads to secondary demyelination, with spinal tracts in the ventromedian and dorsolateral funiculi being most severely affected (Fig. 8–9B). The

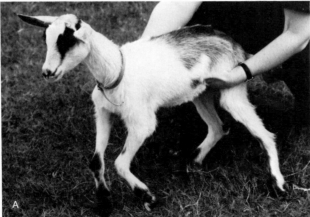
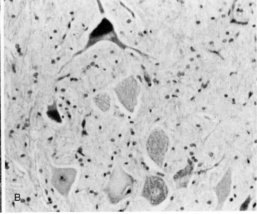

Figure 8–9. Caprine swayback–like syndrome. A, This 3 month old Alpine kid became recumbent and was examined 11 days later. There was tetraplegia with hyporeflexia and muscle atrophy in all limbs. Cerebrospinal fluid analysis was unremarkable. There was no response to oral $CuSO_4$ supplementation for 1 month; however, the lesions seen were similar to those associated with copper deficiency. B, Reactive chromatolytic neurons and neuronal necrosis in the lumbar ventral horn cells. There was also myelin pallor in ventromedial and dorsolateral spinal cord tracts, motor nerve fiber degeneration, and neurogenic-type muscle atrophy.

variation in lesions between congenital and delayed swayback is believed to reflect the affected animal's stage of central nervous system development at the time of copper deficiency.[78] Cerebral myelination and cerebellar cellular differentiation largely occur in utero, whereas spinal cord myelin is produced after birth. The lesions of swayback are due to dysfunction of copper-containing enzymes such as cytochrome oxidase, superoxide dismutase, and ceruloplasmin. In the absence of these enzymes, oxygen free radicals may cause myelin lipid peroxidation.[157] However, the exact mechanisms responsible for swayback are not clear. Copper supplementation (1.5 gm orally) may lead to improvement in mildly affected animals. Herds should be supplemented via regular injections of copper salts or inclusion of copper in fertilizers.

Enzootic ataxia in deer is similar to the disease in sheep and is associated with low copper status of animals in herds where cases occur.[183]

Selenium–Vitamin E Deficiency

Vitamin E and selenium-containing enzymes, such as glutathione peroxidase, scavenge peroxides that otherwise would oxidize proteins and lipids of muscle and nervous tissue.[104] Selenium–vitamin E deficiency causes a degenerative myopathy (white muscle disease) in most animal species (see Chapter 14). Chickens with vitamin E deficiency also may develop encephalomalacia, with white matter of the cerebellum being most severely affected.[131]

Vitamin A

Cats fed a diet composed primarily of liver may develop hypervitaminosis A, with associated bony exostoses on the cervical vertebrae, ribs, and long bones of the thoracic limbs.[72] Compression of the cervical spinal cord in these cats may lead to hyperesthesia and tetraparesis. Affected cats usually recover when they are given a proper diet.

Hypovitaminosis A may occur in young ruminants on summer pastures. Affected animals have increased intracranial pressure because of reduced absorption of cerebrospinal fluid across the arachnoid villi.[24] Retardation of endochondral ossification also may cause defective development of the cranial cavity, leading to brain compression and entrapment of the optic nerves at the optic foramina. Neurologic clinical signs

seen in affected animals, therefore, may include blindness, confusion, ataxia, and seizures. These signs may be partially reversed by vitamin A supplementation.

REFERENCES

1. Adams LG, Dollahite JW, Romane WM, et al: Cystitis and ataxia associated with Sorghum ingestion by horses. JAVMA 155:518, 1969.
2. Allen TA: Canine hypoglycemia. In Kirk RW (ed): Current Veterinary Therapy VIII. Philadelphia, WB Saunders Co, 1983, p 845.
3. Alsupp TN and Wharton MH: Gamma benzene hexachloride (gamma BHC) toxicity in calves. Vet Rec 80:583, 1967.
4. Anderson DC and Cranford RE: Corticosteroids in ischemic stroke. Stroke 10:68, 1979.
5. Austad R and Bjerkas E: Eclampsia in the bitch. J Small Anim Pract 17:793, 1976.
6. Badiali L, Abou-Youssef MH, Radwan AI, et al: Mouldy corn poisoning as the major cause of an encephalomalacia syndrome in Egyptian equidae. JAVMA 29:2029, 1968.
7. Bailey EM: Emergency and general treatment of poisoning. In Kirk RW (ed): Current Veterinary Therapy VIII. Philadelphia, WB Saunders Co, 1983, p 82.
8. Bardens JW: Glycogen storage disease in puppies. Vet Med Small Anim Clin 61:1174, 1966.
9. Basson PA, Kellerman TS, Albl P, et al: Blindness and encephalopathy caused by Helichrysum argyrosphaerum DC (Compositae) in sheep and cattle. Onderstepoort J Vet Res 42:135, 1975.
10. Bath ML: Hexachlorophene toxicity in dogs. J Small Anim Pract 19:241, 1978.
11. Berenyi KJ, Wolk M, and Killip T: Cerebrospinal fluid acidosis complicating therapy of experimental cardiopulmonary arrest. Circulation 52:319, 1976.
12. Bergman EN: Glucose metabolism in ruminants as related to hypoglycemia and ketosis. Cornell Vet 63:341, 1973.
13. Birchard SJ: Surgical management of portosystemic shunts in dogs and cats. Comp Cont Ed Small Anim Pract 6:795, 1984.
14. Blitzer BL: Fulminant hepatic failure. A rare but often lethal coma syndrome. Postgrad Med 68:153, 1980.
15. Blood DC, Henderson JA, and Radostits OM: Veterinary Medicine. A Textbook of the Diseases of Cattle, Sheep, Pigs and Horses, 5th ed. Philadelphia, Lea & Febiger, 1979, p 439, 827, 840, 849, 936, 971, 989, 1078.
16. Bourke CA: Staggers in sheep associated with the ingestion of Tribulus terrestris. Aust Vet J 61:360, 1984.
17. Breitschwerdt EB, Loar AS, Hribernik TN, and McGrath RK: Hypoglycemia in four dogs with sepsis. JAVMA 178:1072, 1981.
18. Breznok EM: Surgical manipulation of portosystemic shunts in dogs. JAVMA 174:819, 1979.
19. Brierley JB: Cerebral hypoxia. In Blackwood W and Corsellis JAN (eds): Greenfield's Neuropathology. London, Edward Arnold (Publishers) Ltd, 1976, p 43.
20. Bulger RJ, Schrier RW, Arend WP, and Swanson AG: Spinal-fluid acidosis and the diagnosis of pulmonary encephalopathy. N Engl J Med 274:433, 1966.
21. Burrows GE: Nitrate intoxication. JAVMA 177:82, 1980.

22. Burrows GE: Lead poisoning in the horse. Equine Pract 4:30, 1982.
23. Byars TD: Chronic liver failure in horses. Comp Cont Ed Small Anim Pract 5:S423, 1983.
24. Calhoun MC, Hurt HD, Eaton HD, et al: Rates of formation and absorption of cerebrospinal fluid in bovine hypovitaminosis. A J Dairy Sci 50:1486, 1967.
25. Carson TL: Organophosphate and carbamate insecticide poisoning. In Kirk RW (ed): Current Veterinary Therapy VIII. Philadelphia, WB Saunders Co, 1983, p 116.
26. Caywood DD, Wilson JW, Hardy RM, and Shull RM: Pancreatic islet cell adenocarcinoma: Clinical and diagnostic features of six cases. JAVMA 174:714, 1979.
27. Charlton KM, Pierce KR, Storts RW, and Bridges CH: A neuropathy in goats caused by experimental Coyotillo (Karwinskia humboldtiana) poisoning. V. Lesions in the central nervous system. Pathol Vet 7:435, 1970.
28. Chew DJ and Meuten DJ: Disorders of calcium and phosphorus metabolism. Vet Clin North Am 12:411, 1982.
29. Chrisman CL: Postoperative results and complications of insulinomas in dogs. J Am Anim Hosp Assoc 16:677, 1980.
30. Chrisman CL: Problems in Small Animal Neurology. Philadelphia, Lea & Febiger, 1982, p 164.
31. Christian RG and Tryphonas L: Lead poisoning in cattle: Brain lesions and hematologic changes. Am J Vet Res 32:203, 1971.
32. Church DB: Diabetes mellitus. In Kirk RW (ed): Current Veterinary Therapy VIII. Philadelphia, WB Saunders Co, 1983, p 838.
33. Clowers GHA Jr and O'Donnell TF: Heat stroke. N Engl J Med 291:564, 1974.
34. Cordy DR: Enzootic ataxia in California lambs. JAVMA 158:1940, 1971.
35. Cornelius LM, Thrall DE, Halliwell WH, et al: Anomalous portosystemic anastomoses associated with chronic hepatic insufficiency in six young dogs. JAVMA 167:220, 1975.
36. Costrini AM, Pitt HA, Gustafson AB, and Uddin DE: Cardiovascular and metabolic manifestations of heat stroke and severe heat exhaustion. Am J Med 66:296, 1979.
37. Davies TS, Nielsen SW, and Kircher CH: The pathology of subacute methylmercurialism in swine. Cornell Vet 66:32, 1976.
38. deLahunta A: Veterinary Neuroanatomy and Clinical Neurology. Philadelphia, WB Saunders Co, 1977, p 141.
39. Demopoulos HB, Flamm E, and Ransohoff J: Molecular pathology and CNS membranes. In Jobsis FF (ed): Oxygen and Physiological Function. 60th FASEB Annual Meeting. Dallas, Professional Information Library, 1977.
40. Dickie CW and James LF: Kochia scoparia poisoning in cattle. JAVMA 183:765, 1983.
41. Diemer NH: Glial and neuronal changes in experimental hepatic encephalopathy. Acta Neurol Scand (Suppl 71) 58:9, 1978.
42. Divers TJ, George LW, and George JW: Hemolytic anemia in horses after ingestion of red maple leaves. JAVMA 180:300, 1982.
43. Divers TJ, Warner L, Vaala WE, et al: Toxic hepatic failure in newborn foals. JAVMA 183:1407, 1983.
44. Eales FA, Gilmour JS, Barlow RM, and Small J: Causes of hypothermia in 89 lambs. Vet Rec 110:118, 1982.
45. Edwards AJ, Mount ME, and Oehme FW: Buckeye toxicity in Angus calves. Bovine Pract 1:18, 1980.
46. Edwards DF, Richardson DC, and Russell RG: Hypernatremic, hypertonic dehydration in a dog with diabetes insipidus and gastric dilatation-volvulus. JAVMA 182:973, 1983.
47. Edwin EE, Markson LM, and Jackman R: The aetiology of cerebrocortical necrosis: The role of thiamine deficiency and of deltapyrrolinium. Br Vet J 138:337, 1982.
48. Edwin EE, Markson LM, Shreeve J, et al: Diagnostic aspects of cerebrocortical necrosis. Vet Rec 104:4, 1979.
49. Elisalde GS, Wooldridge JB, Steel EG, and Elisalde MH: Treatment of a seizuring hypoparathyroid dog. Canine Pract 7(5):14, 1980.
50. Estrada RV, Moreno J, Martinez E, et al: Pancreatic encephalopathy. Acta Neurol Scand 59:135, 1979.
51. Evans ETR, Evans WC, and Roberts HE: Studies on bracken poisoning in the horse. Br Vet J 107:364, 399, 1951.
52. Farrell RK, Sande RD, and Lincoln SD: Nigropallidal encephalomalacia in a horse. JAVMA 158:1201, 1971.
53. Feig PU and McCurdy DK: The hypertonic state. N Engl J Med 297:1444, 1977.
54. Feldman EC and Peterson ME: Hypoadrenocorticism. Vet Clin North Am 14:751, 1984.
55. Finberg L, Luttrell C, and Redd H: Pathogenesis of lesions in the nervous system in hypernatremic states. II. Experimental studies of gross anatomic changes and alterations of chemical composition of the tissues. Pediatrics 23:46, 1959.
56. Finco DR, Duncan JR, Schall WD, et al: Chronic enteric disease and hypoproteinemia in 9 dogs. JAVMA 163:262, 1973.
57. Finco DR, Duncan JR, Schall WD, and Prasse KW: Acetaminophen toxicosis in the cat. JAVMA 166:469, 1975.
58. Fischer JE and Bower RH: Nutritional support in liver disease. Surg Clin North Am 61:653, 1981.
59. Florentin RA and Nam SC: Dietary-induced atherosclerosis in miniature swine: I. Gross and light microscopy observations: Time of development and morphologic characteristics of lesions. Exp Mol Pathol 8:263, 1968.
60. Fowler ME: Nigropallidal encephalomalacia in the horse. JAVMA 147:607, 1965.
61. Gay CC, Blood DC, and Wilkinson JS: Clinical observations of sheep with focal symmetrical encephalomalacia. Aust Vet J 51:266, 1975.
62. Gentz J, Bengtsson G, Hakkavainen J, et al: Metabolic effects of starvation during neonatal period in the piglet. Am J Physiol 218:662, 1970.
63. Graham D and Gonatas NK: Triethyltin sulfate-induced splitting of peripheral myelin in rats. Lab Invest 29:627, 1975.
64. Gulick BA, Knight HD, and Rogers QR: Use of plasma amino acid patterns in liver disease of the horse. Calif Vet 33:21, 1979.
65. Guyton AC: Basic Human Physiology: Normal Function and Mechanisms of Disease. Philadelphia, WB Saunders Co, 1977, p 714, 806.
66. Guyton AC: Textbook of Medical Physiology. Philadelphia, WB Saunders Co, 1981, p 977.
67. Harding JDJ, Lewis G, and Done JT: Experimental arsanilic acid poisoning in pigs. Vet Rec 83:560, 1968.
68. Harrison LH, Colvin BM, Stuart BP, et al: Paralysis in swine due to focal symmetrical poliomalacia: Possible selenium toxicosis. Vet Pathol 20:265, 1983.

69. Hartley WJ: Polioencephalomalacia in dogs. Acta Neuropathol 2:271, 1963.

70. Harvey JW and Kornick HP: Phenazopyridine toxicosis in the cat. JAVMA 169:327, 1976.

71. Harvey JW, Sameck JH, and Burgard FJ: Benzocaine-induced methemoglobinemia in dogs. JAVMA 175:1171, 1979.

72. Hayes KC: Nutritional problems in cats: Taurine deficiency and vitamin A excess. Can Vet J 23:2, 1982.

73. Hemingway RG, Ritchie NS, Brown NA, and Peart JN: Effects of grazing management on plasma calcium and magnesium concentrations of ewes in early lactation. J Agric Sci Camb 64:109, 1965.

74. Herigstad RR, Whitehair CK, Beyer N, et al: Chronic methylmercury toxicosis in calves. JAVMA 160:173, 1972.

75. Herigstad RR, Whitehair CK, and Olson OE: Inorganic and organic selenium toxicosis in young swine: Comparison of pathologic changes with those in swine with vitamin E-selenium deficiency. Am J Vet Res 34:1227, 1973.

76. Hooper PT, Best SM, and Campbell A: Axonal dystrophy in the spinal cords of cattle consuming the Cycad palm Cycas media. Aust Vet J 50:146, 1974.

77. Hossman K-A and Zimmerman V: Resuscitation of the monkey brain after one hour's ischemia. I. Physiological and morphological observations. Brain Res 81:59, 1974.

78. Howell JMcC and Pass DA: Swayback lesions and vulnerable periods of development. In Gawthorne JM, Howell JMcC, and White CL (eds): Trace Element Metabolism in Man and Animals. Berlin, Springer-Verlag, 1981, p 298.

79. Huhnke MR and Monty DE: Physiologic responses of preparturient and postparturient Holstein-Friesian cows to summer heat stress in Arizona. Am J Vet Res 37:1301, 1976.

80. Huxtable CR and Dorling PR: Poisoning of livestock by Swainsona spp.: Current status. Aust Vet J 59:50, 1982.

81. Huxtable CR and Farrow BRH: Functional neoplasms of the canine pancreatic-islet β-cells: A clinico-pathological study of three cases. J Small Anim Pract 20:737, 1979.

82. Jack EJ: Possible hexachlorophene poisoning in calves. Vet Rec 90:198, 1972.

83. Jackson RF, Bruss ML, Growney PJ, and Seymour WG: Hypoglycemia-ketonemia in a pregnant bitch. JAVMA 177:1123, 1980.

84. Jacobson S and Bell B: Recognition and management of acute and chronic hepatic encephalopathy. Med Clin North Am 57:1569, 1973.

85. Johnson RK: Insulinoma in the dog. Vet Clin North Am 7:629, 1977.

86. Johnson RK and Atkins CE: Hypoglycemia in the dog. In Kirk RW (ed): Current Veterinary Therapy VI. Philadelphia, WB Saunders Co, 1977, p 1010.

87. Jones KL, Oyler JM, and Goetsch DD: In vitro enzymatic activity and ^{14}C-glucose metabolic studies with caprine and canine brain homogenates. Am J Vet Res 32:1659, 1971.

88. Jubb KVF, Saunders LZ, and Coates HV: Thiamine deficiency encephalopathy in cats. J Comp Pathol 66:217, 1956.

89. Keenan DM: Acute arsanilic acid intoxication in pigs. Aust Vet J 49:229, 1973.

90. Kingsbury JM: Poisonous Plants of the United States and Canada. Englewood Cliffs, NJ, Prentice-Hall, Inc, 1964, p 23, 38.

91. Kornegay JN, Greene CE, Martin C, et al: Idiopathic hypocalcemia in four dogs. J Am Anim Hosp Assoc 16:723, 1980.

92. Kornegay JN, Oliver JE, and Gorgacz EJ: Clinicopathologic features of brain herniation in animals. JAVMA 182:1111, 1983.

93. Kowalczyk DF: Lead poisoning in dogs at the University of Pennsylvania Veterinary Hospital. JAVMA 168:428, 1976.

94. Krebs HA: Bovine ketosis. Vet Rec 78:187, 1966.

95. Kronfeld DS: Hypoglycaemia in ketotic cows. J Dairy Sci 54:949, 1971.

96. Krum SH and Osborne CA: Heatstroke in the dog: A polysystemic disorder. JAVMA 170:531, 1977.

97. Lampert PW and Schochet SS: Electron microscopic observations on experimental spongy degeneration of the cerebellar white matter. J Neuropathol Exp Neurol 27:210, 1968.

98. Langfitt TW: Increased intracranial pressure and the cerebral circulation. In Youmans JR (ed): Neurological Surgery, vol 2. Philadelphia, WB Saunders Co, 1982, p 846.

99. Leifer CE and Peterson ME: Hypoglycemia. Vet Clin North Am 14:873, 1984.

100. Levesque DC, Oliver JE Jr, Cornelius LM, et al: Congenital portacaval shunts in two cats: Diagnosis and surgical correction. JAVMA 181:143, 1982.

101. Lewis G, Terlecki S, and Parker BNJ: Observations on the pathogenesis of delayed swayback. Vet Rec 95:313, 1974.

102. Loew FM and Dunlop RH: Induction of thiamine inadequacy and polioencephalomalacia in adult sheep with amprolium. Am J Vet Res 33:2195, 1972.

103. Loew FM, Dunlop RH, and Christian RG: Biochemical aspects of an outbreak of bovine polioencephalomalacia. Can Vet J 11:57, 1970.

104. Maas JP: Diagnosis and management of selenium-responsive diseases in cattle. Comp Cont Ed Small Anim Pract 5:S393, 1983.

105. Maddison JE: Portosystemic encephalopathy in two young dogs: Some additional diagnostic and therapeutic considerations. J Small Anim Pract 22:731, 1981.

106. Manning PJ: Thyroid gland and arterial lesions of beagles with familial hypothyroidism and hyperlipoproteinemia. Am J Vet Res 40:820, 1979.

107. Markson LM: Cerebrocortical necrosis: An encephalopathy of ruminants. In Grunsell CSG and Hill FWG (eds): The Veterinary Annual (20th ed). Bristol, John Wright and Sons, Ltd, 1980, p 180.

108. Mason MM and Whiting MG: Caudal motor weakness and ataxia in cattle in the Caribbean area following ingestion of Cycads. Cornell Vet 58:541, 1968.

109. McClymont GL and Setchell BP: Ovine pregnancy toxaemia. 1. Tentative identification as a hypoglycemia encephalopathy. Aust Vet J 31:53, 1955.

110. McGilvery RW: Biochemistry. A Functional Approach. Philadelphia, WB Saunders Co, 1979, p 401, 529.

111. McGuirk SM and Butler DG: Metabolic alkalosis with paradoxic aciduria in cattle. JAVMA 177:551, 1980.

112. Menzies JS, Bridges CH, and Bailey EM: A neurological disease of cattle associated with Solanum dimidiatum. Southwest Vet 32:45, 1979.

113. Meyer DJ: Primary hypoparathyroidism. In Kirk RW (ed): Current Veterinary Therapy VIII. Philadelphia, WB Saunders Co, 1983, p 1000.

114. Meyer DJ, Strombeck DR, Stone EA, et al: Ammonia tolerance test in clinically normal dogs and in dogs with portosystemic shunts. JAVMA 173:377, 1978.

115. Miller SI, Wallace RJ, Musher DM, et al: Hypogly-

cemia as a manifestation of sepsis. Am J Med 68:649, 1980.

116. Molyneux RJ and James LF: Loco intoxication: Indolizidine alkaloids of spotted Locoweed (Astragalus lentiginosus). Science 216:190, 1982.

117. Morris ML, Teeter SM, and Collins DR: The effects of the exclusive feeding of an all-meat dog food. JAVMA 158:477, 1971.

118. Nordstrom CH and Siesjo BK: Cerebral metabolism. In Youmans JR (ed): Neurological Surgery, vol 2. Philadelphia, WB Saunders Co, 1982, p 765.

119. Norton S: Toxic responses of the central nervous system. In Doull J, Klaassen CD, and Amdur MO (eds): Toxicology. The Basic Science of Poisons. New York, Macmillan Publishing Co, Inc, 1980, p 179.

120. Noxon JO: Accidental hypothermia associated with hypothyroidism. Canine Pract 10(1):17, 1983.

121. Oehme FW: Veterinary toxicology. In Casarett LJ and Doull J (eds): Toxicology. The Basic Science of Poisons. New York, Macmillan Publishing Co, Inc, 1975, p 701.

122. Oliver JE Jr and Lorenz MD: Handbook of Veterinary Neurologic Diagnosis. Philadelphia, WB Saunders Co, 1983, p 331.

123. O'Sullivan BM: Humpy back of sheep. Clinical and pathological observations. Aust Vet J 52:414, 1976.

124. Osweiler GD: Strychnine poisoning. In Kirk RW (ed): Current Veterinary Therapy VIII. Philadelphia, WB Saunders Co, 1983, p 98.

125. Osweiler GD and Van Gelder GA: Epidemiology of lead poisoning in animals. In Oehme FW (ed): Toxicity of Heavy Metals in the Environment. Part I. New York, Marcel Dekker, Inc, 1978, p 143.

126. Padovan D: Polioencephalomalacia associated with water deprivation in cattle. Cornell Vet 70:153, 1980.

127. Palmer AC and Walker RG: The neuropathological effects of cardiac arrest in animals: A study of five cases. J Small Anim Pract 11:779, 1970.

128. Palmer AC and Woodham CB: Derrengue, a paralysis of cattle in El Salvador ascribed to ingestion of Melochia pyramidata. Vet Rec 96:547, 1975.

129. Palmer JS and Danz JW: Tolerance of Brahman cattle to organic phosphorus insecticides. JAVMA 144:143, 1964.

130. Panciera RJ, Dahlgren RR, and Rinker HB: Observations on septicemia of cattle caused by a Haemophilus-like organism. Vet Pathol 5:212, 1968.

131. Pappenheimer AM, Goettsch M, and Jungherr E: Nutritional encephalomalacia in chicks and certain related disorders of domestic birds. Storrs Agr Exper Sta Bul 229, 1939.

132. Parker AJ, O'Brien D, and Musselman EE: Diazoxide treatment of metastatic insulinoma in a dog. J Am Anim Hosp Assoc 18:315, 1982.

133. Payne JM: Metabolic Diseases in Farm Animals. London, William Heinemann Medical Books Ltd, 1977, p 84.

134. Payne JM, Rowlands GJ, Manston R, and Dew SM: A statistical appraisal of the results of metabolic profile tests on 75 dairy herds. Br Vet J 129:370, 1973.

135. Pienaar JG, Kellerman TS, Basson PA, et al: Maldronksiekte in cattle: A neuronopathy caused by Solanum kwebense N. E. Br. Ondestepoort J Vet Res 43:67, 1976.

136. Pierson RE and Jensen R: Polioencephalomalacia in feedlot lambs. JAVMA 166:257, 1975.

137. Plum F and Posner JB: The Diagnosis of Stupor and Coma. Philadelphia, FA Davis Co, 1980, p 256, 258.

138. Plum F and Siesjo BK: Recent advances in CSF physiology. Anesthesiology 42:706, 1975.

139. Powell HC, Swarner WO, Gluck L, and Lambert PW: Hexachlorophene myelinopathy in premature infants. Pediatrics 82:976, 1973.

140. Pritchard D, Eggleston GW, and Macadam JF: Mardoo fern and polioencephalomalacia. Aust Vet J 54:204, 1978.

141. Raskin NH and Fishman RA: Neurologic disorders in renal failure (Part 1). N Engl J Med 294:143, 1976.

142. Raskin NH and Fishman RA: Neurologic disorders in renal failure (Part 2). N Engl J Med 294:204, 1976.

143. Read DH, Jolly RD, and Alley MR: Polioencephalomalacia of dogs with thiamine deficiency. Vet Pathol 14:103, 1973.

144. Redding RW: Diagnosis and therapy of seizures. J Am Anim Hosp Assoc 5:79, 1969.

145. Riet-Correa F, Mendez M del C, Schild AL, et al: Intoxication by Solanum fastigiatum var. fastigiatum as a cause of cerebellar degeneration in cattle. Cornell Vet 73:240, 1983.

146. Rosenthral T, Shapiro Y, Seligsohn U, and Ramot B: Disseminated intravascular coagulation in experimental heatstroke. Thromb Diath Haemorrh 26:417, 1971.

147. Rothuizen J and ven den Ingh TSGAM: Arterial and venous ammonia concentrations in the diagnosis of canine hepato-encephalopathy. Res Vet Sci 33:17, 1982.

148. Schaer M: A clinicopathologic survey of acute pancreatitis in 30 dogs and 5 cats. J Am Anim Hosp Assoc 15:681, 1979.

149. Schall WD: Heat stroke. In Kirk RW (ed): Current Veterinary Therapy VIII. Philadelphia, WB Saunders Co, 1983, p 183.

150. Schalm OW: Hematology of lead poisoning in the dog. Canine Pract 7:55, 1980.

151. Schenker S, Breem KJ, and Hayumpa AM: Hepatic encephalopathy: Current status. Gastroenterology 66:121, 1974.

152. Seawright AA: Animal Health in Australia, vol 2, Chemical and Plant Poisons. Canberra, Australia, Australian Government Publishing Service, 1982, p 1.

153. Sherding RG: Hepatic encephalopathy in the dog. Comp Contin Ed Small Anim Pract 1:55, 1979.

154. Sherding RG, Meuten DJ, Chew DJ, et al: Primary hypoparathyroidism in the dog. JAVMA 176:439, 1980.

155. Sjaastad O, Gjessing L, Ritland S, et al: Chronic relapsing pancreatitis, encephalopathy with disturbance of consciousness, and CSF amino acid aberration. J Neurol 220:83, 1979.

156. Smith DLT: Poisoning by sodium salt—a cause of eosinophilic meningoencephalitis in swine. Am J Vet Res 18:825, 1957.

157. Smith RM, King RA, Osborne-White WS, and Fraser FJ: Copper and the pathogenesis of enzootic ataxia. In Gawthorne JM, Howell JMcC, and White CL (eds): Trace Element Metabolism in Man and Animals. Berlin, Springer-Verlag, 1981, p 294.

158. Smith RP and Olson MV: Drug-induced methemoglobinemia. Semin Hematol 10:253, 1973.

159. Sorell M and Rosen JF: Ionized calcium: Serum levels during symptomatic hypocalcemia. J Pediatr 87:67, 1975.

160. Staley EE: An approach to treatment of locoism in horses. Vet Med Small Anim Clin 73:1205, 1978.

161. Storry JE and Rook JAF: The magnesium nutrition of the dairy cow in relation to the development of hypomagnesaemia in the grazing animal. J Sci Food Agric 13:621, 1962.

162. Strombeck DR, Krum S, Meyer D, and Kappesser RM: Hypoglycemia and hypoinsulinemia associated with hepatoma in a dog. JAVMA 169:811, 1976.

163. Strombeck DR, Meyer DJ, and Freedland RA: Hyperammonemia due to a urea cycle enzyme deficiency in two dogs. JAVMA 166:1109, 1975.

164. Strombeck DR and Rogers Q: Plasma amino acid concentrations in dogs with hepatic disease. JAVMA 166:1105, 1975.

165. Strombeck DR, Rogers Q, Freedland R, and McEwan LC: Fasting hypoglycemia in a pup. JAVMA 173:299, 1978.

166. Strombeck DR, Weiser MG, and Kaneko JJ: Hyperammonemia and hepatic encephalopathy in the dog. JAVMA 166:1105, 1975.

167. Surawicz B: Relationship between electrocardiogram and electrolytes. Am Heart J 73:814, 1967.

168. Suzuki K and Kikkawa Y: Status spongiosus of CNS and hepatic changes induced by cuprizone. Am J Pathol 54:307, 1969.

169. Todd JR: Magnesium metabolism in ruminants. Review of current knowledge. In Trace Mineral Studies with Isotopes in Domestic Animals. Vienna, Int Atom Energy Ag, 1969, p 131.

170. Tripier MF, Berard M, Toga M, et al: Hexachlorophene and the central nervous system. Toxic effects in mice and baboons. Acta Neuropathol (Berl) 53:65, 1981.

171. Udall ND: The toxicity of the molluscicides metaldehyde and methiocarb to dogs. Vet Rec 93:420, 1978.

172. Valgamott JC, Turnwald GH, King GK, et al: Congenital portacaval anomalies in the cat: Two case reports. J Am Anim Hosp Assoc 16:915, 1980.

173. Van Gelder GA: Chlorinated hydrocarbon insecticide toxicosis. In Kirk RW (ed): Current Veterinary Therapy VI. Philadelphia, WB Saunders Co, 1977, p 141.

174. Van Kampen KR: Sudan grass and Sorghum poisoning of horses: A possible lathyrogenic disease. JAVMA 156:629, 1970.

175. Waldenlind L: Studies on thiamine and neuromuscular transmission. Acta Physiol Scand (Suppl) 459:1, 1978.

176. Walsh FB and Murray R: Ocular manifestations of disturbances in calcium metabolism. Am J Ophthalmol 36:1657, 1953.

177. Walvoort HC: Glycogen storage diseases in animals and their potential value as models of human disease. J Inherit Metab Dis 6:3, 1983.

178. Ward BC, Jones BD, and Rubin GJ: Hexachlorophene toxicity in dogs. J Am Anim Hosp Assoc 9:167, 1973.

179. Ware AJ, D'Agostino AN, and Combes B: Cerebral edema: A major complication of massive hepatic necrosis. Gastroenterology 61:877, 1971.

180. Watson ADJ: Lead poisoning in a cat. J Small Anim Pract 22:85, 1981.

181. Whipple AO: The surgical therapy of hyperinsulinism. J Int Chir 3:237, 1938.

182. Wilson BJ, Maronpot RR, and Hildebrandt PK: Equine leukoencephalomalacia. JAVMA 163:1293, 1973.

183. Wilson PR, Orr MB, and Key EL: Enzootic ataxia in Red Deer. NZ Vet J 27:252, 1979.

184. Wolf AM: Canine uremic encephalopathy. J Am Anim Hosp Assoc 16:735, 1980.

185. Zaki FA and Nafe LA: Ischaemic encephalopathy and focal granulomatous meningoencephalitis in the cat. J Small Anim Pract 21:429, 1980.

186. Zenoble RD and Hill BL: Hypothermia and associated cardiac arrhythmias in two dogs. JAVMA 175:840, 1979.

187. Zenoble RD and Myers RK: Severe hypocalcemia resulting from ethylene glycol poisoning in the dog. J Am Anim Hosp Assoc 13:489, 1977.

188. Zieve L and Nicoloff DM: Pathogenesis of hepatic coma. Annu Rev Med 26:143, 1975.

189. Zook BC, Carpenter JL, and Leeds EB: Lead poisoning in dogs. JAVMA 155:1329, 1969.

190. Zook BC, Carpenter JL, and Roberts RM: Lead poisoning in dogs: Occurrence, source, clinical pathology, and electroencephalography. Am J Vet Res 33:891, 1972.

191. Zook BC, Kopito L, Carpenter JL, et al: Lead poisoning in dogs: Analysis of blood, urine, hair, and liver for lead. Am J Vet Res 33:903, 1972.

Neoplasia

Neoplasia of the nervous system is no longer considered rare in animals.[13, 20, 25] Indeed, nervous system tumors occur in dogs with a frequency and variety similar to those in humans.[20]

Primary tumors originate from neuroectodermal, ectodermal, or mesodermal cells normally present in, or associated with, brain, spinal cord, or peripheral nerves. Secondary tumors affecting the nervous system may originate from surrounding structures, such as bone and muscle, or may result from hematogenous spread from a primary tumor in another organ. Tumor emboli can lodge and grow anywhere in the brain, meninges, choroid plexus, and spinal cord. In animals, primary tumors rarely metastasize outside the cranial cavity and vertebral canal.[9, 22, 26]

A classification of neoplasia in domestic animals is presented in Table 9–1 and is based on criteria used to classify human tumors.[5, 6, 20, 22] Although many of the animal neoplasms have characteristics analogous with those of corresponding tumors in humans, 15 to 20% of neuroectodermal tumors (especially gliomas) remain unclassified.

In contrast to age and breed, sex is not a predisposing factor for any nervous system tumor type.[10, 22]

CLINICOPATHOLOGIC CORRELATES

Accurate clinicopathologic correlations are frequently not possible with intracranial tumors.[31] The true location of the tumor may be masked by secondary effects. Apart from brain tissue actually infiltrated by a tumor, a mass lesion within the nonexpansible cranial cavity often leads to local necrosis, edema, subfalcial herniation of the cingulate gyrus, subtentorial herniation of the occipital lobes, compression of the hypothalamus, and coning of the cerebellum. Herniation, together with attenuation of the ventricular system, especially at the level of the mesencephalic aqueduct, leads to hydrocephalus and elevated intracranial pressure. Ischemic necrosis of herniated tissue may ensue.[29–31]

Pathologic behavior, topographic pattern, growth characteristics, and secondary changes seen within and surrounding the tumor vary with any given neoplasm of nervous tissue. In general, primary tumors have a slowly progressive growth pattern. Secondary, highly malignant, metastatic tumors and bone tumors frequently have a more acute progression.[23, 33]

INCIDENCE

Nervous system neoplasia in domestic animals has been observed with varying frequency at different institutions. Most available data relate to the dog, in which the incidence of intracranial tumors is 1 to 3% of all canine tumors.[4, 25] Except for lymphosarcomas and neurofibromas in cattle, all tumors involving the nervous system are rare in large animals.

Brain Tumors

Primary tumors of the nervous system in dogs and cats are found more commonly in brain than in spinal cord or peripheral nerve.[6, 21, 22, 25, 42] The most common brain tumors in dogs are meningiomas (Fig. 9–1), gliomas (astrocytomas [Fig. 9–2], oligodendrogliomas), and undifferentiated sarcomas. Primary reticulosis (focal form of granulomatous meningoencephalomyelitis), pituitary adenomas (Fig. 9–3), and plexus papillomas (Fig. 9–4) are also commonly reported.[6, 7, 44] Older (over 5 years) brachycephalic dogs of common ancestry, namely boxer,

Table 9–1. CLASSIFICATION OF NEOPLASIA OF THE NERVOUS SYSTEM OF DOMESTIC ANIMALS[4–7, 10, 11, 13, 15, 19–24, 26, 27, 31, 36, 41–44]

	Predilection Sites	Species (Breed)	Incidence
	Primary Tumors		
Tumors of nerve cells			
Ganglioneuroma	Variable (cerebellum, cranial nerve roots, eye, cervical region)	Dogs, pigs, horses, cattle	Rare
Tumors of neuroepithelium			
Ependymoma	Ependymal surfaces	Dogs, cats, horses, cattle	Uncommon
Neuroepithelioma	Meninges to thoracolumbar spinal cord	Dogs	Uncommon
Plexus papilloma	Fourth ventricle	Dogs, horses, cattle	Common (dogs)
Tumors of glia			
Astrocytoma	Piriform area, convexity of cerebral hemispheres, thalamus, hypothalamus	Dogs (brachycephalic), cats, cattle	Common (dogs)
Oligodendroglioma	Cerebral hemispheres	Dogs (brachycephalic)	Common (dogs)
Glioblastoma	As for astrocytoma	Dogs (brachycephalic), cattle, pigs	Uncommon
Spongioblastoma	Variable (ependymal surfaces, cerebellum, optic nerve/tract)	Dogs (brachycephalic)	Rare
Medulloblastoma	Cerebellum	Dogs, cats, pigs, calves	Common (dogs)
Gliomas, unclassified	Periventricular areas, especially subependymal plate	Dogs (brachycephalic), cattle, horses, sheep, pigs	Common (dogs)
Tumors of peripheral nerves and nerve sheaths			
Neurinoma (schwannoma)	Peripheral nerves	Dogs, cattle	Uncommon
Neurofibroma	Peripheral nerves	Dogs, cattle, horses, pigs, sheep	Common (dogs, cattle)
Neurofibrosarcoma	Peripheral nerves	Dogs, cats, horses	Common (dogs, cattle)
Tumors of the meninges, vessels, and other mesodermal structures			
Meningiomas	Falx cerebri	Dogs (dolichocephalic), cats, horses, cattle, sheep	Common (dogs, cats)
Angioblastoma	Variable (cerebral hemispheres, choroid plexus), medulla, spinal cord	Dogs, horses, pigs	Rare
Sarcoma	Variable (meninges, brain, spinal cord)	Dogs, cats, horses, cattle, sheep	Common (dogs, cats)
Focal granulomatous meningoencephalomyelitis (reticulosis)	Cerebral hemispheres, brain stem	Dogs, cats, horses, cattle	Common (dogs)
Tumors of the pineal and pituitary glands and of the craniopharyngeal duct			
Pinealoma	Pineal body	Dogs, horses, cattle	Rare
Pituitary adenoma	Pituitary gland	Dogs (brachycephalic), cats, horses, cattle, sheep	Common (dogs, horses)
Craniopharyngioma	Hypophyseal-infundibular areas	Dogs	Rare
Tumors of heterotopic tissues (malformation tumors)			
Epidermoid, dermoid, teratoma	Variable (fourth ventricle and cerebellopontine angle for epidermoid)	Dogs, horses, cattle, sheep	Rare
	Secondary Tumors		
Metastatic tumors			
Mammary gland adenocarcinoma, pulmonary carcinoma, chemodectoma, prostatic carcinoma, hemangiosarcoma, fibrosarcoma, malignant melanoma, salivary gland adenocarcinoma	Variable	Dogs, cats, cattle, horses, sleep	Common
Lymphosarcoma	Spinal cord	Cats, cattle, dogs	Common (cattle, cats)
Primary tumors from surrounding tissues			
Osteoma, osteosarcoma, chondroma, chondrosarcoma, hemangioma, hemangiosarcoma, fibrosarcoma, calcifying aponeurotic fibromatosis, epidermoid cyst, lipoma	Variable (brain, spinal cord)	Dogs, cats, horses, cattle, pigs	Common (dogs, cats)

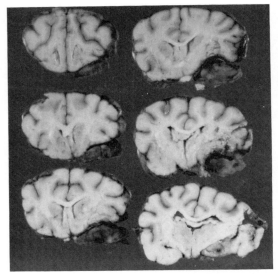

Figure 9–1. Coronal section of right-sided ventral meningioma in 8 year old, male golden retriever. (Courtesy of Dr EJ Hoff.)

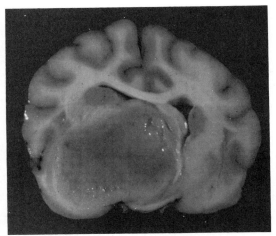

Figure 9–2. Coronal section of astrocytoma in 9 year old, male Boston terrier. (Courtesy of Dr EJ Hoff.)

English bulldog, and Boston terrier, have the highest incidence of brain tumors among domestic animals; of these tumors, the gliomas (including unclassified gliomas) are the most numerous.[6, 11, 22] The common locations of glial tumors are outlined in Table 9–1. Pituitary adenomas are frequently reported in brachycephalic breeds, whereas meningiomas tend to occur more commonly in dolichocephalic breeds (eg, German shepherd, collie). One review reported that 58% of meningiomas occurred on the ventral aspect of the brain.[2] Metastatic tumors are also found (Figs. 9–5 and 9–6).

In the cat, the most commonly reported primary brain tumors are meningiomas.[27] Common locations include tela choroidea of third ventricle and supratentorial meninges.[19, 43] Multiple meningiomas are common in cats.

Spinal Cord Tumors

In dogs and cats, the incidence of primary nervous system tumors is much less in spinal cord than in brain. In dogs, the most common tumor types are extradural, primary, malignant bone tumors (osteosarcoma, fibrosarcoma, hemangiosarcoma) and metastatic tumors to bone and soft tissues.[22, 23, 33, 41] The incidence of primary nervous system tumors is low, being only

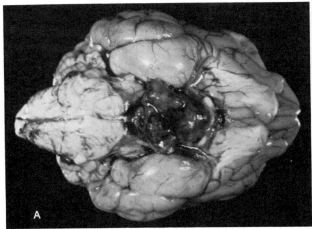
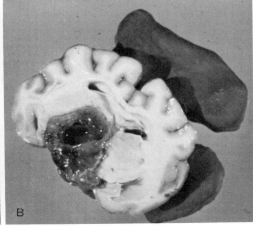

Figure 9–3. Pituitary chromophobe adenoma in 10 year old, female boxer. A, Ventral surface. B, Coronal section.

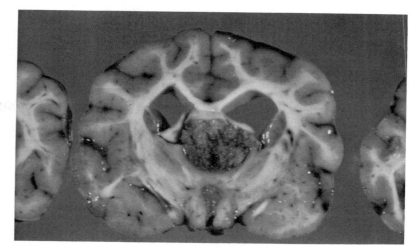

Figure 9–4. Coronal section of choroid plexus papilloma in third ventricle of 6 year old, male Samoyed.

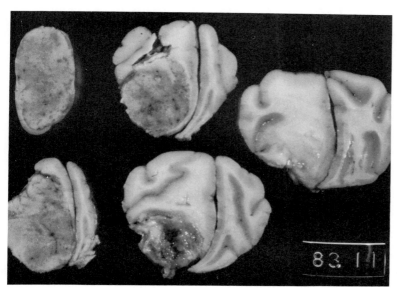

Figure 9–5. Coronal sections of metastatic nasal adenocarcinoma in 5 year old, female (spayed) collie mix. (Courtesy of Dr EJ Hoff.)

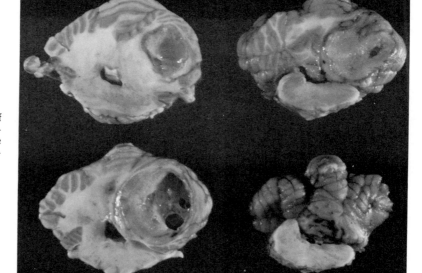

Figure 9–6. Coronal section of metastatic mammary adenocarcinoma in 10 year old, female (spayed) standard poodle. (Courtesy of Dr EJ Hoff.)

15% in one study.[33] In another study, approximately 30% of spinal tumors were primary, with intramedullary sarcomas being most prevalent.[23] A primary tumor that has a predilection for the T10-L1 cord segments in young dogs, especially German shepherds, is a neuroepithelioma. These tumors have an intradural-extramedullary position.

In cats, pigs, and cattle, epidural lymphosarcomas are the most common spinal tumors.[22, 33] Metastatic tumors reaching the spinal cord are unusual in animals;[22, 23, 33, 37] however, an incidence of 16% has been reported in the dog.[41]

The mean age of small animals with spinal tumors is between 5 and 6 years. Age alone does not eliminate a diagnosis of spinal tumor because 8 of 29 animals (30%) in one study were 3 years of age or less.[23] In this same study, approximately 90% of spinal tumors occurred in larger breeds of dogs.

Peripheral Nerve Tumors

Horses and cattle are at a greater risk for developing peripheral nerve tumors than glial or mesenchymal tumors of the central nervous system.[10, 22] Neurofibroma is the most common peripheral nerve tumor in cattle.[22] The most frequent sites involved are the brachial plexus, uni- or bilateral intercostal nerves, and cardiac nerves.

Tumors of cranial and spinal nerves and roots are not common in the dog. The terminology for these tumors has been confusing because of differences in opinion regarding the cell of origin of these neoplasms. Although schwannoma and neurofibroma are accepted and used interchangeably, the designation of peripheral nerve sheath tumor may be more applicable until the neurohistologic issue is settled. In dogs, these tumors are found mainly involving roots of cranial nerve V, brachial plexus, or cervical-thoracic nerve roots. They may extend along peripheral nerves, resulting in intradural-extramedullary spinal cord compression.[3, 7, 23, 33, 41] Brain stem compression has also been reported.[7, 39] Lymphosarcoma may occasionally involve nerve roots or nerves in dogs, cats, horses, and cattle.[1, 22, 24, 35]

CLINICAL SIGNS

Clinical signs will vary according to the location of the tumor and any secondary effects.[15,] [24, 25, 27, 29, 30, 32] Signs associated with various brain, spinal cord, and peripheral nerve syndromes are tabulated (Table 9–2). Onset of clinical signs may be acute or insidious, and the course may be rapidly or slowly progressive.

Table 9–2. CLINICAL SIGNS ASSOCIATED WITH VARIOUS BRAIN, SPINAL CORD, AND PERIPHERAL NERVE SYNDROMES

Syndrome	Clinical Signs
Cerebral or diencephalic	Behavioral or mental status change (apathy, disorientation, hyperexcitability, aggression) Abnormal posture or movement (circling, pacing, head pressing, pleurothotonos) +/− Visual impairment, seizures, papilledema, hypothalamohypophyseal syndrome (pituitary)
Cerebellar	Dysmetria (usually hypermetria) Intention tremor (head, body) Wide based stance Truncal ataxia +/− Menace deficit, eye tremors
Vestibular	Head tilt Circling, falling, rolling Nystagmus Vestibular strabismus
Cervical (C1–C5)	Hemiparesis to tetraplegia Upper motor neuron signs* in thoracic and pelvic limbs Cervical pain, +/− cervical rigidity
Cervicothoracic (C6–T2)	Hemiparesis to tetraplegia Lower motor neuron signs† in thoracic limbs Upper motor neuron signs in pelvic limbs Absent panniculus reflex (C8–T1) +/− Horner's syndrome (T1–T2) (miosis, ptosis, enophthalmos, prolapse of third eyelid)
Thoracolumbar (T3–L3)	Upper motor neuron signs in pelvic limbs Hypalgesia to analgesia caudal to lesion site Spastic paraparesis to paraplegia
Lumbosacral (L4–S3. . .Cd)	Flaccid paraparesis to paraplegia Dilated anal sphincter, urine retention Lower motor neuron signs in pelvic limbs
Neuropathic	Flaccid weakness to paralysis of muscle innervated Significant skeletal muscle atrophy Hyporeflexia, hypotonia, +/− hypalgesia

*UMN signs include spastic paresis or paralysis, hyperreflexia, and hypertonia.
†LMN signs include flaccid paresis or paralysis, hyporeflexia, and hypotonia.

In a recent study of spinal cord tumors in the dog and cat,[23] intramedullary tumors had the shortest duration of clinical signs (1.7 weeks), whereas the extradural tumors had a mean duration of 3.4 weeks. Intradural-extramedullary tumors had the longest mean duration (5.7 weeks). A temporal clinical course for various brain tumors in animals, although seemingly feasible from a retrospective study, is presently unknown.

DIAGNOSIS

Diagnosis of nervous system tumors is based on age, breed, and diagnostic aids including plain film radiography, contrast radiography (myelography, ventriculography, cerebral sinus venography, cerebral angiography), or radioisotopic brain scans (scintigraphy)[14] (see Figs. 4–24, 4–25, 4–28, 4–30, and 4–32). Plain film radiography will detect evidence of bone neoplasia or proliferation or lysis of bone secondary to neoplasms. Intracranial meningiomas may be radiodense because of calcification in the tumor. In some cats, increased or decreased density of the skull may be seen at the site of the tumor.[16]

Tumors in the vertebral canal may cause a loss of bone density, which appears as a widening of the vertebral canal (see Fig. 4–6). Neurofibromas of the nerve roots may cause enlargement of the intervertebral foramen.[28] Myelography should outline spinal tumors and may help differentiate extradural, intradural-extramedullary, and intramedullary neoplasms[23, 33] (see Figs. 4–11, 4–13, and 4–14). In cats, radionuclide imaging has proved inconsistent, and cerebral angiography is not possible, as the lumen of the proximal two thirds of the internal carotid artery becomes obliterated soon after birth. Computed tomography (CT), however, represents an accurate method of localizing brain tumors.[8, 17, 18] Unfortunately, few institutions have computed tomography capability. Abnormalities in the electroencephalographic tracing may localize a focal abnormality. Peripheral nerve disorders can be diagnosed using electrophysiologic techniques (electromyography, nerve conduction velocity determinations) and surgical biopsy or removal of tumor with histopathologic evaluation. Collection of cerebrospinal fluid may reveal an increase in CSF pressure, and examination of CSF may indicate an elevation in protein content; however, these are variable findings. Tumor cells in CSF are rarely encountered.[23, 34, 40]

PROGNOSIS AND TREATMENT

Prognosis for animals with tumors of the nervous system is guarded to poor. Inability to localize accurately a tumor mass in the brain at an early stage usually precludes surgical intervention. However, surgical removal of intracranial meningiomas, and occasionally other types of tumors, is becoming more frequent. Although spinal cord tumors can be localized more definitively, intramedullary masses are not surgically resectable, and extradural tumors are either primary bone tumors (removal of which often results in decreased vertebral stability, subluxation, or pathologic fractures) or metastatic, with possible sites elsewhere.

Although intradural-extramedullary tumors have been considered by some workers to be benign, well encapsulated, and surgically correctable,[33] others have reported that only a small percentage are completely resectable and that recurrence rate is high.[3]

Peripheral nerve or nerve root tumors may be resected; however, it may be necessary to remove the nerve or root affected. Resection with anastomosis of the nerve is possible if the tumor is not too large. If more than one root is involved, or atrophy of all muscle groups is extreme (as may occur with a tumor of the brachial plexus), complete amputation of the limb may be required. The role of radiotherapy and chemotherapy in nervous system tumor management has been extremely limited in veterinary medicine. A report of four dogs with brain tumors diagnosed by CT scan and treated with external beam, megavoltage radiation is encouraging.[38] The median survival time was 322 days compared with 56 days for eight other dogs with brain tumors treated symptomatically. Corticosteroids may ameliorate signs by reducing edema around the tumor and may produce temporary regression of lymphoid and reticulohistiocytic tumors.

REFERENCES

1. Allen JG and Amis T: Lymphosarcoma involving cranial nerves in a cat. Aust Vet J 51:155, 1975.
2. Andrews EJ: Clinicopathologic characteristics of meningiomas in dogs. JAVMA 163:151, 1973.
3. Bradley RL, Withrow SJ, and Snyder SP: Nerve sheath tumors in the dog. J Am Anim Hosp Assoc 18:915, 1982.
4. Dahme M and Schiefer B: Intracranielle Geschwulste bei Tieren. Zentralbl Veterinarmed 7:341, 1960.
5. Fankhauser R: Tumoren des Zentralnervensystems beim Tier. Bull Schweiz Akad Med Wiss 24:168, 1968.

6. Fankhauser R, Luginbuhl H, and McGrath JT: Tumors of the nervous system. Bull WHO 50:53, 1974.
7. Fankhauser R and Vandevelde M: Zur klinik der tumoren des Nervensystems bei Hund und Katze. Schweiz Arch Tierheilkd 123:553, 1981.
8. Fike JR, Le Couteur RA, Cann CE, and Pflugfelder CM: Computerized tomography of brain tumors of the rostral and middle fossas in the dog. Am J Vet Res 42:275, 1981.
9. Gieb LW: Ossifying meningioma with extracranial metastasis in a dog. Pathol Vet 3:247, 1966.
10. Hayes HM, Priester WA, and Pendergrass TW: Occurrence of nervous-tissue tumors in cattle, horses, cats and dogs. Int J Cancer 15:39, 1975.
11. Hayes KC and Schiefer B: Primary tumors in the CNS of carnivores. Pathol Vet 6:94, 1969.
12. Helfer DH and Stevens DR: Spinal neurofibroma in a sheep. Vet Pathol 15:784, 1978.
13. Innes JRM and Saunders LZ: Comparative Neuropathology. New York, Academic Press, 1962.
14. Kallfelz FA, deLahunta A, and Allhands RV: Scintigraphic diagosis of brain lesions in the dog and cat. JAVMA 172:589, 1978.
15. Kay WJ: Diagnosis of intracranial neoplasms. Vet Clin North Am 7:145, 1977.
16. Lawson DC, Burk RL, and Prata RG: Cerebral meningioma in the cat: Diagnosis and surgical treatment of ten cases. J Am Anim Hosp Assoc 20:333, 1984.
17. Le Couteur RA, Fike JR, Cann CE, and Pedroia VG: Computed tomography of brain tumors in the caudal fossa of the dog. Vet Radiol 22:244, 1981.
18. Le Couteur RA, Fike JR, Cann CE, et al: X-Ray computed tomography of brain tumors in cats. JAVMA 183:301, 1983.
19. Luginbuhl H: Studies on meningiomas in cats. Am J Vet Res 22:1030, 1961.
20. Luginbuhl H: A comparative study of neoplasms of the central nervous system in animals. Acta Neurochirurg (Suppl) 10:30, 1964.
21. Luginbuhl H: Oligodendrogliomas in animals. Acta Neurochirurg (Suppl) 10:173, 1964.
22. Luginbuhl H, Fankhauser R, and McGrath JT: Spontaneous neoplasms of the nervous system in animals. Prog Neurol Surg 2:85, 1968.
23. Luttgen PJ, Braund KG, Brawner WR, and Vandevelde M: A retrospective study of twenty-nine spinal tumours in the dog and cat. J Small Anim Pract 21:213, 1980.
24. Mayhew IG and MacKay RJ: The nervous system. In Mausmann RA, McAllister ES, and Pratt PW (ed): Equine Medicine and Surgery, 3rd ed. Santa Barbara, CA, American Veterinary Publications, 1982.
25. McGrath JT: Neurologic Examination of the Dog, 2nd ed. Philadelphia, Lea & Febiger, 1960.
26. Moulton JM: Tumors in Domestic Animals. Los Angeles, University of California Press, 1961.
27. Nafe LA: Meningiomas in cats: A retrospective clinical study of 36 cases. JAVMA 174:1224, 1979.
28. Oliver JE Jr and Lorenz MD: Handbook of Veterinary Neurologic Diagnosis. Philadelphia, WB Saunders Co, 1983.
29. Palmer AC: Clinical and pathological features of some tumours of the central nervous system in dogs. Res Vet Sci 1:36, 1960.
30. Palmer AC: Clinical signs associated with intracranial tumours in dogs. Res Vet Sci 2:326, 1961.
31. Palmer AC: Tumours of the central nervous system. Proc Coll Med 69:49, 1976.
32. Palmer AC, Malinowski W, and Barnett KC: Clinical signs including papilloedema associated with brain tumors in twenty-one dogs. J Small Anim Pract 15:359, 1974.
33. Prata RG: Diagnosis of spinal cord tumors in the dog. Vet Clin North Am 7:165, 1977.
34. Roszel JF: Membrane filtration of canine and feline cerebrospinal fluid for cytologic evaluation. JAVMA 160:720, 1972.
35. Schaer M, Zaki FA, Harvey HJ, and O'Reilly WH: Laryngeal hemiplegia due to neoplasia of the vagus nerve in a cat. JAVMA 174:513, 1979.
36. Sokale EOA and Ladds PW: Multicentric ganglioneuroma in a steer. Vet Pathol 20:767, 1983.
37. Sorjonen DC, Braund KG, and Hoff EJ: Paraplegia and subclinical neuromyopathy associated with a primary lung tumor in a dog. JAVMA 180:1209, 1982.
38. Turrel JM, Fike JR, Le Couteur RA, et al: Radiotherapy of brain tumors in dogs. JAVMA 184:82, 1984.
39. Vandevelde M, Braund KG, and Hoff EJ: Central neurofibromas in two dogs. Vet Pathol 14:470, 1977.
40. Vandevelde M and Spano JS: Cerebrospinal fluid cytology in canine neurologic disease. Am J Vet Res 38:1827, 1977.
41. Wright JA, Bell DA and Clayton-Jones DG: The clinical and radiological features associated with spinal tumours in thirty dogs. J Small Anim Pract 20:461, 1979.
42. Zaki FA: Spontaneous central nervous system tumors in the dog. Vet Clin North Am 7:153, 1977.
43. Zaki FA and Hurvitz AI: Spontaneous neoplasms of the central nervous system of the cat. J Small Anim Pract 17:773, 1976.
44. Zaki FA and Nafe LA: Choroid plexus tumors in the dog. JAVMA 176:328, 1980.

Chapter 10   *JE Oliver, Jr, DVM, MS, PhD*

Seizure Disorders and Narcolepsy

SEIZURES

Seizure, fit, and ictus are synonyms describing the sterotyped alteration in behavior resulting from paroxysmal abnormal brain function. Convulsion usually refers to a seizure with generalized tonic and clonic muscle activity and loss of consciousness. One or more of the following behavioral changes are present in a seizure: (1) loss or derangement of consciousness or memory (amnesia); (2) alteration of muscle tone or movement; (3) alteration of sensation, including hallucinations of special senses; (4) disturbances of autonomic function; and (5) other psychic manifestations or abnormal thought processes or moods.[44] Epilepsy is a disorder of the brain characterized by *recurring* seizures. Narcolepsy (see below) is a disorder of the brain characterized by recurring episodes of sleep and cataplexy.

The terminology of seizure disorders is confusing. The term epilepsy is used to refer to a clinical sign, a syndrome, or a disease, depending on the author. It will be used here to describe a syndrome of recurring seizures, regardless of cause. This definition has limitations. For example, an animal having multiple seizures over a 3 day period caused by acute encephalitis would not be considered an epileptic. If the same animal recovered and continued to have seizures episodically over a long period of time, it would be an epileptic. Because of this confusion of terminology, I will attempt to be specific in the terms used.

A seizure has several components. Before the seizure starts, there may be an *aura*. The aura is a subjective phenomenon, but descriptions from people with seizures indicate that there may be apprehension, anxiety, and various sensory phenomena preceding the actual seizure. The animal often acts restless and seeks attention or, conversely, tries to hide. The aura usually lasts a few minutes, but some dogs seem to have a behavioral change for hours prior to a seizure. The most visible part, the *ictus*, is the most important. The ictus generally lasts 1 to 2 minutes, but there is considerable variation. Following the seizure there is a postictal phase, which lasts from minutes to days. The animal may be confused, anxious, blind, disoriented, or lethargic or pace compulsively. The pre- and postictal phases are not related to the cause of the seizures. These phases are important to the owner, because they are upsetting and sometimes prolonged. A goal of treatment will be to reduce the pre- and postictal phases, as well as the frequency and severity of the ictus.

Incidence

Seizures may occur in any species. Among the domestic animals, the dog most commonly exhibits seizures. The incidence of seizures in the population of any of the domestic species is not known. Most reports on frequency are from teaching hospital or research laboratory populations. These figures do suggest that seizures are a relatively common problem in dogs. Holliday et al[35] reported an incidence of 1% at the teaching hospital of the University of California, Davis. Bunch[9] reported a frequency of 2.3% of sick dogs and 1% of sick cats at the Cornell University teaching hospital.

Seizures without a specific etiologic diagnosis were tabulated from the diagnostic file at the University of Georgia. Based on all admissions, not just sick animals, they accounted for 0.9% in 1980 and 0.5% in 1982 in the small animal clinic, and 0.01% and 0.08% respectively, in the large animal clinic. Seizures also account for a large portion of the problems related to the nervous system. Croft[16] found 260 dogs with a presenting complaint of seizures of 570 dogs with suspected central nervous system disorders.

Beagles in research colonies have been shown to have an inherited form of epilepsy. Biefelt[6] reported an incidence of 5.7% in a large colony. Another colony had an incidence of 11.9%.[54]

Pathophysiology

Considerable progress has been made in understanding the basic cellular mechanisms associated with epilepsy. A comprehensive description is not yet possible. However, future major discoveries are likely to revolutionize therapy.[90]

The basic cellular event in any seizure is a paroxysmal neuronal discharge. This has been called the seizure focus. An epileptic seizure may have one focus or many.[66] The epileptic neurons are capable of a large depolarization of the membrane (20-50 mV) that lasts 50 to 100 msec.[67, 72] The large prolonged depolarization leads to multiple action potentials in a short time. The large depolarization is called the paroxysmal depolarizing shift. Following the paroxysmal depolarizing shift the membrane becomes hyperpolarized (afterhyperpolarization

potential [AHP]), making the membrane resistant to further depolarization. The spike seen on surface electroencephalogram correlates with the paroxysmal depolarizing shift, whereas the slow wave correlates with the afterhyperpolarization potential (Fig. 10–1). Most evidence suggests that the paroxysmal depolarizing shift is a result of synaptic events, a giant excitatory postsynaptic potential (EPSP). However, this is not true of all neuronal populations. Some, such as the hippocampus, may be caused by intrinsic neuronal changes.[67] The evidence is less clear for the afterhyperpolarization potential, with some support for a synaptic mechanism and some for intrinsic ionic mechanisms. The afterhyperpolarization potential is of considerable interest, because it helps terminate the seizure activity. Pharmacologic manipulation of the AHP could lead to effective control of seizures.

A second abnormality may explain why seizure activity affects surrounding neurons. Action potentials apparently arise from dendrites of the neuron, rather than from the junction of the cell body and its axon. These ectopic spike potentials propagate to the neuron of origin and then spread back out in the normal direction, causing repetitive activation at the original focus and to other neurons.

Alterations in inhibitory neurotransmitters, especially γ-aminobutyric acid (GABA), have also been implicated.[80]

The paroxysmal depolarizing shift as a primary event in the seizure focus is established. Its genesis appears to be multifaceted.

Spread of seizure activity from a focus is

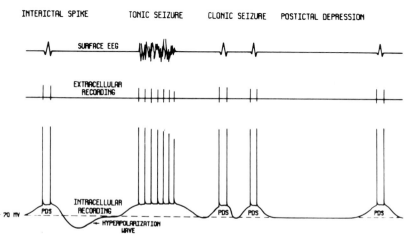

Figure 10–1. Schematic representation of simultaneous surface EEG, extracellular, and intracellular recordings from an epileptic focus. The paroxysmal depolarization shift (PDS) is seen as a spike on the surface EEG. A prolonged PDS with multiple discharges causes a tonic seizure, whereas shorter, repetitive PDS causes a clonic seizure. (From Russo ME: The pathophysiology of epilepsy. Cornell Vet 71:221, 1981.)

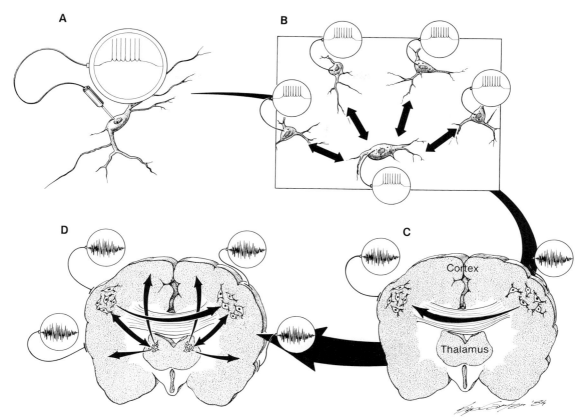

Figure 10–2. Spread of seizure activity from a focal area to the entire cerebrum. A, Paroxysmal depolarization shift in a neuron. B, Spread of activity to surrounding neurons. C, Propagation of seizure activity to other cortical areas by axonal conduction. D, Generalization of seizure activity through the diencephalon.

necessary for a seizure to occur. Cortical neurons are normally surrounded by inhibitory activity. The activity can spread both locally to adjacent neurons as ectopic spike potentials and to other areas by axonal propagation (Fig. 10–2B and C). Repetitive stimulation of a normal group of neurons eventually leads to the development of another focus. This phenomenon has been studied extensively by direct stimulation of neurons and is called kindling.

The basic mechanisms of the spread of the excitation are not known. It appears that there must be a critical mass of epileptic neurons in a focus before the activity will spread. Seizures often occur during sleep. Sleep is characterized by decreased cortical activation through the reticular activating system (RAS) and the thalamus. Experimentally, decreasing the output of the RAS increases seizure activity. The cortical focus is still the origin, but interactions among cortex, thalamus, and RAS are important for generalization (Fig. 10–2D).

Termination of seizure activity and the importance of the afterhyperpolarization potential have been described. Subcortical areas are also important in the termination of seizures. Inhibitory feedback circuits from cerebellum, thalamus, caudate nuclei, and possibly other areas tend to limit the seizure activity. Older theories of "metabolic exhaustion" of the neurons are probably not valid.[87]

Finally, it should be recognized that there is a variability of susceptibility to seizure activity. Some populations of neurons, such as those of the hippocampus, more easily develop seizure activity. Some individuals within a species are more susceptible. Any animal can have a seizure, but some have a lower threshold than others. The reasons are unknown, but they probably account for a genetic predisposition to seizures.

A variety of internal and external factors can affect the seizure threshold in susceptible individuals. Many seizures occur while an animal is asleep. The decrease in activity of the reticular formation apparently releases the mechanism responsible for the spread of seizure activity.[72] Hormonal influences, especially estrogens, may be important in some individuals. Some animals have more seizures during estrus. Progestins have been useful as an adjunct to therapy, and neutering is frequently recommended.

Classification of Seizures

Numerous classifications of seizures have been proposed. For clinical purposes, those based on clinical signs and etiology are most useful.[43, 57-60]

Clinical Signs

The international classification of human epilepsy is used with some modifications[32] (Table 10–1). Seizures should be classified as generalized or partial. Generalized seizures involve the entire body at once. Consciousness is lost in generalized seizures. Partial seizures are also called focal seizures. Only a portion of the brain is involved in the seizure; therefore, the animal shows focal signs. Partial seizures may generalize secondarily, however, so unless the seizure is seen from the onset, localizing signs may be missed. Partial seizures are always caused by a focal, and therefore acquired, brain lesion, hence the importance to the clinician.

There are two general kinds of seizures in each category (Table 10–1).

GENERALIZED SEIZURES

Generalized tonic-clonic seizures are also called major motor or grand mal seizures. The sequence is usually loss of consciousness, extensor tonus of the limbs, and opisthotonos, followed by the clonic phase consisting of paddling movements of the limbs. Visceral activity, including urination, defecation, pupillary dilation, salivation, and piloerection, may occur in tonic or clonic phases.

Generalized tonic-clonic seizures may be caused by extracranial factors, such as metabolic disorders or toxins, or by abnormality in the brain, including a variety of pathologic changes. Generalized tonic-clonic seizures may also be seen in animals with no demonstrable pathologic change in the brain. This is called idiopathic epilepsy and may be inherited.

Absences, or petit mal seizures, are not commonly seen in animals.[33, 34] They are characterized by a brief loss of consciousness, often lasting only seconds. In children, there may be a small motor component, usually movements of the face, and even some autonomic activity. Children with this form of epilepsy have a characteristic 3 Hz spike-wave complex on the EEG. (See Figure 5–11 from a 3 year old poodle seen by Redding,[33] which had frequent brief episodes of staring. The spike-wave complexes are at a frequency of 4 Hz.)

Table 10–1. CLASSIFICATION OF SEIZURES: CLINICAL SIGNS

Clinical Manifestation	EEG	Etiology	Anatomic Location
Generalized Seizures, Bilateral Symmetric Seizures, or Seizures Without Local Onset			
Tonic-clonic (grand mal, major motor)	Generalized dysrhythmia from onset, symmetric, often normal interictal unless they are activated or have organic or toxic origin	1. Genetic predisposition 2. Diffuse or multiple organic lesions 3. Toxic or metabolic	1. Unlocalized 2. Diencephalic (centrencephalic)
Absences with or without motor phenomena (petit mal)—rare or rarely recognized in animals	Generalized 3 per second spike and wave dysrhythmia, symmetric (human)	Usually genetic (human)	1. Unlocalized 2. Diencephalic (centrencephalic)
Partial Seizures or Seizures Beginning Locally			
Partial motor (may generalize to tonic-clonic seizure)—signs depend on site of discharge	Focal dysrhythmia (spikes, slow waves), may generalize secondarily	Acquired organic lesion; see Tables 10–2 and 10–3	Focal cortical or subcortical
Psychomotor (may generalize or appear as complex behavioral change—running, fear, aggression)	Dysrhythmia related to temporal lobe (unproven in animals)	Acquired organic lesion; see Tables 10–2 and 10–3	Limbic system (hippocampus, temporal or piriform lobe)

*Modified from Oliver JE Jr: Seizure disorders in companion animals. Comp Cont Ed Small Anim Pract 2:77, 1980.

PARTIAL SEIZURES

Partial seizures with elemental symptomatology will be called *partial motor seizures* for simplicity. These seizures appear as a turning of the head or body, tonus or clonus (or both) of one or both limbs on one side, or other movements affecting only a part of the body. Partial motor seizures may generalize secondarily. It is important to recognize the focal nature of the seizure, because it signifies a focal lesion that relates to the movement produced.

Partial seizures with complex symptomatology will be called *psychomotor seizures*. Animals with this type of seizure manifest an inappropriate, uncontrolled behavior. Examples include chewing, licking, screaming, running, aggressiveness, fright, and flybiting.[13] Visceral activities such as vomiting, diarrhea, and abdominal discomfort, which were thought to be caused by lesions in the limbic system, have been reported.[6]

Etiology

Seizures may be caused by anything that alters the function of neurons. The most common causes of seizures are listed in Tables 10–2 and 10–3 (along with reference to the chapter in which these diseases are discussed in detail). Only primary generalized epilepsy will be discussed here.

Primary Generalized Epilepsy. Primary generalized epilepsy may be either generalized tonic-clonic seizures or absence attacks. Tonic-clonic seizures are common in animals, but absence attacks are rare. Primary generalized epilepsy is also called idiopathic epilepsy because there is no demonstrable pathologic cause. The term secondary generalized epilepsy is used if there are pathologic changes in the brain or a metabolic cause can be established. Primary generalized epilepsy may be inherited. There is substantial evidence for an inherited tendency for epilepsy in some breeds. Other

Table 10–2. CAUSES OF SEIZURE DISORDERS OF DOGS AND CATS

Classification	Most Frequent Causes	Diagnostic Tests*
Genetic	Genetic	Breed, age, history
Idiopathic	Unknown	Exclusion
Degenerative (Ch 6)	Storage disease	
	Glycoprotein (Lafora's)	Breed, biopsy
	Lipids	Breed, biopsy
Anomalous (Ch 6)	Hydrocephalus	PE, EEG, ventriculography
	Lissencephaly	Breed, PE, EEG
	Porencephaly	Ventriculography
Infectious (Ch 7)	Viral: canine distemper, rabies, feline infectious peritonitis	History, EEG, CSF analysis
	Bacterial: any type	CSF analysis
	Mycotic: cryptococcosis	CSF analysis
	Protozoal: toxoplasmosis	CSF analysis, titer
Metabolic (Ch 8)	Electrolyte: hypocalcemia	Serum calcium level
	Carbohydrate: hypoglycemia, functional insulinoma	Fasting blood glucose levels
	Cardiovascular: arrhythmia, vascular	EKG, arteriography
	Renal	PE, BUN, UA
	Hepatic: cirrhosis,	PE, BSP, SGPT levels, serum NH₃ levels
	portocaval shunt	Same + angiography
Neoplastic (Ch 9)	Primary: gliomas, meningioma	NE, EEG, radiography
	Secondary: metastatic	Same
Nutritional (Ch 8)	Thiamine	History, treatment
	Parasitism (multiple factors)	PE, treatment
Toxic (Ch 8)	Heavy metal: lead	History, blood lead levels
	Organophosphates	History, NE
	Chlorinated hydrocarbon	History, NE
	Strychnine	History, NE
	Tetanus	
Traumatic (Ch 11)	Acute—immediately after head injury	History, PE
	Chronic—weeks to years after head injury	History, EEG

*PE, Physical examination; EEG, electroencephalography; CSF, cerebrospinal fluid; BUN, serum urea nitrogen; UA, urine analysis; BSP, Bromsulphalein test; SGPT, serum alanine transaminase; NE, neurologic examination.

Modified from Oliver JE Jr: Seizure disorders in companion animals. Comp Cont Ed Small Anim Pract 2:77, 1980.

Table 10–3. CAUSES OF SEIZURE DISORDERS OF LARGE ANIMALS

Classification	Most Frequent Cause	Diagnostic Tests*
Genetic	Genetic (bovine)	Breed, age, history
Idiopathic	Unknown (equine)	Exclusion
Degenerative (Ch 6)	Storage disease (bovine)	Breed, biopsy
Anomalous (Ch 6)	Hydrocephalus	Breed, PE, EEG
Inflammatory (Ch 7)	Pseudorabies (bovine, swine)	History, PE, CSF analysis
	Rabies (all)	
	Thromboembolic meningoencephalitis (bovine)	
	Hog cholera	
	Viral encephalitis (equine)	
	Bacterial meningoencephalitis (all)	
	Aberrant parasites (all)	
	Equine protozoal myeloencephalitis	
Metabolic (Ch 8)	Electrolytes: hypocalcemia, hypomagnesemia	Serum calcium and magnesium levels
	Carbohydrate: ketosis (bovine)	Ketones
	Pregnancy toxemia (ovine)	History
	Water intoxication (bovine, swine)	History
	Salt poisoning (swine)	History
	Hepatic encephalopathy	PE, BSP, Serum NH_3 levels
Neoplastic (Ch 9)	Primary (primarily equine, rare)	NE, CSF analysis
	Secondary: metastatic	
Nutritional (Ch 8)	Thiamine (ruminants)	History, treatment
Toxic (Ch 8)	Heavy metals: lead, arsenic	History, blood lead levels
	Organophosphates	
	Chlorinated hydrocarbons	
	Toxic plants	
	Clostridium perfringens type D enterotoxemia (ruminants)	
	Escherichia coli enterotoxemia (swine)	
Traumatic (Ch 11)	Acute (all)	History, PE, NE
Vascular	Intracarotid injections	History
	Neonatal maladjustment syndrome	
	Parasitic thromboembolism	

*PE, Physical examination; EEG, electroencephalography; CSF, cerebrospinal fluid; BSP, Bromsulphalein test; NE, neurologic examination.

Modified from Oliver JE Jr and Lorenz MD: Handbook of Veterinary Neurologic Diagnosis. Philadelphia, WB Saunders Co, 1983.

cases are frequently diagnosed as idiopathic epilepsy, but careful studies of the inheritance have not been done. These two groups are listed in Table 10–4. In a study at the University of Pennsylvania, there was no evidence of an increased incidence of epilepsy in any breed. The incidence of seizures in all breeds closely matched the frequency of admission to the hospital for all problems.[24] The diagnosis of primary generalized epilepsy does not prove inheritance. Only careful breeding studies can prove a genetic trait.

Dogs with primary generalized epilepsy usually have their first seizure between 1 and 3 years of age. Seizures that begin prior to 6 months of age or after 5 years of age are more likely to be secondary.[15, 20, 33, 34, 60]

Seizures are generalized from the onset. An aura is unusual. The tonic phase appears first and lasts seconds to 2 to 3 minutes. It is followed by the clonic phase, which usually lasts a similar

Table 10–4. BREEDS WITH PRIMARY GENERALIZED EPILEPSY

Genetic Factor Likely
Beagle[6]
Dachshund[35]
German shepherd (Alsatian)[23]
Keeshond[86]
Tervuren (Belgian) shepherd[85]
Brown Swiss cattle[1]
Aberdeen Angus cattle[4]
Swedish Red cattle[14]

High Incidence of Seizures[15, 20, 33, 57, 58, 60]
Arabian foals
Cocker spaniel
Collie
Golden retriever
Irish setter
Labrador retriever
Miniature schnauzer
Poodles (standard and miniature)
Saint Bernard
Siberian huskies
Wire haired fox terriers

length of time. Urination, defecation, and salivation are common. Postictal signs are usually mild.

Some dogs, especially German shepherds, Irish setters, and Saint Bernards, frequently have clusters of seizures. Postictal depression is more common following a cluster of seizures. Seizures in these dogs are difficult to control with medication.

Primary generalized epilepsy with no evidence for an inherited basis has been reported in Arabian foals.[20, 50]

An inherited epilepsy has been reported in Brown Swiss and Swedish Red cattle.[1] Seizures and progressive cerebellar ataxia occur in purebred and crossbred Aberdeen Angus cattle.[4] The seizures start in calves and decline in frequency in those that survive.[3]

Diagnosis

Data Base. A problem specific data base for animals with recurring seizures is outlined in Table 10–5.[54, 55, 57] The data base has been formulated on the assumption that the causes of seizures can be grouped into three major categories: (1) extracranial abnormalities, such as metabolic, toxic, and nutritional problems; (2) intracranial diseases, such as encephalitis, brain tumors, degenerative diseases, anomalies, and traumatic injuries; and (3) idiopathic or primary generalized epilepsy.

The minimum data base will usually identify extracranial causes and any intracranial causes that result in neurologic deficits in the interictal period (Table 10–5). It is relatively inexpensive to complete and involves no risk for the patient. The more complete data base and tests for focal brain disease are reserved for animals that have indications of intracranial disease. These tests may require anesthesia, are more expensive, and, in part, may be available only at referral centers.

Plan for Management

The majority of small animals with epilepsy will ultimately be classified as having idiopathic epilepsy because of negative findings on the diagnostic tests. Recently, Knecht et al[39] reviewed the diagnostic results in 70 animals (65 dogs, 5 cats) evaluated because of seizures. The cause of seizures could not be determined in 53 animals (76%). Not all recommended tests were done on all of the animals. The likelihood

Table 10–5. DATA BASE FOR SEIZURE DISORDERS

Minimum Data Base: One or more seizures without previous therapy
Patient profile
  Species, breed, age, sex
History
  Immunizations
  Environment
  Previous illness
  Description of seizures
    Age of onset, frequency, precipitating factors
    Partial or generalized
    Behavioral changes
    Abnormality
Physical examination
  General, with special attention to cardiovascular system
  Funduscopic examination
Neurologic examination
  Complete examination. Note time of last seizure. If it was within 24–48 hours and neurologic examination is abnormal, repeat in 24 hours
Clinical pathology*
  CBC
  Urinalysis
  Chemistries including at least:
    BUN, ALT (SGPT) ALP, calcium, fasting blood glucose levels (GGT, SDH in large animals)
    Others if indicated
    e.g., blood lead level, Coggins' test

More Complete Data Base: If seizures are not controlled with medication, or there is evidence of CNS disease
CSF analysis: cell count, total and differential; protein levels
Skull radiograph
EEG

Focal Brain Disease Suspected
Contrast radiography
Brain scans: nuclear, CAT

*CBC, Complete blood count; BUN, serum urea nitrogen; ALT, serum alanine transaminase; ALP, alkaline phosphatase; GGT, γ-glutamyltransferase; SDH, sorbitol dehydrogenase.

of a procedure contributing to a positive diagnosis was as follows: physical examination, 6 of 70 (8.5%); neurologic examination, 7 of 70 (10%); fundic examination, 0 of 29 (0%); complete blood count, 7 of 57 (12%); serum chemistries, 3 of 54 (6%); electroencephalography, 10 of 46 (22%); radiology of the skull, 5 of 17 (30%); cerebrospinal fluid analysis, 1 of 24 (4%); electrocardiography, 2 of 32 (7%); and immunologic tests, 1 of 10 (10%). Therefore, a plan for management, including a staged diagnostic and therapeutic plan, is recommended (Fig. 10–3).

Animals that have had only one seizure, especially if it is mild, are given a physical and neurologic examination. If no abnormalities are found, the owners are instructed to watch carefully for signs of additional seizures. The first

Minimum Data Base

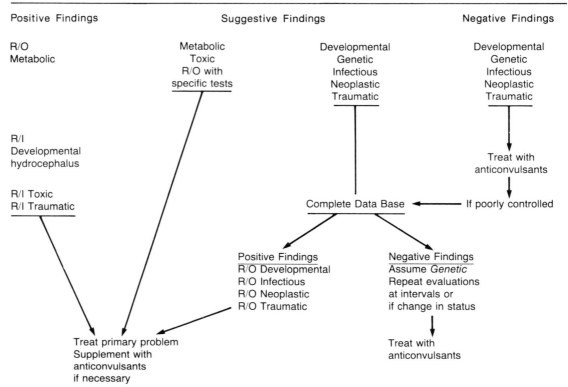

Figure 10–3. Plan for the diagnosis and management of a patient with seizures. R/O, Rule out: Positive findings confirm the diagnosis; negative findings eliminate the diagnosis. R/I, Rule in: Positive findings confirm the diagnosis; negative findings are *not* adequate for diagnosis. (Modified from Oliver JE Jr: Protocol for diagnosis of seizure disorders in companion animals. JAVMA 172:824, 1978.)

examination must include a careful history. Seizure syndromes are episodic, and the veterinarian may never see the signs described by the owner. Other episodic events may be mistaken for a convulsion. The most common of these are syncope, acute vestibular attacks, and narcolepsy (see below). Syncope, or fainting, is a transient loss of consciousness, usually caused by a cardiovascular problem or hypoglycemia. Vestibular attacks usually leave some residual signs such as a head tilt. If the animal has had more than one seizure, a minimum data base is completed (Table 10–5). There are three possible outcomes: positive findings yielding a definitive diagnosis, suggestive findings that require further tests to confirm, or negative findings (Fig. 10–3).

Positive findings include evidence of metabolic or toxic disease, such as a low blood glucose level, or neurologic abnormality, such as the obvious hydrocephalic puppy. These animals are treated for the primary disease if possible and placed on anticonvulsants if necessary.

Suggestive findings include some metabolic abnormalities, such as low serum urea nitrogen (BUN) and low serum albumin levels, which indicate liver disease. Neurologic deficits may suggest primary brain disease but not define the cause. These problems are pursued with appropriate tests to make a definitive diagnosis. Again, the primary disease is treated if possible and anticonvulsants are used if necessary.

Negative findings are common. This does not necessarily mean that there is no primary disease; rather, there is no disease detectable. For small animals, the author recommends that they be placed on anticonvulsant medication and evaluated periodically for signs of progressive disease. Most of them will not progress, and the seizures can be controlled with medication. If any subsequent examination reveals new data, they are pursued as described. If anticonvulsants are not effective, the complete data base should be performed (Fig. 10–3).

Recurrent generalized seizures in food animal patients will usually necessitate euthanasia. Horses with epilepsy should be treated for concurrent disease. Foals can be placed on phenobarbital for several weeks prior to a slow reduction in dosage until discontinuance. Maintaining adult horses on anticonvulsants is a profound undertaking, and such animals should not be ridden. Therefore, much thought should go into initiating such therapy.

Failure to control seizures with anticonvulsant medication is usually evidence of progressive disease, refractory epilepsy, or failure of the owner to follow an adequate treatment plan. Progressive disease should be identified on subsequent examinations. Epilepsy that is refractory to medication is most common in large breed dogs such as the German shepherd, Saint Bernard, and Irish setter. Client education is imperative to assure compliance and will be discussed in the next section.

Treatment

Three anticonvulsant drugs are used routinely and several newer drugs are now available. Phenobarbital, primidone, and phenytoin are commonly used. Valproic acid, diazepam, paramethadione, and carbamazepine have been used occasionally, but large clinical studies are not available. Prolonged treatment of epilepsy in large animals is unusual.

Pharmacologic principles including drug absorption, distribution, elimination, and half-life are important in planning anticonvulsant therapy. The pharmacology of some of these drugs in animals is different from that reported in human beings. Pharmacodynamic studies have been done for several of the drugs in the dog, a few in the cat, and two in the horse.

Drug absorption varies with the drug and species. Absorption is much faster when the stomach is empty. Different formulations of the same drug vary widely in their absorptions.

Anticonvulsant drugs are generally lipid soluble and distribute readily to all tissues including the nervous system. Blood concentrations are usually reasonable indicators of tissue concentrations.

Protein binding also affects availability to the tissues. Some drugs that have less protein binding may be effective at blood concentrations that are lower than reported for humans.

The half-life of a drug, the time required to remove half of the active drug from the body, is one of the most important factors to be considered. The half-life of anticonvulsants varies widely among species. The half-life determines the frequency of administration, the time to reach a steady state, and the time to effectively eliminate the drug. A drug with a long half-life, such as phenobarbital, may be given once or twice a day, require several days to reach a steady state, and persist in the body after medication is stopped. Table 10–6 outlines some of the characteristics of anticonvulsant drugs.

Although pharmacokinetic studies have been done, there are few reports correlating blood concentrations and efficacy. Based on reported and anecdotal experience, the pharmacodynamics of a drug does not directly correlate with efficacy.

The objectives of therapy are to eliminate seizures without producing any side effects. Therefore, the minimal dose to maintain control is desirable. Unfortunately, complete control is often not possible. Realistic expectations are described below and in Table 10–7.

Phenobarbital. Phenobarbital is an effective anticonvulsant in animals, especially for partial motor and generalized tonic-clonic seizures. It is low in cost; is easily administered; comes in tablet, liquid, and injectable formulations; and has minimal side effects. It is safe to use in cats in contrast to the other common anticonvulsants.

Phenobarbital protects against electrically or chemically induced seizures experimentally. It enhances synaptic inhibition, probably through γ-aminobutyric acid (GABA)–mediated mechanism.[51, 89, 90]

Phenobarbital is metabolized in the liver and excreted by the kidneys. It stimulates microsomal enzymes in the liver, increasing the rate of its own metabolism, as well as that of other drugs such as phenytoin. The half-life of phenobarbital in dogs is relatively long (30-70 hours); however, it is extremely variable among dogs, and even in the same dog at different times[25, 31, 79, 91] (see Table 10–6). Animals that are not responding to recommended doses should be monitored by checking serum levels. The time required to reach steady state and to develop effective brain concentrations is relatively long, so rapid results should not be expected. The shorter half-life and apparently consistent pharmacokinetics of phenobarbital in foals makes it a more predictable drug in these patients.[82]

Table 10–6. PHARMACOLOGIC PROPERTIES OF ANTICONVULSANT DRUGS

Drug	Half-Life (Hours ± SE)*	Time to Steady State (days)†	Bioavailability (%)	Protein Binding (%)	Enzyme Induction	References
Phenobarbital	70 ± 16 (M)	10–18	91	45–46	yes	31, 31a, 46
	32 ± 4.8 (B)					31
	40.9 (M)	7				91
	12.8 ± 2.1 (F)					82
Primidone	9–12 (M)	6–8		19–23		31, 31a, 46
	4–6 (B)					31
	1.85 ± 0.3					91
Metabolites						
PEMA	10–16 (M)			6–7		31, 31a
	5–12 (B)					31
	7.1 ± 1.45					91
Phenobarbital (see above)						
Phenytoin	4.4 ± 0.78	0.5–1	36 (19–68)	77	Pronounced	29, 31, 46
	3		40			75
	3					71
	3.65					65
	4.5					75
	24–108 (cat)					71
	41.5 (cat)					84
	α 0.2 (H)		23–44			40
	β 1.5 (H)					
Na valproate	1.7 ± 0.4	6–10 hours	80–90	60–80 (lower with high doses)		31, 45, 46, 48
	2.8–3.1		95			47
Oxazolidinediones						
Trimethadione				6.5–9		46
Dimethadione				7–8		46
Carbamazepine	1.1–1.9	4–12 hours	Liquid better than tablets	71–72	Pronounced	30, 31a, 43
Metabolite						
C-epoxide	1.6–3.1	5–18 hours		40		
Ethosuximide	18 ± 5.1		90	<10		31

*M, Mixed breed dog; B, beagle; F, foals; H, horses.
†Calculated as 3.3–6 times half-life[66, 84] or as published.

The dosage of phenobarbital currently recommended for dogs and cats is 1.5 to 5 mg/kg given twice daily. Serum concentrations should be greater than 10 μg/ml. Serum concentrations above 40 μg/ml produce sedation and ataxia.[25, 77, 79, 91] Phenobarbital may be used in horses and food animals at doses of 0.5 to 2.0 mg/kg twice a day.[14, 50] However, it appears that doses up to 9 mg/kg three times daily may actually be necessary, at least in foals, to achieve anticonvulsant serum concentrations.[82] Adult large animals may have slower metabolism of phenobarbital and require lower doses.

The most common side effects of phenobarbital are CNS depression, polyphagia, polydipsia, and polyuria. They are dose dependent and are eliminated when the dosage is reduced. Most animals that are depressed initially will revert to normal in less than 2 weeks as the liver metabolism increases. If seizures are not too severe or too frequent, low doses can be used initially followed by increasing doses as the animal adapts. Elevated liver enzyme levels are seen in animals treated with phenobarbital, but severe liver disease is unusual.[10] Vitamin K–dependent coagulation defects have been reported in cats.[81] However, these cats were given 10 to 40 mg/kg/day. Abrupt withdrawal of phenobarbital may precipitate seizures, even in normal animals. Any change in medication should be done gradually.

In summary, phenobarbital is a safe, effective anticonvulsant drug. It is recommended as the first choice in most animals. Serum levels should be checked for assessment of an adequate dose before changing to other drugs.

Table 10–7. RECOMMENDED DOSAGE AND SERUM CONCENTRATIONS OF ANTICONVULSANT DRUGS

Drug	Dosage (mg/kg)	Serum Concentration (μg/ml)	Notes	References
Phenobarbital	1.5–5 bid (dog, cat)	15 10–30	Considerable variability in absorption, excretion, and metabolism. May need to monitor serum levels, 40 μg/ml causes CNS depression	25, 28, 31a 91
	10–20 IV, then 5–10 PO, tid (foal)	10–50		82
Primidone	10–15 tid (dog)	15 (phenobarbital)	Serum concentrations of primidone and PEMA decrease with repeated dosing. 40 μg/ml phenobarbital caused side effects	28, 91
	13–77 daily, divided bid or tid	6–37 (phenobarbital)		77
		25–40 (phenobarbital) 7 hours after dose		18
		5–15 (primidone—human)		42
		4–20 (PEMA—human)		
Phenytoin	35 tid (dog)	10	Considerable variability in absorption, excretion, and metabolism. Need to monitor serum levels	75
	20 tid	10		65
	5 tid	1.5–3		64
		10–20 (human)		42
	3–8 tid (horse)	5 (horse)		40
	6–16 tid (horse)	10 (horse)		40
Na valproate	60 tid (dog)	40–100 (human)	Probably should be used in combination with phenobarbital	47
	30–100/day Divided tid			55
		>50 (human)		66
Oxazolidinediones				
Trimethadione		9–80 (human)		46
Dimethadione		600–800 (human)		46
Paramethadione	10–60/day (dog) Divided tid			63
	16 tid			76
Carbamazepine	Not recommended	5–12 (human)		42
Ethosuximide	40 initial dose, 15–25 tid maintenance		Not reported for clinical use in animals. Primarily for absence seizures in humans	31, 31a
		40–100 (human)		42

Primidone. Primidone is an effective anticonvulsant in dogs, but it is not approved for use in cats. Although it has been used, its efficacy in large animals is not known.[50] It is beneficial in partial motor, generalized tonic-clonic, and psychomotor seizures.

Primidone is metabolized to phenobarbital and phenylethylmalonamide (PEMA), with small amounts of unmetabolized primidone remaining.[28] All three components have anticonvulsant activity, although it has been estimated that 85% of the total anticonvulsant activity is from the phenobarbital.[28] Both primidone and PEMA have short half-lives, necessitating administration of the drug three times daily if it is to be effective (Table 10–6). Clinical experience indicates that primidone has efficacy beyond that of phenobarbital alone. However, a recent study found improvement in only 1 of 15 dogs given primidone when they were not controlled on phenobarbital.[26] Measurement of serum phenobarbital level is adequate for monitoring the dose of primidone.

The recommended dose of primidone is from 5 to 15 mg/kg three times daily. When converting a dog from phenobarbital to primidone, 250 mg of primidone should be given for each 65 mg of phenobarbital to maintain a similar serum concentration of phenobarbital.[25] Serum concentrations of phenobarbital should be greater than 10 μg/ml. Primidone is not licensed for use in horses or food animals. It has been used in foals at doses of 0.75 to 1 gm twice daily.[49]

Primidone has most of the side effects of phenobarbital. In addition, liver problems, including elevated liver enzyme levels, necrosis, and cirrhosis, have been reported.[10, 11, 36, 52] Elevated enzyme concentrations are common in animals treated with many of the anticonvulsants, but clinical signs of hepatic disorders have been rare in the author's experience. Adverse reactions to primidone when other medications are administered should also be considered. Chloramphenicol given to a dog on primidone produced severe CNS depression.[12] Chloramphenicol inhibits the microsomal enzyme system, reducing the rate of metabolism of primidone. Other drugs that may produce similar problems include phenytoin, various narcotics, cortisol, diazepam, phenylbutazone, digitalis glycosides, and phenothiazine tranquilizers.[12, 41]

In summary, primidone is an effective anticonvulsant in dogs. It seems to be the most effective drug for controlling psychomotor seizures. Liver function tests should be performed periodically on animals on long-term therapy. Drugs that may alter liver metabolism should be used with caution.

Phenytoin. Phenytoin (diphenylhydantoin) is the most commonly used anticonvulsant drug in humans. It is safe for dogs and not recommended for cats, and little is known of its effects in large animals. It is authorized for use only in dogs in the United States.

Pharmacokinetic studies have clarified some of the problems experienced with phenytoin in dogs, cats, and horses. The half-life of phenytoin in the dog is short (3–4 hours), whereas it is long in the cat (24–100 hours).[29, 31, 65, 71, 73, 75, 84] The half-life in humans is between these extremes. The pharmacokinetics of phenytoin in the horse appear to follow a two compartment model with α half-life of about 0.2 hour and β half-life of about 1.5 hours.[40] Absorption and metabolism are extremely variable among animals, and even in the same animal from day to day. Continued therapy causes a more rapid metabolism of the drug, making it difficult to achieve therapeutic concentrations.[29] The therapeutic serum level is not clearly established either. In humans and most experimental models, 10 to 20 μg/ml of plasma is considered the appropriate therapeutic level. One clinical study reported efficacy at plasma levels of 1.5 to 3 μg/ml.[64] In another study, only 3 of 77 dogs had control of sizures using phenytoin.[25] Of these three, two were also receiving phenobarbital. The one dog controlled on phenytoin alone had serum concentrations of 2.3 μg/ml. Other drugs such as phenobarbital increase the metabolism of phenytoin even more. Combinations of phenytoin and phenobarbital have been used commonly. Current evidence suggests that any efficacy of this combination is primarily from the phenobarbital.

Recommended dosage of phenytoin for dogs is 30 to 50 mg/kg three times daily. Plasma concentration should be 10 to 20 μg/ml. Further clinical trials are needed to see if this elevated dose is reasonable. Phenytoin has been used in foals at 1 to 5 mg/kg twice a day.[68] However, in adult horses, to achieve mean serum concentrations of 5 and 10 μg/ml, doses of 3 to 8 mg/kg and 6 to 16 mg/kg, orally three times daily, respectively, are required.[40]

Phenytoin has rarely caused toxic reactions, probably because it has been used at much lower doses than those currently recommended. It interacts with chloramphenicol similarly to primidone.[74] Liver toxicity is also reported.[56] Gingival hyperplasia, a common side effect in humans, was seen in one dog.[70] Because of the extremely slow metabolism of phenytoin in cats, it is not recommended in that species. A case of dermal atrophy in a cat treated with phenytoin has been reported.[5] In the horse, head and facial twitching and temporary recumbency with fixed dilated pupils have been reported at peak serum concentrations of 16 μg/ml.[40]

In summary, phenytoin is not recommended as a primary anticonvulsant in animals. The necessity for high doses administered three times daily makes it expensive and inconvenient. The one study reporting efficacy at lower doses needs further documentation.

Sodium Valproate. Several new anticonvulsant drugs have become available recently. Of these, sodium valproate (valproic acid) seems to have the most promise. Limited clinical trials suggest that it may be effective in animals refractory to other medication.[55] Because of its short half-life it has been used in conjunction with other drugs.

Sodium valproate is metabolized completely, but several of the metabolic products have anticonvulsant activity.[47, 48] Plasma protein binding of sodium valproate is lower in the dog than in humans, which may allow higher central nervous system levels at lower plasma levels.[45, 46] The half-life is reported as 1.7 to 3.1 hours. Therapeutic levels in humans are 40 to 100 μg/ml.[47]

More clinical trials, including measurement of plasma levels, are needed to establish appropriate dosage schedules. Currently, 60 mg/kg three times daily is recommended as an adjunct to phenobarbital in refractory epilepsy.

Side effects of sodium valproate included alopecia and vomiting.[55] Vomiting was controlled by giving the medication with a meal. Side effects in humans include blood dyscrasias, hepatic necrosis, and tremor.[87]

In summary, sodium valproate should be considered as an adjunct to other anticonvulsants in dogs refractory to standard regimens. Several cases of refractory seizures in large breed dogs were improved following the addition of sodium valproate to their schedule.

Oxazolidinediones (Paramethadione). This group of drugs, including trimethadione, dimethadione, and paramethadione, is used in humans for absence attacks. Successful treatment of generalized tonic-clonic seizures in dogs using paramethadione has been reported.[63, 76] Holliday[34] reported on a dog in which paramethadione seemed to precipitate seizures.

There is little information available on dos-age, therapeutic concentrations, metabolism, or clinical efficacy other than the two brief reports.[46, 63, 76] In both clinical reports the drug was effective in dogs uncontrolled with other medication. It was necessary to use paramethadione in conjunction with primidone in one case.[76] No toxic effects were observed other than vomiting, which could be controlled by administering the drug with food. Hepatic and renal diseases were listed as contraindications.

Further clinical trials and pharmacodynamic studies are needed to define the role of these drugs in veterinary medicine.

Succinamides (Ethosuximide). The succinamides are also used for absence attacks in humans. Some data are available on the pharmacokinetics of ethosuximide in dogs (Table 10–6).[31] The author has not found reports of its use in clinical veterinary medicine. The long half-life and excellent bioavailability make ethosuximide a potentially useful drug in dogs if it has efficacy against generalized tonic-clonic seizures.

Carbamazepine. Pharmacodynamic studies and limited clinical trials indicate that carbamazepine is not useful in dogs, the only species other than humans evaluated.[30, 31, 46] In limited clinical trials, there has been no benefit from this drug. There is one report of liver failure following use of carbamazepine.

Benzodiazepines (Diazepam). The benzodiazepines include diazepam, clonazepam, and lorazepam. The use of diazepam in the treatment of status epilepticus has been reported frequently. It has not been used for chronic control of epilepsy except in rare instances, primarily in cats. The short duration of action is a major disadvantage. Longer acting benzodiazepines are available (e.g., clonazepam, lorazepam), but tolerance to their anticonvulsant effect develops within days to weeks.[31a]

Diazepam is also useful as a tranquilizer in epileptic animals that cannot be given the phenothiazepine-type tranquilizers.

Client Education

Client education about management of an epileptic animal is as important as selecting an appropriate treatment. If the drugs are not administered correctly, they will be ineffective.

Both the veterinarian and the owner should agree on what constitutes successful therapy. Seizures are rarely completely eliminated. If the seizures have been occurring for an extended period of time, the probability of being able to discontinue medication is low. Successful treatment means that seizures are reduced in frequency and that they are less severe. Complete elimination of seizures may be possible, but it should not be expected.

In primary generalized epilepsy the possibility of inheritance should be discussed. For this reason, and because of the effect of estrogens on seizure threshold, neutering should be considered, especially in females.[69]

The plan for administration of medication should be clearly explained. The owner must be certain that the animal actually gets the medication and that it is given according to the proper schedule. Every animal responds individually to medication; finding the correct drug, dose, and schedule may take time, especially if the seizures are not frequent. Medication must be given continuously, not just when seizures occur. Any change in medication must be done slowly. Normal animals on anticonvulsants may have a seizure if medication is withdrawn suddenly.[34] The medication must be given long enough to reach its steady state before deciding it is ineffectual. Even then, blood levels should be measured to assure that an adequate dose is being used.[42]

The owner should know that stimulants, such as amphetamines, and phenothiazine derivatives, such as tranquilizers, lower the seizure threshold.

Care of the animal during a seizure should be discussed. Preventing the animal from injuring itself on surrounding objects or steps is usually all that is necessary. Forcible restraint and placing objects in the mouth to prevent biting the tongue are not of benefit and may be dangerous. If a seizure lasts more than 3 minutes, the animal should be taken to a veterinarian.

The decision to start the animal on medication must be made by the owner with the advice of the veterinarian. The author currently uses the following guidelines: An animal having only one seizure is examined carefully. If there is no evidence of disease the owner is advised to observe carefully for signs of additional seizures. If the animal has had more than one seizure, the minimum data base is completed. If findings are negative, anticonvulsant medication is recommended. Early treatment to prevent seizures reduces the odds of seizures occurring with increasing fequency. Each seizure makes additional seizures more likely (see Pathophysiology).

Ultimately, the decision to use anticonvulsants must be made by the owner. If daily administration of medication is more of a prob-lem than seizures at infrequent intervals, he or she is unlikely to comply, especially with large animal clients. A Saint Bernard that lives in an apartment and has seizures once a week is obviously more of a problem than a small dog that stays outside and only has seizures once every 6 months. The veterinarian can make a recommendation based on good medical practice, but the owner is faced with the real problem.

Status Epilepticus

Status epilepticus is the condition of recurring seizures without periods of consciousness between the seizures. *Clusters* of seizures are several in a relatively short time (e.g., 1 day) but with some normal periods between seizures. Animals that have clusters of seizures may need immediate attention, because they can progress to status epilepticus. Animals in status epilepticus are a true emergency. The repeated seizures can cause permanent brain damage or death.[54, 61]

Successful management of status epilepticus includes stopping the seizures, maintaining homeostasis, and finding the cause, if possible.

Stop the seizures. Diazepam, 10 to 50 mg (0.05–0.4 mg/kg in large animals) intravenously in 10 mg boluses, should be administered and repeated as needed. Diazepam often stops the seizures, at least temporarily, without anesthetizing the animal. If diazepam is ineffective pentobarbital is usually given intravenously (3–15 mg/kg) to effect. Intravenous administration of phenobarbital has been recommended, but its effect is often delayed. Phenobarbital is used for all subsequent injections as the animal recovers from the initial dose of pentobarbital. Ultrashort barbiturates and phenothiazine tranquilizers are not used because they potentiate seizure activity. Xylazine, glyceryl guaiacolate, and phenobarbital are probably of use in large animals.

Maintain ventilation. As soon as the seizures are controlled, adequate ventilation must be assured. If the animal is unconscious or anesthetized, an endotracheal catheter is inserted and ventilation controlled with oxygen administration. Ventilation is critical to prevent brain deterioration.

Establish a venous catheter. Easy access to a vein will be needed to administer further medication and to draw blood samples. A blood sample should be obtain immediately for a profile. Serum calcium and blood glucose levels should be determined as rapidly as possible. A lactated Ringer's drip maintains patency of the vein.

Give 50% dextrose (2–3 ml for toy dogs and cats, 50 ml for giant breed dogs). Hypoglycemic seizures are not common, but the dextrose will not hurt. Hypoglycemia usually causes depression in horses.[50] Young food animals may be given 2 to 3 ml/kg of body weight.

Ruminants should be given thiamine intravenously in 0.5 to 1 g doses, repeated several times in 24 to 48 hours.[14, 20]

Give calcium intravenously if there is reason to suspect hypocalcemia, such as heavy lactation. The heart rate is monitored carefully during calcium administration.

Evaluate the patient. Once the seizures are under control, ventilation is adequate, blood samples have been submitted, and glucose is given, a careful history and examination should be completed. The history is most important because a meaningful neurologic examination cannot be done. If a specific cause, such as toxicity, can be identified specific treatment is started.

Monitor body temperature. Seizures generate considerable muscle energy. If the temperature reaches 105°F, the animal should be cooled with ice to a temperature of 103°F. The temperature is then maintained in a normal range.

Continue to control the seizures. As the animal recovers, intravenous phenobarbital is administered until oral medication can be used. The normal movements of recovery from anesthesia should not be mistaken for seizures.

Successful management of an animal in status epilepticus is a challenge but can be rewarding.

NARCOLEPSY

Narcolepsy is a pathologic disorder of the sleep mechanism of the brain.[92] Four aspects are described in humans: excessive daytime sleepiness, cataplexy, sleep paralysis, and hypnagogic hallucinations. Sleep paralysis and hypnagogic hallucinations are subjective phenomena that cannot be described in animals. Excessive sleeping and cataplexy have been demonstrated in animals with narcolepsy. Cataplexy is sudden loss of muscle tone resulting in collapse of the animal.

Pathophysiology

Normal sleep patterns in dogs include two components, rapid eye movement (REM) and nonrapid eye movement (NREM) sleep. NREM sleep consists of light slow wave sleep and deep slow wave sleep. Studies using EEG and EMG recordings have defined the normal patterns of sleep in the dog (Table 10–8).

Periods of REM sleep during the normal sleep cycle usually start after about 90 minutes of NREM sleep and recur intermittently thereafter.[88] The narcoleptic animal has REM sleep without the preceding NREM sleep.

Monoaminergic neurons of the reticular formation are responsible for normal sleep mechanisms. Biochemical studies indicate that narcoleptic dogs have a decreased concentration and turnover of serotonin, a decreased turnover of norepinephrine, and a decreased concentration of dopamine.[2] Cholinergic mechanisms have been implicated in cataplexy.[21]

Incidence

The frequency of narcolepsy in the population of dogs or other animals is unknown. It was first described in animals in 1973 and numerous cases have been seen in various parts of the

Table 10–8. BEHAVIORAL AND ELECTROENCEPHALOGRAPHIC FEATURES OF STATES OF CONSCIOUSNESS IN THE DOG[88]

State of Consciousness (%)	Behavior	EEG Features
Wakefulness (43–46%)	All normal behaviors	Low voltage–mixed frequency
Light slow wave (NREM) sleep (17–21%)	Lying on ventral surface or on side, eyes closed	Higher voltage, at least one 10–14 Hz spindle/30 sec
Deep slow wave (NREM) sleep (23–28%)	Lying on ventral surface or on side, eyes closed	High voltage–slow waves (4Hz). Spindle usually present
REM sleep (11–13%)	Postural muscles are atonic. Occasional fasciculation of distal and facial muscles. Eyes may be partially open, rapid eye movements present	Low voltage–mixed frequency
Cataplexy in narcoleptics (0.1–25%)	Collapses in any position. Muscles atonic	Low voltage–mixed frequency (similar to REM sleep)

*Percentage of time spent in that state.

world since then.[7, 19, 37, 38, 53] Narcolepsy has been noted most often in dogs, but there are reports of several affected horses and ponies, one bull, and a cat.[2, 21, 53, 62, 78, 83]

Etiology

Narcolepsy has been reported in humans following head injury or encephalitis, but most cases are idiopathic.[92] Breeding trials by a group of scientists studying sleep at Stanford University indicate genetic transmission of the trait in Doberman pinschers and Labrador retrievers.[2, 27] It appears to be an autosomal recessive mode of transmission in the Doberman pinscher. Studies in other breeds, including beagles and miniature poodles, have yielded negative results to date.

Diagnosis

Although electroencephalographic and electromyographic studies have been useful in defining the syndrome, they are not necessary for diagnosis.[27] These tests may be helpful for eliminating other disorders, however.

The diagnosis can be established by observation of the animal during normal activity and provocative testing. Severely affected animals have cataplectic episodes frequently. Food usually elicits cataplectic attacks. This may be used as a test by providing several small bites of food and observing for the attack. Foutz et al describe a quantitative food provocation test.[27] Mildly affected animals may be tested with physostigmine. Physostigmine salicylate, 0.05 to 0.1 mg/kg, increases the frequency of cataplectic attacks in 5 to 15 minutes. Low doses should be used initially to avoid side effects of salivation and diarrhea. Atropine can be given if these occur.

Narcolepsy must be differentiated from epilepsy and episodic weakness caused by neuromuscular disease. The cataplectic attacks are not accompanied by autonomic activity, such as salivation, defecation, and urination, whereas epileptic seizures usually are. The musculature is flaccid, whereas tonic-clonic muscular activity occurs in convulsions. Myasthenia can be ruled out by repetitive electric stimulation of a nerve or by use of peripherally acting anticholinesterase drugs (see Chapter 14). Animals with narcolepsy have normal serum electrolyte levels.

Treatment

Narcolepsy is an incurable disorder. Treatment is designed to reduce the severity of the problem. Owners must understand that treatment must be continued for the life of the animal and it will probably not totally eliminate the cataplectic episodes.

Treatment may be aimed at decreasing the excessive somnolence or the cataplectic episodes or both. Somnolence is not a severe problem in most pets, so most effort is directed at reducing cataplexy.

General stimulants, such as methylphenidate (Ritalin, 0.25 mg/kg), also reduce cataplexy. It is beneficial for short-term therapy but appears to lose its effect over time. The tricyclic antidepressants, such as imipramine (Tofranil) and protriptyline (Vivactil), may also be effective. A starting dose for imipramine is 0.05 mg to 1 mg/kg three times daily. Imipramine causes impotency in the human male.[2, 27]

Monoamine oxidase inhibitors, such as pargyline and phenelzine, were once used in humans but have been discontinued because of serious cardiovascular effects. Narcoleptic dogs are also susceptible to these effects, so this group of drugs is not recommended.[2]

As in the selection and use of anticonvulsant drugs in epilepsy, treatment of narcoleptic animals must be individualized. The appropriate combination of drugs, dose, and dosage schedule must be determined for each animal.[60] Treatment of a narcoleptic quarter horse has been described by Sweeney.[83] This horse responded to imipramine in a manner similar to that of dogs. Intravenous imipramine at a dose of 0.5 mg/kg relieved cataplexy for an average of 5 hours. Oral administration was less predictable. A trial of dextroamphetamine appeared to suppress cataplectic attacks in a 2 month old Shetland pony, although the colt was still subject to attacks of sleepiness.[22]

REFERENCES

1. Atkeson FW, Ibsen HL, and Eldridge E: Inheritance of an epileptic type character in Brown Swiss cattle. J Hered 34:45, 1944.
2. Baker TL, Mitler MM, Foutz AS, and Dement WC: Diagnosis and treatment of narcolepsy in animal. In Kirk RW (ed): Current Veterinary Therapy VIII. Philadelphia, WB Saunders Co, 1983.
3. Barlow RM: Morphogenesis of cerebellar lesions in bovine familial convulsions and ataxia. Vet Pathol 18:151, 1981.
4. Barlow RM, Linklater KA, and Young GB: Familial

convulsions and ataxia in Angus calves. Vet Rec 83:60, 1968.

5. Barthold SW, Kaplan BJ, and Schwartz A: Reversible dermal atrophy in a cat treated with phenytoin. Vet Pathol 17:469, 1980.

6. Biefelt SW, Redman HC, and McClellan RO: Sire and sex-related differences in rates of epileptiform seizures in a purebred beagle dog colony. Am J Vet Res 32:2039, 1971.

7. Blauch BS, and Cash WC: A brief review of narcolepsy with presentation of two cases in dog. J Am Anim Hosp Assoc 11:467, 1975.

8. Breitschwerdt EB, Breazile JE, and Broadhurst JJ: Clinical and electroencephalographic findings associated with ten cases of suspected limbic epilepsy in the dog. J Am Anim Hosp Assoc 15:37, 1979.

9. Bunch SE: Anticonvulsant drug therapy in companion animals. In Kirk RW (ed): Current Veterinary Therapy VIII. Philadelphia, WB Saunders Co, 1983.

10. Bunch SE, Baldwin BH, Hornbuckle WE, and Tennant BC: Compromised hepatic function in dogs treated with anticonvulsant drugs. JAVMA 184:444, 1984.

11. Bunch SE, Castleman WL, Hornbuckle WE, and Tennant BC: Hepatic cirrhosis associated with long-term anticonvulsant drug therapy in dogs. JAVMA 181:357, 1982.

12. Campbell CL: Primidone intoxication associated with concurrent use of chloramphenicol. JAVMA 182:992, 1983.

13. Casey WC, and Blauch BS: Jaw snapping syndrome in eight dogs. JAVMA 175:709, 1979.

14. Chrisman CL: Epilepsy and seizures. In Howard JL (ed): Current Veterinary Therapy: Food Animal Practice. Philadelphia, WB Saunders Co, 1981.

15. Chrisman CL: Problems in Small Animal Neurology. Philadelphia, Lea & Febiger, 1982.

16. Croft PG: Fits in dogs: A survey of 260 cases. Vet Rec 77:438, 1965.

17. Croft PG: Fits in the dog. Vet Rec 88:118, 1971.

18. Cunningham JG, Haidukewych D, and Jensen HA: Therapeutic serum concentrations of primidone and its metabolites, phenobarbital and phenylethylmalonamide, in epileptic dogs. JAVMA 182:1091, 1983.

19. Darke PGG and Jessen V: Narcolepsy in a dog. Vet Rec 101:117, 1977.

20. deLahunta A: Veterinary Neuroanatomy and Clinical Neurology, 2nd ed. Philadelphia, WB Saunders Co, 1983.

21. Delashaw JB Jr, Foutz A, Guillemnault C, and Dement WC: Cholinergic mechanisms and cataplexy in dogs. Exp Neurol 66:745, 1979.

22. Dreifuss FE, and Flynn DV: Narcolepsy in a horse (letter). JAVMA 184:131, 1984.

23. Falco MJ, Barker J, and Wallace ME: The genetics of epilepsy in the British Alsatian. Small Anim Pract 15:685, 1974.

24. Farnbach GC: Seizures in the dog. Part I. Basis, classification, and predilection. Comp Cont Ed Pract Vet 6:569, 1984.

25. Farnbach GC: Serum concentrations and efficacy of phenytoin, phenobarbital, and primidone in canine epilepsy. JAVMA 184:1117, 1984.

26. Farnbach, GC: Efficacy of primidone in dogs with seizures unresponsive to phenobarbital. JAVMA 185:867, 1984.

27. Foutz AS, Mitler MM, and Dement WC: Narcolepsy. Vet Clin North Am Small Anim Pract 10:65, 1980.

28. Frey HH, Gobel W, and Loscher W: Pharmacokinetics of primidone and its active metabolites in the dog. Arch Int Pharmacodyn 242:14, 1979.

29. Frey HH and Loscher W: Clinical pharmacokinetics of phenytoin in the dog. Am J Vet Res 41:1635, 1980.

30. Frey HH and Loscher W: Pharmacokinetics of carbamazepine in the dog. Arch Int Pharmacodyn 243:180, 1980.

31. Frey HH and Loscher W: The dog as a model in epilepsy research: Comparative pharmacokinetics. Vet Res Commun 7:307, 1983.

31a. Frey HH, Loschen W: Pharmacokinetics of anti-epileptic drugs in the dog: A review. J Vet Pharmacol Ther 8:219, 1985.

32. Gastaut H: Clinical and electroencephalographical classification of epileptic seizures. Epilepsia (Suppl) 10:512, 1969.

33. Hoerlein BF: Canine Neurology, 3rd ed. Philadelphia, WB Saunders Co, 1978

34. Holliday TA: Seizure disorders. Vet Clin North Am 10:3, 1980.

35. Holliday TA, Cunningham JG, and Gutnick MJ: Comparative clinical and electroencephalographic studies of canine epilepsy. Epilepsia 11:281, 1971.

36. Jennings PB, Utter WF, and Fariss BL: Effects of long-term primidone therapy in a dog. JAVMA 164:1123, 1974.

37. Katherman AE: A comparative review of canine and human narcolepsy. Comp Cont Ed Pract Vet 2:818, 1980.

38. Knecht CD, Oliver JE, Redding R, et al: Narcolepsy in a dog and a cat. JAVMA 162:1052, 1973.

39. Knecht CD, Sorjonen DC, and Simpson ST: Ancillary tests in the diagnosis of seizures. J Am Anim Hosp Assoc 20:455, 1984.

40. Kowalczyk DF and Beech J: Pharmacokinetics of phenytoin (diphenylhydantoin) in horses. J Vet Pharmacol Ther 6:133, 1983.

41. Kutt H: Interactions of antiepileptic drugs. Epilepsia 16:393, 1976.

42. Kutt H: Anticonvulsant blood levels in the management of epileptic patients. Clin Neuropharm 3:1, 1978.

43. Lawson DC and Kay WJ: Seizures. In Ettinger SJ: Textbook of Veterinary Internal Medicine, 2nd ed. Philadelphia, WB Saunders Co, 1983.

44. Lennox WG: Epilepsy and Related Disorders. Boston, Little, Brown & Co, 1960.

45. Loscher W: Serum protein binding and pharmacokinetics of valproate in man, dog, rat, and mouse. J Pharmacol Exp Ther 204:255, 1978.

46. Loscher W: A comparative study of the protein binding of anticonvulsant drugs in serum of dog and man. J Pharmacol Exp Ther 208:429, 1979.

47. Loscher W: Plasma levels of valproic acid and its metabolites during continued treatment in dogs. J Vet Pharmacol Ther 4:111, 1981.

48. Loscher W and Esenwein H: Pharmacokinetics of sodium valproate in dog and mouse. Arznemittalforsch 28:782, 1978.

49. May CJ and Greenwood RES: Recurrent convulsions in a thoroughbred foal: Management and Treatment. Vet Rec 101:76, 1977.

50. Mayhew IG: Seizure disorders. In Robinson NE (ed): Current Therapy in Equine Medicine. Philadelphia, WB Saunders Co, 1983.

51. McDonald RL and McLean MJ: Cellular bases of barbiturate and phenytoin anticonvulsant drug action. Epilepsia 23 (Suppl 1):S7, 1982.

52. Meyer DJ and Noonan NE: Liver tests in dogs receiving anticonvulsant drugs (diphenylhydantoin and primidone). J Am Anim Hosp Assoc 17:261, 1981.

53. Mitler MM, Soave O, and Dement WC: Narcolepsy in seven dogs. JAVMA 168:1036, 1976.

54. Montgomery DL, and Lee AC: Brain damage in the epileptic beagle dog. Vet Pathol 20:160, 1983.

55. Nafe LA, Parker A, and Kay WJ: Sodium valproate: A preliminary clinical trial in epileptic dogs. J Am Anim Hosp Assoc 17:131, 1981.

56. Nash AS, Thompson H, and Bogan JA: Phenytoin toxicity: A fatal case in a dog with hepatitis and jaundice. Vet Rec 100:280, 1977.

57. Oliver JE: Protocol for the diagnosis of seizure disorders in companion animals. JAVMA 172:822, 1978.

58. Oliver JE Jr: Seizure disorders in companion animals. Comp Cont Ed Small Anim Pract 2:77, 1980.

59. Oliver JE Jr and Hoerlein BF: Convulsive disorders of dogs. JAVMA 146:1126, 1965.

60. Oliver JE Jr and Lorenz MD: Handbook of Veterinary Neurologic Diagnosis. Philadelphia, WB Saunders Co, 1983.

61. Palmer AC: Pathological changes in the brain associated with fits in dogs. Vet Rec 90:167, 1972.

62. Palmer AC, Smith GF, and Turner SJ: Cataplexy in a Guernsey bull. Vet Rec 106:421, 1980.

63. Parker AJ: A preliminary report on a new anti-epileptic medication for dogs. J Am Anim Hosp Assoc 11:437, 1975.

64. Pasten TJ: Diphenylhydantoin in the canine: Clinical aspects and determinations of therapeutic blood levels. J Am Anim Hosp Assoc 13:247, 1977.

65. Pedersoli WM, Redding RW, and Nachreiner RF: Blood serum concentrations of orally administered diphenylhydantoin in dogs and pharmacokinetic values after an intravenous injection. J Am Anim Hosp Assoc 17:271, 1981.

66. Penry JK and Porter RJ: Epilepsy: Mechanisms and therapy. Med Clin North Am 63:801, 1979.

67. Prince DA: Neurophysiology of epilepsy. Annu Rev Neurosci 1:395, 1978.

68. Rossdale PD and Leadon D: Equine neonatal disease: A review. J Reprod Fertil (Suppl) 23:685, 1975.

69. Rosciszewaka D: Analysis of seizure dispersion during menstrual cycle in women with epilepsy. Epilepsy: A Clinical and Experimental Research. Monogr Neural Sci 5:280, 1980.

70. Rost DR and Baker R: Gingival hyperplasia induced by sodium diphenylhydantoin in the dog: A case report. Vet Med Small Anim Clin 73:585, 1978.

71. Roye DB, Serrano EE, Hammer RH, and Wilder BJ: Plasma kinetics of diphenylhydantoin in dogs and cats. Am J Vet Res 34:947, 1973.

72. Russo ME: The pathophysiology of epilepsy. Cornell Vet 71:221, 1981.

73. Sanders JE and Yeary RA: Serum concentrations of orally administered diphenylhydantoin in dogs. JAVMA 172:153,1978.

74. Sanders JE, Yeary RA, Fenner WR, and Powers JD: Interaction of phenytoin with chloramphenicol or pentobarbital in the dog. JAVMA 175:177, 1979.

75. Sanders JE, Yeary RA, Powers JD, and deWet P: Relationship between serum and brain concentrations of phenytoin in the dog. Am J Vet Res 40:473, 1977.

76. Schulman J: Epileptic seizures controlled with paramethadione/primidone. Vet Med Small Anim Clin 76:827, 1981.

77. Schwartz-Porsche D, Loscher W, and Frey HH: Treatment of canine epilepsy with primidone. JAVMA 181:592, 1982.

78. Sheather AL: Fainting in foals. J Comp Pathol Ther 37:106, 1924.

79. Skinner SF, Robertson LT, Artro M, and Gerding RK: Longitudinal study of phenobarbital in serum, cerebrospinal fluid, and saliva in the dog. Am J Vet Res 41:600, •1980.

80. Snead OC: On the sacred disease: The neurochemistry of epilepsy. Int Rev Neurobiol 24:93, 1983.

81. Solomon GE, Hilgartner MW, and Kut H: Phenobarbital induced coagulation defects in cats. Neurology 24:920, 1974.

82. Spehar AW, Hill MR, Mayhew IG, and Hendeles L: Preliminary studies on the pharmacokinetics of phenobarbital in the neonatal foal. Equine Vet J 16:368, 1984.

83. Sweeney CR, Hendricks JC, Beech J, and Morrison AR: Narcolepsy in a horse. JAVMA 183:126, 1983.

84. Tobin T, Dirdjosudjono S, and Baskin SI: Pharmacokinetics and distribution of diphenylhydantoin in kittens. Am J Vet Res 34:951, 1973.

85. Van der Velden A: Fits in Tervuern shepherd dogs: A presumed hereditary trait. J Small Anim Pract 9:63, 1968.

86. Wallace ME: Keeshonds: A genetic study of epilepsy and EEG readings. J Small Anim Pract 16:1, 1975.

87. Ward AA, Penry JK, and Purpura DP (ed): Epilepsy, Research Pub: Assoc Res Nerv Mental Dis, vol 61. New York, Raven Press, 1983.

88. Wauquir A, Verheyen JL, Van Den Broeck WAE, and Janssen PAJ: Visual and computer-based analysis of 24H sleep-waking patterns in the dog. EEG Clin Neurophys 46:33, 1979.

89. Wilder BJ and Bruni J: Seizure Disorders: A Pharmacological Approach to Treatment. New York, Raven Press, 1981.

90. Woodbury DM, Kemp JW, and Chow SU: Mechanisms of actions of antiepileptic drugs. In Ward AA, Penry JK, Purpura DP (ed): Epilepsy, Research Pub: Assoc Res Ner Mental Dis, vol 61. New York, Raven Press, 1983.

91. Yeary RA: Serum concentrations of primidone and its metabolites, phenylethylmalonamide and phenobarbital, in the dog. Am J Vet Res 41:1643, 1980.

92. Zarcone V: Narcolepsy. N Engl J Med 288:1156, 1973.

Chapter 11

IR Griffiths, BVMS, PhD, FRCVS

Central Nervous System Trauma

Central nervous system trauma is a frequent occurrence and results in a wide variety of clinical problems, ranging from minor signs to paralysis, loss of consciousness, and death. It provides both a diagnostic and a management challenge to the clinician, which is reinforced by the need to make correct decisions quickly in most circumstances. The major subdivisions of brain and spinal cord injuries will be discussed.

BRAIN INJURIES

Pathology and Pathophysiology

Brain trauma following head injury is usually associated with road traffic accidents, falls, kicks, running into stationary objects, or occasionally penetrating missile injuries. Injury can also cause skull fractures, which may be linear (nondisplaced) or depressed. The latter are likely to produce contusion of the underlying brain. It must be emphasized that severe or fatal brain damage can occur in the absence of skull fracture and, conversely, minimal brain damage can be present in cases with fractures. Various experimental studies in primates[1, 2] have established the importance of angular acceleration of the head in producing brain trauma, particularly those forms unassociated with fractures. Under certain conditions it was possible to regularly reproduce a type of damage known as diffuse axonal injury (see below) without any object striking the skull, ie, purely the effect of angular acceleration.

Brain trauma may be focal or diffuse and can be immediate (ie, at the time of injury) or delayed. Immediate damage commonly takes the form of contusions and/or brain stem hemorrhage. Contusions are usually superficial on the cerebral gyri and vary from multiple petechiae to larger confluent hemorrhages with necrosis and edema.[22] They are sometimes classified as *coup* injuries, occurring under the area of impact, and *contrecoup*, occurring in a diametrically opposite location. Small contusions are probably of little significance in determining the prognosis.

Brain stem hemorrhages, especially in the midbrain and pons, are not uncommon[35] and range from multifocal petechiae to large confluent hemorrhages (Fig. 11–1). The brain tissue, particularly in the central tegmentum, is often necrotic with fibrinoid necrosis and/or thrombosis of parenchymal vessels (Fig. 11–2). If large, the necrotic area is replaced in time by a cyst. In humans and primates brain stem hemorrhages may be part of diffuse axonal injury, in which numerous axonal retraction balls are present throughout the white matter. Diffuse axonal injury is a major cause of severe brain damage in humans[1] but it is not known whether it occurs in dogs and if the brain stem hemorrhages referred to above[35] are part of this phenomenon. Lesions within the brain stem commonly involve areas of the ascending reticular activating system and are likely to produce disturbances of consciousness, including stupor and coma. Other vital centers controlling respiration and cardiovascular functions are located in the pontomedullary portion of the reticular formation. Consequently, brain stem injury is potentially serious.

Concussion is a term used to imply an immediate but brief loss of consciousness unasso-

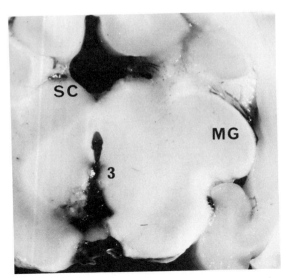

Figure 11–1. Coronal slice through midbrain of a dog involved in a road traffic accident 3 weeks previously. The animal had been comatose/stuporous for 1 week with mid-position fixed pupils. Complete consciousness was never recovered. A central hemorrhagic area extends ventrally from the cerebral aqueduct. 3, Position of oculomotor nucleus; MG, medial geniculate body; SC, rostral (superior) colliculus.

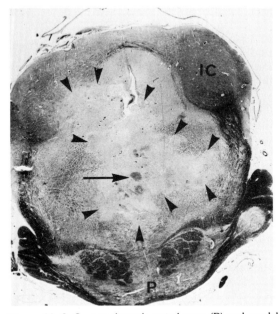

Figure 11–2. Section through rostral pons (P) and caudal (inferior) colliculus (IC) from a dog that died without regaining consciousness 2 days after a dog fight. Small hemorrhages (arrow) are evident in the central tegmentum, some of which are associated with necrotic vessels. The pale area (outlined by arrowheads) is completely necrotic. The area of hemorrhagic necrosis extended rostrally to involve the oculomotor nucleus, causing fixed dilated pupils.

ciated with gross structural damage. The mechanisms of production and underlying cellular pathologic changes are uncertain, but it is thought that the difference between temporary and more serious, permanent damage is one of degree rather than completely separate pathologic forms.

Delayed brain damage takes the form of intracranial hematomas or generalized brain swelling and may be complicated by the development of shifts of brain tissue and herniation. Epidural and subdural hematomas are relatively rare. Although some hemorrhage may occur, this seldom progresses to an expanding mass lesion and brain compression. Following any trauma to the brain there is a degree of local edema with swelling mainly resulting from extravasation of plasma from "leaky" blood vessels.[5] This is termed vasogenic edema. After some injuries a more diffuse brain swelling can arise, affecting one or both hemispheres and causing a rise in intracranial pressure.

Hypercarbia and hypoxia cause cerebral vasodilation and can result from depressed respiration or a partially occluded airway after trauma. If there was brain damage with some degree of swelling, concurrent vasodilation would result in a further increase in intracranial pressure. Raised intracranial pressure is extremely important in humans but its incidence in animals with brain trauma is unknown as pressure is rarely monitored continuously. One serious, and often fatal, complication of raised intracranial pressure caused by brain swelling or an expanding hematoma is shifts of brain tissue, the most important of which is the tentorial hernia. The ventral portion of the occipital lobe herniates through the tentorial opening, compressing the brain stem and oculomotor nerve (Fig. 11–3) and causing parenchymal hemorrhage in the midbrain. The situations leading to tentorial herniation are inevitably serious and life-threatening and the herniation itself usually fatal.

Clinical Signs

There may be evidence of injury to the head with lacerations, bruising, and so on. Deformities of the zygomatic, frontal, or parietal crests suggest an underlying fracture. Particular note should be made of the patency of the airway, especially if the animal is unconscious. The usual post-traumatic checks for shock and thoracic, abdominal, and limb injuries must be

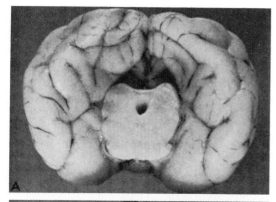
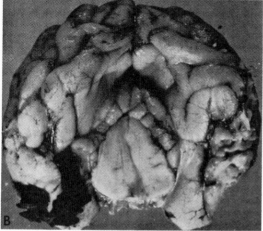

Figure 11–3. Slice through midbrain (looking rostrally) leaving cerebral hemispheres unsectioned. A, Normal brain showing open cerebral aqueduct and relationship of medial occipital lobe to the midbrain. B, Bilateral tentorial herniation (due to severe cerebral edema). The medial occipital lobe has herniated through the tentorial incisure, causing compression and distortion of the midbrain with obliteration of the mesencephalic aqueduct. (From Oliver JE Jr: Neurologic emergencies in small animals. Vet Clin North Am 2:341 , 1972.)

made. Shock or anoxic hypoxia can markedly exacerbate signs of brain trauma.

The clinical signs of brain damage may be focal or diffuse. Full details of performing the neurologic tests are given in Chapter 2, but an outline is presented below. The state of consciousness both at the time of examination and in the intervening period from the injury must be known. Most injured animals are either hyperexcitable, or conversely, lethargic and apathetic. However, excessive drowsiness, stupor, and coma following injury are indicative of brain trauma. Stupor and coma may be due to diffuse hemispheric damage but are more likely to result from brain stem injury. It is important to

know if the state of consciousness is static, worsening, or improving. Vision; the equality, size, and reactivity of the pupils; the position of the eyeballs; and the ability to induce vestibular nystagmus by rotating the head (if neck trauma is not suspected) should be assessed (see Chapter 2). Palpebral, corneal, and swallowing reflexes should be tested. Muscle tone, local limb reflexes, and conscious pain perception can also be examined. If possible, motor function and proprioception should be tested.

A wide variety of post-traumatic syndromes are possible; the commoner are described below.

Hemispheric damage to the cerebral cortex or subcortical white matter may cause loss of consciousness if diffuse, but this is usually temporary. It is more likely for subsequent signs to reflect a lateralization. The animal commonly circles to the affected side and shows mild paresis and proprioceptive defects in the contralateral limbs. If the optic radiation is involved a contralateral homonymous hemianopia with intact photomotor reflexes is present. Contralateral facial hypalgesia may be detected. Such injuries may also cause loss of training and personality changes, which are noted at a later stage. Focal injury, particularly to the motor cortex, commonly following depressed cranial fractures may lead to post-traumatic epilepsy, which can occur some time (weeks or months) after the injury.

Brain stem injuries are invariably serious. Commonly, there is disturbed consciousness often causing stupor or coma, which is usually present from the time of impact.[35] The main localizing signs are indicated in Table 11–1. Of particular importance in the diagnosis are the size and reactivity of the pupils, the muscle tone, and the presence or absence of vestibular eye movements. The exact combination of signs will vary with the location and extent of the damage as indicated in Table 11–1. Compression of the brain stem may also occur as a result of tentorial herniation due to an expanding mass (eg, hematoma) or diffuse brain swelling in the rostrotentorial compartment. The signs usually indicate a progressive dysfunction with a deteriorating level of consciousness and loss of pupillary light reflexes with dilated pupils. Decerebrate rigidity occurs, followed terminally by flaccidity and failing respiration (Tables 11–2 and 11–3). The major differentiating features of brain stem injury and compression due to herniation are listed in Table 11–4.

Head injury can damage the cerebellovestibular system (ie, the cerebellum, areas of me-

Table 11–1. SIGNS CHARACTERISTIC OF FOCAL BRAIN STEM INJURY AT ONE LEVEL

Level	Consciousness	Pupils	Eye Movement	Motor Function	Autonomic Responses
Diencephalon	Apathy to stupor	Small but reactive	Normal	Hemiparesis to tetraparesis	Normal to Cheyne-Stokes respiration
Midbrain	Stupor to coma	Bilaterally dilated or midposition unresponsive	Ventrolateral strabismus bilateral	Decerebrate rigidity	Hyperventilation (variable)
Pons	Coma	Midposition unresponsive	Vestibular eye movements absent	Decerebrate rigidity to paralysis	Rapid shallow respiration, loss of micturition reflex
Medulla	Coma	Midposition dilated terminally	Absent	Paralysis with decreased muscle tone	Irregular to apnea

Modified from Oliver JE Jr: Intracranial injury. *In* Kirk RW: Current Veterinary Therapy VII. Philadelphia, WB Saunders Co, 1980.

dulla associated with the vestibular nuclei and their projections, and the peripheral vestibular receptors).[38] The exact combination of clinical signs will vary with the extent of the damage. There may be predominantly cerebellar signs, usually indicating a unilateral rather than a diffuse lesion. Typically the animal shows truncal ataxia with loss of equilibrium, swaying, and falling to one side. Ipsilateral ataxia takes the form of limb hypermetria and dysmetric head movements. Tremor is not so commonly seen following head injury. Involvement of the flocculonodular lobe of the cerebellum or its vestibular connections can result in nystagmus. Because of the acute onset, the effects of trauma on the cerebellum are similar to those of surgical ablation (see Holliday[25] for a review of this subject).

Other cases may indicate combined cerebellovestibular damage. A unilateral syndrome is characterized by a gross disturbance of equilibrium with falling and a head tilt to the damaged side. If the animal can stand it adopts a wide based stance. Spontaneous horizontal nystagmus away from the affected side and an ipsilateral downward strabismus are usual. There is often hemiparesis, proprioceptive defects, and loss of the hopping reflex ipsilaterally. Disturbances in body tone cause the animal to curve to the affected side when held off the ground in a head-down, vertical position. Cerebellar dysfunction is indicated by dysmetria of the limbs and often the head and neck. Vision and pupillary light reflexes are intact, and consciousness is not impaired. Other cranial nerves such as CN V and CN VII may also be involved if the brain stem is damaged.

Although not strictly brain trauma, head injury can result in damage to the receptors of the utriculus, sacculus, and semicircular canals located in the petrous temporal bone, producing a peripheral type of vestibular dysfunction. The animal is severely imbalanced, falling to the affected side and exhibiting an ipsilateral

Table 11–2. SIGNS CHARACTERISTIC OF PROGRESSIVE UNILATERAL TENTORIAL HERNIATION

Level	Consciousness	Pupils	Eye Movements	Motor Function	Autonomic Responses
CN III	Normal to stupor	Ipsilateral dilation	Normal to slight lateral strabismus	Normal to hemiparesis	Normal
Rostral midbrain	Stupor	Ipsilateral to bilateral dilation	Ipsilateral ventrolateral strabismus	Hemiparesis, ipsi- or contralateral	Normal
Caudal midbrain	Coma	Dilated bilaterally to fixed midposition	Ventrolateral strabismus to fixed midposition	Decerebrate rigidity	Hyperventilation
Pons	Coma	Midposition unresponsive	Vestibular eye movements absent	Paralysis	Rapid shallow respirations
Medulla	Coma	Midposition, dilated terminally	Absent	Paralysis	Irregular to apnea, pulse slowing

From Oliver JE Jr and Lorenz MD: Handbook of Veterinary Neurologic Diagnosis. Philadelphia, WB Saunders Co, 1983.

Table 11–3. SIGNS CHARACTERISTIC OF PROGRESSIVE BILATERAL TENTORIAL HERNIATION

Level	Consciousness	Pupils	Eye Movements	Motor Function	Autonomic Responses
Early diencephalic	Apathy	Small but reactive	Normal	Hemiparesis	Normal to irregular response
Late diencephalic	Stupor	Small but reactive	Normal	Hemiparesis to tetraparesis	Cheyne-Stokes respiration
Midbrain	Coma	Dilated bilaterally	Poor vestibular eye movements	Decerebrate rigidity	Hyperventilation
Pons	Coma	Midposition unresponsive	Vestibular eye movements absent	Flaccid paralysis	Rapid, shallow response
Medulla	Coma	Midposition, dilated terminally	Absent	Flaccid paralysis	Irregular to apnea, pulse slowing

From Oliver JE Jr and Lorenz MD: Handbook of Veterinary Neurologic Diagnosis. Philadelphia, WB Saunders Co, 1983.

head tilt. There is spontaneous horizontal nystagmus to the contralateral side and an ipsilateral downward strabismus. Hopping and placing reactions and proprioception are usually intact. Damage to the postganglionic sympathetic fibers passing through the petrosal bone in small animals will produce an ipsilateral Horner's syndrome. The motor component of CN VII can be involved also, causing a facial paralysis (Figs. 11–4 and 11–5). Examination of the external ear may reveal hemorrhage in the external auditory meatus.[10] Epistaxis from hemorrhage into the guttural pouch in horses may also be evident.

Temporal Relationship of Signs. In the majority of cases the signs are at their most severe within a short time of the injury. A worsening

Table 11–4. COMPARISON OF ACUTE BRAIN STEM INJURY WITH TENTORIAL HERNIATION FOLLOWING HEAD INJURY

	Brain Stem Injury	Tentorial Herniation
Onset	Early	Delayed
Course	Static to progressive	Progressive
Pupil dilation	Constricted early, dilated late	Unilateral dilation, progressing to bilateral dilation
Consciousness	Stuporous to comatose	Alert or apathetic, progressing to coma
Muscle tone	Decerebrate rigidity or paralysis	Normal or weak, progressing to decerebrate rigidity and then to flaccid paralysis
Cranial nerve and spinal reflexes	Usually symmetric	Often unilateral asymmetry

From Oliver JE Jr and Lorenz MD: Handbook of Veterinary Neurologic Diagnosis. Philadelphia, WB Saunders Co, 1983.

clinical state usually indicates a hematoma (unusual) or brain swelling, either of which can lead to tentorial herniation. Prolonged impaired consciousness with no improvement, or incomplete return of mental status, suggests a brain stem lesion. Cases with cortical or subcortical damage or cerebellovestibular injury often show marked improvement over a period of time. The most marked recovery usually occurs within 3 to 4 weeks and can be remarkable, particularly in young animals.

Diagnosis

This is usually straightforward and is based on evidence of brain dysfunction in an animal known to have suffered an injury. Lack of a history of head injury does not rule it out, however, especially in large animals. Almost invariably some signs are present immediately after the trauma. Skull fracture can be diagnosed radiographically, although it may be impossible to position the animal satisfactorily without anesthesia or sedation. This is usually undesirable, particularly when the information from plain radiographic examination may not be essential in the management of the case.

Differential Diagnosis

This is not usually a problem except when the presumed trauma was not actually observed or when signs develop some time after a known incident. Owners often relate signs of illness to known events, such as injuries that have occurred some time previously and may have no connection with the animal's current problem. Other conditions causing stupor and coma include metabolic encephalopathies such as

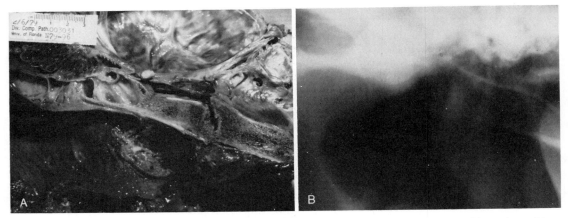

Figure 11–4. A, Basilar skull fractures, such as this one through the junction of the basioccipital and basisphenoid bones and the petrosal bones, occur in horses that fall over backwards, striking their occipital protuberance. Signs will include evidence of vestibular and facial nerve abnormalities and degrees of depression, tetraparesis, and other cranial nerve involvement if the medulla oblongata is traumatized. B, Confirmation of such fractures on radiographs can be difficult as shown by the radiograph of the basilar skull region of the same horse. (Courtesy I. G. Mayhew.)

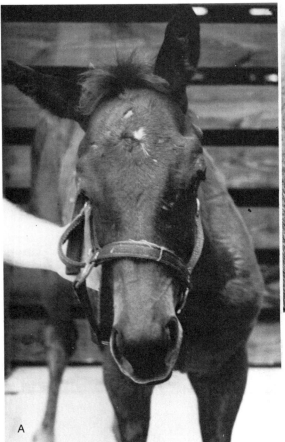

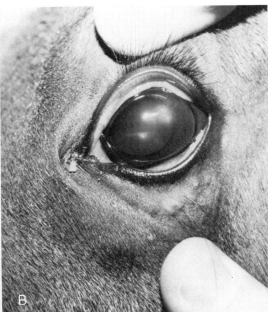

Figure 11–5. A, This foal suffered head injury and probably fractured the right temporal bone. There was a period of unconsciousness with bleeding from the right ear and nose. On recovery of consciousness, the foal was depressed and evidenced a right head tilt, ventral deviation of right eye, and right facial paresis. Often horses will recover from such a syndrome if they retain vision to help in accommodating to the vestibular system deficit. B, This foal, however, had also damaged both optic nerves as they exit the calvarium within the optic foramen, resulting in blindness with dilated pupils that were unresponsive to light. The signs of vestibular damage persisted and traumatic lesions were detected in the right facial and vestibulocochlear nerves and in both optic nerves at postmortem examination. (Courtesy I. G. Mayhew.)

hypoglycemia and hyperammonemia or intoxications from substances such as barbiturates (see Chapter 8). These conditions can be diagnosed by the appropriate biochemical or toxicologic tests.

Cases of cerebellovestibular injury should be differentiated from idiopathic vestibular syndrome when signs of medullary involvement such as paresis, loss of hopping or placing reactions, depression, and cerebellar signs are absent[13, 36] (see Chapter 14).

Cerebrovascular accidents (CVA), such as ischemic encephalopathy of cats and strongyle thromboembolism or intracarotid injections in horses (see Chapter 7), occur infrequently. However, in the absence of a proper history, they could be difficult or impossible to differentiate from some cases of cerebral trauma. These conditions have an acute onset and can have similar signs. External evidence of injury or cardiovascular signs in CVA may not be present. Fortunately, the treatment for both conditions is likely to be similar.

Treatment

In all instances, but particularly when the patient is unconscious, airway patency must be established. Blood, saliva, and so on must be cleared from the oropharynx by swabs or suction. Pulling the tongue forward may relieve respiratory obstruction in unconscious animals. If this fails an endotracheal tube can be inserted to alleviate any upper airway problems. When there is pharyngeal or laryngeal trauma a tracheotomy tube can be inserted to maintain the airway. Oxygen should be administered unless it is established that the animal is not hypoxic. Some authorities also recommend hyperventilation[16] to reduce arterial pCO_2 and promote cerebral vasoconstriction and reduction in intracranial pressure. Arterioles within damaged areas are usually unresponsive to changes in pCO_2, but the procedure can be used in unconscious animals in an attempt to limit brain swelling, provided a ventilator is available.

As some degree of brain edema, either focal, or as a more generalized swelling, occurs in all brain trauma cases with clinical signs, glucocorticosteroids should be administered intravenously as soon as possible. Further details of the rationale are given under Spinal Cord Injuries and in Chapter 15. A soluble glucocorticoid, such as methylprednisolone sodium succinate (10 mg/kg three times daily) is recommended as the initial treatment. Dimethyl sulfoxide (DMSO; 1 gm/kg, 10% in D5W, IV, b.i.d.) is recommended in large animals. Betamethasone or dexamethasone (1 to 2 mg/kg) may be substituted after the first treatment. If the animal is improving, glucocorticoids may be stopped to avoid side effects. If the condition of the animal is worsening despite glucocorticoid or DMSO therapy, then mannitol should be given, though not in animals in shock.[40] Such deteriorating cases must be monitored for developing tentorial herniation. It is unlikely that animals with severe brain stem trauma from the time of injury will respond to any treatment.

Plasma expanders, blood, and crystalloid solutions should be given for shock as indicated. Unconscious animals and those with severe nonneural injuries will require fluid maintenance, and an intravenous catheter should be placed in any animal requiring prolonged medication. Antibiotics need only be given in animals with open wounds or that remain unconscious, particularly if endotracheal tubes or urinary catheters are inserted.

If the stuporous or comatose animal is to be maintained, nutrients must be given in addition to fluid maintenance. If the animal can be roused it may swallow material placed in its mouth. This must be done carefully to avoid aspiration. If the procedure is impossible, a stomach tube can be passed to allow various purées, custards, milk products, forage slurries, or commercial foods to be administered.

In the majority of cases treatment is medical. Surgery is indicated if there is evidence of developing herniation and in these cases must be an emergency procedure (see Chapter 18). Surgery is also indicated for the elevation of depressed skull fractures (Chapter 18) but should be performed when the general and neurologic condition will permit anesthesia.

Because of the risk of focal seizures in dogs it is wise to place them on prophylactic anticonvulsants for a period of 4 to 6 weeks. Any other animals that develop seizures should also be treated (see Chapter 10). A résumé of the management of head injuries is given in Table 11–5.

Prognosis

This depends on the severity of the immediate brain damage and the development of any secondary complications, such as brain hernias.

Those with mild signs, brief or no loss of

Table 11–5. MAJOR STEPS IN THE MANAGEMENT OF ACUTE HEAD INJURY

Procedure	Purpose
1. Brief clinical examination	Determine shock, non-neural trauma, and patency of airway
2. Clear airway obstruction if present	Maintain brain oxygenation
3. Initial neurologic examination	Check consciousness, pupil size, and reactivity and position of eyeballs. Assess muscle tone and motor function if applicable
4. Give high dose glucocorticosteroids IV (and/or DMSO IV in large animals)	Reduce local traumatic edema and help prevent brain swelling
5. Move to clinic and monitor	Determine if condition is improving, stable, or worsening
6. Possible radiography but not if necessary to anesthetize for positioning	Check for skull fractures

If condition worsens with indication of herniation consider surgery. Otherwise management is likely to be medical.

consciousness, and a generally improving clinical status usually have an excellent prognosis. Cases with focal cerebrocortical and subcortical injuries are usually included in this category, although the tendency to circle may continue for several weeks and highly trained working dogs may lose some of their training. Cerebellovestibular injuries also tend to improve, although some residual dysfunction is likely. It is virtually impossible to be precise in the prognosis at the initial assessment, but the majority of functional recovery will have occurred in 3 to 4 weeks.

Most cases of brain stem injury have a poor prognosis, particularly if there is a prolonged period of stupor or coma. Although some improvement may well occur, a satisfactory recovery is unlikely. Long-term maintenance of stuporous or comatose animals is not usually attempted. The longer the period of impaired consciousness without improvement, particularly if other signs of brain stem dysfunction are present, the poorer is the prognosis. A 1 week period would be a reasonable time in such circumstances, and with no change in the clinical status the owner could be advised of the unlikely recovery.

Cases showing worsening of signs, particularly those of brain stem compression, must be given a poor to bad prognosis.

SPINAL CORD INJURIES

Pathology and Pathophysiology

Types of Injury

Most, but not all, spinal cord injuries result from, or are concurrent with, vertebral damage. Trauma to the vertebral column can cause fractures, dislocations, combined fractures and dislocations, and traumatic disc protrusions (in small animals). Vertebral fractures may result in gross separation of the two major fragments (transverse fracture) or compression of the centrum so that its length is reduced. In immature animals epiphyseal separations are not uncommon. The odontoid process of the axis may be fractured from the body. The cervical region is more frequently involved than the thoracolumbar region in adult large animals (Fig. 11–6 and 11–7).

Luxations follow tears of the anulus fibrosus, with involvement of the dorsal diarthrodial joints. Displacement of the vertebrae may be maintained or a degree of reduction may occur. Depending on the degree of initial displacement, the various vertebral ligaments may also be ruptured. Atlantoaxial subluxation may occur with trauma but is often associated with underlying congenital deformities (see Chapter 6).

Traumatic disk protrusion is the forcible and rapid compression of an intervertebral disk at the time of injury, resulting in rupture of the anulus fibrosus and the almost explosive ejection of the nucleus. This usually occurs in a dorsomedian or dorsolateral position, causing spinal cord injury.

In young animals the nucleus pulposus is of a gel-like consistency (not degenerate) and is found lying in the extradural space.

It is important to recognize that severe spinal cord injury can occur in the absence of any bony, diskal, or ligamentous damage. This form of injury may be called spinal cord concussion,[26] but the terminology should not necessarily imply a mild or temporary dysfunction.

Pathologic Changes of the Spinal Cord

No standard pathologic changes occur in spinal cord injuries; similar vertebral injuries can cause vastly different spinal cord lesions.

Complete anatomic severance of the spinal cord and meninges may occur in some fractures or luxations, but it is more common for the dura to remain intact, even if the enclosed nervous tissue has been lost at the site of

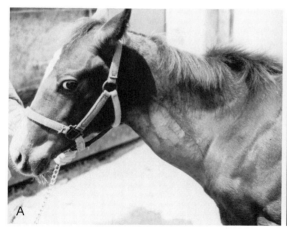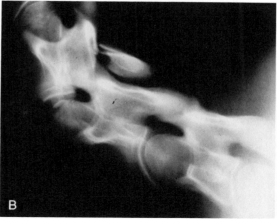

Figure 11–6. A, This 4 month old quarter horse filly was found with a deformed neck and weakness 3 days after being weaned. Tetraplegia developed over several days. B, Radiographs revealed fractured C4 and C5 vertebrae with a traumatic laminectomy of C4. The filly improved with antiinflammatory therapy and 18 months later has a normal gait, slightly deformed neck, and fused C4 and C5 vertebrae on radiographs. (Courtesy I. G. Mayhew.)

damage, so that the spinal cord resembles a tube whose contents have been squeezed out. The commonest type of spinal cord lesion associated with trauma is necrosis, which may be total or subtotal within the transverse plane of a segment. Hemorrhage is usually found within both the spinal cord and the meninges, and thrombosed vessels are not uncommon. Sometimes the necrosis is localized to a vascular territory and constitutes an infarct. The extent and severity of necrosis tends to be more severe when a static compression (from a fracture or luxation) is maintained compared with those cases in which the compression is only transient.[19]

Transient spinal cord compression, usually due to subluxation followed by a degree of reduction, constitutes a form of impact injury and is often associated with a central hemorrhagic necrosis, which is most severe in the gray and central white matter. The peripheral white matter tends to be better preserved (Fig. 11–8).

Traumatic disk protrusions cause an impact injury rather than a maintained compression of the cord as the nucleus disperses along the extradural space. Histologically the spinal cord may show any of the changes described above. In the cervical area it is common for the protrusion to be dorsolateral in location, causing a heminecrosis of the cord.[17]

Pathogenesis of the Spinal Cord Lesion

Although the study of naturally occurring spinal cord trauma is useful, it provides little

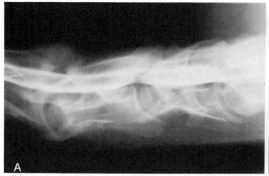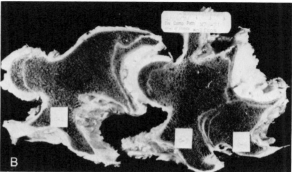

Figure 11–7. Equine cervical vertebrae that are fractured and then heal can remodel to a great degree. A young thoroughbred colt broke its neck 12 months previously. The colt became tetraplegic over several weeks, and radiographs revealed six vertebral bones in the neck. A, In fact, C5 and C6 had fused to become one bone, and remodeled bone and soft tissue were demonstrated by myelography to be compressing the spinal cord between C4 and the fused C5–C6 vertebral bone. B, A dorsal view of a dorsal plane section of the vertebrae shows C5 and C6 fused into one bone.

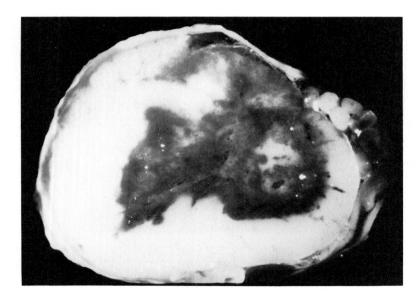

Figure 11–8. C2 segment of spinal cord from a dog that fractured the axial body 2 days previously. The most severe damage is located in the central areas of the spinal cord. This type of lesion is typical of transient impact injuries. (From Griffiths IR: Spinal cord injuries: A pathological study of naturally occurring lesions in the dog and cat. J Comp Pathol 88:303, 1978.)

information on the development of the lesion, as the damage is established by the time necropsy is performed. Experimental studies have provided information on the early events,[11] and some aspects of these are reviewed here. A commonly used model of impact injuries employs a small weight dropped from a known height on to the exposed dura. The resultant lesion is more severe in the center of the cord and closely resembles the natural form illustrated in Figure 11–8. Other models have used focal clipping of the cord or vertebral distraction to mimic various natural injuries. (Experimental spinal cord compression caused by extradural balloons are more relevant to mass lesions and will not be considered here.)

The sequence of events is initiated at the time of impact, although changes will evolve temporally. Immediately on impact there is hemorrhage and extravasation of plasma, mainly from vessels in the gray matter. These events are augmented by the hypertensive episode that accompanies spinal cord injury.[4]

Much of the gray matter and central white matter rapidly becomes necrotic,[6] probably as the result of a severe reduction in spinal cord blood flow.[18] Leakage of plasma continues at a declining rate over several hours and spreads centrifugally and longitudinally, constituting what is termed vasogenic edema.[21] In addition to this protein-rich fluid, there is a more gradual and persistent edema with raised water content and elevated sodium ion and decreased potassium ion concentrations.[31, 34]

In the more severely injured white matter, axonal swellings (retraction balls or reactive axons)[9] appear within 3 hours and many fibers have periaxonal swellings.[7, 14] In less severely involved areas, fibers commonly show either partial or full thickness demyelination.[20]

Reactive changes develop quickly with infiltrates of hematogenous cells, initially neutrophils and then increasing numbers of monocytes, which will act as macrophages. Vascular proliferation occurs, and the central necrotic area breaks down to form a cyst. Connective tissue increases, initially in the perivascular spaces and pia, but in more severe lesions can become extensive.

Reparative changes also occur. Remyelination is evident by 3 weeks.[20] Regenerating axonal sprouts are also found within the spinal cord; however, many of these derive from injured dorsal nerve root fibers. Although intrinsic spinal cord neuronal fibers are capable of regeneration, this seldom becomes a marked feature. Regeneration within the CNS has been reviewed by Berry.[8] Recent experimental studies to promote regeneration have used peripheral nerve grafts to replace the irreparably damaged spinal cord segments.[29, 30]

Clinical Signs

As the majority of affected animals have been involved in severe injury, problems other than those directly related to the spinal cord may be present. These can include thoracic or abdominal injuries, fractures of bones other than the vertebrae, and hypovolemic shock. Generalized shock can exacerbate the signs of primary neurologic damage. It is, therefore, essential in relation to both the differential diagnosis and assessment of the neurologic damage to perform a full examination.

Fractures or dislocation of the thoracic or lumbar vertebrae may produce external evidence of vertebral malalignment.

The neurologic signs of spinal cord injury depend principally on the location and severity of the damage, so that a range of clinical signs is possible. Pain is frequently present and may be severe, particularly in the acute injury. Indeed, in some instances, such as odontoid fractures, pain may be the major or only sign. However, pain is not usually a feature of traumatic disk protrusions.[17]

The following clinical categories of spinal cord injury apply best to the dog, although they are pertinent to all species. In large animals, the evaluation of spinal reflexes, limb tone, and areas of hypalgesia in recumbent patients is difficult and hinders precise localization of the lesion.

Cranial Cervical Segments (C1–C5). Motor signs are typically upper motor neuron (UMN) in nature and commonly affect both thoracic and pelvic limbs, producing quadriplegia or paresis. In impact injuries causing a predominantly central spinal cord lesion (as discussed in Pathology and Pathogenesis) the weakness may be more severe in the thoracic limbs because the motor tracts to the thoracic limbs lie more centrally than those to the pelvic limbs. Cervical dorsolateral disk protrusions or infarctions typically produce hemiplegia or asymmetric tetraplegia.

Cranial cervical trauma causing tetraplegia usually causes an adult large animal to have difficulty raising its head and neck off the ground. Therefore, it often remains in lateral recumbency, as opposed to a sternal position. Local cervical and cervicofacial reflexes are often disrupted.

Sympathetic dysfunction may be manifest by Horner's syndrome and/or skin hyperthermia. It is more usual to recognize ipsilateral dysfunction, particularly with dorsolateral disk protrusions or infarctions. Bladder dysfunction may be present but is not usually found in the case of dorsolateral disk protrusions. Loss of conscious pain sensation is unusual, as spinal cord trauma of such magnitude is likely to cause respiratory failure. Damage of respiratory pathways to the phrenic nucleus (C6) and intercostal muscle lower motor neurons with resultant apnea is the most likely cause of death in these patients.

Special cervical problems are the dorsolateral traumatic disk protrusion, odontoid fractures, and atlantoaxial subluxations. The clinical findings of the disk injury are almost pathognomonic. These are ipsilateral hemiplegia or asymmetric tetraplegia, sympathetic dysfunction (as above), and positional dystonia in which limb tone is normal when the animal is lying on the affected side, but extensor tone increases markedly when it is turned to the unaffected side. Neck pain is not a feature, and bladder control and pain sensation are usually intact.[17] Infarctions produce a similar syndrome (see Chapter 7).

With odontoid fractures and atlantoaxial subluxations, pain is often the predominant sign and motor signs are minimal or absent.

Cervical Enlargement (C6–T1). Damage to these segments typically results in a lower motor neuron (LMN) type of lesion in the thoracic limbs and an upper motor neuron (UMN) type in the pelvic limbs. Different muscle groups in the thoracic limbs may be more severely affected depending on the segmental involvement. Sympathetic dysfunction, Horner's syndrome, and skin hyperthermia (with sweating horses) are commonly seen. If segments C8 and T1 are involved the panniculus reflex is absent on one or both sides. Bladder control may or may not be lost, depending on the severity of the injury. Affected recumbent horses may lift their heads and necks from the ground but usually cannot remain sternal.

Cranial Thoracic Segments (T2–T4/5). Motor function may well be retained in the thoracic limbs, although a Schiff-Sherrington phenomenon is commonly seen in dogs, particularly those with more severe damage. The pelvic limbs usually demonstrate an upper motor neuron type of motor loss. Horner's syndrome is not present, but skin hyperthermia (and sweating in horses) may be found caudal to the lesion. The panniculus reflex is lost at the caudal border of the last intact dermatome. Bladder control may be absent and conscious pain sensation lost below the lesion. Although the phrenic nucleus is functional these animals commonly demonstrate paradoxic respiration due to intercostal muscle paralysis. A dog-sitting posture will frequently be seen with severe thoracolumbar lesions in large animals.

Remainder of Thoracic Segments and Cranial Lumbar Segments (T4/5–L3). This area of the spinal cord is most frequently affected by injury in dogs. Animals typically demonstrate an upper motor neuron type of dysfunction in the pelvic limbs with a loss of panniculus reflex at the caudal border of the last intact derma-tome, provided the lesion is cranial to L1 seg-ment. Caudal to L1 segment the panniculus reflex is intact. Skin hyperthermia of the hind-quarters may also be present, particularly with more cranial segment damage. With damage caudal to about T13–L1 segment this effect becomes much less noticeable or absent. Blad-der control and pain sensation may also be lost.

Lumbosacral Cord (L4 to Caudal Segments). Damage to these segments produces either lower motor neuron or combined upper and lower motor neuron dysfunction of the pelvic limbs, anus, and tail. Nerve roots are commonly involved in addition to the spinal cord (see Chapter 14). Loss of the anal reflex, loss of bladder control, and sensory loss of a dermato-mal type in the limbs are likely with damage to this area.

The possible variations of clinical signs due to lesions in this area are complex (for further details, see Chapter 14).

Effect of Time on Clinical Signs

Although the effect of spinal shock tends to be minimal in domestic animals compared with primates, it is common for hyporeflexia to occur below acute, severe injuries for a period of hours (rarely for a few days). This is most often seen with thoracolumbar lesions producing de-pressed pedal and patellar reflexes and hypo-tonia in the pelvic limbs and is seldom found with minor cord injuries. Hyporeflexia associ-ated with the acute lesion is usually followed by hyperreflexia after a short interval (usually a few days).

Animals with chronic, severe spinal injuries may demonstrate other late onset signs such as mass reflexes and reflex walking (spinal walk-ing).

In the vast majority of instances the maximum severity of dysfunction occurs immediately or within a short time of injury. In severe cases there may be no obvious improvement with time, but many animals with mild injuries show some restitution of function (even without treat-ment). Occasionally the severity of signs wors-ens with time. This feature is usually associated with unstable fractures or subluxations allowing continued damage to the spinal cord or caused by ascending-descending hemorrhagic myelo-malacia (see Chapter 7). Exuberant callus for-mation can result in progression of spinal cord compression weeks to months following verte-bral trauma. This does appear to occur with cervical injury in horses somewhat frequently.

Diagnosis and Differential Diagnosis

The clinical signs described above will indi-cate the location of the lesion and provide information on the severity of the damage. In the majority of instances the clinical examina-tion will not identify the cause of the problem, although with a dorsolateral cervical disk pro-trusion the clinical syndrome may be quite distinctive. Ancillary examinations such as ra-diography are required.

An animal presenting with a spinal cord prob-lem after known or presumed injury is likely to have spinal cord trauma. The conditions to be considered are the following:
1. Vertebral fractures.
2. Vertebral luxations and subluxations.
3. Combined fractures and luxations.
4. Traumatic disk protrusions.
5. Spinal cord concussion.

In the vast majority of instances plain radiog-raphy will positively identify conditions 1, 2, 3, and 4. A lateral position will usually suffice for the diagnosis, occasionally a ventrodorsal view is also required, but no other diagnostic test is usually necessary for these conditions.

In spinal cord concussion or infarction no significant abnormality will be seen on plain radiography. Myelography is not usually under-taken for the diagnosis of conditions 1, 2, 3, and 4; although if decompressive surgery is contemplated, it might be used to define the site and extent of spinal cord compression. Myelography will almost invariably indicate a blockage of the subarachnoid space, due to cord swelling, in the case of spinal cord concussion.

Examination of cerebrospinal fluid is not gen-erally indicated for diagnostic purposes. Sam-ples may be grossly normal or slightly blood tinged to xanthochromic, depending on the time interval from the injury. Gross subarach-noid hemorrhage is not common following trauma. Results of routine laboratory examina-tion of CSF may again be normal or show mild increases in levels of cells and protein.

The history and radiologic findings usually suffice for differential diagnosis, but occasionally other diseases must be considered. These are necessarily conditions with acute onset of signs and include the following:
6. Spinal cord infarction and ischemia.
7. Spontaneous intramedullary and sub-arachnoid hemorrhage.
8. Degenerative disk protrusions.
9. Vertebral collapse due to neoplasia, in-fection, or osseous dystrophies.
10. Aortic and/or iliac thromboembolism.

11. Parasitic thromboembolism and infarction.

12. Some peracute infections.

Spinal cord infarction (see Chapter 7) cannot be positively diagnosed clinically, but there is not usually a history of injury and the animal is not painful. Infarction can be differentiated from conditions 1, 2, 3, and 4 by the absence of plain radiographic findings. Myelography is likely to be normal in infarction, allowing differentiation from cord concussion.

Spontaneous intramedullary and subarachnoid hemorrhage (see Chapter 7) is not usually associated with trauma. Severe pain and sometimes pyrexia may be present. Plain radiographic findings are normal, and diagnosis is made by demonstrating blood in CSF.

The neurologic signs caused by degenerative disk protrusions at the thoracolumbar junction may be preceded by a period of spontaneous pain. Severe trauma is not usually implicated in the etiology, and the majority can be positively diagnosed by plain radiography.

Vertebral collapse (pathologic fractures) can be caused by neoplasia (either primary or secondary), osteomyelitis, or osseous dystrophies. The collapse can occur spontaneously or be associated with mild trauma. In all three conditions the neurologic signs may be preceded by spontaneous pain. Systemic signs may be seen with neoplasia or osteomyelitis (see Chapters 7 and 9). Osseous dystrophies, which will also affect bones other than vertebrae, are likely to be seen in growing animals but may be associated with primary hyperparathyroidism (see Chapter 8).

Thromboembolism of the aorta or its major branches can produce peracute paraplegia or paraparesis and most often occurs in cats, and occasionally in dogs and horses. In dogs and horses, the condition may produce exercise induced paresis, pain, and stiffness of the pelvic limbs. For further details consult Chapter 7, but it is worth emphasizing that in every case of acute onset pelvic limb neurologic disease the presence or absence of the femoral pulses should be determined.

Parasitic thromboembolism, with or without parasite migrations, can produce acute onset of spinal cord disease with or without progression of signs (see Chapter 7). At times, peracute infectious processes affecting the spinal cord can mimic traumatic spinal cord injury. Two examples of this are equine protozoal myeloencephalitis and equine herpesvirus I myelitis (see Chapter 7).

Other conditions are occasionally confused with spinal cord trauma. Acute onset polyneuropathies and myopathies, in particular, must be excluded from the diagnosis (see Chapter 14). Bilateral limb fractures, pelvic fractures (with or without sciatic nerve dysfunction), and bilateral acute cranial cruciate ligament ruptures can all superficially resemble paraplegia caused by spinal cord trauma. These conditions can be excluded by a thorough physical examination.

Assessment of the Severity of Spinal Cord Injury

This is an extremely important judgment based largely on the clinical findings. Basically, the spinal cord serves to transmit information between somatic and visceral organs and the brain. The white matter conducts impulses in a longitudinal direction. The gray matter acts, in part, as a distribution center for information to and from the periphery. Certain areas of gray matter, those in the cervical and lumbar enlargements supplying limbs, bladder, and respiratory muscles, in particular, are of greater importance than those supplying neck or abdominal wall musculature, which usually have a multiple innervation.

In estimating the severity of damage, these aspects must be appreciated. Examination of motor function, bladder control, and various sensory modalities can be used to assess the conducting ability of white matter. Table 11–6 indicates how these functions can be used to grade the severity of the injury to white matter. The Schiff-Sherrington phenomenon, usually

Table 11–6. ESTIMATION OF THE SEVERITY OF DAMAGE TO WHITE MATTER BASED ON CLINICAL ASSESSMENT OF ITS CONDUCTING ABILITY

	Group	Function Tested	Result	Prognosis
Increasing severity of damage	1	Motor function below lesion	Paresis	Good
	2	Motor function below lesion	Paralysis	Good
	3	Motor function below lesion	Paralysis	Guarded
		Bladder control*	Loss	
	4	Motor function below lesion	Paralysis	Very poor
		Bladder control*	Loss	
		Conscious pain sensation below lesion	Absent	

*May be difficult to assess in acute lesion.

found with cranial thoracic lesions, is often associated with more severe spinal cord damage.[15]

Recent work in acute experimental spinal cord trauma in cats has shown that the results of spinal evoked potentials (SEP) correlate closely with the degree of clinical recovery. From this work and from research in progress, the spinal evoked potentials may be a prognostic aid when the clinician must decide whether prompt surgery has a reasonable chance of success in a compressive cord injury.[24a]

Grading of gray matter damage is more variable but depends mainly on the degree of denervation of the structures supplied from the affected segments. Impairment of motor function, depression of local spinal reflexes, and the eventual development of muscle atrophy are the major clinical signs. As the majority of muscles are innervated from more than one segment, paralysis of a group usually indicates involvement of several segments and implies a severe injury.

Great care must be taken in any attempt to correlate radiologic appearances with severity of injury and prognosis. Although there is a general correlation between the degree of reduction in canal diameter and severity of cord injury,[15] the converse need not be true and severe cord injury can occur with no or minimal displacement. The degree of displacement on a radiograph represents the *least* displacement there has been.

Treatment

Treatment of acute spinal cord trauma may be medical, surgical, or a combination of both. Over the past decade a large number of experimental studies have examined therapies to reduce the rapid progression of the cord lesion. The results are somewhat confusing and difficult to apply to the clinical situation.

Many of these therapies have been based on the belief that various bioactive substances released or produced in injury (eg, noradrenaline or serotonin) were responsible for the progression of the lesion. The treatments have sought to nullify their effects. Other drugs have been used to decrease vascular permeability, decrease cord edema, maintain cellular integrity, or improve spinal cord blood flow. Among the drugs examined either singly or in combinations have been α-methyltyrosine, reserpine, levodopa,[37] phenoxybenzamine,[23] methysergide,[27] dimethyl sulfoxide (DMSO),[24, 28, 41] ϵ-aminoca-

proic acid (EACA),[41] vasodilators,[42] several hyperosmolar agents[24, 39] (eg, mannitol), and various glucocorticosteroids. It is probably true that the benefits advanced by one group have been denied by another. Although some of these drugs have been employed in clinical therapy,[32] the only group to be regularly used are the glucocorticosteroids.

GLUCOCORTICOSTEROIDS

These drugs[21, 24, 31, 47] have been the subject of numerous experimental studies and their role in veterinary neurology has been presented.[33] The main rationale for use in spinal cord injury has been to reduce post-traumatic edema. Other studies have indicated a role in preventing disturbances of certain electrolytes, such as potassium and calcium.[31] High doses of glucocorticosteroids have been reported to reduce or prevent the reduction of blood flow in white matter.[47] From these and other studies, it appears that they have a rational role in management of spinal cord trauma. Good clinical studies evaluating the use of these drugs in spinal cord trauma are scarce.

It is not uncommon for a clinical improvement to follow glucocorticosteroid therapy in cases with incomplete post-traumatic spinal cord lesions or compressions. One gains the impression that this is related to the therapy, but it is quite possible that an equal (if perhaps slower) recovery would have occurred without therapy. There appears little, if any, clinical evidence that glucocorticosteroid therapy will convert a previously irrecoverable injury into one that will recover.

Recent controlled studies in the treatment of acute experimental spinal cord trauma in the cat at L2 have shown a general lack of efficacy of mannitol, DMSO, naloxone, thyrotropin releasing hormone, and dexamethasone given 45 minutes after spinal cord trauma.[24, 24a] Cats that received these agents scored no better than untreated or saline treated controls. However, under the same experimental protocol, the use of the highly soluble and fast acting methylprednisolone sodium succinate produced a rapid sparing action on the spinal cord and the cats were generally ambulatory within a week after trauma.[24a]

These studies indicate that recovery will be enhanced and accelerated with the immediate administration of a highly soluble steroid such as methylprednisolone sodium succinate, 30 mg/kg divided into three daily doses, followed by diminishing doses for 10 days or after a few days substitution of diminishing doses of dexamethasone. Recent experimental work with cats also used a dose of methylprednisolone up to 30 mg/kg.[47] Highly utilizable glucocorticosteroids should be administered as soon as possible after trauma, prior to examination and other procedures.[24a]

SURGICAL TREATMENT

The reasons for surgery are to stabilize an unstable vertebral column and to decompress a compressed spinal cord. Surgical treatment is usually combined with therapy to reduce spinal cord swelling[32, 43] (see glucocorticosteroids above and Chapter 15). In the majority of instances, surgery should be performed as soon as possible, particularly in the more severe injuries. Experimental work has indicated that there is an inverse relationship between the severity of injury and the time for successful decompression.[45] The surgical techniques are described in Chapter 17.

Besides the stabilization and decompressive measures, myelotomy and hypothermic or normothermic perfusion of the spinal cord have also been advocated.[3, 46]

Diagnostic Plan for and Management of Suspected Acute Spinal Cord Injuries

Because the animal is likely to be in pain and frightened, steps should be taken to prevent anyone being bitten or injured by a violent struggling patient, and the animal must be handled gently.

Before any analgesics are administered, a clinical examination should be performed to determine other traumatic damage and shock. A rectal examination can usually be performed at this stage in large animals of suitable size. A limited neurologic examination will give some indication of the site and severity of any cord injury. Although it is unwise to encourage walking at this stage, it should be possible to gain some impression of whether motor function is present in the limbs and tail. Local limb reflexes and anal and panniculus reflexes can be rapidly checked and any area of skin hypersensitivity noted during the last procedure. Pain sensation should be tested from the feet and tail and the presence of paradoxic respiration or the Schiff-Sherrington phenomenon noted. The functional status of the bladder cannot usually be ascertained at this stage. An estimation of the site and the severity of the lesion is now possible.

At this stage analgesics can be given if necessary. Intravenous glucocorticosteroids (see above), and antibiotics if indicated, should be administered with blood or plasma expanders if necessary. The animal may now be moved on a rigid support, preferably without any bending or sudden jerks being applied to the vertebral column, for radiography. Details of radiologic diagnosis are given in Chapter 4. Radiographic quality may have to be sacrificed for patient well-being. The body should be manipulated as little as possible during radiography until any vertebral damage is defined. It is better not to anesthetize animals for radiography, as protective muscle spasm is abolished and further spinal cord trauma may occur.

Deciding on the Method of Treatment. Following the accurate diagnosis of the injury (see Diagnosis and Differential Diagnosis above) a decision regarding further treatment is made (see Treatment). Cases with complete functional loss (group 4, Table 11–6) are probably unlikely to respond to any treatment. There is a small possibility that in some of these cases the severe signs have been exacerbated by hypovolemic or spinal shock. Restoration of blood volume and the elapse of 24 hours will usually clarify the position. The continuation of complete functional loss confirms the poor prognosis.[15, 35] Any surgery or medical therapy should be undertaken only at the owner's insistence once he or she is fully aware of the facts. Most clinicians are aware of animals that recovered, but this should not detract from the generally gloomy outlook.

The major question is whether to operate on cases with incomplete cord lesions (ie, evidence of some remaining conduction across the site of damage). There are few published controlled studies comparing treatments of clinical injuries, and individual clinicians will tend to adopt procedures they believe produce good results. The major reasons for considering surgery have been presented above. There appears little point in operating on traumatic disk protrusions, as the damage constitutes an impact injury rather than compression and the vertebral column is not unstable. Similarly, cord concussion is unlikely to benefit from surgery.

Cases in which the clinical signs are worsening, usually due to persistent vertebral instability, require surgical stabilization. If instability can be demonstrated on initial examination, vertebral stabilization is also indicated to prevent further cord trauma and exacerbation of signs.

In the remaining cases, those with incom-

Table 11–7. MAJOR STEPS IN THE MANAGEMENT OF ACUTE SPINAL INJURIES

Procedure	Purpose
1. Brief clinical examination	Determine presence of shock and presence of non-neural trauma
2. Preliminary neurologic examination	Check for motor function, local reflexes, panniculus reflex, and pain sensation. Initial assessment of location and severity of injury
3. Administer high dose glucocorticosteroids IV. Give analgesics if necessary	Reduce cord edema, maintain cord blood flow, and stabilize cell and organelle membranes
4. Move animal to clinic and repeat (1) and (2) if necessary	
5. Radiography (plain) of vertebrae	Determine if vertebral or disk damage is present
6. In exceptional instance myelography and CSF examination may be necessary	If no obvious abnormality on plain radiography, ? cord concussion, ? vascular accident
By this stage clinician should know if there is cord injury or associated vertebral damage. The lesion should have been localized and its severity estimated.	
7. Decide on further management	Is surgical or medical therapy indicated?

plete cord lesions and with no definite vertebral instability demonstrated, the decision to operate or not becomes a personal judgment. Some clinicians would operate on the majority of such cases, particularly if some degree of compression is demonstrated radiographically. Experience has shown that many such cases will improve markedly or recover completely with medical and nursing therapy. A résumé of the management of spinal cord injuries is given in Table 11–7.

Prognosis of Spinal Cord Injuries. The prognosis is based on the severity of the initial injury and the time interval between injury and any improvement. It is, therefore, not a static determination but may need revision as developments do or do not occur. At the time of initial injury the presence or absence of conscious pain sensation is a good guide to the severity of most cord lesions.[35] (This parameter must be used with some care in caudal lumbosacral injuries affecting cord and/or nerve roots.) Animals with loss of pain sensation will probably fall into group 4 of Table 11–6, and the majority have an unfavorable prognosis for any reasonable recovery. Minor improvements and even recovery are occasionally seen in such cases, but the longer the time over which no improvement occurs, the more certain is the gloomy prognosis.

Developing a prognosis for the remaining cases, groups 1 to 3, can be difficult but the less severe the initial damage (ie, group 1) the better the prognosis.

Many cervical cord injuries have a reasonably good prognosis. The ratio of canal to cord diameter is greatest in the cervical region, so that a greater vertebral displacement can be tolerated. Animals with severe complete cervical injuries usually have a rapid demise, owing to respiratory failure, but in the remainder the outlook is generally good[12, 44] if the correct surgical or medical treatment is given.

In thoracic or lumbar injuries, one can be optimistic about good recoveries in groups 1 and 2 (Table 11–6). In group 3 one would have to give a cautious indication of recovery (50–60%) which may not be complete.

In all situations the parameters are checked at intervals and return or lack of return of functions may alter the prognosis accordingly. In general one would expect some clinical evidence of a returning function within about a 10 day period. For example, in a paraplegic dog in group 2, some evidence of motor function (not necessarily the ability to walk) would be expected within 10 days. The longer the time after this without return of that function, the poorer is the prognosis. Some recovery may still occur, but the longer the interval the less likely it is to be complete. Of necessity, prognosis can only be based on probabilities and most clinicians are aware of cases that astounded everyone by recovering against all the indications otherwise.

Nursing of Acute Spinal Injuries. Regardless of whether surgery is used, the nursing is of critical importance. Unnecessary movement is avoided, and with small patients it is helpful to have some firm but movable base to the bed so that the animal can be maneuvered in and out. Bed sores are a likely complication in paralyzed animals. To prevent this, regular turning and suitable bedding are required. A synthetic fleecy bedding causing minimum skin pressure and also allowing urine to pass through and maintain dryness is suitable for smaller patients. Skin ulceration can occur from urine scalds.

Regular turning also minimizes respiratory problems that may occur particularly in quadriplegic or paretic animals.

Care of Urinary Tract in CNS Trauma. In certain spinal cord or brain trauma cases, loss of bladder control may occur (see Chapter 13). If there is urinary retention, the bladder must be emptied. This can be done by manual pressure on the abdomen or by catheterization. Manual expression is usually satisfactory if it can be performed easily. In other cases or if urine scalding of the skin occurs a catheter must be used. It is probably best to place an indwelling catheter attached to the vulva or prepuce by a "sticky tape" butterfly and suture. Continuous drainage can then occur into a collecting system such as a discarded plastic fluid infusion set. Antibiotics must be given in these circumstances to prevent urinary tract infection. Such an arrangement prevents urine stasis and keeps the animal and bedding dry. If any slight leakage of urine causes wetting of the preputial or vulval area, scalding can be prevented by waterproofing with petrolatum.

REFERENCES

1. Adams JH, Gennarelli TA, and Graham DI: Brain damage in non-missile head injury: Observations in man and subhuman primates. *In* Thomas-Smith W and Cavanagh JB (ed): Recent Advances in Neuropathology 2. Edinburgh, Churchill Livingstone, 1982.
2. Adams JH and Graham DI: The pathology of blunt head injuries. *In* Critchley M, O'Leary JL, and Jennett B (ed): Scientific Foundations of Neurology. London, Heineman, 1972.
3. Albin MS, White RJ, Acosta-Rua G, et al: Study of functional recovery produced by delayed localised cooling after spinal cord injury in primates. J Neurosurg 29:113, 1968.
4. Alexander S and Kerr FWL: Blood pressure responses in acute compression of the spinal cord. J Neurosurg 21:485, 1964.
5. Bakay L, Lee JC, Lee GC, and Peng JR: Experimental cerebral concussion. Part 1. An electron microscopic study. J Neurosurg 47:525, 1977.
6. Balentine JD: Pathology of experimental spinal cord trauma. 1. The necrotic lesion as a function of vascular injury. Lab Invest 39:236, 1978.
7. Balentine JD: Pathology of experimental spinal cord trauma. 11. Ultrastructure of axons and myelin. Lab Invest 39:254, 1979.
8. Berry M: Regeneration in the central nervous system. *In* Thomas-Smith W and Cavanagh JB (ed): Recent Advances in Neuropathology. No 1. Edinburgh, Churchill Livingstone, 1979.
9. Bresnahan JC: An electron microscopic analysis of axonal alterations following blunt contusion of the spinal cord of the rhesus monkey (Macaca mulatta). J Neurol Sci 37:59, 1978.
10. Chrisman CL: Vestibular diseases. Vet Clin North Am 10:1, 1980.
11. Collins WF and Kauer JS: The past and future of animal models used for spinal cord trauma. *In* Popp AJ, Bourke RS, Nelson LR, and Kimelberg HK: Seminars in Neurological Surgery. Neural Trauma. New York, Raven Press, 1979.
12. Denny HR: Fractures of the cervical vertebrae in the dog. Vet Annu 23:236, 1983.
13. deLahunta A: Veterinary Neuroanatomy and Clinical Neurology. Philadelphia, WB Saunders Co, 1977.
14. Dohrmann GJ, Wagner FC, and Bucy PC: Transitory traumatic paraplegia: electron microscopy of early alterations in myelinated nerve fibres. J Neurosurg 36:407, 1972.
15. Feeney DA and Oliver JE Jr: Blunt spinal trauma in the dog and cat: Neurologic, radiologic and therapeutic correlations. J Am Anim Hosp Assoc 16:664, 1980.
16. Fenner WR: Seizures and head trauma. Vet Clin North Am Small Anim Pract 11:1, 1981.
17. Griffiths IR: A syndrome produced by dorso-lateral "explosions" of the cervical intervertebral discs. Vet Rec 87:737, 1970.
18. Griffiths IR: Spinal cord blood flow after acute experimental cord injury in dogs. J Neurol Sci 27:247, 1976.
19. Griffiths IR: Spinal cord injuries: A pathological study of naturally occurring lesions in the dog and cat. J Comp Pathol 88:303, 1978.
20. Griffiths IR and McCulloch MC: Nerve fibres in spinal cord impact injuries. Part 1. Changes in the myelin sheath during the initial 5 weeks. J Neurol Sci 58:335, 1983.
21. Griffiths IR and Miller RM: Vascular permeability to protein and vasogenic oedema in experimental concussive injuries to the canine spinal cord. J Neurol Sci 22:291, 1974.
22. Gurdjian ES and Gurdjian ES: Cerebral contusions: Reevaluation of the mechanism of their development. J Trauma 16:35, 1976.
23. Hedeman LS and Sil R: Studies in experimental cord trauma. Part 2: Comparison of treatment with steroids, low molecular weight dextran and catecholamine blockade. J Neurosurg 40:44, 1974.
24. Hoerlein BF, Redding RW, Hoff EJ, and McGuire JA: Evaluation of dexamethasone, DMSO, mannitol and solcoseryl in acute spinal cord trauma. J Am Anim Hosp Assoc 19:216, 1983.
24a. Hoerlein BF, Redding RW, Hoff EJ, and McGuire JA: Evaluation of naloxone, crocetin, thyrotropin releasing hormone, methylprednisolone, partial myelotomy, and hemilaminectomy in the treatment of acute spinal cord trauma. J Am Anim Hosp Assoc 21:67, 1985.
25. Holliday TA: Clinical signs of acute and chronic experimental lesions of the cerebellum. Vet Sci Commun 3:259, 1980.
26. Holmes G: The Goulstonian Lectures on spinal injuries of warfare. Br Med J 2:769, 1915.
27. Howitt WM and Turnbull IM: Effect of hypothermia and methysergide on recovery from experimental paraplegia. Can J Surg 15:179, 1972.
28. Kajihara K, Kawanago H, de la Torre JC, and Mullan S: Dimethylsulphoxide in the treatment of experimental acute spinal cord injury. Surg Neurol 1:16, 1973.
29. Kao-CC, Bunge RP, and Rejer PJ: Spinal Cord Reconstruction. New York, Raven Press, 1983.
30. Kao-CC, Chang LW, and Bloodworth JMB: Axonal regeneration across transected mammalian spinal cords. An electron microscopic study of delayed microsurgical nerve grafting. Exp Neurol 54:591, 1977.
31. Lewin MG, Hasenbout RR, and Pappius HM: Chemical characteristics of traumatic spinal cord edema in

cats. Effects of steroids on potassium depletion. J Neurosurg 40:65, 1974

32. Mendenhall HV, Litwak P, Yturraspe DJ, et al.: Aggressive pharmacologic and surgical treatment of spinal cord injuries in dogs and cats. JAVMA 108:1026, 1976.

33. Metz SR, Taylor SR, and Kay WJ: The use of corticosteroids for treatment of neurologic disease. Vet Clin North Am 12:1, 1982.

34. Nemecek St RP, Suba P, Rozsival V, and Melka O: Longitudinal extension of oedema in experimental spinal cord injury—evidence for two types of post-traumatic oedema. Acta Neurochirug 37:7, 1977.

35. Oliver JE Jr: Neurologic emergencies in small animals. Vet Clin North Am 2:341, 1972.

36. Oliver JE Jr and Lorenz MD: Handbook of Veterinary Neurologic Diagnosis. Philadelphia, WB Saunders Co, 1983.

37. Osterholm JL: The pathophysiological response to spinal cord injury. The current status of related research. J Neurosurg 40:5, 1974.

38. Palmer AC: Pathogenesis and pathology of the cerebellovestibular syndrome. J Small Anim Pract 11:167, 1970.

39. Parker AJ, Park RD, and Stowater JL: Reduction of trauma-induced edema of spinal cord in dogs given mannitol. Am J Vet Res 34:1355, 1973.

40. Parker AJ: Blood pressure changes and lethality of mannitol infusion in dogs. Am J Vet Res 34:1523, 1973.

41. Parker AJ and Smith CW: Lack of functional recovery from spinal cord trauma following dimethylsulphoxide and epsilon amino-caproic acid therapy in dogs. Res Vet Sci 27:253, 1979.

42. Rivlin AS and Tator CH: Effect of vasodilators and myelotomy in recovery after acute spinal cord injury in rats. J Neurosurg 50:349, 1979.

43. Rucker NC, Lumb WV, and Scott RJ: Combined pharmacologic and surgical treatments for acute spinal cord trauma. Am J Vet Res 42:1138, 1981.

44. Stone EA, Betts CW, and Chambers JN: Cervical fractures in the dog: A literature and case review. J Am Anim Hosp Assoc 15:463, 1979.

45. Tarlov IM: Spinal Cord Compression. Mechanisms of Paralysis and Treatment. Springfield, IL, Charles C Thomas, 1975.

46. Tator CH: Spinal cord cooling and irrigation for treatment of acute cord injury. In Popp AJ, Bourke RS, Nelson LR, and Kimelberg HK: Seminars in Neurological Surgery. Neural Trauma. New York, Raven Press, 1979.

47. Young W and Flamm ES: Effect of high-dose corticosteroid therapy on blood flow, evoked potentials and extracellular calcium in experimental spinal injury. J Neurosurg 57:667, 1982.

Chapter 12
BF Hoerlein DVM, PhD

Intervertebral Disk Disease

HISTORY

The protruding or extruded intervertebral disk that compresses the spinal cord and causes a clinical neurologic deficit is the most common central nervous system disorder in the dog encountered by the practicing veterinarian. The neurologic signs of pain, paresis, and paralysis from disk disease have been recognized in humans and some animals for several hundred years, but the true nature of disk involvement was not established until the current century. In the early 1500s, Vesalius descibed the intervertebral disk and differentiated the anulus fibrosus and the nucleus pulposus. Further anatomic studies of the intervertebral disk were made in 1857 by Virchow and in 1858 by Von Luschka.[39] In 1929, Dandy[18] operated on two cases of intervertebral disk protrusion. In 1932, Mixter and Barr[61] started a series of publications concerning the true nature of disk protrusions and their pathologic importance in humans; they demonstrated that so-called chondromas are actually intervertebral disk herniations and not neoplasms.

The recognition of intervertebral disk disease in the dog began in the late nineteenth century by European veterinarians. It is extremely difficult to credit veterinary scientists with their respective contributions through the years. (For further historical data, consult the discussions and references below.)

ANATOMY OF THE DISK

The function of the vertebral column is to provide a rigid structure for the attachment of muscles and bones and to protect delicate structures, especially parts of the nervous system, while being pliable enough to allow movement with maximal efficiency. These objectives are attained by a series of vertebrae connected by two types of intervertebral joints. The intervertebral disk is an important component in one of these types of articulations[68] (Fig. 12–1).

The disk structures in humans and the dog are similar.[51] Excluding the caudal area, intervertebral disks in the dog (numbering 26) represent about 18% of the length of the vertebral column (25% in humans and 12% in the cat and horse).[95] The disks are amphiarthrodial joints in the intervertebral articulations and are widest in the cervical and lumbar regions. The cartilaginous end plates of the vertebral epiphyses and the intercapital ligament are closely related to the disk both structurally and physiologically. The intercapital ligament is present between the second and eleventh thoracic vertebrae, largely replaces the dorsal anulus fibrosus, and is primarily responsible for lack of disk protrusions in this area. The cartilaginous end plates form the cranial and caudal boundaries of the disk and are composed of thin layers of hyaline cartilage that cover the vertebral body epiphyses. The vertebrae on each side of the disk have a specialized plate of dense, smooth bone termed the vertebral end plate. These plates are perforated by numerous small canals that are related to the underlying marrow spaces and function in the nutrition of the disk.[90]

Each disk consists of a central soft gelatinous substance called the nucleus pulposus and a multilayered fibrous envelope called the anulus fibrosus. The inner portion of the anulus, termed the transitional zone, is composed of a somewhat fibrocartilaginous matrix. The nucleus occupies the middle to dorsal third of the disk and is highly specialized tissue originating

321

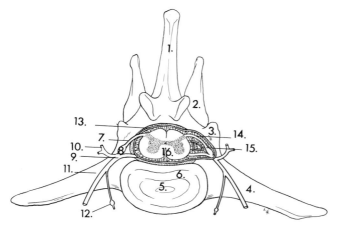

Figure 12–1. Intervertebral disk and associated structures. 1, Spinous process; 2, articular process; 3, accessory process; 4, transverse process; 5, nucleus pulposus; 6, anulus fibrosus; 7, dorsal root; 8, dorsal root ganglion; 9, ventral root; 10, dorsal branch; 11, ventral branch; 12, ramus communicans and sympathetic trunk ganglion; 13, epidural space; 14, dura mater and arachnoid; 15, subarachnoid space; 16, spinal cord.

from the embryonic notochord. Newborn feline and canine disks contain large numbers of notochordal cells.[8, 9]

The anulus is a fibrocartilaginous tissue consisting of bands of parallel fibrous lamellae that run obliquely between the adjacent vertebrae, crossing each other at angles of 100 to 120° in a lacelike fashion. The inner lamellae attach to the cartilaginous end plates, whereas outer layers attach to the vertebral end plates. The ventral portions of the anulus are from 1.5 to 3 times thicker than the dorsal area, which explains why most extruded disks are dorsal (against the spinal cord).

The additional supporting structures of the disk are the dorsal and ventral longitudinal ligaments. The dorsal longitudinal ligament is strongly attached to the median ridge of bone on the floor of the vertebral canal and spreads laterally to intermingle with the outer layers of the anulus of the disk. The ventral longitudinal ligament is situated in similar fashion on the ventral aspects of the vertebrae[60] (Fig. 12–2).

The nutrition of the disk is largely by diffusion of fluids and nutriments from the cartilaginous end plates and the vessels adjacent to the anulus.[4] The diffusion of metabolites and removal of cellular wastes from the disk is facilitated by normal vertebral movement. Additionally, the long chain polyanions of the proteoglycan complexes are believed to have an integral function in disk nutrition. Because vertebral fusion results in significant compositional changes in the canine disk matrices, it is felt that the loss of proteoglycans and mechanical failure of the nucleus pulposus profoundly affect disk nutrition.[9]

The anulus of the disk is supplied with sensory fibers, which may account for some of the pain associated with stretching or tearing of the anulus.[15, 19, 80] In dogs, sensory fibers are much more extensive in the dorsal longitudinal ligament than in the anulus. The nucleus pulposus contains no nerve fibers.[20a] No meningeal ramus could be found in dogs, so the exact source of these nerves is unknown. The nerves to one disk originated from four to five consecutive dorsal root ganglia. Pain arising from the anulus would likely be referable to an area four to five segments long.[20a]

PATHOPHYSIOLOGY OF THE DISK

Physiologically, the intervertebral disk forms an elastic cushion between the bony vertebrae

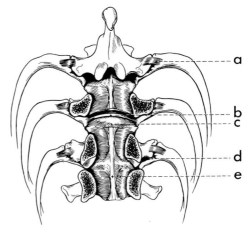

Figure 12–2. Ligaments of vertebral column and ribs, dorsal aspect. a, Costotransverse ligament; b, intercapital ligament; c, intervertebral disk; d, ligament of neck; e, dorsal longitudinal ligament. (From Evans HE and Christensen GC: Miller's Anatomy of the Dog, 2nd ed. Philadelphia, WB Saunders Co, 1979.)

to allow movement, to minimize trauma and shock, and to unite the segments into a column.[1] In the dog, the most important center of mobility is the region at, and around, the so-called anticlinal vertebra (T11), which marks the transition from the caudally to the cranially sloping spinous processes. Disk protrusions occur most frequently immediately caudal to this area.[90]

When the vertebral column is placed in the vertical position and thereafter loaded, the pressure on the anulus is three to five times greater in a tangential direction than in a vertical direction. Therefore, the normal anulus in an animal has to withstand a more severe stress through tension than through pressure. This ability to withstand severe stress is mechanically great, because violent physical strain more often results in fractures than in ruptured disks (at least in the nonchondrodystrophoid groups of dogs).[36, 90]

The intradiskal pressure depends chiefly on two factors, the water binding properties of the nucleus and the power of resistance and elasticity of the surrounding structures, particularly the anulus. Disk functions are largely dependent on the histochemical components and their changes in the aging process.

PATHOGENESIS

Disk disease in the dog appears in two morphologically distinct forms, one in dogs of the chondrodystrophoid (ChD) breeds (dachshund, French bulldog, Pekingese) at a comparatively early age, and another in aged dogs of all other nonchondrodystrophoid (non-ChD) breeds. The degeneration begins as a fibroid or chondroid metamorphosis or change at the periphery of the nucleus pulposus, and progresses centrally. In chondrodystrophoid animals this process takes the chondroid metaplastic form and occurs at 8 months to 2 years of age, whereas in nonchondrodystrophoid animals the change is fibroid and occurs at 8 to 10 years of age. Chondroid metamorphosis or changes at the center of the disk in chondrodystrophoid dogs might be interpreted as a the result of deferral of the final embryologic stages because of the abnormally slow differentiation. Degeneration of the anulus fibrosus accompanies or possibly precedes the nuclear changes. As nuclear metamorphosis progresses, it loses its useful elasticity and thus the ability to act as an efficient shock absorber. A possible decrease in nuclear nutrition may result from an ineffective pumping mechanism potentiating further degeneration. As the nucleus continues to degenerate, a resulting diffuse disintegration occurs, leading to homogeneous calcification.[34, 35]

In chondrodystrophoid dogs at the age of 1 year, 75 to 100% of all nuclei have been transformed into chondroid tissue and 30 to 60% show macroscopic signs of degeneration, largely in the form of calcification. When dachshunds (at a mean age of 2 years) were surveyed radiographically, nearly 90% showed disk calcification. When such dogs reach 6 or 7 years of age probably all will show macroscopically observable signs of disk degeneration, and about 75% will have developed a prolapse to some degree. Disk degeneration and signs of small hard protrusions occur proportionate to age in nonchondrodystrophoid dogs and in cats, clinical disease being infrequent in cats and an occasional problem in large breeds of dogs.[34, 35, 36]

Braund and workers[8, 9, 27] established that the systemic disk degeneration in the chondrodystrophoid group of dogs is related to biochemical and morphologic changes, which occur much earlier in chondrodystrophoid than in nonchondrodystrophoid breeds. Commensurate with morphologic nucleus pulposus transmutation, collagen levels approach 30 to 40% of dry weight within 6 to 12 months. Extraordinary changes in all other biochemical parameters occur during the first 1.5 to 3 years. Total hexosamines, sialic acid, noncollagenous protein, and galactosamine values in the nucleus pulposus are 30 to 50% lower in chondrodystrophoid dogs than in nonchondrodystrophoid dogs of similar age. These changes contribute to loss of water content; the nucleus loses its ability to adequately deform and distribute the movement and loading forces placed on the vertebral column and its disk. This mechanical failure of the nucleus ultimately results in disruption of annular fibers in the weakest portion of the disk, which is the dorsal area (50% less fibers than the ventral anulus). Although injury does not appear to play a major role in the chondrodystrophoid disk degeneration, it would seem to be a factor in the precipitation of an extruded nucleus after the normal mechanical efficiency of the disk is impaired.

Because of the pronounced morphologic and biochemical changes in the so-called chondrodystrophoid breeds that occur early in life and predispose the disk to protrusion and extrusion, the question of heredity arises. It is significant that the chondrification process takes place only in the vertebral column and is not a generalized disturbance of connective tissue development, such as in menisci and articular cartilages.[8, 9] There are various degrees of so-called hypochondroplasia, varying from complete dwarfism to involvement of only long bone growth. Types of short limb dwarfism in animals are seen in so-called creeper chickens, Kerry-Dexter type cattle, the Alaskan malamute, and certain foxhounds.[95] Means of transmission in some of these cases have been determined.

About 20% of all dachshunds in teaching hospitals are admitted for disk disease. These same hospitals report that from 48 to 70% of cases of disk disease are found in dachshunds.[42] Ball et al[3] studied pedigrees of 536 registered dachshunds with intervertebral disk disease and found patterns of occurrence consistent with a genetic model involving the cumulative effect of several genes with no dominance or sex linkage, subject to environmental modification. In 2 families studied, there were 52 cases among 85 dachshunds in 15 litters—a prevalence of 62% as compared with a breed prevalence of 19%. It was concluded that lineages with high prevalence of disk disease should be considered high risk genetically and breeders should avoid using them in breeding.[3, 42]

Hormones, such as estrogen, androgen, thyroid hormones, and glucocorticoid, may be involved in the pathogenesis of disk disease.[67] In one study involving 100 dogs with signs of intervertebral disk disease, T3 and T4 examinations demonstrated that 10 to 20% had suspicious findings and 39 to 59% were considered hypothyroid.[30] However, resting T3 and T4 values are not necessarily indicative of hypothyroidism, especially in animals on medication or in those with other problems.

Most authorities agree that active, well-conditioned dogs have fewer problems with disk disease than the house pet. It must probably be concluded that the underlying complexities of disk disease are multifactorial, and clarification in areas of molecular biology and breed and lineage genetics awaits further research.

Types of Disk Protrusions

Disk protrusions assume two main forms, which Hansen[34, 36] classified as types 1 and 2. Hansen's type 1 usually refers to a massive extrusion or prolapse of the nucleus resulting from a rupture of the anulus and is due to the chondroid degeneration occurring in chondrodystrophoid group of dogs (see above). The senile or type 2 fibroid degeneration seen in nonchondrodystrophoid breeds is caused by a partial rupture of the anulus and results in a round domelike bulging of the dorsal surface of the disk. This type 2 disk degeneration has certain similarities to spondylosis deformans. Type 1 prolapses are caused by more or less broad, linear ruptures of the anulus and are large in a vertical or horizontal direction; their shape is irregular and their consistency brittle and grainy. Type 2 prolapses are usually smaller and smooth and are cushion shaped, hemispheric, or dome shaped at or around the disk itself[34] (Figs. 12–3 to 12–7).

In the acute type 1 disk prolapse the rupture is accompanied by epidural hemorrhage, the volume of which may exceed that of the protruded material. The extruded nuclear material is gritty, cheeselike, hemorrhagic, or slate gray in appearance; it can be a somewhat circumscribed vertical mass or a widespread, horizontal, carpetlike mass extending around the sides of the spinal cord. An inflammatory reaction occurs, causing a fibrinous adhesion between the protruding mass and the dura. The protru-

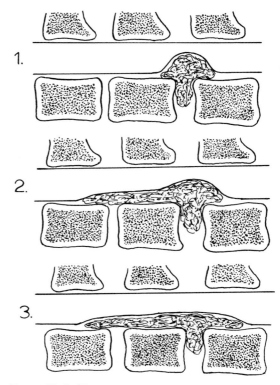

Figure 12–3. The stages of a ruptured disk, showing its distribution in the extradural space and subsequent spinal cord pressure. 1, Initial stage of ruptured disk and protrusion. 2, Migration of extruded nucleus pulposus. 3, Note that nucleus may extend 1 to 3 vertebral lengths.

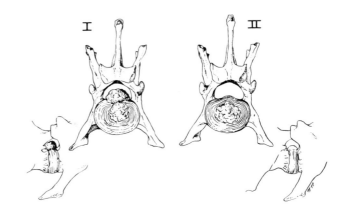

Figure 12–4. Hansen's classification of disk protrusions. Type I is the clinical ruptured disk with a massive extrusion of the nucleus and a compressive mass on the cord. This type is characteristic of the chondrodystrophoid group of dogs. Type II is typically a small round dome-shaped protrusion seen in older dogs and generally produces mild clinical signs or none. This type is characteristic of nonchondrodystrophoid groups of dogs.

sion is composed of polymorphonuclear leukocytes, red cells, fibroblasts, large mononuclear cells, polynuclear giant cells, occasional chondrocytes, and much nondescript necrotic tissue debris.[42] The inflammation is like that caused by a foreign body and is initiated by the irritating nucleus and the forceful ejection ("dynamic force" of Olsson) of the nucleus.[66] The body tries to absorb the foreign material and frequently does so more or less completely. Incomplete absorption leaves a mass that organizes into a fibroid, cartilaginous, and frequently calcific protrusion. A subsequent rupture in the same disk creates a larger residual mass that is fairly characteristic of cervical or caudal lumbar disk disease. The thoracolumbar junction is frequently afflicted with a severe rupture of the anulus in which the degenerated nucleus is driven against the spinal

cord with dynamic force. Such a "blowout" causes severe neurologic signs and occasionally a progressive hemorrhagic malacia of the spinal cord, which results in progressive respiratory paralysis and death.[41, 42]

Type 1 disk lesions occur primarily in fairly young smaller breeds of dogs such as dachshund, toy poodle, Pekingese, beagle, and cocker spaniel. The disk degeneration occurs early, such as at 2 to 9 months of age, whereas the clinical signs generally develop at 3 to 6 years. Type 2 disk changes develop in larger breeds such as German shepherd, Labrador retriever, and Doberman pinscher and at older ages, 5 to 12 years of age. Type 1 disk disorders are much more frequent and important in clinical practice. The usual type of disk lesion seen in old cats is similar to type 2 and is rarely a clinical disorder.[42, 52, 54]

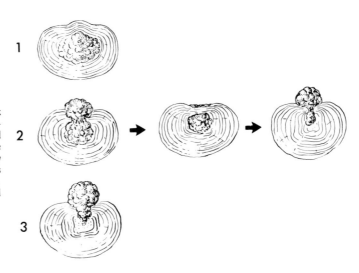

Figure 12–5. A sequence in a clinical disk (Hansen's type I). 1, A partial rupture or stretching of the inner anular fibers, causing a small herniation of the nucleus. 2, A complete rupture of the anulus, which may be phagocytized by scavenger cells; the anulus heals with fibrous tissue only to rupture again under clinical stress. 3, A massive compression of the spinal cord results.

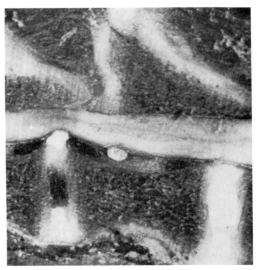

Figure 12–6. This is a sagittal section through the vertebrae of a dachshund with posterior paresis, showing a calcified disk protrusion. Notice the compression mass caudal to the protruding disk. (From Gage, EP and Hoerlein BF: The vertebral column. *In* Canine Surgery, 2nd Archibald ed. Santa Barbara, CA, American Veterinary Publications, Inc., 1974.)

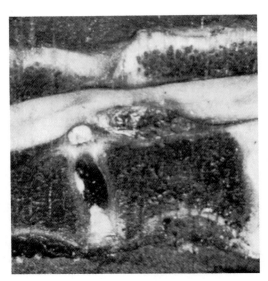

Figure 12–7. An epidural deposit of ruptured disk material and necrotic mass (2 mm lateral to the part of the spine shown in Figure 12–6). (From Gage EP and Hoerlein BF: The vertebral column. *In* Canine Surgery, 2nd Archibald ed. Santa Barbara, CA, American Veterinary Publications, Inc., 1974.)

Pathologic Changes in the Spinal Cord

Compressive Myelitis

The spinal cord consists of soft compressible tissue and compensates remarkably well for pressure, especially if the pressure develops slowly, as occurs frequently in disk protrusions. If the pressure continues to progress, the spinal cord reaches a point of noncompensation and serious clinical and pathologic signs develop. However, in the acutely ruptured disk the extruded mass is large and develops suddenly. The spinal cord cannot compensate because of acute vascular embarrassment, vascular leakage of protein, and degenerative tissue changes. The spinal cord changes depend on the size and rate of compression, with lesions varying from slight demyelination to total necrosis of both gray and white matter. The major forces in compressive disk disease are mechanical disruption of neuronal tissue and hypoxic changes resulting from pressure on the vascular system in the spinal cord. The vascular changes include blockage of the longitudinal sinuses and possible collapse of the thin walled meningeal veins, resulting in decreased drainage, stasis, edema, hypoxia, and finally necrosis of spinal cord tissue[94] (Fig. 12–8).

The most extensive damage to the spinal cord is adjacent to the compressive mass and force,

which would involve the white matter initially and most frequently. The clinical signs in most disk compressions are upper motor neuron in character because of the white matter involvement. Depending on the size and rate of development, the changes progress from demyelination, necrosis of myelin and axons, to massive malacia. Macrophages infiltrate the damaged area and remove the axonal and mye-

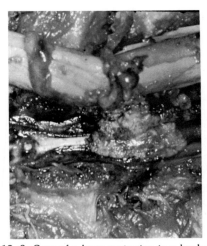

Figure 12–8. Case of a large protrusion in a lumbar disk. The disk probably suffered from several partial ruptures and protrusions, which organized into a mass, gradually increasing in size after each episode. Periodic attacks of pain occurred, and paraplegia eventually resulted.

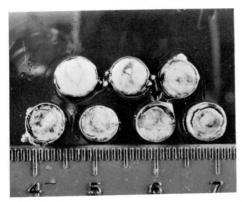

Figure 12–9. Cross sections of the spinal cord at various levels demonstrate medullary as well as subarachnoid hemorrhage. (From Hoerlein BF: Intervertebral disc protrusions in the dog. Vet Scope 4, Fall, 1959.)

lin debris. The microvasculature becomes activated, and astrocytes gradually fill up the defect.

Even though changes in the white matter predominate, severe disruption of the white matter can cause alterations in the gray tissue, in which hypoxia causes necrosis. If these gray matter changes occur in the brachial or lumbar intumescences, lower motor neuron signs predominate.[32, 42, 94, 97]

Progressive Malacia

The suddenly extruded disk may cause acute compressive disease characterized by sudden total loss of neuronal function as evidenced in lower motor neuron disease. This disorder may be called hemorrhagic myelomalacia or, improperly, hematomyelia. The cord characteristically shows hemorrhage in extradural, sub-

arachnoid, and intramedullary tissue. The parenchymal bleeding is due to ischemic and hemorrhagic infarction, leading to sudden and massive occlusion of all the microvasculature to the cord parenchyma, which may also be influenced by histochemical, enzymic, and metabolic changes (see Chapters 7 and 11). The myelomalacia first starts at the disk extrusion site, then descends or ascends through the cord. Rarely the malacia may skip a segment of spinal cord in its progression cranially or caudally. If the hemorrhagic malacia ascends it may cause a total quadriplegia and death from respiratory paralysis. Microscopically the cord changes include hemorrhagic infiltration, demyelination, degenerative neurons, polymorphonuclear infiltrations, and cavitations. On occasion, similar myelomalacia may be seen in the absence of evidence of spinal compressive diseases and is associated with trauma[32, 42, 94] (see Chapter 11) (Figs. 12–9 and 12–10).

INCIDENCE

The incidence of intervertebral (IV) disk disease has been covered extensively in the literature[33, 42, 48, 73, 86] and will therefore be treated briefly in this discussion. The Veterinary Medical Data Retrieval Program (VMDP)* used the "251 code" to reword a broad range of pathologic observations (eg, radiographic, surgical, and necropsy examinations) of any portion of the intervertebral disks.[42] Even though this category might include cases in which the abnormal disk was not producing a

*American Association of Veterinary Medical Data Program Participants, Inc., New York State College of Veterinary Medicine, Cornell University, Ithaca, NY.

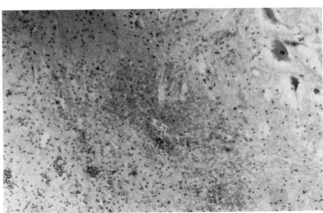

Figure 12–10. A histopathological section of the spinal cord shown in Figure 12–9 shows evidence of hemorrhage, aggregations of polymorphonuclear cells, demyelination, and necrosis. (From Hoerlein BF: Intervertebral disc protrusions in the dog. Vet Scope 4, Fall, 1959.)

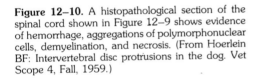

Table 12–1. FREQUENCY OF DISK DISEASE WITHIN CANINE BREEDS*

Breed	Frequency (%)	1–2 yr	2–4 yr	Age (%) 4–7 yr	7–10 yr	10–15 yr	Sex (%) Female	Male
Dachshund	24.51	3.63	25.36	45.32	26.98	9.04	53.3	46.8
Standard	26.21	4.91	27.25	46.4	27.13	10.14	51.1	48.9
Miniature	22.81	2.35	23.47	44.24	26.83	7.94	55.4	44.6
Pekingese	8.13	5.38	15.12	13.17	7.72	3.02	49.6	50.4
Welsh corgi	6.92	1.68	3.28	15.16	11.01	4.76	51.6	48.4
Beagle	5.41	0.71	6.11	12.02	9.83	3.61	51.4	48.6
Lhasa apso	4.78	2.37	9.74	7.92	2.50	3.20	47.1	52.9
Poodle, small	2.74	0.61	3.64	4.87	3.29	1.86	38.7	61.3
TOTAL	11.0	2.8	12.7	20.5	12.6	4.9	49.3	50.7

*Compiled data from VMDP (American Association of Veterinary Medical Data Program Participants).

neurologic syndrome, it was felt that this retrieval was appropriate for a comparative study, especially in the dog. Of 878,658 canine case histories, in 17,746 cases intervertebral disk disease was diagnosed, for a 2.02% frequency. It is recognized that almost any dog regardless of breed can have a disk protrusion, however, the chondrodystrophoid breeds are highly susceptible and by far are the most important breeds seen with clinical disk disease. As noted in Table 12–1, the latest statistics from the VMDP show the standard and miniature dachshund frequency of disk disease within the breed to be 26.2 and 22.8%, respectively, whereas the next highest five frequencies were noted for Pekingese, 8.1%; Welsh corgi, 6.9%; beagle, 5.4%; Lhasa apso, 4.8%, and miniature poodle, 2.7%. Past and current frequency of breeds actually treated for disk disease in the Auburn Clinic place the dachshund at 65%, mixed breeds at about 13%, and the small poodles, Pekingese, beagles, and cocker spaniels declining from approximately 8% to 2%, respectively.[42]

The VMDP retrieval for noncanine disk disease (code 251) produced 107 cases out of 650,361 mammals (0.02%). Of these 107 cases, 56 were observed in the cat from a population of 274,535 (0.02%) and 19 in the horse from a total of 226,546 diagnoses (0.008%). Additional species noted were bovine, 8 (0.007%); porcine, 9 (0.008%); caprine, 2 (0.002%); and miscellaneous other mammalian, 10 (0.09%). Two of 865 rabbits (hares), for 0.2% frequency, were reported in the retrieval. Although as many as 107 cases of disk disease were reported in noncanine mammals, the overall incidence of 0.02% is extremely low when compared with an overall incidence of 2.02% in all breeds of dogs. One would conclude that intervertebral disk disease primarily affects the dog in veterinary medicine and is a frequent disorder in susceptible breeds.

The age incidence for disk disease in most chondrodystrophoid breeds has been established by investigators to be highest at 3 to 7 years, with the overall average being about 5 years[23, 29, 42, 73, 79] (Table 12–2). From the VMDP data for the six breeds selected in Table 12–1, the female average was 49.3%, whereas the male incidence was 50.7%. In the VMDP noncanine disk retrieval, the incidence in males was 54% in cats and 63% in horses.

In analyzing 2395 cases from the Auburn Clinic, the frequency of lesion locations was approximately 14% in the cervical area (C2–C3 and C3–C4 being most affected), about 55% in the T9–T10 through T13–L1 area, and some 30% in the lumbar area. About 65% of all disk lesions occurred in the T11–T12 to L1–L2 areas[42] (Table 12–3).

Clinical disk disease in the cat is infrequent and has not been a major problem in feline practice. Because lymphosarcoma can be seen epidurally in the cat[84, 99] and may cause neurologic signs similar to those of disk protrusions, one must take care not to confuse neoplasia with disk etiology. In necropsy surveys, Hansen type 2 disk lesions may be seen in clinically

Table 12–2. FREQUENCY OF CANINE DISK DISEASE BY AGE (2377 cases) (Auburn University, 1952–1975)

Age in Years	Number	Percentage	
1 and under	26	1.1	
2	110	4.6	
3	338	14.2	
4	463	19.5	73.1
5	571	24.0	
6	366	15.4	
7	239	10.1	
8	141	5.9	
9	61	2.6	
10 and over	62	2.6	

From Hoerlein BF: Canine Neurology, 3rd ed. Philadelphia, WB Saunders Co, 1978.

Table 12–3. SITE OF CANINE DISK LESIONS
(2620 disks, 2395 cases)
(Auburn University, 1952–1975)

Vertebral Space	Number of Cases	Percentage
Cervical		
2–3	160	6.1
3–4	85	3.2
4–5	49	1.9
5–6	48	1.8
6–7	15	0.6
C7–T1	6	0.2
TOTAL	363	13.9
Thoracic		
9–10	2	0.1
10–11	21	0.8
11–12	259	9.9
12–13	598	22.8
T13–L1	574	21.9
TOTAL	1454	55.5
Lumbar		
1–2	287	11.0
2–3	183	7.0
3–4	165	6.3
4–5	124	4.7
5–6	33	1.3
6–7	10	0.4
L7–S1	1	—
TOTAL	803	30.6
Thoracolumbar junction		
T11–T12 to L1–L2	1718	65.6

From Hoerlein BF: Canine Neurology, 3rd ed. Philadelphia, WB Saunders Co, 1978.

normal cats, especially those 6 years of age and older. The incidence of these lesions parallels an increase in age, which is similar to survey reports for type 2 lesions in humans and in nonchondrodystrophoid breeds of dogs. In the cat, the highest number of protrusions was seen in the cervical area, the next highest in the midlumbar area, and next at the thoracolumbar junction. However, the highest incidence of *degeneration* in any form was in the T1–T10 area, which coincided with the presence of the intercapital ligament, the lowest area for disk protrusion occurrence.[11, 33, 37, 42, 48, 53, 86, 90]

CLINICAL SIGNS

The protruding or extruded nucleus pulposus causes a localized compressive cord lesion unless the ruptured anulus and extruded nucleus occur suddenly and with great force, in which event more diffuse spinal cord damage is accomplished. Because much of the damage from the more common chronic disk lesion is to the white matter and is located in the regions C1–C5 or T3–L3, the signs would be characteristic of upper motor neuron deficits. If the lesions involve the cervical and lumbar intumescences (C6–T2, L4–S2) and are affecting the gray matter, lower motor neuron deficits may be seen. However, both types of deficits could occur at the same time, eg, brachial LMN and T13–L1 UMN lesions[2] (Fig. 12–11).

The types of clinical signs most frequently seen in characteristic disk lesions are pain, paresis, and paralysis. Pain is caused by the extruded material irritating the nerve roots (radicular pain), the meninges, and possibly the disk structures. Dogs with extruded *cervical* disks usually show extreme pain as evidenced by the head and neck being held low and rigid. The patient may refuse to eat and drink because these actions accentuate the pain. The owner describes the dog as "bowing its neck" or "standing on its head." With disk disease involving the *thoracolumbar* area, pain may be evidenced by "arching" the back, tensing of the abdominal muscles, and carefully walking on tiptoes. Abdominal pain could be confused with that from acute pancreatitis or peritonitis. Manipulation of the neck and muscular palpation along the thoracolumbar spine will accentuate the pain in mild cases in which signs are not so obvious. Pin pricking or pinching the skin, especially in the thoracolumbar area, elicits the panniculus reflex and a painful response at or cranial to the lesion, whereas the response is diminished or lost caudal to the lesion. When the pain response is marked, a localization of the lesion can be made to within one or two vertebral spaces cranial to the protrusion, depending on the spinal location. Testing the limb dermatomes for peripheral nerve analgesia by pinching or pricking the skin may be helpful in localizing the lesion. Intermittent pain is the primary sign in cervical disk disease, whereas pain in the thoracolumbar area may rapidly advance to paresis or paralysis of the pelvic limbs.[41, 42]

Paresis or weakness may be accompanied by degrees of ataxia and is evidence of marked cord damage. Generally the paresis (paraparesis in pelvic limbs) is bilaterally symmetric, but if the compression predominates on one side a scoliosis in the thoracolumbar segment may occur with monoparesis, curling of the toe, and ataxia. An upper motor neuron monoparesis of a pelvic limb is more likely to be caused by a spinal cord infarction than a compressive lesion (see Chapter 7). Paresis may occur with pain or may be part of a progressive syndrome preceding paralysis. Frequently paraparesis may be evident in lieu of thoracic limb signs in marked compressions of the cervical spinal cord.[41, 42]

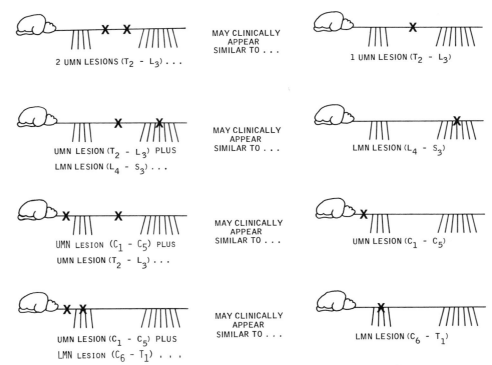

Figure 12–11. Multiple spinal cord lesions that can clinically resemble spinal cord lesions. UMN, upper motor neuron; LMN, lower motor neuron. (From Bailey CS and Holliday TA: Diseases of the spinal cord. In Ettinger SJ: Textbook of Veterinary Internal Medicine. Philadelphia, WB Saunders Co, 1975.)

Paralysis of the limbs is evidence of severe spinal cord damage and may occur suddenly in cases of a thoracolumbar lesion without the sequence of pain and paresis. Frequently the owner reports that the dog was normal at night but was found paralyzed the following morning with no evidence of trauma. In other cases, the dog had been showing pain and weakness for several days or even weeks, had improved, but became paraplegic with an unusual stimulus or mild trauma. The clinical signs are characteristic of upper motor neuron deficits (unless the C7–T2 or L4–S2 sites are involved). In paraplegia and quadriplegia urinary retention is a constant sign. The crossed extensor reflex is a rather constant sign in advanced spinal compression (UMN) in the cat but is not as reliable a reflex sign in the dog. An important prognostic sign in both species is the ability to consciously perceive deep pain in the limb. If there is no behavioral response on pinching the base of the toenail, the prognosis for recovery is unfavorable. Because the motor fiber tracts in the dog are more vulnerable to compressive damage than the pain tracts, loss of pain in addition to motor dysfunction indicates serious cord damage and probable permanent loss of function.

When lower motor neuron signs occur in the limbs the prognosis is grave unless the lesion is a compression of the cauda equina at the lumbosacral junction[32, 42, 44] (Figs. 12–12 and 12–13).

The clinical signs in progressive myelomalacia resulting from an acute ruptured disk or acute trauma can be distinguished from those of localized disk compression because of the profound lower motor neuron signs of atonia, areflexia, and loss of sensation. When the malacia descends in the spinal cord, the abdomen becomes flaccid and distended; the bladder is distended, is incontinent, and is easily expressed because of an atonic sphincter; the limbs and tail have no sensory or motor function; and the anus is dilated, and frequently the feces are tarry. As the malacia ascends, the head and neck are extended dorsally and are hypertonic, the thoracic limbs are hypertonic and rigid, and normal balance in the pectoral limbs is impaired. As the cranial progression continues, the intercostal, limb, and neck muscles become paralytic. The animal generally becomes recumbent and succumbs in 3 to 6 days. Occasionally the malacia progresses in only one direction and stops. In the early stages

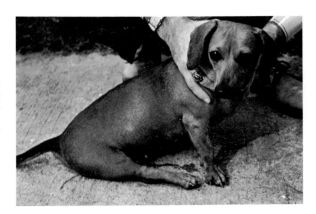

Figure 12–12. Characteristic case of a local compression myelitis resulting from a terminal thoracic or lumbar disk protrusion. The pelvic limbs are rigid, hyperflexic, and urinary and fecal retention is common. The front limbs, neck, and head are normal. If pain is not too severe, the animal may eat and may generally feel well.

of progressive hemorrhagic myelomalacia the clinician must frequently make a decision as to the value of surgical therapy. In such cases, the wheelbarrow test is a reliable aid. Poor prognosis is indicated when the animal is unable to move and maintain balance on its thoracic limbs when the pelvic limbs are elevated and the animal is gently propelled forward and sidewards. Serial evaluation of the level of cutaneous sensation over a 24 hour period is a reliable method for detecting progressive myelomalacia. The author is not aware of progressive myelomalacia in the cat as the result of a ruptured disk.[31, 42]

DIAGNOSIS

The diagnosis of disk disease is based on the assessment of the clinical signs, a knowledge of a typical history of breed involvement, frequency of recurrences, the results of a carefully executed physical and neurologic evaluation, and a proper radiographic examination.

The radiographic examination will usually confirm the diagnosis of disk disease or demonstrate other types of spinal compressive disorders. For the radiographic examination to be optimally diagnostic, careful positioning of the suspected disk space with the animal under heavy sedation or anesthesia is necessary. Radiographic lesions are typically a narrow or wedged-shaped disk space, a small and/or cloudy intervertebral foramen ("horse's head"), abnormally spaced articular processes, and an opaque or calcified disk and/or a disk protrusion mass in the canal. Occasionally a myelogram is necessary to confirm the diagnosis and precisely locate the lesion.[42] (See Chapter 4 and Figs. 4–1 to 4–4, 4–10, 4–11, 4–16 for details on the radiographic examination.)

Other aids in diagnosis may involve a paravertebral electromyogram,[14, 82] spinal evoked potentials for prognosis,[45] nerve conduction studies,[7, 77] electroencephalograms for determining brain disease,[76, 78] and possibly dermal thermograms.[74] If available, plain and computer assisted tomography can aid in diagnosis of spinal compressive disease.

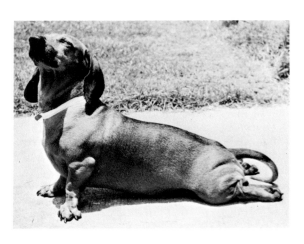

Figure 12–13. Dog with a progressive hemorrhagic myelomalacia resulting from an acute rupture of the disk. The pelvic limbs are flaccid, the anal sphincter is relaxed, and the reflexes are either diminished or absent. The pectoral limbs are becoming rigid or spastic, the head and neck are rigid, the eyes are "glassy," and the animal does not feel well. (From Hoerlein BF: Intervertebral disc protrusions in the dog. Vet Scope 4, Fall, 1959.)

Comparison of Disk Disease in Humans and Dogs

There are differences in the disk syndromes that occur in humans and dogs.[1, 44, 57] Some of the variations in clinical manifestations are due to anatomic differences. The length of the vertebral column is 71 cm in the average man and 109 cm in a 40 pound shepherd-type dog. The vertebral canal in humans is triangular in shape, whereas in the dog it is oval. The spinal cord occupies about 80% of the cross-sectional area of the canal in the dog (a much greater percentage than that in humans). This means that an extradural mass will compress the spinal cord more readily and more seriously in dogs than in humans.

One of the primary differences is that the spinal cord terminates in the cranial lumbar area in humans and that the usual disk lesion in humans is seen in the terminal lumbar area, caudal to the spinal cord termination. In the dog the spinal cord terminates in the caudal lumbar area, and the most prevalent disk lesions are seen in the thoracolumbar junction. Therefore, the disk compresses a nerve root in humans and a nerve root and spinal cord in the dog. The vertebral column in human beings has been compared to a truss with its joints of support at the two pairs of extremities. In the dog and other quadrupeds the mechanism that serves to bend or straighten the column is compared to a bow and string—the bow being represented by the vertebrae and the string by the sternum and abdominal muscles. Being usually in the upright position, humans have more disk pressure in a vertical direction (compression), whereas in the dog the disk stress is in a tangential direction (tension).

The age changes in the disk are similar in humans, the cat, and the nonchondrodystrophoid breeds of dogs owing to the gradual loss of water, the chemical changes, and nuclear fibrosis. However, these changes differ greatly from the early chondroid changes seen in the disk of the chondrodystrophoid group of dogs. The highest incidence of clinical disk disease in men occurs between 20 and 60 years of age, whereas in women the disorder tends to occur later in life and the incidence between 60 and 95 years of age is twice that in men. In the human, 64% of the disk cases are seen in men, whereas in the dog there seems to be little sex predilection.

Because there is a marked difference in lesion site and cord terminations between humans and dogs, there is a vast difference in clinical manifestations. The profound paralysis early in the course of the disease in the dog differs from the usual pain syndrome with minimal paresis seen in humans. In the dog the incidence at paralysis mandates more frequent surgical correction early in the course of the clinical signs. However, the pain syndrome associated with cervical disk protrusion, the thoracolumbar lesions in older nonchondrodystrophoid breeds of dogs, and especially lumbosacral protrusions causing radicular pain are similar to the syndrome seen in humans. It is concluded that the thoracolumbar disk pain and/or paresis or paralysis syndrome seen in the chondrodystrophoid group of dogs is a much more severe disorder than that seen in humans, which is predominantly one of pain.[44]

TREATMENT

The veterinary literature portrays such a variety of therapy that many clinicians are dismayed as to which is the best course to follow. The fairly frequent incidence of spontaneous improvement and occasional long-term recovery is due to the resorption of the extruded disk material, formation of a stable fibrosis in the offending disk, and the compensatory ability of the spinal cord to accommodate pressure. However, the so-called spontaneous recovery may be temporary and subsequent attacks frequently follow, usually with more intense damage. If one is aware that the usual source of pain is meningeal or nerve root irritation, and that motor deficits result from nerve root or spinal cord compression, the neurosurgeon should be prepared to treat either surgically or nonsurgically. The decision should be based on the individual case, considering the breed involved, age and history (eg, recurrences, duration of signs), clinical signs, and radiographic evidence of lesions.

During the author's 30 years of clinical experience, the following criteria for *nonsurgical* therapy have been helpful:

1. Pain and little or no motor deficit.
2. Pain and/or paresis, first attack.
3. Any compressive disk case with pain, paresis, or paralysis that because of other medical disorders is not a reasonably good surgical risk.
4. A major motor deficit (paralysis) that is found in a patient with no conscious perception of deep pain and that is more than a few days in duration. Any such case is not a good surgical candidate regardless of duration.
5. Cases of progressive myelomalacia.[42]

It easily follows then which cases should be candidates for *surgical* and postsurgical supportive medical therapy, such as:

1. Any pain and/or paresis case that does not respond to conservative care or has experienced recurrent episodes.

2. Profound neurologic deficit (such as paralysis from a UMN lesion of a reasonably short duration), conscious perception of deep pain, and a definable radiographic lesion. These cases should be operated on as soon as possible to obtain prompt relief.[42]

Overall Care

The medical and postsurgical management of animals with disk protrusion involves general good nursing care. Proper nutrition, administration of vitamins and minerals if indicated, maintenance of urine and fecal elimination, and particularly rest are of prime importance. Confinement in a small area, such as a cage, an infant's playpen, or a large transportation crate, in a quiet surrounding can be used. Careless handling by animal caretakers should be avoided. The patient must be properly handled frequently to promote a good psychologic status. The patient must be responsive to at least one hospital person who becomes its friend, if a favorable outcome is to be achieved.[42]

The patient must be kept clean, and every effort must be made to avoid pressure on decubital sores and other cutaneous irritations in recumbent patients. A warm sitz soak administered twice daily for 10 to 15 minutes in water to which antiseptic detergent (such as povidone) has been added will help keep the animal clean, as well as diminish muscle spasms, promote a setting for proper passive exercise, and give the patient a mental boost. Various cushion materials in the cage, such as synthetic fleece or lambs' wool blankets and foam rubber pads, should be used. The prolonged presence of urine and feces on the skin must be avoided. The use of frames or ambulatory carts in the cage for short periods of time can be helpful in relieving the characteristic pressure sores seen in the pelvic region of paraplegics.

Care of the urinary bladder is not only important to avoid development of cystitis and cutaneous lesions, but also to ensure return of normal bladder, as well as ambulatory function, which is hindered by prolonged distention of the bladder. Complete bladder emptying must be accomplished at least three times daily by manual expression and/or aseptic catheterizations. After catheterization, flushing the bladder with warm saline should be considered in many cases. Systemic antibiotics may be necessary to combat infections. (The neurogenic bladder is discussed in Chapters 13 and 15.)

Supervised exercise is important in any case of intervertebral disk disease with motor deficits. Exercise of the limbs may be employed in the sitz soak by restraining the toes of the pelvic limbs on the floor of the tub with one hand and forcefully flexing the limbs by pushing down on the pelvic area with the other hand. Exercise can be gradually increased in intensity and duration only after the acute pain has subsided. Exercising the animal in a yard or on a nonslippery surface by supporting the tail or by using a belly band can be performed in the rehabilitative stages of patient care. Swimming in a child's wading pool can be helpful therapy.

The care of a paralytic involves a great deal of time and patience. In most cases, paralytics will require intensive nursing by clinical personnel for a few days after surgery. In addition to the nursing care discussed, it is important that the personnel establish a human–companion animal bond in the owner's absence. The owner may be unable to furnish the initial care needed because of distance or employment status. The cooperation of the owner should be solicited as soon as possible, but great care should be taken in training the owner in the proper procedures.[42]

The *medicinal* therapy[42] for the usual disk protrusion causing pain and weakness is not complicated. These patients do not need a great deal of medical therapy other than rest and good nursing care. If pain is excessive, analgesic or anti-inflammatory agents such as phenylbutazone, the salicylates, and low doses of glucocorticosteroids (dexamethasone, 0.2 mg/kg twice daily) may be used (see Chapter 15). The key therapy is rest. Local applications of moist heat or warm sitz soaks are usually adequate nonmedical analgesics. One must also bear in mind that all these drugs can be toxic. One of the chief problems in veterinary practice is that *rest* is not enforced at home when dexamethasone is administered. The complete relief of the beneficial self-limiting pain and resultant overactivity may cause increased extruded disk material and a worsening of neurologic dysfunction. Excessive pain should be lessened with medication, but not completely relieved in the outpatient.

In any sudden profound paralysis, whether the cause is an acutely ruptured disk or other spinal injury, a soluble glucocorticosteroid should be administered intravenously in adequate dosage as soon as possible—preferably within 30 to 45 minutes after injury. Agents such as methylprednisolone sodium succinate (Solu-Medrol), given at 30 mg/kg daily dosage rate, gain high concentration in the injured spinal cord and do much to protect the neuronal cells from the diminished circulation and hypoxic changes produced by the injury. This medication should be administered at least three times daily until a more residual effect can be obtained from agents such as dexamethasone. Although many surgeons use large doses of dexamethasone (2 mg/kg) as the sole source of steroids in acute spinal trauma or surgery, the results of recent research dictate the initial use of a soluble corticosteroid.[46] Mannitol infusions in a 20 to 25% solution have been used routinely by some surgeons in disk surgery. Recent investigations have demonstrated that mannitol solutions given in acute spinal injury could be injurious.[45] Disk extrusion cases of this nature will recover sooner and at a high percentage rate if prompt surgical relief is provided.[40, 42]

The high dosage administration of glucocorticosteroids should be diminished gradually and preferably stopped within 6 days to avoid the development of gastrointestinal inflammation and ulceration. Administration of antacids or gastrointestinal protective agents may aid in prevention of such sequellae.[5, 47, 63, 92]

Other reported medical treatments of disk disease include glucocorticosteroids epidurally, B complex vitamins, vitamin E and selenium, muscle relaxants such as methocarbamol (Robaxin), chlorphenesin carbonate (Maolate), and chymopapain enzyme injections into the disk (also known as diskolysis). Chymopapain has been approved in the United States for use in humans with herniated disks. Since Widdowson's[96] inconclusive results with chymopapain in 1967, diskolysis will no doubt be given further trials in veterinary medicine. Diskolysis in the dog using collagenase injected with the aid of computed tomography has been proposed.[16]

The treatment of progressive myelomalacia strictly entails good nursing and does not involve surgery. The use of an agent such as methylprednisolone[46] given as soon as possible, followed by dexamethasone, is the basic therapy. Bladder care, nutritional maintenance, and frequent turning of the recumbent patient to forestall pneumonia are additional nursing requirements.

The various means of physical therapy used with or without the addition of surgery are ultrasound,[85] traction and manipulation,[17, 62] thermal therapy, massage, exercises and stretching, and electric stimulation of muscles to prevent atrophy.[50] Trusses, corsets, braces, and casts have been used to promote rest and immobility of the vertebral column. The use of mobile carts or ambulatory devices has been tried for many years, but these should be used sparingly to encourage walking, not in lieu of walking.[42]

In conclusion, the key to nonsurgical treatment of disk protrusions is rest and general nursing care, employing analgesics only for excessive pain. Supervised exercise and hot water baths are helpful. The initial use of highly soluble glucocorticosteroids in the acute injury followed by a more residual steroid preparation such as dexamethasone in less severe cases (with or without surgery) should be considered. Care should be used with steroids to prevent gastrointestinal sequelae or exacerbation of neurologic damage when rest is not enforced. Proper care of the urinary bladder is a complete necessity in successful patient management.

Results of Therapies (Surgical and Nonsurgical)

In a disorder such as the disk protrusion, which involves a rather high incidence of spontaneous improvement, the analysis of data concerning the efficacy of various treatment methods is most difficult. Rest and maintenance of normal body metabolism and elimination are most important; one should not interfere with the natural course of improvement frequently seen in mild disk protrusions. For the sizable number of protrusions that are not mild and produce severe neurologic dysfunction, surgical intervention should be considered.

The indications for nonsurgical and surgical therapies have been presented and the details of the surgical procedures in prevalent use will be discussed in Chapter 17. Briefly, the hemilaminectomy involves the removal of the lateral lamina on one side of the vertebrae; the bony defect should extend from the floor to the roof (arch) of the vertebral canal and as far cranial and caudal as necessary to afford decompression of the cord and removal of the extruded disk mass.[24, 25, 40, 42, 75] The dorsal laminectomy and its modifications involve the removal of the roof of the canal extending craniocaudad at least three vertebral lengths.[21, 38, 42, 71, 93] Disk fenestration and its modifications generally utilizes a ventral midline approach in the cervical region,[40, 42, 66] and a dorsolateral,[66] lateral,[20, 64, 87, 98] or ventrolateral approach in the thoracolum-

Table 12-4. RESPONSE TO A SURVEY OF VETERINARY NEUROSURGEONS ON THE PREFERENCE OF SURGICAL PROCEDURES

Clinical Signs	Surgical Procedures for Clinical Thoracolumbar Disc Protrusions								
	Fenestration, All Types	Dorsal Laminectomy (Funkquist B)	Modified Dorsal Laminectomy	Deep Dorsal Laminectomy	Hemilaminectomy	Hemilaminectomy and Fenestration	Durotomy	Myelotomy	No Surgery
Recurrent pain	++++*	–	–	–	–	++	–	–	–
Paresis, first or recurrent attack	+++	–	–	+	++	+++	–	–	–
Sudden paraplegia with pain	–	–	+	+	++	+++	++	–	–
Recurrent paraplegia with pain	+	–	+	+	++	++++	++	–	–
Sudden paraplegia with no pain	–	–	++	++	++	+++	+++	+	+
Chronic paraplegia with no deep pain	–	–	+	+	+	–	++	–	+++

	Surgical Procedures for Clinical Cervical Disk Protrusions							
	Ventral Fenestration	Ventral Slot, No Graft	Ventral Slot, Graft	Dorsal Laminectomy	Hemilaminectomy	Durotomy	Myelotomy	No Surgery
Acute pain, first attack	++++	++	–	–	–	–	–	++
Acute pain, recurrent attacks	++++	++	–	–	–	–	–	–
Chronic pain	++++	++++	–	–	–	–	–	–
Pain with motor deficits	++	++++	+	+++	–	–	–	–

Frequency of Responses

	Grade
0–4	–
5–9	+
10–19	++
20–29	+++
30–above	++++

From Hoerlein BF: The status of the various intervertebral disk surgeries for the dog in 1978. J Am Anim Hosp Assoc 14:563, 1978.

Table 12–5. SUMMARY OF DISK SURGERY

Procedure	Indications	Advantages	Disadvantages	References
Thoracolumbar Surgery				
A. Fenestration				
1. Dorsolateral	Pain Slight paresis Prophylaxis	Less cord trauma, as surgery does not involve cord Easily combined with hemilaminectomy	No means of observing lesion Probably more surgically traumatic than muscle separation procedures	65
2. Dorsolateral muscle separation	Same as A (1)	Less cord trauma Probably less traumatic to spinal musculature	No observation of lesion Not easily combined with decompressive surgery	98
3. Lateral muscle separation	Same as A (1) Flo[20] also advocates this for paraplegia	Same as A (2)	Same as A (2)	20, 87
4. Ventrolateral fenestration	Lumbar disk problems Pain, paresis	Same as A (2)	No observation of lesion No data on clinical cases Traumatic to spinal nerves	64
5. Ventral—paracostal or intercostal	Same as A (1)	No cord trauma Least traumatic to spinal musculature	No observation of lesion Decompressive surgery requires separate approach Need two body wall incisions for most thoracolumbar fenestrations	56, 81
B. Decompressive surgery				
1. Dorsal laminectomy	Resistant pain Paresis Paraplegia	Provides good vision for other pathologic lesions Good for durotomy and myelotomy	Cannot remove protruding mass Prophylactic fenestrations not described—recurrences frequent Leaves cosmetic and structural defects	21
2. Modified dorsal laminectomy	Same as B (1)	Provides good observation of lesion Good for durotomy Can remove compressive mass but not the disk	Prophylactic fenestrations not described Leaves cosmetic and structural defects	93
3. Hemilaminectomy and disk fenestration	Same as B (1)	Provides good observation of lesion Durotomy–not as good as B (1 & 2) Good decompression Effective prophylactic fenestration Cosmetically and structurally sound	Not good for myelotomy Venous sinus hemorrhage is possible	40, 42

Table 12–5. SUMMARY OF DISK SURGERY *Continued*

Procedure	Indications	Advantages	Disadvantages	References
Thoracolumbar Surgery *Continued*				
4. Hemilaminec-tomy—lateral muscle separation approach	Same as B (1)	Less traumatic to spinal musculature Decompressive area to disk and floor of canal Same advantages as other hemilaminectomies	Same as other hemilaminectomies	13, 42
Cervical Disk Surgery				
A. Fenestration				
1. Ventral	Pain Paresis	Easily performed with little postoperative reaction	Adequate removal of massive calcific protrusion is not possible If protrusion is large, recovery may be slow or may not occur	40, 42, 65
B. Decompressive surgery				
1. Partial spondylectomy and diskectomy without graft (ventral slot)	Resistant pain Paresis and paralysis	Affords good removal of protruding mass and usually adequate decompression Moderate to slight postoperative reaction	Venous sinus hemorrhage is possible in removing mass	91
2. Partial spondylectomy and diskectomy with graft	Same as B (1)	Same as B (1) Moderate postoperative reaction Possibly provides greater stability from graft	Same as B (1), although author does not stress it Surgical time is longer owing to graft procedures, therefore there is more chance of sepsis or shock	70, 72
3. Dorsal laminectomy (Funkquist B)	Same as B (1)	Good exposure of cord for lesions other than disk problems Good decompression	No provision for removing protruding mass and causative disk lesion Severe postoperative reaction frequently occurs	21
4. Hemilaminectomy	Same as B (1)	Good exposure of cord Good decompression Possible to remove protruding mass	Difficult to remove causative disk lesion by fenestration Approach is more difficult than that of dorsal laminectomy Moderate postoperative reactions	42, 69

From Hoerlein BF: Canine Neurology, 3rd ed. Philadelphia, WB Saunders Co, 1978.

bar disk.[56, 81] Fenestration involves the curettage of as much of the disk as possible. The ventral fenestration combined with a ventral midline vertebral slot, frequently called a partial spondylectomy and diskectomy, is generally confined to decompressing an extruded cervical disk.[13, 70, 72, 91]

In 1977–1978 a questionnaire designed to determine the use of the various surgical procedures among practicing veterinary surgeons was distributed to existing North American veterinary schools, two private teaching hospitals, and surgeons in private practice who were members of the American Veterinary Neurology Association. Of the estimated 70 to 90 persons contacted, 50 surgeons from 20 institutions and 7 practitioners responded. Table 12–4 records the results. It is noted that fenestration methods were used primarily for pain and/or mild paresis, whereas the decompressive surgeries were used for cases with marked neurologic damage in both cervical and thoracolumbar lesions. The survey was made several years ago; however, it is anticipated that, although current responses might indicate a slightly different choice of the individual surgeries used, the decompressive modes would be most prevalent in animals with marked motor deficits[43] (Table 12–4).

As noted in the aforementioned survey,[43] there are several methods for fenestration and decompression. In addition, there are variations of each procedure peculiar to the surgeon and his or her capabilities. Some surgeons prefer the dorsal laminectomy and possible durotomy for thoracolumbar[10, 26, 38, 59, 71, 93] and cervical disk extrusions.[49] Others prefer hemilaminectomy of thoracolumbar disks with concomitant fenestration of highly susceptible or slightly affected disks.[24, 40, 42, 55] Most surgeons recognize the value of the decompressive partial spondylectomy and diskectomy for extruded cervical disks in chondrodystrophoid and large nonchondrodystrophoid breeds that have persistent pain and/or motor signs.[13, 70, 72, 89, 91] The original descriptions of the ventral cervical decompressive procedure employed a bone graft stabilization,[70, 72] which has now been shown to be unnecessary in the routine case of intervertebral disk disease.[91] In the few reported disk extrusions in the cat, the decompressive hemilaminectomy or dorsal laminectomy has been employed.[28, 37, 42, 88]

There is general agreement that if there are serious motor deficits, prompt surgical decompression results in maximal and prompt recovery.[38, 40, 42] A few reports of delayed surgery in such cases have been cited.[55, 58] There is also consensus that when the conscious perception of deep pain is absent, along with profound motor deficits, the prognosis is guarded to unfavorable regardless of the type of treatment used. Many surgeons prefer fenestration-type surgeries for less severe cases[6, 20, 98] and will prophylactically perform fenestration of additional susceptible disks during decompression.[24, 42, 43, 55] A few surgeons believe that recurrences involving other disks are not frequent enough to warrant so-called prophylactic fenestrations.[71] However, prophylactic fenestrations do not require a great amount of time and are a worthwhile effort.

It is difficult to accurately compare the success of nonsurgical with surgical care in the disk syndrome because the competent practitioner will use various methods on different types of cases. Frequently the chronic disk disease that does not respond to nonsurgical care is subjected to surgery. Nonsurgical recoveries are reported to range from 30 to 50%.[21, 42] Many authors concur that at least one third of the so-called recoveries in nonsurgically treated cases are followed by recurrences; generally the recurrence results in greater neurologic damage.[42]

Most of the statistical reports on the various surgical procedures indicate success rates in the vicinity of 75 to 90% when the aforementioned principles of case selection are followed.[38, 42, 71] The most extensive long-term evaluation of surgical results has been reported by Hoerlein and coworkers[42] and involved 1184 dogs seen from 1950 to 1975 at the Auburn Clinic. Forty per cent of these animals were observed from 3 to 5 years after surgery. Good surgical results were acquired in 87% of paralytics, 90.5% of paretics, and 82.7% of the pain cases. In a smaller number of nonsurgical cases, 22.4%, 29.7%, and 37.5% of the paralytics, paretics, and pain cases, respectively, showed good results.

To update the disk disease status at the Auburn Clinic, a random survey (approximately 10%) of the surgical cases seen from 1975 to 1983 was performed. In cases of thoracolumbar disk disease (50% were paraplegics), 92.9% of the surgeries performed involved the combined hemilaminectomy-fenestration procedure. Whereas the aforementioned results were based on follow-up evaluations, in this survey the motor ability was evaluated at the end of the hospitalization stay, which averaged 9.4 days. At this time, 63.5% were walking well, 23.7% were fair, and 12.8% were poor. Most of the "fair" category should improve to the category of walking "well" with additional time. On this premise, about 86% would be walking well when judged on the same basis as the previous surveys (1950–1975). Of the cervical disk surgeries, 78.4% involved the combination fenestration and ventral slot procedure. Evaluation at the end of the hospital stay found 85.7% good results. These surgical results parallel the findings of the more extensive survey performed in the 1950–1975 era.

Obviously, the results of the various surgical procedures used in disk cases may be fairly consistent. Surgeons are most proficient with the methods they use routinely. For those choosing a method, Table 12–5 summarizes the author's opinions about the advantages and disadvantages of the basic surgical procedures.

REFERENCES

1. Armstrong JR: Lumbar Disc Lesions, 2d ed. Edinburgh, E and S Livingstone Ltd, 1958.
2. Bailey, CS and Morgan, JP: Diseases of the spinal cord. In Ettinger SJ: Textbook of Veterinary Internal Medicine. 2nd ed. Philadelphia, WB Saunders Co, 1983, p 532.
3. Ball MU, McGuire JA, Swaim SF, and Hoerlein BF: Patterns of occurrence of disc disease among registered dachshunds. JAVMA 180:519, 1982.
4. Beadle OA: The intervertebral discs: Observations on their normal and morbid anatomy and relation to certain spinal deformities. Medical Research Council, Special Report Series No 161. London, His Majesty's Stationery Office, 1931.
5. Bellah JR: Colonic perforation after corticosteroid and surgical treatment of intervertebral disk disease in a dog. JAVMA 183:102, 1983.
6. Bojrab MJ: Current Technique in Small Animal Surgery I. Philadelphia, Lea & Febiger, 1975, p 404.
7. Bowen JM: Peripheral nerve electro-diagnostics, electromyography, and nerve conduction velocity. In Hoerlein BF: Canine Neurology, 3rd ed. Philadelphia, WB Saunders Co, 1978.
8. Braund KG: Acute spinal cord traumatic compression. In Bojrab MJ (ed): Pathophysiology in Small Animal Surgery. Philadelphia, Lea & Febiger, 1981, p 220.
9. Braund KG, Ghosh P, Taylor TK, and Larsen LH: Morphological studies of the canine intervertebral disc. The assignment of the beagle to the achondroplastic classification. Res Vet Sci 19:167, 1975.
10. Brown NO, Helphrey ML, and Prata RG: Thoracolumbar disk disease in the dog: A retrospective analysis of 187 cases. J Am Anim Hosp Assoc 13:665, 1977.
11. Butler WF and Smith RN: The nucleus pulposus of the intervertebral disc in newborn cats. Res Vet Sci 5:71, 1964.
12. Butler WF and Smith RN: Age changes in the intervertebral disc. Res Vet Sci 6:280, 1965.
13. Chambers JN, Oliver JE, Kornegay JN, and Malnati GA: Ventral decompression for caudal cervical disk herniation in large- and giant-breed dogs. JAVMA 180:410, 1982.
14. Chrisman CL, Burt JK, Wood PK, and Johnson EW: Electromyography in small animal clinical neurology. JAVMA 160:311, 1972.
15. Cloward RB: The clinical significance of the sinuvertebral nerve of the cervical spine in relation to the cervical disc syndrome. J Neurol Neurosurg Psychiatry 23:321, 1961.
16. Coin CG, Coin JT, and Garrett JK: Canine disc herniation diagnosis by computed tomography. Scientific exhibit, Am Vet Med Assoc Convention, Salt Lake City, UT, July, 1982.
17. Cottle LW: Traction in the treatment of canine spinal disorders. J Am Anim Hosp Assoc 8:332, 1972.
18. Dandy WE: Loose cartilage from intervertebral disk stimulating tumor of the spinal cord. Arch Surg 19:660, 1929.
19. Dohn DF: Anterior interbody fusion for treatment of cervical disk conditions. JAMA 197:897, 1966.
20. Flo GL and Brinker WO: Lateral fenestration of thoracolumbar discs. J Am Anim Hosp Assoc 11:619, 1975.
20a. Forsythe WB and Ghoshal NG: Innervation of the canine thoracolumbar vertebral column. Anat Rec 208:57, 1984.
21. Funkquist B: Decompressive laminectomy in thoracolumbar disc protrusion with paraplegia in the dog. J Small Anim Pract 11:445, 1970.
22. Funkquist B: Investigations of the therapeutic and prophylactic effects of disc evacuation in cases of thoraco-lumbar herniated discs in dogs. Acta Vet Scand 19:441, 1978.
23. Gage ED: Incidence of clinical disc disease in the dog. J Am Anim Hosp Assoc 11:135, 1975.
24. Gage ED: Modifications in dorsolateral hemilaminectomy and disc fenestrations in the dog. J Am Anim Hosp Assoc 11:407, 1975.
25. Gage ED and Hoerlein BF: Hemilaminectomy and dorsal laminectomy for relieving compressions of the spinal cord in the dog. JAVMA 152:351, 1968.
26. Gambardella PC: Dorsal decompressive laminectomy for treatment of thoracolumbar disc disease in dogs: A retrospective study of 98 cases. Vet Surg 9:24, 1980.
27. Ghosh P, Taylor TKF, Braund KG, and Larsen LH: The collagenous and non-collagenous proteins of the canine intervertebral disc and their variation with age, spinal level, and breed. Gerontology 22:124, 1976.
28. Gilmore DR: Extrusion of a feline intervertebral disk. Vet Med Small Anim Clin 78:207, 1983.
29. Goggins JE, Li AS, and Franti CE: Canine intervertebral disk diseases; characterization by age, breed, and anatomical site of involvement. Am J Vet Res 9:1687, 1970.
30. Greene JA, Knecht CD and Roesel OF: Hypothyroidism as a possible cause of canine intervertebral disk disease. J Am Anim Hosp Assoc 15:199, 1979.
31. Griffiths IR: The extensive myelopathy of intervertebral disc protrusions in dogs (ascending syndrome). J Small Anim Pract 13:425, 1972.
32. Griffiths IR: Some aspects of the pathogenesis and diagnosis of lumbar disk protrusion in the dog. J Small Anim Pract 13:439, 1972.
33. Haley JC and Perry JH: Protrusions of intervertebral disc. Am J Surg 80:394, 1950.
34. Hansen HJ: A pathologic-anatomical interpretation of disc degeneration in dogs. Acta Orthop Scand 20:280, 1951.
35. Hansen HJ: A pathologic-anatomical study on disc degeneration in dogs. Acta Orthop Scand (Suppl 11) 1952.
36. Hansen HJ: Pathogenesis of disc degeneration and rupture. In Pettit GO (ed): Intervertebral Disk Protrusions in the Dog. New York, Appleton-Century-Crofts, 1966 p 24.
37. Heavner JE: Intervertebral disc syndrome in the cat. JAVMA 159:425, 1971.

38. Henry WB Jr: Dorsal decompressive laminectomy in the treatment of thoracolumbar disc disease. J Am Anim Hosp Assoc 11:627, 1975.

39. Higley HG: The Intervertebral Disc. Webster City, Ia, National Chiropractic Assoc, 1960.

40. Hoerlein BF: The treatment of intervertebral disc protrusions in the dog. Proc Am Vet Med Assoc 206, June 23–26, 1952.

41. Hoerlein BF: Intervertebral disc protrusions in the dog. I. Incidence and pathological lesions. II. Symptomatology and clinical diagnosis. III. Radiological diagnosis. Am J Vet Res 19:260, 1953.

42. Hoerlein BF: Canine Neurology, 3rd ed. Philadelphia, WB Saunders Co, 1978.

43. Hoerlein BF: The status of the various intervertebral disk surgeries for the dog in 1978. J Am Anim Hosp Assoc 14:563, 1978.

44. Hoerlein BF: Comparative disk disease; man and dog. J Am Anim Hosp Assoc 15:535, 1979.

45. Hoerlein BF, Redding RW, Hoff EJ Jr, and McGuire J: The evaluation of dexamethasone, DMSO, mannitol, and solcoseryl in acute spinal cord trauma. J Am Anim Hosp Assoc 19:221, 1983.

46. Hoerlein BF, Redding RW, Hoff EJ Jr, and McGuire JA: Evaluation of naloxone, crocetin, thyrotropin releasing hormone, methylprednisolone, partial myelotomy, and hemilaminectomy in the treatment of acute spinal cord trauma. J Am Anim Hosp Assoc 21:67, 1985.

47. Hoerlein BF and Spano JS: Non-neurological complications following decompressive spinal cord surgery. Arch Am Coll Vet Sug 4:11, 1975.

48. Horwitz T: Lesions of the intervertebral disc and ligamentum flavum of lumbar vertebrae; an anatomic study of 75 human cadavers. Surgery 6:410, 1939.

49. Hurov L: Dorsal decompressive cervical laminectomy in the dog: Surgical considerations and clinical cases. J Am Anim Hosp Assoc 15:301, 1979.

50. Jadeson WJ: Rehabilitation of dogs with intervertebral disc lesions by physical therapy methods. JAVMA 138:411, 1961.

51. King AS and Smith RN: A comparison of the anatomy of the intervertebral disc in dog and man with reference to herniation of the nucleus pulposus. Br Vet J 111:135, 1955.

52. King AS and Smith RN: Disc protrusions in the cat: Distribution of dorsal protrusions along the vertebral column. Acta Orthop Scand 72:335, 1960.

53. King AS and Smith RN: Disc protrusions in the cat: Age incidence of dorsal protrusions. Acta Orthop Scand 72:381, 1960.

54. King AS and Smith RN: Degeneration of the intervertebral disc in the cat. Acta Orthop Scand 34:139, 1964.

55. Knecht CD: The effect of delayed hemilaminectomy in the treatment of intervertebral disc protrusion in dogs. J Am Anim Hosp Assoc 6:71, 1970.

56. Leonard EP: Orthopedic Surgery of the Dog and Cat, 2d ed. Philadelphia, WB Saunders Co, 1971.

57. Lindgren S: Some problems concerning herniated intervertebral disc from the clinical point of view. JAMA 142:445, 1950.

58. Martin JG: The feasibility of delayed surgery in intervertebral disc protrusions causing paraplegia or paresis. 36th Annual Meeting, Am Anim Hosp Assoc 409, 1969.

59. Mendenhall HV, Litwak P, Yturraspe DL, et al: Aggressive pharmacological and surgical treatment of spinal cord injuries in dogs and cats. JAVMA 168:1036, 1976.

60. Evans HE and Christensen GC: Miller's Anatomy of the Dog. 2nd ed. Philadelphia, WB Saunders Co, 1979.

61. Mixter WJ and Barr JS: Rupture of the intervertebral disk with involvement of the spinal canal. N Engl J Med 211:210, 1934.

62. Moltzen H: Manipulation as a method of therapy for spinal disorders in dogs and cats. J Am Anim Hosp Assoc 7:242, 1971.

63. Moore RW and Winthrow SJ: Gastrointestinal hemorrhage and pancreatitis associated with intervertebral disk disease in the dog. JAVMA 180:1443, 1982.

64. Northway RB: A ventrolateral approach to lumbar intervertebral disc fenestration. Vet Med Small Anim Clin 60:884, 1965.

65. Olsson SE: Observations concerning disc fenestration in dogs. Acta Orthop Scand 20:349, 1951.

66. Olsson SE: The dynamic factor in spinal cord compression. A study on dogs with special reference of cervical disc protrusions. J Neurosurg 15:308, 1958.

67. Paatsama S, Rissanen P, and Rokkanen P: Effect of estradiol, testosterone, cortisone acetate, somatotropin, thyrotropin, and parathyroid hormone on the lumbar intervertebral disc in growing dogs. J Small Anim Pract 10:351, 1969.

68. Pettit G: Intervertebral Disc Protrusion in the Dog. New York, Appleton-Century-Crofts, 1966.

69. Pettit GD and Whitaker RP: Hemilaminectomy for cervical disc protrusions in a dog. JAVMA 143:379, 1963.

70. Popovic NA, Vander Ark G, and Kempe L: Ventral approach for surgical treatment of cervical disk disease in the dog. Am J Vet Res 32:1155, 1971.

71. Prata RG: Neurosurgical treatment of thoracolumbar disks: The rationale and value of laminectomy with concomitant disk removal. J Am Anim Hosp Assoc 17:17, 1981.

72. Prata RG and Stoll SG: Ventral decompression and fusion for the treatment of cervical disc disease in the dog. J Am Anim Hosp Assoc 9:462, 1973.

73. Priester WA: Canine intervertebral disk disease—occurrence by age, breed, and sex among 8117 cases. Theriogenology 6:293, 1976.

74. Purohit RC, Kircher IM, Redding RW, and Swaim SF: Thermography as a diagnostic aid in localization of intervertebral disk disease in the dog. J Thermog, 1986, in press.

75. Redding RW: Laminectomy in the dog. Am J Vet Res 12:123, 1951.

76. Redding RW: Canine electroencephalography. In Hoerlein BF: Canine Neurology, 3rd ed. Philadelphia WB Saunders Co, 1978,

77. Redding RW and Ingram JT: Sensory nerve conduction velocity of cutaneous afferents of the radial, ulnar, peroneal, and tibial nerves of the cat: Reference values. Am J Vet Res 45(5):1042, 1984.

78. Redding RW and Knecht CD: Atlas of Electroencephalography of the Dog and Cat. New York, Praeger Publishers, 1984.

79. Riser WH: Posterior paralysis associated with intervertebral disc protrusion in the dog. North Am Vet 27:633, 1946.

80. Roofe PG: Innervation of annulus fibrosus and posterior longitudinal ligament. Arch Neurol Psychol 44:100, 1940.

81. Ross GE: Surgical treatment of intervertebral disc disease. 36th Annual Meeting, Am Anim Hosp Assoc 409, 1969.

82. Rowe NF: Electromyographic study of the paraspinal muscles of the dog in clinical intervertebral disc disease. Thesis (MS), Auburn University, Auburn, AL, 1975.

83. Russell WW and Griffiths RC: Recurrence of cervical

disc syndrome in surgically and conservatively treated dogs. JAVMA 153:1412, 1968.

84. Schappert HR and Geib LW: Reticuloendothelial neoplasms involving the spinal canal of cats. JAVMA 150:753, 1967.

85. Schirmer RC: Ultrasound therapy. *In* Kirk RW: Current Veterinary Therapy III. Philadelphia, WB Saunders Co, 1968.

86. Schmorl G: Zur pathologischen Anatomie der Virbelsaule. Klin Wochenschr 8:1243, 1929.

87. Seemann CW: Lateral approach for thoracolumbar disc fenestration. Mod Vet Pract 49:73, 1968.

88. Seim HB and Nafe LA: Spontaneous intervertebral disk extrusion with associated myelopathy in a cat. J Am Anim Hosp Assoc 17:201, 1981.

89. Seim HB and Prata RG: Ventral decompression for the treatment of cervical disk disease in the dog: A review of 54 cases. J Am Anim Hosp Assoc 18:233, 1982.

90. Smith RN: Anatomy and physiology. *In* Pettit GD (ed): Intervertebral Disc Protrusion in the Dog. New York, Appleton-Century-Crofts 1966.

91. Swaim SF: Ventral decompression of the cervical spinal cord in the dog. JAVMA 162:276, 1973.

92. Toombs JP, Caywood DD, Lipowitz AJ, and Stevens JB: Colonic perforation following neurosurgical procedures and corticosteroid therapy in four dogs. JAVMA 177:68, 1980.

93. Trotter EJ: Modified dorsal laminectomy and selective regional spinal cord hypothermia in the treatment of thoracolumbar disk disease. *In* Bojrab JJ (ed): Current Techniques in Small Animal Surgery I. Philadelphia, Lea & Febiger, 1975, p 406.

94. Vandevelde M: Spinal cord compression. *In* Bojrab M (ed): Pathophysiology in Small Animal Surgery. Philadelphia, Lea & Febiger, 1981, p 228.

95. Verkeijen J and Bouw J: Canine intervertebral disc disease: A review of etiologic and predisposing factors. Vet Quart 4:125, 1982.

96. Widdowson WL: Effects of chymopapain in the intervertebral disc of the dog. JAVMA 150:608, 1967.

97. Wright F and Palmer AC: Morphological changes caused by pressure on the spinal. cord. Pathol Vet 6:355, 1969.

98. Yturraspe DJ and Lumb WV: A dorsolateral muscle-separating approach for thoracolumbar intervertebral disk fenestration in the dog. JAVMA 162:1037, 1973.

99. Zaki FA and Hurvitz AI: Spontaneous neoplasms of the central nervous system of the cat. J Am Anim Pract 17:773, 1974.

Disorders of Micturition

Micturition is the physiologic process of storage and complete voiding of urine.[4] Abnormal micturition includes inappropriate voiding, inadequate voiding with overflow of urine, increased frequency, or reduced capacity. Only abnormalities related to neurologic dysfunction will be considered here.[34]

There are no data on the incidence of problems related to micturition in animals. Some degree of voiding difficulty is present in every paraplegic animal, most animals with moderate to severe spinal cord or cauda equina disease, and some animals with other parts of the nervous system affected.[33] Although some paralyzed animals have problems with constipation, the ability of the gastrointestinal tract to function virtually independent of the central nervous system (CNS) makes this a minor problem in management. The neurogenic bladder, on the other hand, can be life threatening.[37]

PATHOPHYSIOLOGY

Micturition is accomplished through a complex integration of parasympathetic, sympathetic, and somatic components of the nervous system (Fig. 13–1). Some details of this organization are still unknown.[4, 11, 13]

The fundamental process in micturition is the detrusor (bladder muscle) reflex. As the bladder fills, there is little increase in intravesical pressure. The stretch of the smooth muscle is in part passive, but inhibition by the sympathetic nerves is probably important also.[14] When the bladder nears its capacity, tension receptors are activated in the bladder wall.[20] The receptors initiate impulses through sensory fibers in the

342

pelvic nerve to the sacral spinal cord.[9, 11] The sensory discharge ascends in the spinal cord to the reticular formation of the pons. Integration at this level results in a volley of impulses descending the spinal cord to activate parasympathetic preganglionic neurons in the sacral spinal cord.[29, 35] The parasympathetic neurons synapse on postganglionic neurons in the pelvic plexus and bladder wall. Postganglionic neurons activate the detrusor muscle, causing a contraction of the bladder. The long-routing of the reflex to the pons is necessary for a sustained, coordinated reflex. Lesions of any portion of this pathway, including the spinal cord, abolish the detrusor reflex.[4, 10, 13, 25]

Normal voiding requires a sustained contraction of the bladder and opening of the outflow tract, the urethra. Continence is maintained by the resistance to flow in the urethra. A combination of several mechanisms maintains this resistance. A passive component includes the resting length and diameter of the urethra, its natural softness that allows it to collapse, elastic fibers in the wall, and possible pressure from blood vessels in the urethra.[3, 7, 17] The major resting pressure is exerted from smooth muscle in the urethra. It is innervated by both sympathetic and parasympathetic nerves and is continuous with the detrusor muscle.[13, 16, 23] There is no distinct anatomic "internal sphincter muscle." Sympathetic nerves in the urethral smooth muscle apparently are most important for the resting tone. Striated muscle around the urethra is innervated by the pudendal nerve, a somatic nerve.[30] The striated muscle contributes to resting tone, but is even more important in reflexes and voluntary contraction.[11, 13] Some investigators have suggested sympathetic inner-

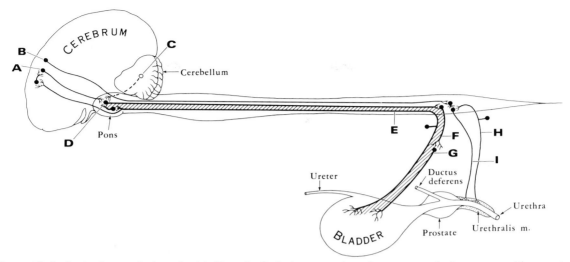

Figure 13–1. Anatomic organization of micturition. A, Cortical neurons for voluntary control of micturition; B, cortical neurons for voluntary control of sphincters; C, cerebellar neurons that have an inhibitory influence on micturition; D, pontine reticular neurons that are necessary for the detrusor reflex; E, afferent (sensory) pathway for the detrusor reflex; F, preganglionic pelvic (parasympathetic) neurons to the detrusor; G, postganglionic pelvic (parasympathetic) neurons to the detrusor; H, afferent (sensory) neurons from the urethral sphincter, pudendal nerve; I, efferent (motor) neurons to the urethral sphincter, pudendal nerve. (From Oliver JE Jr and Osborne CA: Neurogenic urinary incontinence. *In* Kirk RW (ed): Current Veterinary Therapy VII. Philadelphia, WB Saunders Co, 1980.)

vation of this striated muscle; however, the bulk of the evidence is against this.

During the detrusor reflex, there is direct inhibition of both the sympathetic and the pudendal nerves, allowing for relaxation of the urethra.[10, 17] In addition, contraction of the detrusor muscle shortens the muscle fibers spiraling into the urethra and results in an opening of the proximal urethra. The net result is an increase in intravesical pressure and a decrease in urethral resistance, allowing voiding to occur.

Superimposed on this involuntary reflex system is the ability to initiate or inhibit micturition. This is accomplished by cortical control of the pontine micturition center.[15, 17] Additionally, the cortex has direct pathways (upper motor neurons) to the pudendal nerves, enabling voluntary contraction of the muscles. Lesions of the cerebral cortex do not abolish micturition, but they do eliminate voluntary control. Animals with cortical lesions may begin voiding in the house, for example.

The cerebellum has inhibitory inputs into the pontine micturition center. Its physiologic role is not clear. Lesions of the cerebellum may cause increased frequency of voiding, with a reduced bladder capacity.[17, 32, 33]

Overdistention of the bladder often causes a loss of the contractile response of the muscle.

There are at least two hypotheses for this problem. The motor nerves in the bladder wall innervate many muscle cells through modified neuromuscular junctions. The junctions are characterized by a varicosity of the axon containing synaptic vesicles, a thinning of the Schwann cell layer, and a close apposition to specialized areas of the muscle fibers.[11] All muscle cells are not innervated. Excitation spreads from innervated cells to noninnervated cells by means of "tight junction." It has also been hypothesized that the neurotransmitter spreads through the extracellular space. Overdistention causes a separation of the tight junctions and an increase in extracellular space. Either of these would interfere with the spread of excitation and cause a flaccid, noncontracting bladder. If infection and fibrosis occur, function may not be restored. Early decompression of an overdistended bladder is essential if function is to be restored.[32]

Table 13–1 summarizes the functions of the various components of the micturition reflex and the effects of lesions.

The neurologic problems associated with abnormal micturition primarily cause alterations in the detrusor reflex and in sphincter activity. The detrusor reflex may be absent or decreased, hyperactive or normal. Sphincter activity may

Table 13–1. EFFECT OF LESIONS OF NEUROMUSCULAR SYSTEM

Location of Lesion	Normal Function	Bladder					Sphincter			
		Voluntary Control	Sustained Detrusor Reflex	Tone	Volume	Residual Urine	Voluntary Control	Reflexes (Perineal, Bulbourethral)	Tone	Synergy with Detrusor
Cerebral cortex to brain stem	Voluntary control to detrusor and sphincter	Absent	Normal	Normal	May be larger or smaller than normal	None	Absent	Normal to hyperreflexic	Normal to increased	Normal
Cerebellum	Modulation (inhibition) of detrusor reflex	Normal, but increased frequency	Possibly hyperreflexic	Normal	Small	None	Normal	Normal	Normal	Normal
Brain stem (pons) to sacral spinal cord	Sustained detrusor reflex	Absent	Lost early; small unsynchronized contractions late	Atonic early; possibly increased late	Large	Large	Absent	Normal to hyperreflexic	Normal to increased	Absent
Partial lesions (reflex dyssynergia)	Sustained detrusor reflex	May be present	May be present	Normal to atonic	Large	Small to large	May be normal	Normal	Normal to increased	Absent
Sacral spinal cord or roots	LMN to detrusor and sphincter	Absent	Absent	Atonic	Large	Large	Absent	Absent	Flaccid	Absent
Disruption of tight junctions of detrusor	Spread of excitation in detrusor	Absent	Absent	Atonic	Large	Large	Normal	Normal	Normal	Normal (cannot evaluate, however)

From Oliver JE Jr and Osborne CA: Neurogenic urinary incontinence. In Kirk RW (ed): Current Veterinary Therapy VI. Philadelphia, WB Saunders Co, 1977.

be decreased, increased, or normal. Combinations of these two problems produce most of the syndromes currently described.

Detrusor Areflexia with Sphincter Hypertonus. Lesions from the pons to the L7 spinal cord segments cause a loss of the detrusor reflex. Frequently there is increased tone and exaggerated reflexes in the skeletal muscle of the sphincter. This has been called an upper motor neuron (UMN) bladder, but this term is misleading because the bladder is areflexic, not hyperreflexic. The "automatic" or hyperreflexic bladder seen in humans is rarely, if ever, present in dogs. The author has tried to reproduce it experimentally, so far unsuccessfully. Dogs with complete spinal cord transections have been monitored for over 2 months with no evidence of anything more than small uninhibited bladder contractions. Detrusor areflexia is common in animals with spinal cord lesions resulting from herniated disks, trauma, or tumors. The animal is unable to void, and it is difficult to express the bladder manually because of increased tone in the urethra. Overflow occurs when the bladder pressure exceeds outflow resistance. The perineal reflex is intact.[27, 31]

Detrusor Areflexia with Normal Sphincter Tone. Lesions from the pons to L7 spinal cord may cause detrusor areflexia without an increase in sphincter tone, just as all upper motor neuron lesions do not cause exaggeration of other spinal reflexes (see Chapter 2). In addition, trauma to the pelvis may injure the pelvic nerves without damaging the pudendal nerve. The animal is unable to void, but manual expression is relatively easy. Perineal reflexes are intact.[27, 31]

Detrusor Areflexia with Sphincter Areflexia. Lesions of the sacral spinal cord or sacral roots (cauda equina) cause a loss of the detrusor reflex with a flaccid, areflexic sphincter. The bladder is easily expressed and overflows easily, and the perineal reflex is absent.[3, 27, 31]

Detrusor Areflexia from Overdistention. Prolonged overdistention of the bladder prevents the spread of excitation in the detrusor muscle. The bladder is large and atonic. The sphincter and perineal reflexes are normal. The animal often attempts to void because sensory pathways are intact. Small amounts of urine may be voided by an abdominal press, but residual volume is large.[27, 32]

Detrusor Hyperreflexia. Frequent voiding of small quantities of urine, often without warning, is evidence of detrusor hyperreflexia. It is common with cystitis, occasionally seen with cerebellar disease, and rare otherwise. The bladder is usually small, there is little or no residual urine, and perineal reflexes are intact.[26, 31]

Reflex Dyssynergia. A normal or hyperactive detrusor reflex is accompanied by a hyperreflexic sphincter in this syndrome. The animal initiates voiding, but the stream is abruptly stopped by an involuntary contraction of the urethra.[28] Reflex dyssynergia in humans is supposed to be caused by an upper motor neuron lesion.[17] A number of male dogs have been observed with something like this syndrome, but have not fulfilled the diagnostic criteria. Diagnosis would require documentation of a detrusor reflex followed by contraction of the sphincter. The dogs have been normal neurologically, in contrast to the syndrome in people.

Normal Detrusor Reflex with Decreased Sphincter Tone. Normal voiding but leakage of urine at other times is characteristic of decreased urethral resistance. Lesions of the pudendal nerve may cause this syndrome, but they are rare. Hormone responsive incontinence, in both males and females, is the most common cause.[5, 34, 36] Iatrogenic damage to the urethra, such as may occur in prostatic surgery or in perineal urethrostomies, may also cause decreased sphincter resistance.

Inappropriate Voiding. Animals may suddenly alter their normal behavior patterns, including micturition and defecation. A dog or cat that has been house trained for years and begins voiding in the house may have cerebral disease or a primary behavior disorder.[25] Other neurologic abnormalities are usually present if there is a cerebral lesion. Behavior disorders can be difficult to manage. Several books are available for reference.[6, 12, 18, 21]

Table 13–2 summarizes the signs of abnormal micturition.

DIAGNOSIS

The objective in evaluation of a patient with a voiding disorder is to locate the source and cause of the problem. Neurogenic disorders must be distinguished from non-neurogenic disorders, such as obstructions, cystitis, and malformations.[19, 34] In neurogenic disorders, it is important to determine if the detrusor reflex is normal, hyperactive, or absent, and if the sphincter is normal, hyperactive, or depressed. The recommended minimum data base (Table 13–3) is designed to provide most of this information and to reveal any additional problems that may affect the prognosis.[31] Table 13–4 illustrates the logic of establishing a diagnosis

Table 13–2. SIGNS OF ABNORMAL MICTURITION

Problem	Voiding	Attempts to Void	Expression of Bladder	Residual Urine	Perineal Reflex	Probable Lesion
Detrusor areflexia with sphincter hypertonus	Absent	No	Difficult	Large amount	Present	Brain stem to L7 spinal cord
Detrusor areflexia with normal sphincter tone	Absent	No	Possible, some resistance	Large amount	Present	Brain stem to L7 spinal cord
Detrusor areflexia with sphincter areflexia	Absent	No	Easy, often leaks	Large to moderate amount	Absent	Sacral spinal cord or nerve roots
Detrusor areflexia from over-distention	Absent	Yes	Possible, some resistance	Large amount	Present	Detrusor muscle
Detrusor hyperreflexia	Frequent, small quantity	Yes	Possible, some resistance	None	Present	Brain stem to L7, partial or cerebellum; rule out inflammation of bladder
Reflex dyssynergia	Frequent, spurting, unsustained	Yes	Difficult	Small to large amount	Present, may be exaggerated	Brain stem to L7, partial
Normal detrusor reflex with incompetent sphincter	Normal, but with leakage of urine with stress or full bladder	Yes	Easy	None	May or may not be present	Pudendal nerves, sympathetic nerves, hormone deficiency

based on clinical findings.[34] The specific items of information necessary to follow the algorithm will be discussed.

History

In addition to the usual items in a history, some specific information pertinent to micturition should be obtained. For instance, the pattern of micturition habits should be determined from as early an age as possible. Age at house training, frequency of micturition at various ages, and changes in habits may provide clues

Table 13–3. MINIMUM DATA BASE FOR DIAGNOSIS OF URINARY INCONTINENCE

History
Physical examination
  Includes: Observation of voiding and measurement of residual urine
Neurologic examination
  Includes: Sphincter reflexes
Clinical pathology
  Includes: CBC, urinalysis, BUN or creatinine
Radiology
  Includes: Survey of abdomen and pelvis; contrast cystography and urethrography; intravenous pyelogram

From Oliver JE Jr and Osborne CA: Neurogenic urinary incontinence. In Kirk RW (ed.): Current Veterinary Therapy VI. Philadelphia, WB Saunders Co, 1977.

to the onset of a problem prior to the owner's recognition of its significance.

Signs of abnormality in the nervous system or urinary tract or previous trauma may be important. Previous surgical procedures, especially neurologic, abdominal, or pelvic (eg, ovariohysterectomy), should be analyzed in relation to the onset of the problem.[19]

The onset and chronologic course of signs will allow construction of sign-time graph, which is useful for determining the etiology of the disease (see Chapter 2).

Voluntary control of micturition is often best established by the owner's observation. This can be supplemented and confirmed by direct observation of the animal in natural surroundings (eg, outside on grass). If the animal can volitionally initiate voiding, the detrusor reflex is probably present. Voluntary control also means that micturition can be withheld a reasonable length of time (house training) and can be interrupted if necessary. Interruption of micturition is more difficult to evaluate than voluntary initiation. A dog that is lead trained can be interrupted by a pull on the lead and commanded to come. Individual interpretation of interruption may be subjective.

Reflex dyssynergia will usually appear as normal initiation of voiding followed by narrowing of the stream and sudden interruption of flow. Straining will often continue, and voiding may continue in brief spurts. Dyssynergia must be

Table 13–4. ALGORITHM FOR DIAGNOSIS OF DISORDERS OF MICTURITION

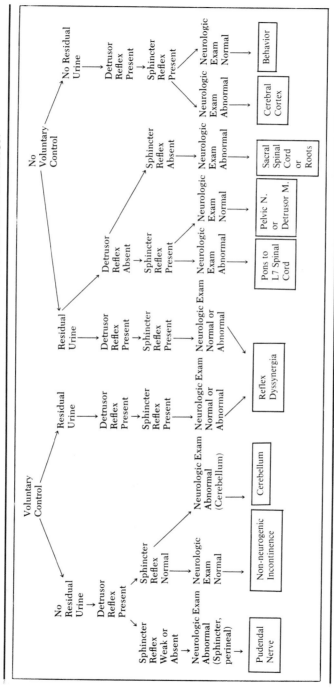

From Oliver JE Jr and Osborne CA: Neurogenic urinary incontinence. *In* Kirk RW (ed.): Current Veterinary Therapy VI. Philadelphia, WB Saunders Co, 1977.

differentiated from partial obstruction (eg, urethral calculi), which is usually recognized by catheterization and/or urethral contrast radiography.

Various types of incontinence may be described by the owner. Precipitate voiding, in which the animal voids suddenly in inappropriate places without apparent warning, is characteristic of cerebellar lesions and some partial spinal cord or brain stem lesions (Table 13–4). Differentiation of precipitate voiding from loss of normal voluntary control as in cortical lesions or behavior changes may be difficult on the basis of the history alone.

Dribbling of urine may be the result of loss of urethral resistance or overflow from an areflexic bladder (Table 13–2).

Physical Examination

Observation of the animal may confirm the characteristics of micturition as described in the history. The differences among the various abnormalities of micturition may be subtle, so it is critical that the problem described by the owner be verified by the examiner.

The presence of a detrusor reflex can be assumed if voiding is sustained (Table 13–4). However, bladder contractions with incomplete voiding are common in neurologic disorders. Such contractions are not the result of a true detrusor reflex; therefore, every animal with a problem associated with micturition should have residual urine measured. After the animal has voided, preferably outside in natural surroundings, the bladder should be catheterized and the residual urine measured. Residual urine should be less than 10% of the normal volume, and most small animals will have less than 10 ml remaining (0.2–0.4 ml/kg).[26]

Obstruction in the urethra usually can be detected when a catheter is passed. The primary exception is a urethral flap, which is rare in small animals, but is normal at the level of the pubis in ruminants. A flap can be confirmed only by excretory urethrography.[34]

Palpation of the bladder before and after voiding provides some information regarding bladder tone. The tone of the detrusor muscle is intrinsic and not directly related to innervation. However, a normally functioning bladder will contract to accommodate the volume of urine present. An overdistended bladder with rupture of the tight junctions will not contract. A chronically infected bladder will often be small and have thickened, fibrotic walls. A small contracted bladder with infection may not be the primary problem, as bladder infection is a common sequela to neurogenic disorders. Some of the non-neurogenic causes of incontinence, such as tumors or calculi, may also be identified by palpation.[34]

Manual expression of the bladder provides some information on the tone of the urethral sphincters. Normally, expression of the bladder is more difficult in the male than in the female. Urethral sphincter tone will be decreased in lesions of the sacral spinal cord, sacral roots, or pudendal nerve (lower motor neuron) and increased in lesions between L7 spinal cord segment and the brain stem. The sacral spinal cord segments lie within the body of the fifth lumbar vertebra, so lesions of the vertebrae from L5-L6 caudally will affect the sacral roots. In large animals, lesions at the level of the midsacrum will affect the sacral segments and nerve roots.

Neurologic Examination

The complete neurologic examination is described in Chapter 2. Reflexes related to the sacral spinal cord segments are especially important in evaluating neurogenic bladder dysfunction.

The anal and urethral sphincters are innervated by the pudendal nerve, primarily from sacral segments 1 and 2, but occasionally with fibers from S3.[30, 35] It is easier to evaluate anal sphincter function because observation and palpation are more convenient.

The anal sphincter can be observed for tone, or it can be palpated with the gloved digit. Two sacral reflexes can also be evaluated. The bulbocavernosus reflex is a sharp contraction of the sphincter in response to a squeeze of the bulb of the penis or the clitoris. The perineal reflex is a contraction of the sphincter in response to a pinch or pin prick of the perineal region. The perineal reflex can also be used to test sensory distribution in the perineal region. Unilateral lesions can be detected in this manner. Lesions of the sacral spinal cord, sacral roots, or pudendal nerves will diminish or destroy these reflexes, and the anal sphincter will be atonic.

The history, physical examination, and neurologic examination should provide sufficient data to differentiate neurogenic from non-neurogenic bladder disorders and to localize the lesion in the nervous system in neurogenic disorders. Additional data are necessary for an etiologic diagnosis and a prognosis.

Clinical Pathology

The minimum data base includes a complete blood count (CBC), urinalysis, and blood urea nitrogen (BUN) or creatinine values. Each of these is essential for prognosis of urinary tract dysfunction and may assist in diagnosis of non-neurogenic problems of micturition.

All animals with neurogenic bladder disorders are likely to have cystitis. Constant surveillance and appropriate treatment, when indicated, are imperative if a favorable outcome is to be expected. Ureteral reflux is also a frequent complication of neurogenic bladder dysfunction. Reflux when cystitis is present may lead to pyelonephritis, uremia, and death.[37]

Radiologic Examination

Radiography is important for differentiating non-neurogenic problems and for evaluating the extent of urinary tract disease, which may be a complication of neurogenic disorders, and the primary neurologic problem.[34]

Contrast cystourethrography, especially when performed in conjunction with cystometry, offers promise of more adequately evaluating the functional morphology of the lower urinary tract. Monitoring the pressure in the bladder during filling and the initiation of the detrusor reflex, with radiographs taken at each stage, provides a more complete assessment.

Urodynamics

Electrophysiologic tests, including cystometry, urethral pressure profiles, flow studies, and electromyography, have not been included in the minimum data base because they are not widely available. Techniques and normal values are described in Chapter 5.

The cystometrogram provides an objective assessment of the presence of a detrusor reflex, estimates the tone of the detrusor muscle, determines the capacity of the bladder, and detects uninhibited contractions.[17, 31] The presence or absence of the detrusor reflex is the most valuable information, and this can usually be determined from careful observation.

The urethral pressure profile measures the resting pressure of the urethra throughout its length. Although this information is beneficial, resting pressures do not always correlate with functional problems. Assessment of urine flow rates during voiding would be more useful, but

the techniques currently available involve significant risk in patients with neurogenic bladder disorders (see Chapter 5).

Electromyography and evoked response studies of the structures innervated by the pudendal nerve can be useful in patients with lower motor neuron disorders.

All of these tests are of value in more precisely defining the location of the problem and monitoring the effects of therapy. At present, they are only available at a few referral centers.

The final diagnosis depends on locating the lesion in the nervous system and establishing the etiology of the lesion, the functional central nervous system deficit, and the functional deficit related to micturition.

TREATMENT

Management of an animal with a disorder of micturition depends on the underlying cause. Specific treatments of nervous system diseases causing the problem are described in other chapters. Functional deficits of micturition may be temporary or permanent, depending on the reversibility of the CNS lesion and the maintenance of integrity of the urinary system. If the bladder becomes severely infected with secondary sclerosis of the bladder wall, normal function will not be restored even if the CNS lesion is corrected.

Management of the neurogenic bladder that is related to the loss of the detrusor reflex is discussed in Chapter 15. Some drugs that may be useful in treating the neurogenic bladder are listed in Table 13–5. Treatment of the functional disorders listed in Table 13–2 will be presented below.

Detrusor Areflexia with Sphincter Hypertonus. Lesions from the pons to L7 spinal cord segments may abolish the detrusor reflex and produce upper motor neuron signs characterized by sphincter hyperreflexia and increased tone. The animal cannot void, and it is difficult, if not impossible, to express the bladder manually.

The primary requirement in all neurogenic bladder disorders is complete evacuation of the bladder at least three times daily. It must be done frequently enough that the bladder is never overdistended. Manual expression is usually ineffective and is often dangerous when urethral tone is increased. Aseptic catheterization is required. Indwelling catheters should be avoided whenever possible because of the in-

Table 13–5. DRUGS USED IN TREATING DISORDERS OF MICTURITION

Drug Action	Drug	Dose	Side Effects
Increase detrusor contractility	Bethanechol (urecholine)	2.5–10 mg tid/sc, 2–15 mg tid orally	Cholinergic: GI hypermotility, hypotension
Decrease detrusor contractility	Propantheline (Pro-Banthine)	15–30 mg tid	Anticholinergic: decreased GI motility, constipation, decreased salivation, tachycardia
	Oxybutynin (Ditropan)	5 mg tid	
Increase urethral resistance	Phenylpropanolamine (Coldecon)	12.5–50 mg tid	Sympathomimetic: Urinary retention, hypertension.
	Diethylstilbestrol (stilbestrol)	0.1–1 mg/day for 3–5 days, then 1 mg/week	Estrogen: Estrus, bone marrow toxicity
	Estradiol cypionate (ECP)	0.1–1 mg parenterally at intervals of weeks to months	Same. Caution must be used as this is potent estrogen
	Testosterone (Depo-Testosterone cypionate)	2.2 mg/kg parenterally at intervals of weeks to months	Androgen: Caution in animals with prostatic hyperplasia perineal hernia and perianal adenoma
Decrease urethral resistance	Phenoxybenzamine (Dibenzyline)	0.5 mg/kg bid or tid	Sympatholytic: Hypotension
	Diazepam (Valium)	2–10 mg tid	Tranquilizer and skeletal muscle relaxant: sedation
	Dantrolene (Dantrium)	1–5 mg tid	Skeletal muscle relaxant: weakness, hepatotoxicity

fection that inevitably occurs. The one exception is detrusor areflexia from overdistention (see below).

Urethral tone may be reduced by administration of an α-adrenergic blocking agent, such as phenoxybenzamine, or a skeletal muscle relaxant, such as diazepam (Table 13–5).[1, 24] Bethanechol, a cholinergic agent, may reduce bladder capacity and increase the contractility of the detrusor muscle, but does not restore the reflex.[36] It is of little benefit in this situation. (See Chapter 15 for more details on management of this group of patients.)

Detrusor Areflexia with Normal Sphincter. Some lesions of the spinal cord and brain stem may abolish the detrusor reflex without producing hypertonus of the urethral sphincter. The bladder can be manually expressed without danger. Manual expression is less likely to produce infection than repeated catheterization, but catheterization should be done periodically after expressing the bladder to assess adequacy of emptying. Other aspects of management are the same as those described previously.

Detrusor Areflexia with Sphincter Areflexia. Lesions of the sacral spinal cord or roots will produce a lower motor neuron deficit of both the bladder and the sphincter. Management of the bladder is the same as that described for normal sphincter tone.

An additional management problem is created by the constant leakage of urine through the incompetent sphincter. More frequent evacuation of the bladder will reduce the problem but not entirely eliminate it. Continual soiling of the skin with urine quickly leads to irritation and formation of decubital ulcers. Frequent hydrotherapy and protective emollients are useful adjuncts.

Long-term management of the patient with paralysis of the sphincter has not been completely successful. Surgical reconstruction of the bladder neck and urethra is sometimes successful in humans but has had no significant trial in animals. Artificial urinary sphincters are being used successfully in humans. They have been employed in experimental studies on dogs with good results. Their use in clinical veterinary medicine will be limited by cost and the necessity for the owner to deflate the cuff each time the animal must void.

Detrusor Areflexia from Overdistention. Severe overdistention of the bladder can produce a separation of the tight junctions between detrusor muscle fibers, thus preventing excitation-contraction coupling. The neural elements may be normal.

The bladder must be treated early if irreversible deficit is to be avoided after overdistention. Complete evacuation of the bladder must be accomplished and maintained for 1 to 2 weeks. Manual expression is not recommended because of the increased stress on the detrusor muscle. Intermittent aseptic catheterization can be performed at least three times daily, but preferably four times a day. Use of an indwelling catheter for the first 5 to 7 days followed by intermittent catheterization, if needed, is the procedure of choice. This is one of the few instances in which an indwelling catheter is recommended. Function should return in 1 to 2 weeks if treatment is successful.

Bethanechol may be of benefit, especially if partial contractions are present.

Antibiotics should be administered throughout the treatment period. Frequent urinalyses, with cultures when indicated, are mandatory. Infection in the overdistended bladder will lead to fibrosis, and adequate function will not be restored.

Detrusor Hyperreflexia. Frequent voiding of small volumes of urine, often without much warning and with little or no residual urine, is characteristic of detrusor hyperreflexia. Partial long tract lesions or abnormalities of the cerebellum may produce these signs. The condition is not usually detrimental to the patient, but it may be an early sign of a progressive disease of the nervous system. Additionally, it is socially unacceptable in the house pet. The condition must be differentiated from the small, contracted, irritable bladder associated with chronic cystitis.

If treatment is desired, anticholinergic medication may be of benefit. Propantheline (Pro-Banthine) has been used in doses of 7.5 to 30 mg three or four times daily. The lowest dose should be tried first and increased in small increments until response is obtained. Overdosage may result in urinary retention in addition to the other side effects characteristic of this group of drugs.[1, 17]

Reflex Dyssynergia. Initiation of a detrusor reflex with voiding followed by an uncontrolled reflex contraction of the urethra is termed reflex dyssynergia. It is well documented in humans with upper motor neuron lesions. It has not been satisfactorily documented in dogs. Dogs with upper motor neuron lesions rarely have a good detrusor reflex. The few dogs that appeared to have dyssynergia clinically were all male and were normal neurologically. The author has not been able to document simultaneous bladder and urethral contractions in these patients. Some have improved with use of phenoxybenzamine, however.[28, 36]

Normal Detrusor Reflex with Decreased Sphincter Tone. The majority of these patients have hormone responsive incontinence or a structural abnormality of the urethra.[20] α-Adrenergic stimulating drugs, such as phenylpropanolamine, may be beneficial.[26, 36] Hormone-responsive incontinence has been seen in both male and female dogs and cats that have been neutered.[5, 36]

REFERENCES

1. Applebaum SM: Pharmacologic agents in micturitional disorders. Urology, 16:555, 1980.
2. Atenburrow DP and James E: Urinary incontinence in a pony mare. Equine Vet J 13:206, 1981.
3. Barrett DM and Wein AJ: Controversies in Neuro-urology. New York, Churchill Livingstone, 1984.
4. Barrington FJF: The nervous mechanism of micturition. Quart J Exp Physiol 8:33, 1914.
5. Barsanti JA and Finco DR: Hormonal responses to urinary incontinence. In Kirk RW: Current Veterinary Therapy VIII. Philadelphia, WB Saunders Co, 1983.
6. Beaver BL: Veterinary Aspects of Feline Behavior. St. Louis, CV Mosby Co, 1980.
7. Bors E and Comarr AE: Neurological Urology. Baltimore, University Park Press, 1971.
8. Bradley WE and Teague CT: Cerebellar influence on the micturition reflex. Exp Neurol 23:399, 1969.
9. Bradley WE and Teague CT: Hypogastric and pelvic nerve activity during the micturition reflex. J Urol 101:438, 1969.
10. Bradley WE and Teague CT: Electrophysiology of pelvic and pudendal nerves in the cat. Exp Neurol 35:378, 1972.
11. Bradley WE and Timm GW: Physiology of micturition. Vet Clin North Am 4:487, 1974.
12. Campbell WE: Behavior Problems in Dogs. Santa Barbara, CA, American Veterinary Publications, 1978.
13. DeGroat WC: Nervous control of the urinary bladder of the cat. Brain Res 87:201, 1975.
14. DeGroat WC and Saum WE: Sympathetic inhibition of the urinary bladder and of pelvic ganglionic transmission in the cat. J Physiol 214:297, 1972.
15. Gjone R and Setekleiv J: Excitatory and inhibitory bladder responses to stimulation of the cerebral cortex in the cat. Acta Physiol Scand 59:337, 1963.
16. Gregg RA, Boyarsky S, and Labay P: Blocking of Beta adrenergic receptors in the urinary bladder using sotalol. South Med J 62:1355, 1969.
17. Hald T and Bradley WE: The Urinary Bladder, Neurology and Dynamics. Baltimore, Williams & Wilkins Co, 1982.
18. Hart BL: Feline Behavior: A Practitioner's Monograph. Santa Barbara, CA, Veterinary Practice Publishing Co, 1978.
19. Holt P: Urinary incontinence in the dog. In Pract 5:162, 1983.
20. Holt PE: Efficacy of emepronium bromide in the treatment of physiological incontinence in the bitch. Vet Rec 114:355, 1984.
21. Houpt KA and Wolski TR: Domestic Animal Behavior for Veterinarians and Animal Scientists. Ames, Iowa State University Press, 1982.
22. Iggo A: Tension receptors in the stomach and the urinary bladder. J Physiol 12:593, 1955.
23. Jonas U and Tanagho EA: Studies on vesicourethral reflexes. Invest Urol 12:357, 1975.
24. Krane RJ and Olsson CA: Phenoxybenzamine in neurogenic bladder dysfunction. II. Clinical consideration. J Urol 110:653, 1973.
25. Langworthy OR and Hesser FH: An experimental study of micturition released from cerebral control. Am J Physiol 115:694, 1936.
26. Moreau PM: Neurogenic disorders of micturition in the dog and cat. Comp Cont Ed Pract Vet 4:12, 1982.
27. Oliver JE Jr: Disorders of micturition. In Hoerlein BF: Canine Neurology, 3rd ed. Philadelphia, WB Saunders Co, 1978.

28. Oliver JE Jr: Dysuria caused by reflex dyssynergia. *In* Kirk RW: Current Veterinary Therapy VIII. Philadelphia, WB Saunders Co, 1983.

29. Oliver JE Jr, Bradley WE, and Fletcher TF: Spinal cord representation of the micturition reflex. J Comp Neurol 137:329, 1969.

30. Oliver JE Jr, Bradley WE, and Fletcher TF: Spinal cord distribution of the somatic innervation of the external urethral sphincter in the cat. J Neurol Sci 10:11, 1970.

31. Oliver JE Jr and Lorenz MD: Handbook of Veterinary Neurologic Diagnosis. Philadelphia, WB Saunders Co, 1983.

32. Oliver JE Jr and Osborne CA: Neurogenic urinary incontinence. *In* Kirk RW: Current Veterinary Therapy VI. Philadelphia, WB Saunders Co, 1980.

33. Oliver JE Jr and Selcer RR: Neurogenic causes of abnormal micturition in the dog and cat. Vet Clin North Am 4:517, 1974.

34. Osborne CA, Oliver JE Jr, and Polzin DE: Nonneurogenic urinary incontinence. *In* Kirk RW: Current Veterinary Therapy VI. Philadelphia, WB Saunders Co, 1980.

35. Purinton PT and Oliver JE Jr: Spinal cord origin of innervation to the bladder and urethra of the dog. Exp Neurol 65:422, 1969.

36. Rosin A and Ross L: Diagnosis and pharmacological management of disorders of urinary continence in the dog. Comp Cont Ed Pract Vet 3:601, 1981.

37. Tribe CR: Renal Failure in Paraplegia. London, Pitman Medical Pub Co, 1969.

Diseases of Peripheral Nerves, Cranial Nerves, and Muscle

NEUROPATHIES

Peripheral neuropathies are common entities in domestic animals, particularly dogs. Apart from those due to trauma, the pathophysiology of most neuropathies is poorly understood. An increasing number have been shown to have a congenital and/or hereditary basis (Table 14–1).

Clinical findings in neuropathies relate to dysfunction of the structures innervated by affected motor nerve fibers and the areas innervated by sensory fibers. Motor nerves represent the *lower motor neuron* because they are the final common pathway between the central nervous system and the target organs. In the voluntary (somatic) nervous system, these organs are skeletal muscles (Figs. 14–1 and 14–2). The target organs of the autonomic nervous system are smooth muscles associated with blood vessels and visceral structures, glands, and cardiac muscle.

The autonomic nervous system includes the cranial parasympathetic outflow in the third, seventh, ninth, and tenth cranial nerves; the sympathetic outflow from all the thoracic and first five lumbar segments of the spinal cord; and the sacral parasympathetic outflow in the sacral cord segments.

Peripheral neuropathies result in lower motor neuron signs, which include flaccid muscle weakness or paralysis, significant muscular atrophy, and reduced or absent muscle tone (hypotonia, atonia) and reflexes (hypo-, areflexia). Because most spinal nerves contain motor and sensory components, a variable degree of sensory loss will be detected in cutaneous (dermatomal) testing. Peripheral neuropathies may involve a single nerve (mononeuropathy) or several (polyneuropathy). The pattern of distribution may be proximal (eg, hereditary spinal muscular atrophy in Brittany spaniels) or distal (eg, giant axonal neuropathy in German shepherds), symmetric or asymmetric. Pelvic limbs usually are affected first in polyneuropathies. Although some neuropathies may be acute (eg, traumatic, ischemic disorders) or subacute (eg, coonhound paralysis) in onset, the majority are insidious and have a chronic course. Signs of autonomic nerve dysfunction are rarely observed in animals with diffuse polyneuropathies. Similarly, cranial nerves are not commonly affected, with the exception of facial nerve (CN VII) paresis in coonhound paralysis and hypothyroid neuropathy, vagus nerve (CN X) dysphagia or megaesophagus in giant axonal neuropathy, and left recurrent laryngeal nerve dysfunction in idiopathic equine laryngeal hemiplegia.

The main pathologic changes observed in peripheral neuropathies, irrespective of etiology, are axonal degeneration and/or demyelination. The former may be characterized by

353

Table 14–1. CLASSIFICATION OF PERIPHERAL NEUROPATHIES

Congenital or Hereditary
Giant axonal neuropathy of German shepherd dogs
Central-peripheral neuropathy in boxer dogs
Inherited hypertrophic neuropathy in Tibetan mastiff dogs
Sensory neuropathy in long haired dachshund dogs
Sensory neuropathy in English pointer dogs
Laryngeal paralysis in dogs, horses
Esophageal hypomotility in dogs, cats, foals
*Hereditary spinal muscular atrophy in Brittany spaniel dogs
*Hereditary neuronal abiotrophy in Swedish Lapland dogs
*Stockard's paralysis in Great Dane × bloodhound and Great Dane × St Bernard dogs
*Hereditary neurogenic amyotrophy in pointer dogs

Inflammatory and Immune Mediated
Coonhound paralysis in dogs
Acute canine idiopathic polyneuropathy
Chronic relapsing polyradiculoneuritis in dogs, cats
Brachial plexus neuropathy in dogs, cats
Ganglioradiculitis and sensory neuronopathy in dogs
Neuritis of the cauda equina in horses
Polyradiculoneuritis in large animals
Labyrinthitis
Guttural pouch mycosis in horses

Metabolic
Diabetic neuropathy in dogs, cats

Toxic or Nutritional
Various in large animals (also see Chapter 8)

Idiopathic
Distal denervating disease in dogs
Distal symmetric polyneuropathy in dogs
Idiopathic facial paralysis
Idiopathic vestibular disease
Trigeminal neuritis
Sensory trigeminal neuropathy
Feline dysautonomia (Key-Gaskell syndrome)
Stringhalt in horses
Pseudoamyloid multiradicular degeneration in a pony

Traumatic
Traumatic neuropathy
Brachial plexus avulsion and compression
Calving paralysis, foaling paralysis
Postnatal quadriceps atrophy in calves

Degenerative
Paraneoplastic neuromyopathy

Vascular
Ischemic neuromyopathy
Aortoiliac thrombosis

Neoplastic
See Chapter 9

*These diseases are discussed under Neuronal Abitrophies in Chapter 6.

Wallerian degeneration, which occurs in the distal stump following nerve transection or injury, is the most common form of axon degeneration (see Chapter 19).

In some disorders, axonal degeneration occurs in distal parts of the nerve and gradually progresses toward the cell body. The underlying mechanisms are incompletely understood. This pathologic change, which is also known as dying back disease and peripheral axonopathy, has been reported in several spontaneous neuropathies in dogs.

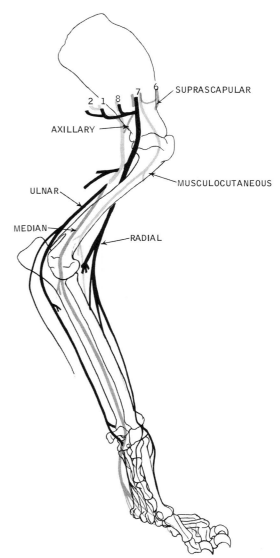

Figure 14–1. A medial view of the thoracic limb of the dog illustrating the relative course and distribution of the major nerves.

fiber loss in cross-sectional studies or presence of linear rows of myelin ovoids or balls in teased nerve preparations. Axonal degeneration may result from diseases of the nerve cell body (neuronopathy) or the axon itself (axonopathy).

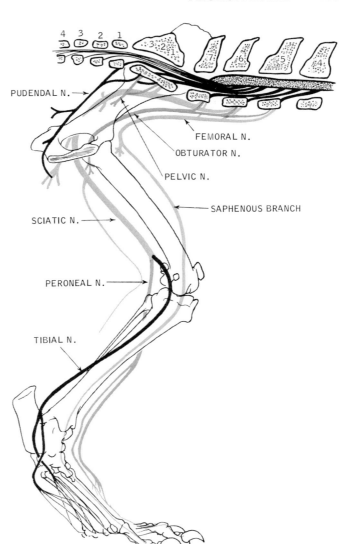

Figure 14–2. A medial view of the pelvic limb illustrating the relative course and distribution of the major nerves.

Demyelination is characterized by the presence of fibers with inappropriately thin myelin sheaths. In teased nerve preparations, demyelination is recognized as regions of nodal lengthening or internodal myelin absence. Short "intercalated" internodes with thin myelin sheaths suggest fiber remyelination. Repeated episodes of demyelination and remyelination result in formation of concentric layers of Schwann cell processes around axons. These structures, known as onion bulbs, may result in thicking of the nerve, producing a hypertrophic neuropathy.

The diagnosis of peripheral neuropathies is based on age, breed, clinical evidence of a lower motor neuron disorder, and electrophysiologic data (electromyography, nerve conduction studies, evoked potentials). Confirmation is made by pathologic evaluation of nerve or muscle biopsy or postmortem samples.

A classification of the neuropathies discussed is given in Table 14–1.

Congenital or Hereditary Disorders

Canine Giant Axonal Neuropathy

Giant axonal neuropathy is a rare neurologic disease of German shepherd dogs, which is inherited as an autosomal recessive trait.[72–75]

The pathogenesis is unknown; however, a slowing or blocking of slow axonal transport in nerves has been suggested.[75] Pathologically the disease is characterized by loss of myelinated nerve fibers and presence of giant axons in myelinated and unmyelinated fibers.[96, 101] The swollen axons contain masses of neurofilaments. Similar changes are found in the central nervous system (CNS). In both peripheral nervous system (PNS) and CNS, lesions predominate at the end of long nerve fibers. The disease exemplifies a "central-peripheral distal axonopathy."[196]

Clinical neurologic signs, which are noted at approximately 14 to 16 months of age, are more obvious in pelvic limbs and are progressive. They are characterized by paresis, proprioceptive loss, diminished patellar reflexes, and pelvic limb hypotonia with atrophy of muscles below the stifles. Conscious perception of pain is gradually reduced in pelvic limbs. Bark may be lost or diminished, and there may be fecal incontinence. Megaesophagus develops after about 18 months, resulting in regurgitation and occasionally inhalation pneumonia. Electrophysiologically, amplitude of evoked compound muscle action potentials is decreased several months prior to clinical evidence of neuropathy.[75] This decrease is progressive. Denervation potentials are demonstrated by electromyography in distal muscles of pelvic limbs and thoracic limbs by 18 months.

Diagnosis is based on signalment, clinical, electrophysiologic, and pathologic (nerve biopsies) data. Prognosis is poor. There is no treatment.

Central-Peripheral Neuropathy in Boxer Dogs

This is a newly described neurologic disease of boxer dogs.[99] The etiology of the disorder is unknown; however, a genetic basis is suspected.

Pathologic changes in nerve roots and peripheral nerves include both axonal degeneration and demyelination or remyelination, suggesting the presence of axonal and Schwann cell defects. Lesions characterized by swollen axons are widespread in the CNS, although there is no apparent tract or distal distribution of the lesions.

Clinical signs usually become apparent at about 6 months of age. There is a progressive ataxia and weakness, initially in pelvic limbs but later involving thoracic limbs. Proprioceptive function, muscle tone, and tendon reflexes are diminished or absent, whereas pedal reflexes and pain sensation are preserved. Muscle atrophy is minimal. Electrodiagnostic studies reveal little spontaneous activity, normal or slight reduction in motor nerve conduction velocities, and smaller amplitude of evoked muscle action potentials than normal.

Diagnosis is suggested by signalment, clinical, electrophysiologic, and nerve biopsy data and is confirmed by pathologic evaluation of the CNS. Prognosis is poor. There is no treatment.

Inherited Hypertrophic Neuropathy in Tibetan Mastiff Dogs

An autosomal recessive neurologic disease has been reported recently in Tibetan mastiff dogs.[53] This disease results in a reduced density of myelinated fibers, widespread demyelination, and primitive onion bulb formation with relatively little axonal degeneration in peripheral nerves and roots. Results of initial studies suggest an inborn defect in the Schwann cell's ability to form or maintain a stable myelin sheath.

Clinical signs appear in animals from 7 to 12 weeks of age and consist of generalized weakness, hyporeflexia, and muscle hypotonia. Severely affected pups may become totally recumbent within 3 weeks after onset, with subsequent development of sternal compression and limb contractures. Some pups may regain the ability to stand and walk. Mild muscle wasting occurs and ambulatory pups have a shuffling, plantigrade gait. Pain perception is normal.

Electrodiagnostic studies reveal moderate to severe reduction in nerve conduction velocities and infrequent denervation potentials. There is inconstant elevation in cerebrospinal fluid protein level.

Diagnosis is based on signalment, clinical, electrophysiologic, and nerve biopsy data. Prognosis is poor. There is no treatment.

Canine Sensory Neuropathies

There have been recent reports of neuropathies in certain breeds of dogs, which are characterized by sensory deficits, namely proprioception and nociception, with or without loss of motor function. These include the following:

Sensory Neuropathy in Long Haired Dachshund Dogs. This is a neurologic disease reported in long haired dachshund puppies, for which a genetic basis is suspected.[78] The pathogenesis is unknown. Pathologic changes occur in distal sensory nerves, and both larger caliber myelinated fibers and unmyelinated fibers show degenerative changes. Less severe, but similar changes occur in mixed nerves. In the CNS, distal degeneration has been observed in the fasciculus gracilis.

Clinical signs are noted in dogs shortly after they begin to ambulate, characteristically loss of proprioception and placing reactions (especially in pelvic limbs), reduction or loss of pain sensation over the whole body in response to superficial and deep pain stimulation, and urinary incontinence. There is no evidence of paresis or muscular atrophy, and patellar reflexes are normal. Results of electromyographic studies and motor nerve conduction velocities are normal. Sensory nerve potential may be reduced or absent.

Diagnosis is based on signalment, clinical, electromyographic, and pathologic (nerve biopsy) data. Prognosis is poor. There is no treatment.

Sensory Neuropathy in English Pointer Dogs. This rare disease, believed to be inherited, has been reported in English pointer dogs.[55, 59]

Pathologically, changes affecting the primary sensory neurons are observed, including small spinal ganglia with reduced numbers of cell bodies, degeneration of unmyelinated and myelinated fibers in the dorsal roots and peripheral nerves, and reduced fiber density in the dorsolateral fasciculus of the spinal cord.

The pathogenesis of this disease is presently unclear; however, a deficiency in growth and/or differentiation of primary sensory neurons may be involved. Fiber degeneration may progress slowly with age to include sensory systems not affected in early postnatal life. The loss of primary sensory neurons is associated with a notable reduction in staining of substance P, an excitatory agent that mediates nociception.[52]

Clinical signs are characterized by loss of nociceptive sensation and acral mutilation. This nociceptive loss is more apparent in distal parts of limbs, so that acral analgesia is replaced by hypalgesia proximal to the carpus and tarsus. No nociceptive loss is detected about the face. Although blunting of digital pain has been detected prior to weaning, clinical signs usually become apparent at 3 to 8 months when the dog suddenly begins to lick and bite its paws. Acral changes include swollen reddened paws, ulcerations, lacerations, paronychia, painless fractures, and autoamputations.

There is no evidence of proprioceptive loss, ataxia, or depressed tendon reflexes. Results of electromyographic studies and sensory and motor nerve conduction studies are normal.

Diagnosis is based on signalment, clinical, and normal electrophysiologic data. Pathologic evaluation of nerve or spinal ganglia biopsy samples may support the clinical diagnosis.

Prognosis is poor because of high potential for osteomyelitis secondary to autoamputation. There is no treatment for the underlying sensory neuropathy.

An apparently similar, recessively inherited entity has been reported in short haired pointer dogs[173, 180, 193] and has been called toe necrosis, hereditary neurotrophic osteopathy, and ulceromutilating acropathy.

Canine Laryngeal Paralysis

Spontaneous laryngeal paralysis has been reported sporadically in dogs. A hereditary form (autosomal dominant) has been documented in Siberian huskies and Bouviers des Flandres either as unilateral or bilateral disease.[175, 212, 213] The acquired disease has been reported in middle aged and old large and giant breed dogs, such as Saint Bernard, Chesapeake Bay retriever, and Irish setter.[159]

The etiology of laryngeal paralysis is unknown. The motor innervation to the muscles of the larynx is derived largely from branches of the recurrent laryngeal nerves, dysfunction of which results in impaired contraction of the dorsal cricoarytenoid muscle, and hence reduced abduction of the vocal cords. Histologic evidence of neurogenic atrophy is found in intrinsic laryngeal muscles. Axonal degeneration, with increase in endoneurial connective tissue and number of Schwann cells, is present in right and left recurrent laryngeal nerves. Changes occur along the entire length of these nerves, suggesting that the primary lesion is in the neurons of origin. Similar degenerative changes have been described occasionally in vagus and sciatic nerves.[159, 213]

Onset of clinical signs in the hereditary form is from 4 to 6 months of age. The acquired form may develop in animals from 1.5 to 13 years of age. Clinical signs reflect respiratory (inspiratory) distress and are characterized by increasing loss of endurance, increasing laryngeal stridor, dyspnea, cyanosis (during episodes of severe dyspnea), and collapse with complete airway obstruction. Clinical signs are usually of several months duration. Pelvic limb weakness and "foot drop" associated with bilateral cranial tibial muscle denervation have also been observed in dogs with hereditary and acquired forms of laryngeal paralysis.

Diagnosis of laryngeal abductor dysfunction is made by laryngoscopy. Recurrent laryngeal paralysis is confirmed by detection of denervation potentials in individual intrinsic laryngeal muscles and by evidence of neurogenic atrophy in biopsy specimens of the cricoarytenoid muscle.

Prognosis is usually favorable with surgical management, such as lateral fixation of the arytenoid cartilage or partial laryngectomy[107, 109] in acquired paralysis, but has been variable in hereditary paralysis. Prevention of the inherited form by breeding control is indicated.

Equine Laryngeal Hemiplegia

This disorder is similar to canine laryngeal paralysis. It is common in the horse, and it has been estimated that up to 5% of all thoroughbreds develop clinical signs related to the condition. Clinical manifestations are usually observed in horses at approximately 6 years of age.[47] The narrowing of the rima glottidis results in inspiratory dyspnea and a "roaring" noise. The etiology and pathogenesis are not known. Neurogenic atrophy occurs in laryngeal muscles. Recent results indicate that adductor muscles may be more severely involved than abductors, especially on the left side. Degenerative changes are found in distal parts of the left recurrent laryngeal nerve and include loss of myelinated nerve fibers and evidence of segmental demyelination or remyelination. A large number of clinically normal horses, with no history of inspiratory dyspnea or noise, have subclinical pathologic changes of the muscles supplied by the left recurrent laryngeal nerve.[46, 77, 104] Diagnosis is usually based on signalment data and clinical signs. Prognosis is fair with surgical management, which is discussed elsewhere.[110] Acquired laryngeal paralysis is associated with other more generalized diseases, such as lead poisoning, hepatoencephalopathy and organophosphate toxicity.[179]

Esophageal Hypomotility

This condition has been termed esophageal achalasia, megaesophagus, and esophageal neuromuscular disease. Both congenital and acquired esophageal dysphagias have been seen in the dog and cat.[42, 108, 177] The congenital form is common in Great Dane, German shepherd, and Irish setter dogs.[202] The condition occurs as an inherited disease in wire haired fox terriers

and miniature schnauzers.[45, 51, 163] In cats, Siamese and Siamese-related breeds may be predisposed.[44] A congenital form has been reported in a 6 month old thoroughbred foal.[16] The congenital form is usually apparent in animals at the time of weaning.

Acquired esophageal hypomotility may occur in any dog or cat at any age. In most cases, the cause is unknown; however, the condition has been observed in association with certain systemic neuromuscular disorders such as myasthenia gravis, hypothyroidism, hypoadrenocorticism, polymyositis, myotonia, and giant axonal neuropathy.[79, 85, 95, 126, 129, 136, 165]

The pathogenesis is unknown, but neural rather than muscular mechanisms are considered to be involved.[91] In the dog, the striated muscle of the esophagus is innervated by fibers that pass from the nucleus ambiguus to the esophagus via the vagus nerves.[116] Electrolytic lesions of the nucleus ambiguus in dogs and of the parasympathetic nucleus of the vagus in cats produce esophageal dysfunction similar to the clinical syndrome.[111] A reduction of the normal number of neuronal cell bodies in the nucleus ambiguus was noted in an affected dog[43] but has not been found in affected cats.[41]

Clinical features are postprandial regurgitation of undigested food, with radiographic evidence of megaesophagus to the level of the diaphragm. Abnormal esophageal motility with failure of the gastroesophageal junction to dilate when swallowing is initiated may be demonstrated by contrast radiography. In most animals there is no true achalasia or primary failure of the gastroesophageal junction to relax.

Prognosis is generally good in young dogs fed with the head in an elevated position.[68, 184, 191] These animals, by the time they mature, appear normal by radiographic, manometric, and clinical examination.

Acquired, idiopathic esophageal hypomotility has a poor prognosis for recovery. Cachexia becomes an important complication, and death is a consequence of aspiration pneumonia.

Inflammatory and Immune Mediated Diseases

Coonhound Paralysis

Coonhound paralysis (CHP) is a rare neurologic disease of dogs, occurring especially in raccoon hunting breeds;[56, 60] however, a similar condition can occur in dogs with no possible exposure to raccoons.[157, 158] The etiology and pathogenesis are unknown. A raccoon bite has been a relatively consistent antecedent in coonhound paralysis. The condition has been reproduced experimentally by injection of raccoon saliva into a dog that had recovered from two earlier spontaneous attacks.[113] Results of this work suggested that raccoon saliva contains the etiologic factor for coonhound paralysis and that only specifically susceptible dogs are at risk when exposed to this factor.

Interest has focused on coonhound paralysis mainly because of its resemblance to Guillain-Barré syndrome in humans and its potential as an elucidating model. Like the human syndrome, coonhound paralysis may have an immunologic pathogenesis, although results of a recent study did not conform with the evidence presented in Guillain-Barré syndrome for an obligatory role of macrophages in initiating myelin damage.[56] However, the observed changes do resemble those reported in immunologic mediated, experimental allergic neuritis.[113, 114]

Pathologic changes are associated with a polyradiculoneuritis, with both segmental demyelination and concurrent degeneration of myelin and axons. Leukocytic infiltration, consisting mostly of cells of the monocyte-macrophage series, and scattered aggregates of lymphocytes and plasma cells are also observed. Changes occur in peripheral nerves and nerve roots, especially in the latter, and more consistently in ventral roots than dorsal roots.

The disease affects dogs of any breed, both sexes, and usually adult age. Clinical signs frequently appear 7 to 11 days after an encounter with a raccoon. Onset is marked by weakness and pelvic limb hyporeflexia. Paralysis progresses rapidly, resulting in a flaccid symmetric tetraplegia. Motor impairment is more pronounced than sensory changes. Many dogs appear to be hyperesthetic to sensory stimuli. Bladder and rectal paralysis are not observed. In severely affected animals there may be complete absence of spinal reflexes, facial weakness, and labored respiration. Death may occur from respiratory paralysis. The duration of paralysis varies from several weeks to 3 months.

Motor nerve conduction velocities may be markedly reduced, and electromyographic studies reveal widespread denervation 6 to 7 days after the onset. Elevated protein levels with normal cell counts ("albuminocytologic dissociation") in cerebrospinal fluid have been reported, especially in samples obtained from lumbar puncture.

Diagnosis is based on historical, clinical, electrodiagnostic, and nerve biopsy data.

Prognosis is usually favorable; however, protection from future attacks is short lived or nonexistent. Treatment is symptomatic. Good nursing care is essential.

Acute Canine Idiopathic Polyneuropathy

A neurologic condition characterized by acute progressive flaccid tetraparesis and hyporeflexia has been reported in dogs.[157, 158] The etiology of this condition is unknown. There is no history of antecedent exposure to raccoons; however, clinical electrophysiologic and pathologic data are similar to findings in coonhound paralysis, suggesting that these disorders may share a common immunopathogenesis.

Affected animals usually recover in about 3 to 6 weeks. Management is the same as for coonhound paralysis.

Chronic Relapsing Polyradiculoneuritis

A chronic neurologic disorder characterized by periodic remission has been reported in a dog.[54] Pathologic findings were a long-standing demyelinating polyradiculoneuritis characterized by symmetric demyelination or remyelination, prominent onion bulb formation, and axonal sprouting. Inflammatory mononuclear infiltrates (including macrophages and plasma cells) were prominent. The etiology of this disorder is not known; however, the pathologic changes are compatible with an autoimmune pathogenesis. Onset of signs was not related to a specific antecedent such as a raccoon bite or urticarial reaction.

Clinical findings include tetraparesis, diminished or absent reflexes, muscle wasting, elevated protein level but normal cell count in CSF, muscle denervation potentials, and slowed peripheral nerve conduction velocities. The progressive course was interrupted by partial remission of signs.

A disorder has been reported in a cat in which the clinical and pathologic changes resemble those in the dog with chronic relapsing polyradiculoneuritis.[87]

The prognosis of chronic relapsing polyradiculoneuritis appears to be poor. Treatment with glucocorticoids has not been effective.

Brachial Plexus Neuropathy

This is a rare neurologic condition, involving the nerves of the brachial plexus, that has been reported in dogs.[3, 61] It has been suggested that this disorder may be the result of an allergic or hypersensitive reaction similar to serum neuritis in humans following prophylactic inoculations, such as with tetanus antiserum. The proposed pathogenesis is that the allergic condition produces spinal nerve swelling and subsequent compression at the level of the intervertebral foramina. Pathologic changes described include severe axonal and myelin degeneration of peripheral nerves of the thoracic limbs.

Clinical signs described in one dog were characterized by acute onset of thoracic limb paresis with depressed or absent reflexes and hypotonia, facial paresis, and neurogenic atrophy in all thoracic limb muscles.

Electromyographic studies revealed denervation potentials and absence of evoked muscle action potentials in the thoracic limbs. Cerebrospinal fluid evaluation was normal.

This dog manifested two allergic episodes with facial edema and generalized urticaria over a 48 hour period prior to development of neurologic signs. Immunologic testing indicated that these signs were related to an all horse meat diet. Three weeks prior to signs the dog was vaccinated with modified live rabies virus.

No improvement was noted in this dog 49 days after onset of clinical signs even with glucocorticoid therapy. In a second dog with brachial plexus neuropathy, slight improvement was reported 4 months after signs first developed.[3]

Brachial plexus neuropathy has been reported in a cat[29] with clinical signs similar to those in the dog. Conspicuous differences include absence of denervation (clinically and electrodiagnostically) and rapid recovery (3 weeks). Vaccination with modified live rabies virus was considered to be related to the neuropathy.

Ganglioradiculitis and Sensory Neuronopathy in the Dog

Three different breeds of dogs were reported to have a nonsuppurative inflammation of the cranial and spinal sensory ganglia and associated nerve roots. There was secondary neuronal fiber degeneration in the ascending spinal and brain stem tracts.[57] A similar disease has been reported as a sensory neuronopathy in four dogs of different breeds.[222] In both reports acute to chronic signs of sensory ataxia were seen with various degrees of hyporeflexia and face and limb hypalgesia. Lesions in the cases of the latter report contained less nonsuppurative inflammatory infiltrate. Whether the syndromes

are all the same disease is not known. Although glucocorticosteroid therapy may be indicated, it was not effective in two dogs in which it was tried.[57]

Neuritis of the Cauda Equina in the Horse

This is a severe, idiopathic polyradiculoneuritis of the cauda equina that produces lower motor neuron disease of adult horses of either sex and of any breed.[73, 150, 190] The cause of neuritis of the cauda equina (NCE) remains unknown. The condition may represent an immunogenic response to a persisting herpesvirus infection[81]; an allergic neuritis in response to antigens released by trauma or infection[93]; or a postinfectious allergic neuritis, comparable to Guillain-Barré syndrome and experimental allergic neuritis.[62]

Pathologic changes may involve spinal and cranial nerves, with most severe lesions being present in the sacral and caudal nerve roots. Changes in intradural roots are characterized by infiltrations of mononuclear cells and macrophages and demyelination. In extradural roots, granulomatous inflammation and axonal degeneration are the predominant lesions reported.[58]

Clinical signs are characterized by urinary and fecal incontinence, inability to retract the penis, paralysis and anesthesia of the tail, and perineal anesthesia. Cranial nerve dysfunction (eg, facial paralysis, masseteric muscle atrophy, and vestibular signs) may also be present. Pelvic limb paresis is often observed.

Examination of cerebrospinal fluid samples obtained by lumbar tap is typified by mononuclear and polymorphonuclear pleocytosis (>100 cells/cu mm) and elevated protein content (100–300 mg/dl).

Diagnosis is based on signalment and clinical data and confirmed by pathologic studies. The differential diagnosis includes especially a sacral (S2) fracture, but also equine herpesvirus type 1 (EHV1) myeloencephalitis, rabies, sorghum intoxication, protozoal myeloencephalitis, and spinal nematodiasis (see Chapters 7 and 8). However, only the sacral fractures regularly result in such a dense motor and sensory deficit (Fig. 14–3). Prognosis is poor. There is no treatment.

Polyradiculoneuritis in Large Animals

Polyradiculoneuritis has been reported in a 6 week old French Alpine goat showing progressive pelvic limb ataxia.[140] Nonsuppurative leptomeningitis with fibrosis was present, along

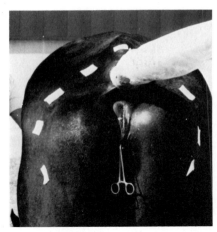

Figure 14–3. Fracture of S2 in this horse resulted in the cauda equina syndrome with slightly asymmetric analgesia, areflexia, hypotonia and muscle atrophy of the tail, anus, and perineum within the tape marks. Obstipation and urinary retention-incontinence were also present. (Courtesy of Dr IG Mayhew.)

with pale staining of nerve roots and nonsuppurative radiculoneuritis. The etiopathogenesis was not determined.

Labyrinthitis

Labyrinthitis or otitis interna refers to an inflammation of the inner ear resulting in dysfunction of the membranous labyrinth. This disorder is usually associated with otitis media. In dogs, the latter is most commonly associated with otitis externa.[182] The nasopharynx is also a source of retrograde infection by way of the eustachian tubes. A third source of infection of the middle and inner ear structures is hematogenous spread. Extension of infection from middle and inner ear areas to the meninges is a potential untoward sequela and occurs more often in pigs, calves, and cats. A detailed study of this so-called otoencephalitis in pigs has been documented.[38]

Most infections are caused by bacteria including staphylococci, α-streptococcus, *Proteus* sp, *Pseudomonas* sp, and *Escherichia coli*. Foreign bodies such as grass awns may initiate inflammation and predispose to secondary microbial infection. Animals predisposed to chronic otitis externa and chronic ear mite infestations would appear to have an increased risk of developing otitis media-interna; however, in a recent survey, no breed was disproportionately represented in the hospital population examined.[182]

Varying degrees of vestibular disturbance will reflect labyrinthine disease. Signs may range from head tilt, nystagmus (horizontal or rotatory), and ataxia, to torticollis, circling, falling, and rolling.[182] Attendant middle ear inflammation may disturb function of the facial and sympathetic nerves, which course through the petrosal bone in small animals, resulting in Horner's syndrome. The facial nerve (CN VII) may be affected in inner ear infection as it courses adjacent to the vestibulocochlear nerve. Another structure commonly involved is the cochlear nerve, dysfunction of which results in deafness. Occasionally, labyrinthitis is bilateral. If the infection spreads to the brain, signs of meningitis, pyrexia, depression, brain stem involvement, and seizures may be observed.

The diagnosis of labyrinthitis is suggested by clinical signs and confirmed by otoscopic examination and skull radiography.[160] Otoscopy may reveal an otitis externa and evidence of erosion, rupture, or bulging of the tympanic membrane. In small animals, fluid in the middle ear produces bulging of the tympanic membrane, which may appear opaque and hyperemic. Fluid and/or inflammatory exudate should be cultivated from the external and middle ear by aspiration if the tympanic membrane has ruptured or by myringotomy. Radiographic examination of the petrous temporal bones using dorsoventral, lateral oblique, and rostrocaudal projections may reveal middle ear inflammation as suggested by fluid density, osteitis, sclerosis, or erosion of the bulla (Fig. 14–4). Normal detail of the bony labyrinth may be lost.

Recently, a cluster of cases of vestibular and facial nerve paralysis was described in calves.[141] Space occupying nodules were detected on the facial and vestibulocochlear nerves at the level of the internal acoustic meatus of these calves. The lesions were granulomatous with inflammatory cells and a fibrous tissue capsule. Several calves had been dehorned recently and one had a postdehorning necrotic-granulomatous lesion that involved the cornual nerve. Similarity of the lesion to neuritis of the cauda equina, histiocytosis, sarcoidosis, and tumors was discussed. The state of the ear cavities was not defined, however, and chronic otitis media-interna with rupture of the granulating inflammation through the internal acoustic meatus seems possible.

Although bacterial otitis media-interna occurs in horses, proof of this in syndromes of vestibular and facial nerve paresis is sparse.[14, 171]

Prognosis is usually favorable with prolonged oral and topical antibiotics chosen on the basis of culture and sensitivity studies.[197, 198] In more chronic cases, surgical débridement and drainage of the middle ear may be required (see

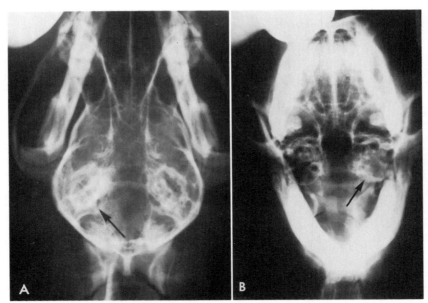

Figure 14–4. Radiographic appearance of two dogs with sclerosis and exudate in the bulla ossea, which produced characteristic clinical signs of otitis media and labyrinthitis. A, Ventrodorsal view. B, Open mouth anteroposterior view.

Chapter 18). In some animals neurologic signs may persist or recur.

Guttural Pouch Mycosis

Guttural pouch mycosis in horses is characterized by a variety of clinical signs, the most prominent of which include epistaxis and dysphagia. The usual site of infection is the dorsal wall of the medial compartment, along which course the internal carotid artery (the source of the epistaxis), the glossopharyngeal nerve, the pharyngeal branch of the vagus nerve, and the cranial cervical sympathetic trunk and ganglion; the spinal accessory nerve and the hypoglossal nerve are also in close proximity. In unusual circumstances the infection can involve the lateral compartment and affect the facial nerve. Mycotic lesions of the tympanic bullae have only rarely led to vestibular problems with this disease. Thus, in addition to dysphagia, clinical neurologic signs may include laryngeal hemiplegia, facial paralysis, vestibular disease, and Horner's syndrome. The prognosis for this condition is poor, but surgical intervention has recently been discussed.[88]

Metabolic Diseases

Diabetic Neuropathy

Spontaneous diabetes mellitus is a well-recognized disorder in dogs for which clinical and biochemical features have been documented. Cases of clinical and subclinical polyneuropathy have been reported in dogs with spontaneous diabetes mellitus.[27, 123, 201]

The etiologic factors and mechanisms by which peripheral nerve fibers degenerate in diabetic neuropathies are not known.[206] It is now believed that vascular factors are unlikely to play an important role in the genesis of the symmetric polyneuropathies associated with diabetes,[205] and interest has focused on metabolic derangement of Schwann cells and on primary axonal disease.[40] This metabolic dysfunction may repesent another peripheral-distal axonopathy or dying back disease.[195, 196]

Pathologic changes reported in dogs range from active fiber degeneration to demyelination or remyelination and axonal regeneration, especially in distal nerves. In cats, demyelination and remyelination are prominent findings.[139]

Clinical signs are extremely variable, ranging from a subclinical condition to one with an acute onset of progressive paraparesis, proprioceptive deficits, muscle atrophy, and depressed spinal reflexes. Cats often assume a plantigrade posture in pelvic limbs. Diabetic cataracts may be present. Electrodiagnostic testing has revealed fibrillation potentials, positive sharp waves and fasciculation potentials in muscles, slow nerve conduction velocities, and decreased amplitudes of evoked muscle action potentials.[201]

Diagnosis is based on clinicopathologic evidence of diabetes mellitus (hyperglycemia, glycosuria, insulin assays) and clinical, neurologic, electrophysiologic, and nerve biopsy data.

Insufficient information is available to establish guidelines for prognosis and therapy; however, insulin management resulted in amelioration of signs of clinical polyneuropathy in one case.[123]

Toxic and Nutritional Disorders

The ingestion of *Melochia pyramidate*, a weed found in the coastal area of El Salvador, is believed to be responsible for a progressive tetraparesis syndrome referred to as derriengue.[164] A distal wallerian degeneration of the sciatic nerves, with associated denervation muscle atrophy, and neuronal fiber degeneration in the rostal portions of the dorsal spinocerebellar tract were documented in some cases. The disease has clinical and pathologic similarities to an ataxia, knuckling of the fetlocks, and goose stepping syndrome associated with ingestion of cycad palms in Australia and the Caribbean. Feedlot cattle in the United States have been reported to have a similar syndrome; affected animals are referred to as knucklers. The lesion in these syndromes may be referred to as a central-peripheral distal axonopathy.[164]

Delayed organophosphate toxicity, arsanilic acid overdosing in pigs, organomercurial toxicity, acute delayed swayback in lambs, and pantothenic acid deficiency in swine are a few other syndromes that include degeneration of sensory or motor nerves. There may be an accompanying spinal cord fiber tract degeneration and sometimes ventral horn cell or cerebellar lesions[164] (see also Chapter 8 and reference 32). Sorghum toxicity in horses (lathyrism) is discussed in Chapter 8.[1]

Idiopathic Diseases

Distal Denervating Disease

A degenerative neuropathy has been reported in dogs in the United Kingdom.[97] In this disorder there is no breed or age predisposition. The etiology and pathogenesis are unknown. Pathologically, there is degeneration of the distal intramuscular axons with collateral sprouting. Skeletal muscle changes are typical of neurogenic atrophy. Proximal and middle portions of peripheral nerves are normal, and there is no evidence of sensory nerve damage.

The rate of onset of clinical signs is variable from 1 week to greater than 1 month. The main presenting sign reported is tetraparesis. The head and neck could not be supported in two dogs. Mastication, swallowing, respiration, and bladder function are unimpaired. Pain sensation is preserved. Muscle atrophy may be prominent, especially involving proximal extensor muscles. There is hypotonia and depressed or absent patellar reflexes. Seventh cranial nerve dysfunction has been observed.

Moderate to marked spontaneous potentials (fibrillations and positive sharp waves) are present in limb, axial, and masticatory and tongue muscles. Motor nerve conduction velocities are in the low normal range. The amplitude of evoked potentials is reduced. Sensory nerve potentials are normal.

The prognosis for full recovery is good, with appropriate nursing care. Most dogs recover within 1 to 5 months of clinical onset of signs.

Distal Symmetric Polyneuropathy in Dogs

A distal symmetric sensorimotor polyneuropathy has been reported in young adult dogs (1.5 to 3 years).[24, 69, 83] This condition is clinically and pathologically different from other reported peripheral neuropathies in dogs. The cause and pathogenesis are not known; however, a dying back process or peripheral axonopathy has been suggested. In one dog, the condition was noted after canine heartworm disease therapy (thiacetarsamide) complicated by disseminated intravascular coagulation.

Pathologic changes characterized by fiber degeneration and loss, especially of large caliber myelinated fibers, are present in distal parts of appendicular and laryngeal nerves. Sensory and autonomic nerves appear to be affected to a lesser degree. No lesions are found in the CNS. There is evidence of neurogenic atrophy in distal skeletal muscles.

Clinical signs include chronic pelvic limb paresis, which progresses to involve thoracic limbs, and bilateral atrophy of distal appendicular and bulbar musculature. A reduced response to painful stimuli has been observed in one dog.

Electrodiagnostic studies indicate fibrillation potentials, positive sharp waves in distal limb muscles (below stifle and elbow), and absence of evoked action potentials.

Diagnosis is based on clinical, electrodiagnostic, and nerve biopsy data. Prognosis is poor. There is no known effective treatment, and the disease appears to progress.

Idiopathic Facial Paralysis

Facial nerve paralysis of acute onset has been reported in mature dogs, with an apparent predisposition for cocker spaniels.[25] The cause of this condition is unknown. The facial paralysis is unrelated to otitis media.

Pathologic studies of facial nerve biopsies reveal active degeneration of myelinated fibers, especially those of larger diameter. Clinical signs are characterized by ear drooping, lip commissural paralysis, sialosis, and collection of food on the paralyzed side of the mouth. The palpebral fissure is usually widened in dogs (see Fig. 2–24) and narrowed in horses. Menace response testing and trigeminofacial and acousticofacial reflexes are absent. Bilateral facial paralysis may be observed. There is no evidence of Horner's syndrome.

Electrodiagnostic testing usually reveals spontaneous denervation potentials in superficial facial muscles. Stimulation of the facial nerve external to the stylomastoid foramen may fail to evoke muscle action potentials. Skull radiographic studies are noncontributory.

Prognosis is guarded. Improvement may take place in a few weeks or months or may never occur. Chronic lip paralysis may result in permanent contracture, and inability to close the eyelids often leads to corneal lesions owing to lack of lacrimal lubrication. Treatment is empiric. The efficacy of steroid therapy is unknown. Artificial tears may ameliorate corneal dryness.

Unilateral or bilateral facial paresis or paralysis in dogs is reportedly caused by a hypothyroid neuropathy, pituitary neoplasia, or both,[67] sometimes accompanied by peripheral vestibular signs. Results of thyroid hormone replacement in such animals have been variable.

In adult horses, facial paralysis has been reported in association with peripheral vestibular disease. Trauma was considered to be the causative factor.[86]

Facial nerve paralysis following recumbency is not uncommon in large animals, particularly the horse,[153] and has been documented in the dog.[176]

Idiopathic Vestibular Disease

An acute vestibular syndrome without evidence of inflammatory lesions is seen in cats and older dogs[67, 160] and possibly in horses.[144] There are signs of peripheral vestibular involvement, including head tilt, asymmetric ataxia, and horizontal or rotatory nystagmus. More severe signs of falling, rolling, and vomiting (especially in the dog) are seen occasionally. The signs appear suddenly, often causing severe incapacitation. In a few days, the animal tends to stabilize and gradually improves for several weeks. Residual deficits, such as a mild head tilt, may be seen.

It is important to exclude an infection as the cause because the idiopathic syndrome and acute labyrinthitis have identical clinical signs. In the idiopathic disease, the external, middle, and inner ear are grossly normal. Results of otoscopic and radiographic examinations are normal. The canine disease must also be differentiated from brain stem disease. The syndrome has been mistaken for an acute vascular accident in the brain stem. The signs of the idiopathic syndrome are only those of peripheral vestibular dysfunction. Postural reactions and other cranial nerves are not affected. In the early stages, postural reactions may be difficult to test, and the peripheral nature of the syndrome may not be obvious until the second or third day (see Chapter 2).

A variety of treatments have been tried, including antibiotics, antiinflammatory agents, antimotion sickness drugs, and others. There is no evidence that any treatment changes the course of the disease. If infection cannot be absolutely excluded, antibiotics are recommended, but aminoglycosides should be avoided.

Trigeminal Neuritis

Bilateral paralysis of muscles of mastication occurs in dogs and cats and is characterized by acute onset of inability to close the jaw. Pathologically, a bilateral nonsuppurative neuritis is found in all motor branches of the trigeminal nerve and ganglion, associated with demyelination and occasional fiber degeneration. Sensory perception of the head is normal. Horner's syndrome may be observed. The disease appears to be self limiting, and recovery usually occurs in 2 to 3 weeks.

Sensory Trigeminal Neuropathy

Sensory trigeminal neuropathy has been reported in a 2 year old rough collie dog.[37] The cause was not determined. Pathologic abnormalities were limited to the three major branches of both trigeminal nerves and the trigeminal ganglia. There was partial loss of myelinated nerve fibers in each branch and also in the spinal tract of the fifth nerve in the brain stem. It was considered that the primary abnormality was in the trigeminal ganglion. Clinical signs of excess salivation, coughing, and dysphagia were believed to be associated with bilateral loss or absence of tactile sensation and deep pain from the face, tongue, and oral mucosa. The condition in this dog remained relatively unchanged over an 18 month period.

Feline Dysautonomia (Key-Gaskell Syndrome)

This disease was reported by Key and Gaskell[124] in cats with an unusual combination of clinical signs. The etiopathogenesis is unknown. Pathologic changes primarily involve neuronal perikarya, especially autonomic ganglia. Lesions are characterized by neuronal degeneration and loss, neuronophagia, and occasionally mild mononuclear perivascular cuffing. Degeneration has been found in many autonomic nerves.[103] Changes are frequently present in dorsal nucleus of the vagus and motor nuclei of cranial nerves III, V, VII, and XII and in the ventral horns and intermediolateral gray matter of spinal cord. Sensory ganglia are affected to a much lesser degree. Clinical signs suggest involvement of the parasympathetic nervous system. The pathologic features resemble those of grass sickness of horses.[12]

Historically, cats begin vomiting or retching and become depressed and anorexic. The third eyelid protrudes, and pupils are dilated. Cats may be febrile, emaciated, and dehydrated. Sneezing may occur, and the nose is often dry. Dried exudate may block the external nares. Occasionally, mild pelvic limb ataxia or more generalized paresis, depressed proprioception, and absent anal reflex have been detected. Megaesophagus is often present, and Heinz bodies have been demonstrated in up to 50% of the red blood cells. Their significance is uncertain.[103, 152]

No specific treatment is available, but supportive therapy is indicated. Prognosis is guarded, especially in cats that have persistent regurgitation and vomiting. Cats that begin to produce secretions and eat and drink have the best prognosis.

Stringhalt in Horses

Stringhalt (archaic "springhalt") refers to a rapid, involuntary flexion of the pelvic limb of a horse (see Fig. 14–5). This may be subtle or profound so that the hoof hits the abdomen, and it may be uni- or bilateral.[169]

Isolated cases involving one pelvic limb are sometimes associated with lesions, often traumatic, in the region of the hock. Endemic and epidemic (Australian) stringhalt usually occurs in a group of horses, it is usually bilateral, and signs may involve the thoracic limbs and even the neck and trunk. Some horses may become "roarers." Muscular hypertonia and, surpris-

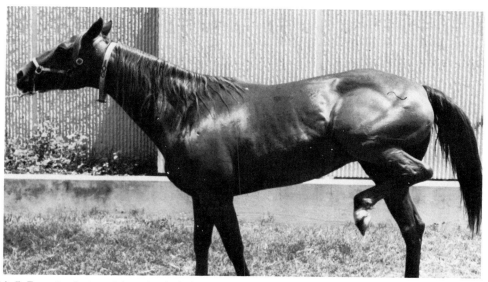

Figure 14–5. Excessive flexion of the pelvic limb during the protraction phase of stride is typical of stringhalt. This horse had an acute onset of signs in both pelvic limbs and had slight hypometria in the thoracic limbs; these findings resemble Australian stringhalt or neurolathyrism. Signs resolved with time. (Courtesy of Dr IG Mayhew.)

ingly, muscle atrophy occur in the affected limbs, especially involving distal muscles. Wallerian degeneration and neurogenic-type muscle atrophy have been found. The lesion may represent a distal, mixed neuropathy that involves sensory fibers more than motor fibers. A plant or fungal toxicosis is suspected, and lathyrism appears to mimic this endemic form.

Removal of affected horses from offending pastures can result in improvement of signs early in the course of disease in endemic stringhalt. Lateral digital extensor tenectomy may be beneficial in monomelic cases, especially if hock trauma is suspected and a period of rest does not result in improvement of signs.

Trauma

Traumatic Neuropathy

Trauma to peripheral nerves, cranial and spinal, represents the most common cause of neuropathies in animals. Nerve injuries may result from mechanical blows, gunshot, fractures, pressure, and stretching (see Brachial Plexus Avulsion and Compression below). Iatrogenic causes include crushing or cutting the nerve, spearing the nerve with an intramedullary pin, compressing by casts or splints, and injecting agents into or adjacent to the nerve.

Nerve damage may be defined in terms of structural damage. Neurotmesis is complete severance of all structures of the nerve with wallerian degeneration (axonal necrosis and myelin fragmentation) of the distal stump. Axonotmesis consists of damage to the nerve fibers resulting in axonal degeneration, however, the endoneurial and Schwann cell sheaths remain intact and provide a framework for axonal regeneration. Neurapraxia is an interruption in the function and conduction of a nerve, without structural damage.

The regenerative ability of a nerve is directly proportional to the amount of continuity of connective tissue structures of the nerve. In neurapraxic and axonotmesic lesions in which the endoneurial connective tissue and Schwann cells remain intact, the potential for axonal regeneration is good. In neurotmesis, axonal regeneration is usually frustrated by lack of connective tissue scaffold or growth tubes. In addition, scar tissue tends to interfere with sprouting axons, resulting in neuroma formation.[28]

Once an axon has grown past the point of injury and penetrated a Schwann tube in the distal nerve stump, remyelination occurs. Axonal regeneration occurs at a rate of 1 to 4 mm per day (see also Chapter 19).

Clinical signs of cranial and spinal nerve dysfunction are outlined in Tables 14–2 and 14–3 and depicted in Figures 14–6 to 14–17.

Diagnosis of traumatic neuropathy is usually based on history and clinical signs. Electrodiagnostic data may be helpful in evaluating nerve integrity and severity of damage, and in monitoring progress of regeneration. Approximately 5 to 7 days (longer in large animals) are required after injury before increased insertional activity and spontaneous potentials (positive sharp waves and fibrillation potentials) are detected. Nerve integrity may be easily assessed by nerve stimulation proximal and distal to the site of the lesion.[215] Exploratory surgery has been advocated as another method for direct evaluation of peripheral nerve damage.[203]

Prognosis is guarded with peripheral nerve injury. Lesions characterized by neurapraxia and axonotmesis have a better prognosis than those of neurotmesis. The closer the nerve injury is to the muscle it must reinnervate, the better the prognosis. Self mutilation can be a major complication of abnormal sensation in an affected area produced by regeneration of sensory nerves.

Treatment may involve surgical anastomosis or neurolysis (see Chapter 19). For nerve damage that is chronic, proximal, or severe, procedures for muscle relocation and muscle tendon transfers have been described.[10, 133] Physical therapy, such as swimming, electric stimulation, manipulation, and whirlpool bath, may help to overcome circulation problems and delay muscle atrophy.

Brachial Plexus Avulsion and Compression

Lesions of the brachial plexus are often encountered clinically in animals, especially dogs, following trauma. Traction of the thoracic limb in dogs has been accepted as the cause of this traumatic disorder. The frequency of root avulsion is believed to be due to the lower resistance of nerve roots to stretch, probably because they lack a perineurium. The ventral roots are more susceptible to traumatic stretch than the dorsal roots.

A syndrome of traumatically induced brachial plexus deficits, with prominent signs of radial nerve involvement, is seen in horses (Fig. 14–18). From the few detailed postmortem studies undertaken, it appears as though the brachial plexus receives impact injury between the scap-

Table 14–2. SPINAL NERVE LESIONS AND THEIR ASSOCIATED DEFICITS (BASED ON THE DOG)

Nerve	Muscles*	Clinical Signs of Dysfunction
Suprascapular (C6–C7)	Supraspinatus Infraspinatus	Loss of shoulder extension (muscle atrophy with prominent spine of scapula). Lateral luxation of shoulder (horse). (Figs. 14–6 and 14–7)
Musculocutaneous (C6–C8)	Biceps brachii Brachial Coracobrachial	Reduced elbow flexion; loss of biceps reflex; reduced sensation over medial surface of forearm. No gait abnormality in horse. (Fig. 14–8)
Axillary (C7–C8)	Deltoid Teres major Teres minor	Reduced shoulder flexion; deltoid atrophy. Minimal gait deficit all species
Radial (C7–T1)	Triceps brachii Extensor carpi radialis Ulnaris lateralis	Reduced extension of elbow, carpus, and digits; loss of extensor postural thrust and limb support (with high radial damage, ie, above elbow); loss of triceps reflex; reduced sensation over dorsal surface of forearm. (Figs. 14–9 and 14–10)
Median (C8–T1)	Flexor carpi radialis Superficial digital flexor	Reduced flexion of carpus and digits. Minimal gait deficit all species. (Fig. 14–16)
Ulnar (C8–T1)	Flexor carpi ulnaris Deep digital flexor	Reduced flexion of carpus and digits; reduced sensation over caudal surface of forearm. Minimal gait deficit all species. (Fig. 14–11)
Femoral (L4–L5)	Iliopsoas Quadriceps Sartorius	Inability to extend stifle and inability to bear weight; loss of patellar reflex; reduced sensation over medial surface of paw, hock, stifle, and thigh, just medial thigh in large animals (saphenous nerve). (Fig. 14–12)
Obturator (L5–L6)	External obturator Pectineal Gracilis	Inability to adduct hip and thigh (animal "does the splits" on smooth surface). (Fig. 14–13)
Sciatic (L6–L7–S1)	Biceps femoris Semimembranous Semitendinous	Loss of ability to flex stifle and other functions along its branches (tibial and common peroneal nerve); loss of flexor reflex. (Figs. 14–14 and 14–15)
Tibial	Gastrocnemius Popliteal Deep digital flexor	Inability to extend hock and flex digits; reduced sensation over plantar surface of foot. (Fig. 14–16)
Common peroneal	Long peroneal Lateral digital extensor Long digital extensor Cranial tibial	Inability to flex hock and extend digits; knuckling of dorsal foot. Reduced sensation over dorsocranial surface of the foot, hock, stifle, minimal in large animals. (Fig. 14–17)
Pudendal (S1–S2–S3)	External anal sphincter Striated urethral muscle	Loss of perineal reflex; loss of bulbocavernosus reflex. (Fig. 14–3)
Pelvic (S2–S3)	Smooth muscle of bladder, rectum	Inadequate bladder contraction, obstipation

*Muscle atrophy of innervated muscles will occur.

Table 14–3. CRANIAL NERVE LESIONS AND THEIR ASSOCIATED DEFICITS (BASED ON THE DOG)

Nerve	Clinical Signs of Dysfunction	Clinical Tests	Normal Response	Abnormal Response
I. Olfactory	Hyposmia or anosmia	1. Smell of food or nonirritating volatile substance	1. Food: interest or attempt to eat. Volatile substance: sniffing, recoil, and nose lick	1. No reaction
II. Optic*	Visual impairment, hesitancy in walking	1. Obstacle test 2. Visual placing test 3. Menace reaction 4. Following movement (ophthalmoscopic examination)	1. Avoidance of obstacle 2. Visual placing of limbs 3. Eye blink 4. Follows motion of objects	1. Bumping objects 2–4. No reaction
	Anisocoria Mydriasis	1. Point source of light in each eye	1. Direct and consensual pupillary reflexes	1. On affected side, direct and consensual pupillary reflexes absent; on unaffected side, direct and consensual pupillary reflexes present
III. Oculomotor	Anisocoria Mydriasis Ptosis Strabismus (ventrolateral)	1. Point source of light in each eye 2. Observation of eye movements when following a moving object in horizontal/vertical planes	1. Direct and consensual pupillary reflexes 2. Normal medial, dorsoventral ocular movement	1. On affected side, direct pupillary reflex absent, consensual reflex present; on unaffected side, direct pupillary reflex present, consensual reflex absent 2. Impaired ocular movement in vertical plane and impaired ocular adduction in horizontal plane (unable to follow upward, downward, or medially)
IV. Trochlear	Strabismus (dorsomedial)	—	—	
V. Trigeminal (motor) (sensory)	Masseteric and temporalis muscle atrophy; inability to open and close jaws	1. Jaw tonus 2. Palpation of masseter and temporalis muscle 3. Palpebral reflex 4. Corneal reflex	1. Resistance to opening jaws 2. Normal contour/muscle resilience 3. Eye blink 4. Globe retraction	1. Lack of resistance or supranormal resistance 2. Hypotonia, atrophy 3–4. No reaction; intense discomfort recoil, vocalization
VI. Abducens	Strabismus (medial)	1. Observation of eye when following moving object in horizontal plane	1. Normal lateral ocular movement	1. Impaired ocular abduction (unable to follow laterally)
VII. Facial	Asymmetry of facial expression, inability to close eyelids, lip commissure paralysis, auricular paralysis	1. Palpebral reflex 2. Menace reflex 3. Handclap 4. Tickle ear	1–3. Eye blink 4. Auricular contraction	1–4. No reaction
VIII. Vestibulocochlear (cochlear)	Deafness	1. Handclap 2. EEG alerting	1. Startle reaction, eye blink, auricular contraction 2. EEG alert recordings	1–2. No reaction
(vestibular)	Circling, head tilt, nystagmus, loss of balance	1. Rapid head movement in horizontal/vertical planes 2. Caloric test 3. Rotatory test 4. Righting reactions	1–2. Physiologically induced nystagmus 3. Postrotatory nystagmus 4. Normal righting	1–4. No reaction; spontaneous, positional nystagmus; strabismus (ventrolateral upon dorsal head extension)
IX. Glossopharyngeal	Dysphagia	1. Gag reflex	1. Swallow	1. No reaction

Table 14–3. CRANIAL NERVE LESIONS AND THEIR ASSOCIATED DEFICITS
(BASED ON THE DOG) *Continued*

Nerve	Clinical Signs of Dysfunction	Clinical Tests	Normal Response	Abnormal Response
X. Vagus	Dysphagia	1. Gag reflex 2. Laryngeal reflex 3. Oculocardiac reflex 4. Endoscopy; slap test	1. Swallow 2. Cough 3. Bradycardia 4. Laryngeal symmetry	1–3. No reaction 4. Laryngeal paralysis, absent slap test
XI. Spinal accessory	Dorsolateral neck muscle atrophy; torticollis	1. Palpation of cervical musculature	1. Normal contour/muscle resilience	1. Hypotonia, muscle atrophy
XII. Hypoglossal	Deviation of tongue (animal licks only affected side)	1. Tongue stretch 2. Tongue inspection	1. Retraction 2. Normal bulk	1. No retraction 2. Atrophy

*The optic nerve is not a true nerve developmentally, structurally, or in its pathology. It is a tract of the central nervous system. It is surrounded by meninges, including a subarachnoid space.

ula and the rib cage. The same may be true of some of the postrecumbency (anesthesia) "radial paralyses" seen in cattle and horses.

Avulsion is usually intradural, and the lesion in dogs is diffuse rather than circumscribed, with involvement of fibers at many different levels.[94] Degenerative changes in dorsal and ventral nerve roots and ventral branches of spinal nerves are characterized by axonal necrosis, myelin fragmentation, and loss of myelinated fibers. Many fibers are damaged where they penetrate the leptomeninges, resulting in

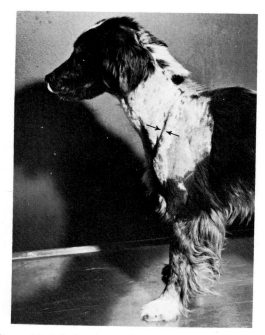

Figure 14–6. Left suprascapular nerve paralysis in a dog 6 months after neurectomy. Notice the prominence of the spine of the scapula from atrophy of the supraspinatus and infraspinatus muscles. Functional deficit is minimal.

neuroma formation. Retrograde changes are observed in the ventral horn cells and are characterized by chromatolysis, cell swelling, and neuronal depletion. Retraction balls may be seen. Dorsal column degeneration occurs only with lesions central to the dorsal root ganglion.

Clinical signs reflect the distribution of damage to nerve roots, branches, and plexal cords and not direct peripheral nerve involvement.[100] Signs may vary from weakness of single muscle groups without sensory loss to paralysis of all thoracic limb muscle groups with accompanying sensory loss (eg, a lesion from C6 to T1–T2). A lesion that involves spinal cord segments C8–T1 may produce ipsilateral loss of the panniculus reflex; whereas involvement of the T1 root, which contains preganglionic sympathetic fibers, frequently results in partial Horner's syndrome and anisocoria, although this apparently has not been seen in the horse, perhaps reflecting the more distal (subscapular) involvement.

Sensory impairment of conscious pain is usually present to a varible degree in all dogs with brachial plexus avulsion. In general, desensitized areas of skin may be detected on lateral, medial, dorsal, and palmar surfaces of the affected thoracic limb but usually do not extend more proximally than the elbow. Hypalgesic areas are detected in large animals, but the deficits are not well demarcated, unless there is C6 or C7 nerve root involvement.

Diagnosis is most commonly based on historical and clinical data. Electrodiagnostic testing is useful for detecting muscle denervation, especially minor degrees that cannot be noted on routine neurologic examination. This information may be helpful when surgical management by muscle tendon transpositions is being considered. Myelography may occasionally demonstrate a contrast outlined diverticulum.

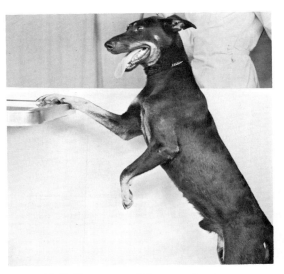

Figure 14–8. Transection of the musculocutaneous nerve paralyzes the flexors of the elbow. The dog cannot lift the limb to the table.

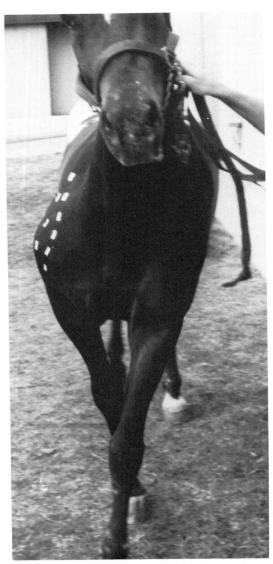

Figure 14–7. Cranial view of a horse with sweeney (suprascapular nerve paralysis) on the right side. With weight bearing on the affected limb there is a lateral subluxation of the shoulder, as shown. This horse ran into a tree and, in addition to damage to the suprascapular nerve, had analgesia over the C8 dermatome on the right (outlined with tape). (Courtesy of Dr IG Mayhew.)

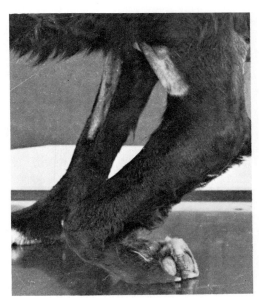

Figure 14–9. The radial nerve has been transected proximal to the triceps muscle in this dog. The dog cannot extend any of the joints except the shoulder and cannot bear weight.

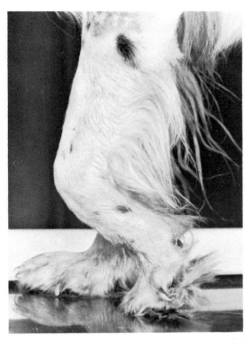

Figure 14–10. The radial nerve has been transected distal to the nerves to the triceps muscle in this dog. Weight bearing can occur, but the carpus cannot be extended actively. Some animals learn to flip the foot forward into a weight-bearing position.

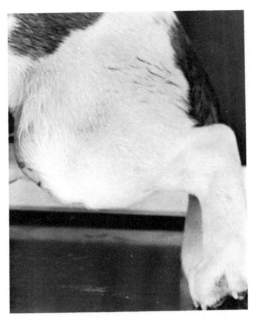

Figure 14–12. In left femoral nerve paralysis, the dog's leg collapses when a step is taken because the stifle can neither be extended nor fixed to bear weight.

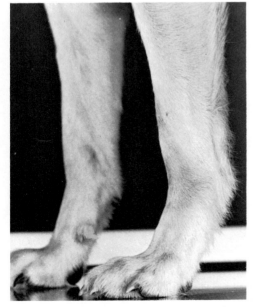

Figure 14–11. Left median and ulnar nerve paralysis in a dog. No lameness is evident other than a slight sinking of the left carpus and fetlock due to a loss of function of the flexors of these joints.

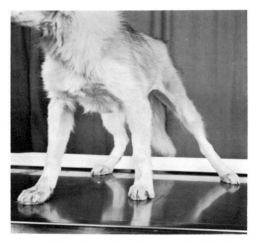

Figure 14–13. A dog with an injury to the left obturator nerve. Abduction of the limb is seen on slick surfaces because the adductor muscles are paralyzed.

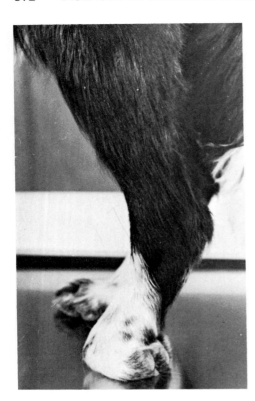

Figure 14–14. With left sciatic nerve paralysis (including both peroneal and tibial nerves), the animal can extend and fix the stifle but knuckles the paw. The hock passively flexes and extends as the weight is shifted.

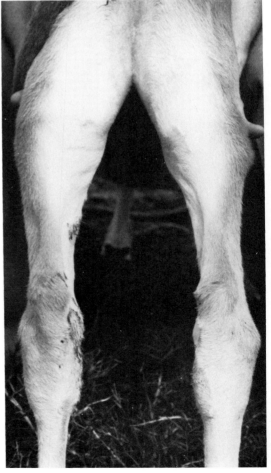

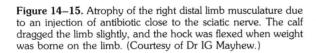

Figure 14–15. Atrophy of the right distal limb musculature due to an injection of antibiotic close to the sciatic nerve. The calf dragged the limb slightly, and the hock was flexed when weight was borne on the limb. (Courtesy of Dr IG Mayhew.)

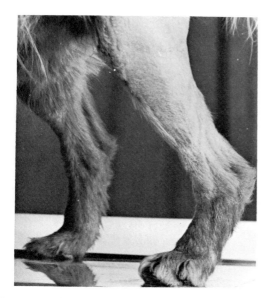

Figure 14–16. Left tibial nerve paralysis causes an exaggerated flexion of the hock.

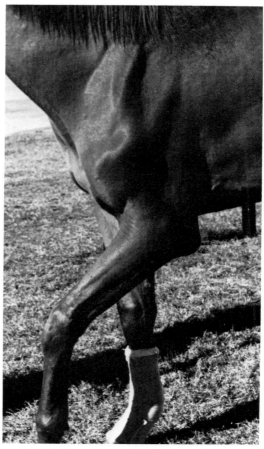

Figure 14–18. This horse had traumatic compression of its left brachial plexus. Little weight bearing was possible, and contracture of the knee and fetlock had occurred several weeks after injury. The dropped elbow and triceps atrophy indicate radial nerve involvement. In addition, there was clinical and EMG evidence of involvement of suprascapular, median, and ulnar components of the brachial plexus, which was confirmed at necropsy examination. (Courtesy of Dr IG Mayhew.)

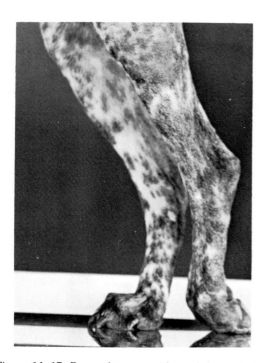

Figure 14–17. Peroneal nerve paralysis of the dog's left pelvic limb results in a straightening of the hocks and a tendency to knuckle the paw because of loss of function of the digital extensor muscles.

The prognosis is guarded to poor. The progress of recovery is slow, requiring many months. Electrophysiologic testing will detect early changes in reinnervation and recovery. Some fibers, following acute injury, may show a temporary conduction block, from which they will recover within a few days. Muscle tendon transpositions have been successful in some dogs with partial avulsion. Amputation of the affected limb may be necessary if it is severely excoriated from dragging or self multilation.

Calving or Foaling Paralysis

Although metabolic derangements (eg, milk fever) and decubital neuromyopathy probably account for more cases of the postcalving, downer cow syndrome, a specific neuropathy does occur at this time resulting in degrees of paraparesis. Particularly with a large calf, a small cow, and a degree of dystocia, the ventral roots of the lumbar nerves can become compressed within the pelvic canal during delivery. This is probably the pathogenesis of the resulting "obturator-sciatic" paresis that characterizes the syndrome.[49]

Similar postpartum paralysis occurs in mares, but the pathogenesis does not appear to be well defined. Sacroiliac subluxation with palpable hemorrhage around both femoral nerves was associated with one case of postfoaling recumbency in a mare. Absent patellar reflexes and analgesia of the medial thigh regions were also present.

Antiinflammatory agents and supportive care should be instituted, although it is hard to predict which cases will improve and which will not.

Postnatal Quadriceps Atrophy in Calves

Following delivery, often assisted, of large calves in anterior presentation there can be a syndrome of femoral paralysis and subsequent quadriceps atrophy (Fig. 14–19). Degrees of quadriceps traumatic myonecrosis and femoral nerve injury are seen at necropsy evaluation.[209] Compression and overextension of these structures are thought to be the cause of the syndrome. Severe cases do not improve, but many calves survive with an acceptable gait and some degree of muscle atrophy. Supportive nursing care is indicated.

Degenerative Disorders

Paraneoplastic Neuromyopathy

Tumor induced organ dysfunction not directly attributable to malignant invasion has been defined by such terms as paraneoplastic, carcinomatous, or remote effects syndrome. Polyneuropathies occurring in dogs with primary and metastatic neoplasia have been reported.[35, 102, 192]

Paraneoplastic neuromyopathy may occur in animals with any form of systemic neoplasia. In people, the highest incidence occurs in patients with small cell anaplastic bronchogenic carcinoma.[210] The veterinary literature probably does not reflect the incidence of paraneoplastic polyneuropathy in animals.

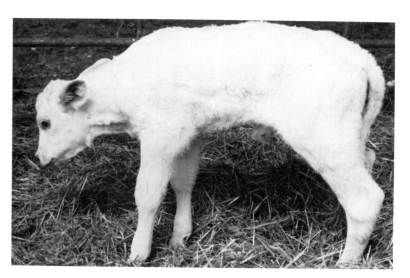

Figure 14–19. Following an assisted delivery, this large Charolais calf had difficulty standing on its pelvic limbs. It postured with its head down and pelvic limbs slightly flexed because of marked pelvic limb extensor weakness. There was atrophy of both quadriceps muscle groups and poor patellar reflexes bilaterally. This case represents the postnatal quadriceps atrophy syndrome associated with birth trauma to the quadriceps musculature and the femoral nerves. (Courtesy of Dr IG Mayhew.)

The pathogenesis of these disorders is not known, although several theories have been suggested:[130] (1) elaboration of primary neuro- or myotoxic factors by the tumor; (2) an influence through alteration of homeostatic endocrine functions secondarily affecting muscle; (3) utilization or trapping of specific nutrients or factors required for normal neuromuscular function; (4) stimulation of a host mechanism generating secondary neuro- or myoactive reactions.

Pathologic changes in nerves include paranodal and segmental demyelination or remyelination and occasionally axonal degeneration. Skeletal muscle changes are observed and include focal myonecrosis, intrafascicular fatty infiltration, internal nuclei, and atrophy of fiber types (especially type 2).

Clinical signs are variable, with the few cases reported being subclinical,[102, 192] as is also reported in people.[181] A paraneoplastic effect should be considered in any older animal with neoplasia that manifests vague neurologic signs.

Electrodiagnostic testing may reveal slow nerve conduction velocities and spontaneous potentials, including fibrillations, positive sharp waves, and high frequency bizarre waves.

Diagnosis may be suggested by detection of a tumor, vague ill defined neurologic signs suggestive of a polyneuropathy, and electrodiagnostic and nerve and muscle biopsy data. Confirmation generally requires postmortem studies.

Prognosis is poor. There is no treatment.

Vascular Disorders

Ischemic Neuromyopathy/Aortoiliac Thrombosis

This is a disorder that occurs with moderate frequency in cats and only occasionally in dogs and horses.

In the cat it is associated with cardiomyopathy.[134, 208] The causes of the disease and of emboli formation in the heart are uncertain. The emboli may be carried to any site within the arterial circulation. Most commonly occlusion occurs at the aortic trifurcation. Thrombi that extend into the iliac arteries are termed saddle thrombi. Vasoactive substances released from the thrombus may be involved in the pathogenesis.[33, 161] Cats of all ages may be affected. There is a predilection for male cats and cats of the Persian breed.[207]

Pathologically, in affected cats, lesions in peripheral nerves begin in the midthigh region, with the central fibers in a fascicle being more susceptible than the peripheral ones. The majority of fibers show changes of wallerian-type degeneration, whereas others have evidence of paranodal or segmental demyelination. In skeletal muscle, ischemic myopathy characterized by focal necrosis, myophagia, internal nuclei hypertrophy, and occasional cellular infiltrates, also contributes to the clinical signs.

Clinical signs are usually acute in onset and include pelvic limb pain, plantigrade stance, paraparesis, or paralysis. Femoral pulse may be weak or absent, the gastrocnemius muscle is firm and often painful, and the limbs are cool. Distal limb muscles below the stifle are particularly affected. Flexion and extension of both hip and stifle joints and the patellar reflex are usually present. Pain sensation is absent in the distal limbs.

Electrodiagnostic studies in cats have revealed absent or reduced evoked potentials from interosseous and cranial tibial muscles. Nerve conduction velocities may be either normal or reduced.[98] Chest radiography may indicate cardiopulmonary disease. Abdominal films may demonstrate the rare occurrence of a radiopaque foreign body located in the aortic lumen.[131] Diagnosis of occlusive vascular disease can be confirmed from an aortogram (Fig. 14–20).

Although the collateral circulation does return in the majority of cases (with return of function to varying degrees within 6 weeks to 6 months), the prognosis is guarded because of the potential of further thromboembolism. Femoral pulses frequently return within 1 to 2 weeks. At present no results show that any therapy produces a significantly better recovery than no therapy. The effectiveness of embolectomy is uncertain.

Thrombosis of the terminal aorta and iliac arteries of the horse is thought to be associated with *Strongylus vulgaris* migration,[89] although trauma[171] and infection have been considered as potential etiologies as well.[89] It has been reported in a calf.[178]

A history of transient, unilateral pelvic limb lameness induced by moderate to strenuous exercise or simply poor racing performance is common, but clinical signs may be peracute with the horse showing evidence of pain and anxiety, sweating, elevated heart and respiratory rate, reluctance to bear weight, or even paraplegia, shock, and death. Profound neurologic defects may accompany the other signs of aortic thrombosis, with complete paralysis of

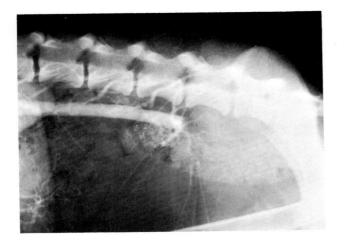

Figure 14–20. A 4 year old pointer with pelvic limb paresis. The limbs were warm and painful. No femoral pulse could be detected in either limb. An aortic occlusion was seen in this lateral aortogram.

the pelvic limbs due to interference with circulation to the nerves and muscles.[144]

Diagnosis is by careful rectal examination of the abdominal aorta and its branches, with evidence of variations in the amplitude of the pulse and asymmetry of the vasculature. Occasionally the amplitude of the pulse in the great metatarsal and digital arteries is reduced, and saphenous vein refill time may be prolonged after exercise.

Some horses will recover in time possibly because of recanalization of the artery or the development of collateral circulation. Chemotherapy has been relatively unsuccessful to date.[171]

Pseudoamyloid Multiradicular Degeneration in Spinal Nerve Roots in a Purebred Shetland Pony

Single reference is made to this congenital disorder of Shetland ponies showing ataxia and tetraparesis. Nerve fiber degeneration and accumulation of pale staining foamy material occurred in spinal nerve roots without any clue as to the pathogenesis of the disorder.[117]

MYOPATHIES

Myopathies are relatively uncommon entities in domestic animals. The most common myopathies in animals are those that occur secondary to peripheral nerve disease. The majority of primary myopathic disorders have been described in dogs, and these usually are congenital or hereditary, metabolic, or traumatic in origin (Table 14–4).

Pathologic changes in muscle may be assessed qualitatively, using routine histologic stains, or quantitatively, using histochemical tests. En-

Table 14–4. CLASSIFICATION OF PRIMARY MYOPATHIES

Congenital or Hereditary
Myotonic myopathy in dogs, horses, goats
X-Linked myopathy in Irish terriers
Muscular dystrophy in Labrador retrievers
? Canine hypotrophic myopathy
Congenital myopathies in lambs, piglets

Immune Mediated
? Masticatory myositis in dogs
? Polymyositis in dogs

Metabolic or Toxic
Hyperadrenocortical myopathy in dogs
Steroid myopathy in dogs
Hypothyroid myopathy in dogs
Exertional myopathy in dogs, horses
Malignant hyperthermia in dogs, cats, horses, pigs
Cassia occidentalis toxicosis in cattle

Idiopathic
Idiopathic feline polymyopathy
Immobilization myopathy in dogs

Infectious
Toxoplasma myositis
Clostridial myositis

Traumatic
? Myositis ossificans in dogs, cats, pigs
? Fibrotic myopathy in dogs, horses
Downer cow myopathy

Nutritional
Vitamin E–selenium responsive myopathy in dogs, horses, cattle, sheep, pigs

Degenerative
Paraneoplastic neuropathy

Vascular
Ischemic neuromyopathy in dogs, cats, horses
Postanesthetic neuromyopathy

? Suggests that the classification is uncertain.

zyme histochemical techniques applied to canine skeletal muscle[22, 23] have resulted in the recognition of three fiber types (I, IIA, and IIC), have demonstrated abnormalities in fibers that appear to be normal by routine staining procedures, and have made possible the diagnosis of specific enzyme deficiencies.

Pathologic alterations in muscles are limited to certain reactions, eg, alteration in size of muscle fibers (atrophy, hypertrophy), changes in fiber type distribution (grouping, predominance, or deficiency of fiber types), degenerative changes (fiber necrosis), cellular reactions (inflammation, fibrosis), and architectural changes ("moth eaten" fibers, fatty infiltration). Skeletal muscle has a considerable regenerative capacity following injury. A grouping of muscle fibers of the same histochemical type in a muscle that normally has a mosaic pattern is strong evidence of past denervation and subsequent reinnervation.

Myopathies tend to be characterized by muscle weakness and fatigue, with reduced exercise tolerance. Muscle strength may return with rest. The gait is often altered as a result of weakness and muscle stiffness. Selected muscles may be increased in size because of inflammation, hypertrophy, or spasm. More frequently, however, muscle mass is reduced as a result of nerve damage (ie, *neurogenic atrophy*). In contrast to generalized or diffuse muscle atrophy that occurs secondary to chronic spinal cord disease or systemic diseases that produce cachexia (which may take several months to develop), neurogenic atrophy occurs only in those muscles innervated by the injured nerve or nerves (*segmental atrophy*) and becomes clinically apparent after 1 to 2 weeks. Chronic neurogenic atrophy may result in fibrosis and limited joint movement from muscular contracture. A dimple contracture in a muscle (eg, limb or tongue) may be elicited in animals with myotonic myopathy by a sudden tap with a percussion hammer. Muscle pain, induced by palpation, is often recorded in animals with polymyositis.

In contrast to neurogenic muscle atrophy, primary myopathies tend to be diffuse, with a bilaterally symmetric distribution. Tendon reflexes are usually preserved, and sensory perception of pain is not impaired.

Diagnosis of myopathies is based on signalment data (many primary myopathies are breed and age specific), clinical signs, laboratory findings (serum enzyme level determination, especially creatine phosphokinase [CPK]), electrodiagnostic testing for spontaneous potentials, and characteristic pathologic findings obtained from muscle biopsy examination.

Congenital Hereditary Disorders

Myotonic Myopathy

Myotonia refers to a state in which active contraction of a muscle persists after cessation of voluntary effort or stimulation. This condition is characterized by muscle spasm (stiffness) and by temporary inability to initiate movement. A severe myotonic myopathy affecting almost all skeletal muscles occurs in immature chow chow puppies and in other breeds, often soon after they become ambulatory.[76, 84, 95, 120, 216] An autosomal recessive inheritance is suspected for this disease in chow chows. The pathogenesis may be associated with a decrease in resting chloride conductance of the muscle membrane, similar to myotonia congenita in humans.[30] The possibility of a multisystem membrane defect associated with low serum cholesterol level has also been considered.[84]

Myopathic changes are mild and consist of occasional angular atrophic fibers, internal nuclei, and marked size variation of type I and type II fibers. A relative increase in number of type II fibers has been reported.[187]

Clinical signs are characterized by stiffness in the first movements after a period of rest, splaying of thoracic limbs, bunny hopping pelvic limb gait, and occasional falling over and remaining rigid in lateral recumbency for up to 30 seconds. Some affected dogs may manifest respiratory difficulty from impaired abduction of vocal cords and regurgitation of food. Stiffness and weakness largely disappear with exercise. Proximal limb and neck muscles and tongue are hypertrophied. Signs are worse in cold weather. In older animals, an increasing period of exercise is necessary for muscle relaxation to occur. Percussion of muscles results in formation of dimples. This reaction is elicited in conscious and anesthetized dogs and in those administered neuromuscular blocking agents.

Serum CPK levels may be slightly elevated. Electromyographic studies are characterized by presence of trains of high frequency, bizarre myotonic potentials producing a "revving motorcycle" sound.

Diagnosis is based on signalment, clinical, and electrodiagnostic data.

Prognosis is guarded. Membrane stabilizing agents (procainamide, quinidine, and phenytoin) have been beneficial in the treatment of myotonia. Results of long-term therapeutic trials are lacking.

A similar disorder occurs in goats and young horses. In goats, the condition is believed to be inherited as either an autosomal dominant or autosomal recessive trait.[31] Decreased chloride conductance of the muscle membrane has been reported.[30] Affected animals may respond to appropriate stimulation (eg, auditory) by falling on their sides with rigidly extended limbs.

In young horses, clinical signs of myotonia consist of mild pelvic limb stiffness and bilateral swellings of the caudal thigh muscles[200] (Fig. 14–21). Trains of bizarre high frequency discharges occur on needle EMG. Signs generally occur within 6 months of birth. No abnormal chloride conductance has been associated with myotonic myopathy in horses.

X-Linked Myopathy in Irish Terriers

This myopathy, believed to be an autosomal recessive sex-linked hereditary condition, has been reported in male Irish terrier puppies.[217]

The pathogenesis is unknown, although mitochondrial changes suggest a defect in oxidative phosphorylation. At necropsy, muscles are

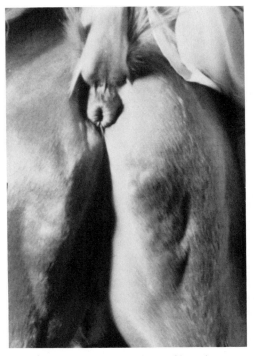

Figure 14–21. Myotonia in a horse. Note the myotonic dimpling in the right thigh muscles. (Courtesy of Dr IG Mayhew, University of Florida.)

pale with white streaks. A patchy distribution of lesions is seen histologically, characterized by considerable fiber size variation with many round, atrophic fibers, phagocytosis, giant cells, and calcification. Histochemical distinction between type I and type II fibers is lost.

A stiff gait and dysphagia develop at 6 to 8 weeks of age. Affected animals are unable to jump or support themselves on their pelvic limbs. The condition may be progressive or remain static, and animals have a low exercise tolerance. Skeletal muscles undergo atrophy and have increased tone, and there is initial resistance to passive joint movements.

Serum CPK and aldolase levels are high. Electromyography reveals continuous, bizarre, high frequency discharges (pseudomyotonia).

Diagnosis is based on signalment, clinical, electrophysiologic, serum muscle enzyme, and muscle biopsy data. Prognosis is poor. There is no treatment.

Identical clinical and pathologic findings are noted in young, male golden retrievers.[67] Breeding trials to determine a possible hereditary basis are lacking.

Muscular Dystrophy in Labrador Retriever Dogs

A severe degenerative myopathy that is inherited as an autosomal recessive trait has been reported in Labrador retriever dogs.[127, 128] The pathogenesis of this condition is unknown. Pathologic findings include increased numbers of central nuclei (sometimes involving 40% of fibers) and pronounced fiber size variation associated with atrophic and hypertrophic fibers. Atrophic fibers are angular, round, or polygonal, often form small groups, and are predominantly type I. Hypertrophic fibers are mainly type II.[189] A deficiency of type II fibers has been reported.[127] Intramuscular and peripheral nerves are normal.

Clinical signs, observed between 2 and 6 months of age, are characterized by exercise and cold intolerance, symmetric wasting of proximal limb and masticatory muscles, stiff or stilted gait, and difficulty in maintaining the head in an erect position. A bunny hopping pelvic limb gait is frequently seen. Signs decrease with rest. The condition appears to be progressive with sporadic exacerbations of clinical signs, during which time CPK levels are elevated.

Variable occurrence of fibrillation potentials, positive sharp waves, and high frequency, bizarre waves of short duration (myotonic potentials) have been recorded with electrodiagnostic testing.

Diagnosis is based on signalment, clinical, and muscle biopsy data. Prognosis is poor. There is no treatment.

Canine Hypotrophic Myopathy

A subclinical myopathy has been reported in pectineus muscles of German shepherd dogs.[34, 36] Hypotrophy of the pectineus muscle is characterized by a retardation in muscle fiber growth, particularly of type II fibers. It has been suggested that hypotrophy of the pectineus muscle may potentially influence the development of the coxofemoral joint; however, additional studies have not substantiated the relationship between pectineal myopathy and subsequent development of hip dysplasia.[138] Indeed, hip dysplasia can still develop in dogs in which the pectineus muscle has been excised.

Congenital Myopathies in Lambs and Piglets

An autosomal recessive, congenital, progressive muscular dystrophy occurs in Merino sheep in Western Australia (McGavin).[35] Affected lambs have marked stiffness in the pelvic limbs, which is accentuated with exercise. The signs generally progress, but affected sheep may survive for years. There is a gross and histologic myopathy of the thigh, particularly the vastus intermedius muscles. The dystrophic lesion is grossly visible as atrophy and fatty replacement of muscle.

Certain Suffolk lambs in Britain with a congenital, degenerative, and necrotic myopathy of neck musculature showed difficulty in lifting the head and rigidity of the neck, with difficulty nursing.[155] Many lambs recovered spontaneously but those that succumbed often had marked flexion-contracture involving the limbs, particularly the thoracic limbs. Necrosis and fibrosis was present in neck musculature, especially the longissimus cervicis muscles. Fibrous contracture of neck musculature appeared to be associated with permanent deformity (wedge shape) of cervicothoracic vertebrae. The cause was not defined.

A few congenital myopathies occur in piglets, the most frequently seen being the asymmetric pelvic limb syndrome and congenital splayleg.[164] The latter causes difficulty in standing up; it is ascribed to myofibrillar hypoplasia and has been associated with *Fusarium* (F_2) mycotoxicosis.

Immune Mediated Disease

Masticatory Myositis

This inflammatory myopathy is the most commonly recognized myositis in dogs. Two forms of the disease are believed to occur:

Acute Form. Eosinophilic myositis is observed most commonly in adult German shepherd dogs.[219] This disease is characterized by recurrent inflammation of muscles, especially those of mastication (masseteric, temporalis, pterygoid), often in association with peripheral blood eosinophilia and the presence of eosinophils in muscle lesions. The etiopathogenesis is unknown. The suggestion that it represents an autoimmune disease remains unconfirmed.

Lesions consist of myonecrosis, hemorrhage, edema, and cellular infiltrates (macrophages, lymphocytes, plasma cells, occasionally neutrophils, and sometimes eosinophils). Clinical signs are characterized by acute onset of painful, swollen masticatory muscles. The jaw is held partially open (pseudotrismus), and passive manipulation is painful. Dogs are often febrile, and tonsils and mandibular lymph nodes may be swollen. The acute phase may last 2 to 3 weeks, with signs reaching a peak by 10 to 14 days. Serum CPK levels are elevated early in the disease and γ-globulin levels may be increased.

Diagnosis is based on signalment, clinical, and muscle biopsy data. Prognosis is guarded. The acute disease is usually responsive to glucocorticosteroids (eg, 0.5–1.0 mg/kg of prednisone twice daily). The dose is reduced after remission and gradually withdrawn using alternate day therapy. Repeated episodes, however, result in muscle atrophy.

Chronic Form. So-called atrophic myositis and cranial myodegeneration[220, 221] is characterized by atrophy of muscles of mastication (Fig. 14–22). This condition, the cause of which is unknown, usually occurs in dogs of any breed without an antecedent acute phase. There is no peripheral or local eosinophilia. The atrophy is accompanied by a state of trismus, which may not be reduced under general anesthesia and which may interfere with eating.

Pathologic studies reveal large numbers of atrophic fibers and increased amounts of perimysial connective tissue. Focal areas of lymphoplasmacytic infiltrates may be seen occasionally in masticatory and other skeletal muscles. Degenerative changes have been reported in terminal portions of the motor trigeminal nerve.

Prognosis of this form is also guarded because

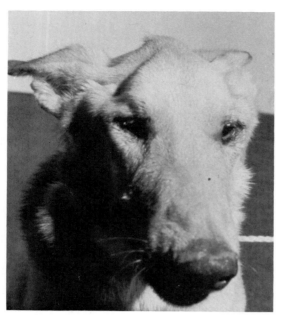

Figure 14–22. Atrophic myopathy in a dog. Note the generalized atrophy of the temporal and masseter muscles. (Courtesy of Dr IG Mayhew, University of Florida.)

of the severe trismus.[82] Spontaneous regression has been observed.

Polymyositis

Polymyositis is a relatively common myopathic disorder in dogs, the cause of which is unknown. It has been suggested that polymyositis, masticatory myositis, and other clinical variations such as pharyngeal-esophageal and focal appendicular myositis may represent different clinical and pathologic expressions of a single primary muscle inflammatory disease.[67] The predilection for masticatory muscles may be related to a difference in susceptibility of these muscles to immune or infectious processes. The muscles innervated by the mandibular branch of the trigeminal nerve have a predominance of type IIC myofibers and a variety of the type I myofiber. Most other muscles in the dog are composed primarily of type I and type IIA and, to a lesser extent, type IIC myofibers.[162]

The responsiveness of the disease to immunosuppressive therapy suggests that the pathogenesis is immune mediated. Histologic findings in skeletal muscle (appendicular and masticatory) are focal, multifocal, or diffuse myonecrosis, phagocytosis and lymphoplasmacytic cellular infiltrates, considerable fiber size variation, and areas of fiber regeneration. Deposition of immunoglobulin G on sarcolemmal membranes has been demonstrated.[126]

Clinical signs are variable and are usually observed in larger breed, mature adults of either sex. Onset of signs may be acute or chronic. Signs include weakness of gait with rapid fatigability, abnormalities of deglutition with esophageal dilation and inhalation pneumonia, shifting lameness or stiffness of gait, muscle swelling and pain, pyrexia, muscle atrophy, voice change, and depression.[4, 126, 185] Neurologic examination findings are normal. Early in the disease, serum CPK and aldolase levels may be elevated.

Electrodiagnostic changes include polyphasic motor unit potentials, positive sharp waves, and fibrillation potentials. Some dogs have hypergammaglobulinemia, positive antinuclear antibodies, and circulating antimuscle antibodies. Polymyositis has been reported in dogs with autoimmune diseases; namely, systemic lupus erythematosus[129] and primary lymphocytic thyroiditis.[67]

Prognosis is usually favorable provided severe damage has not occurred in esophageal and laryngeal muscles. Treatment is similar to that for masticatory myositis.

Metabolic or Toxic Disorders

Hyperadrenocortical Myopathy

An acquired degenerative myopathy has been reported in dogs in association with hyperadrenocorticism.[19, 79, 115] Hyperadrenocorticism (HAC) may be idiopathic or secondary to an anterior pituitary gland adenoma or an adrenal gland adenoma. The pathophysiologic basis for hyperadrenocortical myopathy is unknown, although the changes probably result from excessive circulating glucocorticoids, because identical muscle changes are observed in dogs receiving glucocorticosteroids.[18, 92]

Histologic findings are mild degenerative changes of fiber size variation, focal necrosis and fiber splitting, and fiber atrophy, especially of type II fibers. Fiber grouping may be present, and evidence of demyelination or remyelination has been noted in appendicular nerves.[19]

Clinical signs of hyperadrenocorticism include polydipsia, polyuria, alopecia, and pendulous abdomen. Myopathic signs are characterized by gradual development of a stiff or stilted gait, weakness, and muscular atrophy. Limb rigidity is not unusual.

Electromyographic studies reveal evidence of bizarre, high frequency discharges, often producing a "dive bomber" sound. Myotonic dimpling may also be elicited in some patients.

Diagnosis is based on clinicopathologic evidence of hyperadrenocorticism (plasma cortisol assay, ACTH response testing, dexamethasone suppression test), signalment (mature female poodles may be predisposed), clinical, and electrophysiologic findings.

Prognosis is guarded. Myopathic signs may abate following surgical or medical management of the hyperadrenocorticism.

Steroid Myopathy

This myopathy is associated with exogenous administration of glucocorticoids that results in iatrogenic hyperadrenocorticism. Clinical, electrophysiologic, and pathologic data are identical to those described for spontaneous hyperadrenocorticism.[18, 92]

Hypothyroid Myopathy

A subclinical myopathy has been reported in dogs with primary hypothyroidism.[17] The etiopathogenesis of this endocrine myopathy is unknown. A disturbance in carbohydrate metabolism has been proposed to explain the preferential type II fiber atrophy that occurs in human and canine muscle.[145, 146] Atrophic type II fibers are oval or angular in outline and are distributed throughout all muscle fascicles. A deficiency of type II fibers has been noted in some dogs. No cellular response or myodegeneration is seen, and intramuscular and peripheral nerves are normal. Myopathic changes are considerably more pronounced in muscles of hypothyroid dogs that have concomitant endocrinopathy, such as diabetes mellitus or hyperadrenocorticism.[20]

Bilaterally symmetric flank alopecia and obesity are often associated with the hypothyroidism. Weakness and reduced exercise tolerance in some dogs with chronic hypothyroidism may reflect an underlying myopathy. Electrodiagnostic findings are normal.

Reversal of the myopathy following thyroid hormone replacement has not been determined by clinical trials.

Hypothyroidism may be associated with muscle disease in horses.[214]

Exertional Myopathy

Exertional myopathy (exertional rhabdomyolysis) is a disease that affects many animal species, including humans. It is an important complication commonly arising in newly captured wild animals.[9] In domestic animals exertional myopathy occurs most frequently in racing greyhound dogs and in working and racing horses. It has been reported in a dog as a complication of prolonged convulsive seizures.[194] The pathogenesis is poorly understood. The contribution of stress is largely an unknown and unmeasurable factor inherent in capturing wild animals. In racing greyhounds severe acidosis leading to muscle cell swelling, local ischemia, muscle cell necrosis, and myoglobulinuria with nephropathy has been proposed as a likely sequence of events.[64, 90]

Pathologic findings in muscle include multifocal hemorrhage and myonecrosis.

Clinical signs generally occur during a race or trial and are characterized by extreme distress, hyperpnea, and generalized muscle pain especially over back and hindquarters. Myoglobinuria and death within 48 hours are common in severe, acute cases.

Prognosis depends on the severity of clinical signs. Dogs with hyperacute signs usually die within 48 hours from renal failure. Mortality rate is low in less severe cases that are treated with intravenous fluids, bicarbonate, anabolic steroids, antibiotics, cooling, and rest.

The disorder occurs in working and racing horses that have been resting and consuming a high energy diet and then are exerted.[214] This condition has been called equine paralytic myoglobinuria, azoturia, Monday morning disease, and tying up syndrome. Clinically, the horses develop a stiff gait and are reluctant to move. Muscles of the pectoral and pelvic girdles may be swollen, excessively firm, and tender. Pelvic limbs are often rigidly extended, and there is myoglobinuria. Signs may be as subtle as poor performance, but in severe cases recumbency and death are common.

In severe cases elevated serum muscle enzyme levels (CPK, aldolase, lactate dehydrogenase [LDH], aspartate aminotransferase [AST]) are confirmatory. In mild forms a provocative exercise test can be useful. A resting baseline serum CPK value is obtained, after which the horse is exercised (eg, 20 minutes of lunging). The serum CPK level is checked at 1 hour and 12 to 18 hours after exercise. An unfit horse may have an elevated 1 hour value, but normal and unfit (nonmyopathic) horses will have 12 to 18 hour serum CPK levels that have returned to about twice baseline. Horses with exercise induced rhabdomyolysis will have elevated 1 hour levels and (usually greatly) elevated 12 to 18 hour serum CPK levels.

The respective roles of genetic influences, carbohydrate loading, lactic acidosis, low vitamin E and selenium status, potassium depletion, and hypothyroid status in the etiopathogenesis have been considered.[214] Treatment consists of rest and correction of fluid, acid-base, and electrolyte disturbances. Sedation (eg, with acetylpromazine) and antiinflammatory therapy (eg, phenylbutazone) may be necessary, although glucocorticoid therapy may not be indicated. With continued exercise the condition may often recur.

Malignant Hyperthermia

Malignant hyperthermia is a paradoxic response to certain anesthetic drugs (eg, halothane and succinylcholine), in which muscle is stimulated sufficiently to produce a fatal hypermetabolic response, with a consequent rise in body temperature. Malignant hyperthermia is a rare but well-recognized condition in humans. Only isolated cases have been reported in dogs,[7] cat,[66] and foal.[125]

Malignant hyperthermia occurs most commonly in pigs (in which it is also known as porcine stress syndrome), usually as a result of a variety of different forms of stress, including transportation, fighting, hot weather, and restraint.[204] The disease in pigs is considered to be a valuable model for human malignant hyperthermia. Certain breeds are especially susceptible, including Pietrain, Poland China, and some lines of Landrace pigs. The disorder is a heritable defect in ability to maintain homeostasis so that stress causes excessive stimulation of β-adrenergic receptors with rapid depletion of adenosine triphosphate, rapid muscle glycolysis, and excessive production of muscle lactate. High levels of myoplasmic calcium are believed to initiate this sequence of events.[137]

Clinical signs are characterized by increased muscle tone, affecting the limbs and muscles of the chest particularly, decreasing compliance, and making pulmonary ventilation difficult. Death may occur quickly. Rigor mortis ensues within a few minutes. Postmortem examination may reveal muscle that is pale, soft, and exudative, or dark, firm, and dry.

A halothane test is now available to determine susceptibility in pigs,[80] and a similar test has been used to screen horses.[214]

Malignant hyperthermia in pigs is irreversible, and the prognosis is poor. Treatment with glucocorticoids, sodium bicarbonate, tranquilizers, intravenous fluids, dantrolene Na, and total body cooling is frequently disappointing.

Cassia occidentalis Toxicosis in Cattle

Cassia occidentalis (coffee senna) is a plant indigenous to the southeastern United States. It causes a myopathy in cattle that graze in pastures where it is present, as well as in cattle fed grain or hay contaminated with the plant.[148] The syndrome mimics nutritional (vitamin E–selenium deficiency) myopathy. Usually there is a sudden onset of recumbency, urine is dark, and there is extensive myodegeneration, particularly in the pelvic limbs. Treatment with vitamin E–selenium combination may exacerbate the condition.

Idiopathic Diseases

Idiopathic Feline Polymyopathy

A polymyopathy of unknown cause has been observed in mature cats usually over 1 year of age, without breed or sex predisposition. Histologic findings include myonecrosis, lymphocytic cellular infiltrates, internal nuclei, and fiber degeneration.[5] Clinical signs are characterized by a persistent ventroflexion of the neck, appendicular weakness especially in the thoracic limbs, painful muscles, and exercise intolerance. Serum CPK and aldolase levels are elevated. Electromyography reveals fibrillation potentials, positive sharp waves, and bizarre, high frequency waves.

Prognosis is guarded. Some cats may recover spontaneously, whereas others appear to respond to glucocorticosteroids. Recurrences have been observed.

Immobilization Myopathy

A myopathy in the quadriceps muscle has been reported in dogs following treatment of femoral fractures by limb immobilization in hyperextension for 3 to 7 weeks.[26] The pathogenesis is not well understood. It has been proposed that joint stiffness occurs as a result of fibrous adhesions in and around the stifle while it is maintained in an extended position. Immobilization of muscle induces muscle atrophy. This change is especially influenced by the degree of stretch in which the muscle is held.

Subsequently, the quardriceps muscle group, held in a shortened state, is believed to undergo selective and progressive atrophy.

Pathologic findings in vastus lateralis muscle include fiber size variability, increased perimysial fibrosis and focal necrosis, and pronounced type I fiber atrophy.

The clinical syndrome is characterized by limb hyperextension, generalized muscle atrophy of the affected limb, abducted gait, and limited range of joint motion.

Prognosis is guarded. Breakdown and removal of adhesions by surgical management may result in a return of function of the femorotibial joint and reversibility of the type I fiber atrophy.[186]

Similar clinical signs are seen in dogs and foals with congenital limb contractures.[105, 199]

Infections

Toxoplasma Myositis

This is probably the most commonly reported infectious myositis in small animals, even though the incidence is low.[6, 71, 106, 112, 154] The disease in dogs tends to be more severe in the young. The exact pathogenesis of toxoplasmosis is speculative. Although the predilection for the neuromuscular system is accepted, its myotropism in congenital and chronic infections remains enigmatic. Exacerbations of disease may reflect depression of immune mechanisms. Histologic changes are variation in fiber size as a result of pronounced fiber atrophy, severe multifocal or diffuse myonecrosis, and mononuclear granulomatous inflammation. Free toxoplasma organisms are frequently seen within muscle fibers. Interstitial fibrosis is pronounced in chronic cases.

Toxoplasma myositis results in progressive pelvic limb paresis, synchronous hopping gait, and bilateral rigidity of the pelvic limb extensor muscles (Fig. 14–23). These muscles are nonpainful on palpation and slowly become atrophic. A fulminating disease resulting in tetraplegia within 1 week has been observed in two mature dogs (4 to 5 years of age). Extremely severe myonecrosis and mononuclear cell infiltrations were found in all skeletal muscles. Toxoplasma organisms were identified in muscle and CNS.[21]

Diagnosis is based on clinical data, positive serologic evidence, and on histologic demonstration of the organism in lesions from muscle biopsy samples.

Prognosis is poor when signs of pelvic limb spasticity are observed. Furthermore, many affected animals have concomitant lesions in the central nervous system. Sulfadiazine and pyrimethamine have been used to treat systemic toxoplasmosis.

Clostridial Myositis

True blackleg, or *Clostridium chauvoei* polymyositis, is most common in cattle. Infection

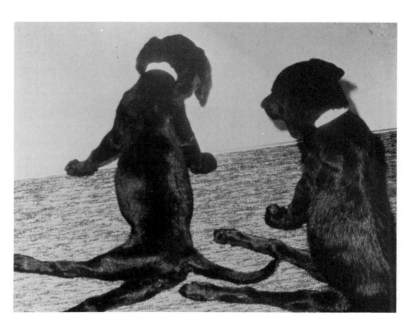

Figure 14–23. Stiff stifle syndrome associated with toxoplasmosis in a litter of puppies.

with other clostridial species, including *C. septicum* and *C. novyi*, can mimic the disease; sheep, and less often horses and other species, can be affected.[15] An episode of muscle damage may promote the growth of the anaerobic organisms, although this may not be necessary in true blackleg in cattle. Exotoxins are produced, and subsequent toxemia often results in death.

Penicillin therapy and débridement of necrotic tissue is indicated. Effective toxoid vaccines are available.

Trauma

Myositis Ossificans

Myositis ossificans is a rare myopathic disorder of animals that is characterized by heterotopic ossification of skeletal muscle and other soft tissues. Local and generalized forms of this disease have been reported in dogs, cats, and pigs.[135, 156, 188] The etiopathogenesis is uncertain. Trauma is often associated with localized myositis ossificans, but it is not a prerequisite. The generalized form in people is suggested to be congenital or hereditary in nature.

Histopathologic lesions vary from mild interstitial fibrosis to complete replacement of muscle by fibrous tissue and heterotopic bone. Clinical signs are variable and include progressive weakness, stiffness, and palpable firm enlargements in affected muscles.

Radiographic studies reveal multiple radiopacities of irregular linear calcification. Prognosis is poor. There is no treatment.

Fibrotic Myopathy

A chronic progressive disorder has been reported in adult working horses[2] and in German shepherd dogs (mainly male, with an age range from 2 to 7 years).[151, 211] The cause of the condition is unknown. Excessive exercise over a long period resulting in tearing and stretching of muscle fibers has been proposed as a causative factor.[211] In dogs the condition is associated with a palpable, thin, fibrous band that extends from the tuber ischii to the tibia within the belly of the semitendinosus muscle. Lameness is observed in the affected limb, resulting from failure to fully extend the limb. In horses, the affected limb is pulled down before the end of the protraction phase of stride, such that the foot is slapped to the ground. Histologically the band consists of an abundance of dense collagenous connective tissue, with a distinct interface between connective tissue and muscle bundles.

Prognosis is poor, as the condition tends to recur within 3 to 8 months following surgical resection of the fibrous band.

Similar fibrous bands have been observed in gracilis and quadriceps muscles in dogs[211] and in semitendinosus, semimembranosus, gracilis, and biceps muscles in horses.[2, 11]

Downer Cow Myopathy

Following primary recumbency in adult cattle, associated with numerous traumatic, metabolic, toxic, nutritional, infectious, and other causes, a secondary stage of recumbency frequently ensues. Ischemic necrosis and inflammation of caudal thigh muscles and the sciatic nerve result from pressure damage, which is akin to the compartment syndrome in humans. Struggling in terminal stages of recumbency frequently results in rupture and crushing of muscles and ligaments.[48] A similar syndrome has been reproduced in cattle with anesthetic induced recumbency of 6 to 12 hours duration.[50] Systemic signs and clinicopathologic findings reflect the profound myonecrosis and enforced recumbency.

Early treatment of underlying perturbations and intensive nursing care are required for successful therapy of affected cattle.

Nutritional Diseases

Vitamin E–Selenium Responsive Myopathy

Vitamin E–selenium responsive myopathies have been reported in sheep, cattle, pigs, horses, poultry, and only rarely dogs.[122, 142, 147] The condition is also known as white muscle disease, stiff lamb disease (because of its prevalence in lambs), nutritional myopathy, and selenium responsive myopathy. This myopathy is associated with low dietary levels of selenium, vitamin E, or both, and sometimes the presence of nutritional oxidants. The pathogenesis of the disorder is unknown. Skeletal muscle lesions tend to be bilaterally symmetric and may affect individual or several muscle groups. Grossly, the affected muscle is paler than normal and may show distinct chalky longitudinal striations. Histologic findings are characterized by necrosis, phagocytosis, proliferation of sarcolemmal nuclei, loss of striation, and fiber regeneration.

Clinical signs include acute death, weakness, dysphagia, sialosis, dysphonia, tachypnea, stiff stilted gait, and difficulty in rising from a recumbent position. Signs may be exacerbated with exercise.

The precise syndrome depends on which muscle groups are affected. Additionally, in foals there is a component of fat necrosis, hemorrhage, and edema of subcutaneous tissues and fat.[15] Resulting swelling and pain are often present about the head, neck, and perineum. Severe cellulitis and myonecrosis can involve the muscles of the head, resulting in dysphagia in horses and foals. In all cases possible involvement of cardiac musculature should be considered because of the potential for sudden death.

Elevated serum muscle enzyme activity and myopathic changes on needle electromyography are most frequently used to confirm a diagnosis of myopathy. Muscle biopsy from affected sites, as well as serum vitamin E and selenium assay in affected animals, herd or litter mates, and control animals, can confirm the diagnosis.

Mildly affected animals can respond dramatically to administration of parenteral vitamin E and selenium. Supplementation of the diet with these nutritional components is indicated.

Degenerative Conditions

Paraneoplastic Neuromyopathy. Skeletal muscle changes in dogs with systemic neoplasia are described under Neuropathies.

Vascular Disorders

Ischemic Neuromyopathy. Skeletal muscle changes in cats and horses with ischemic neuromyopathy resulting from aortic thromboemboli are described under Neuropathies.

Postanesthetic Neuromyopathy

Following long periods of general anesthesia, particularly on hard surfaces, some horses exhibit signs of localized or generalized neuromuscular deficiency.[218] Various syndromes can be related to one muscle group (eg, triceps, gluteal, quadriceps femoris), one peripheral nerve (eg, radial, sciatic), mixtures of muscle groups and peripheral nerves, or generalized signs. The animal is weak, and affected muscles may be swollen and hard or may be flaccid, perhaps reflecting myopathy versus neuropathy, respectively. Areas of skin hypalgesia may be detected.

Serum muscle enzyme activities are elevated, and myoglobinuria may be present.

Primarily type II muscle cell degeneration, followed by frank myonecrosis, is present and likely represents pressure effects and blood flow alterations (ischemia), as in the compartment syndrome in humans and the downer cow myopathy.[50, 218] The presence of at least ischemic neurapraxia is assumed from some of the clinical syndromes.

Horses often recover completely, but some have residual muscle atrophy, and a few exhibit massive areas of ischemic myonecrosis and interfascicular nerve fiber degeneration at postmortem examination.

Therapy is essentially as for nutritional rhabdomyolysis. Short recumbency times, adequate padding, maintenance of good cardiovascular function, and manipulation of limbs, all during anesthesia, may help prevent the syndrome. The use of dantrolene Na as a preanesthetic prophylactic measure is suggested.[218]

JUNCTIONOPATHIES

Certain disorders of the neuromuscular junction (junctionopathies) (Table 14–5), namely, botulism and tick paralysis, will produce signs that mimic those observed in a diffuse peripheral neuropathy. In contrast, the clinical syndrome of myasthenia gravis, another junctionopathy, is similar to that of a diffuse myopathic disorder and is characterized by episodic weakness. Electrodiagnostic testing and nerve and muscle biopsies will help to differentiate junctionopathies from polyneuropathies and primary myopathies.

Table 14–5. CLASSIFICATION OF JUNCTIONOPATHIES

Congenital or Hereditary
Congenital myasthenia gravis*

Immune Mediated
Acquired myasthenia gravis*

Metabolic or Toxic
Botulism
Aminoglycosides
Tetracyclines
Hypocalcemia
Hypercalcemia

*Treatment schedules:
  Tensilon (edrophonium): 0.5–5 mg IV (adults); 0.1–0.5 mg IV (puppies)
  Mestinon (pyridostigmine): 30–60 mg orally bid or tid (adults); 7.5 mg orally sid (puppies).

Botulism

The most common cause of botulism is the ingestion of spoiled food or carrion containing a preformed exotoxin produced by *Clostridium botulinum*. The toxin blocks release of acetylcholine from neuromuscular junctions and cholinergic autonomic synapses.[121] Onset of clinical signs is from hours to several days following ingestion of toxin. Clinical signs reflect a progressive, symmetric, generalized ascending lower motor neuron disorder, ranging from mild weakness to severe flaccid tetraplegia with absent spinal reflexes and evidence of weakness in muscles of the face, jaw, pharynx, and esophagus. Early in the course of the disease or in mildly affected dogs, the gait may be stiff and pelvic limbs may be used in a synchronous fashion (bunny hopping). Large animals frequently tremble or shake violently prior to becoming recumbent.

Electrodiagnostic studies may reveal a reduction in amplitude of evoked potentials and motor unit potentials, normal or decreased nerve conduction velocities, but no denervation potentials.

The differential diagnosis includes tick paralysis, polyradiculoneuritis, and other polyneuropathies. Diagnosis is suggested by historical, clinical, and electrodiagnostic data. It is confirmed by identification of the toxin by neutralization with type specific antitoxin in the material ingested or in serum, feces, or vomitus of an affected animal.[8]

The prognosis is usually favorable in dogs but poor in large animals. Treatment is primarily supportive. Severely affected animals should be monitored closely to avoid the potential complications of decubitus, inhalation pneumonia, and respiratory paralysis. Type specific antisera are expensive and not readily available. The toxin associated with canine disease has been reported to be type C.[8, 13, 63, 172] Types C, E, and particularly B are associated with the disease in horses.[144]

Toxicoinfectious botulism is probably the etiology of "shaker foal syndrome." The toxin is elaborated by *Cl. botulinum* organisms in necrotic tissue of wounds, abscesses of the liver, or the gastrointestinal tract. Rapidly growing foals, 2 to 4 weeks of age, are affected and exhibit a stilted gait, muscle tremors, dysphagia, and the inability to stand for more than a few minutes. The foals also experience constipation, mydriasis, frequent urination, and nasal reflux of milk.[144] The mortality rate is high, although use of antiserum has greatly improved the outlook.

Myasthenia Gravis

In animals, two forms of myasthenia gravis occur: an acquired and a congenital form. Acquired myasthenia gravis is an uncommon disorder characterized by failure of neuromuscular transmission that has been most frequently observed in large breeds of dogs, especially German shepherds, with an average age of onset of 5 years.[166, 183] The condition has been reported in cats.[65, 143] There is no sex predominance. Acquired canine myasthenia gravis is an immune mediated disease caused by production of antibodies directed against acetylcholine receptors of the neuromuscular junction. Reactive antibodies are demonstrable in the sera of 90% of dogs with acquired myasthenia gravis,[132] and immune complexes have been localized at the neuromuscular junction.[168, 170] A deficiency of functional acetylcholine receptors at the neuromuscular junction reduces the sensitivity of the postsynaptic membrane to the transmitter, acetylcholine.

Acquired myasthenia gravis in dogs has also been associated with mediastinal tumors,[166] and in one such case antibodies reactive with muscle striations coexisted with a high titer of autoantibodies to acetylcholine receptor.[132]

Clinical signs are characterized by progressive muscular weakness with exercise. The thoracic limbs are predominantly affected, and the stride becomes progressively shorter. Facial features may droop. The animal may have difficulty in closing its mouth and holding up its head, and the bark may have a high pitch. Dysphagia and regurgitation are common. Most affected dogs have intrathoracic megaesophagus, which can be detected by radiography. Signs are exacerbated by exposure to cold.[165]

Diagnosis is based on clinical signs, electrodiagnostic evidence of decremental response of muscle action potentials after repeated nerve stimulation, serologic testing for autoantibodies, and amelioration of signs following administration of the short acting anticholinesterase edrophonium (Tensilon).

Prognosis is guarded. One potential complication is inhalation pneumonia. Long acting anticholinesterase drugs such as pyridostigmine (Mestinon) may result in clinical control. Overdosage will produce a cholinergic crisis with signs similar to those of undertreatment. Some dogs may recover spontaneously, whereas others become refractory to anticholinesterase therapy after a period of successful treatment. Corticosteroids have been used successfully in people. Anticholinesterase dosage schedules are given in Table 14–5.

Congenital myasthenia gravis occurs in young dogs, usually appearing between the ages of 6 and 9 weeks, with multiple cases in a single litter. Congenital myasthenia gravis has been described in three breeds: Jack Russell terrier,[167] springer spaniel,[119] and smooth fox terrier.[118, 149] Breeding studies suggest that congenital myasthenia gravis is inherited as an autosomal recessive trait.

The physiologic basis of congenital myasthenia gravis is the same as that of the acquired form; however, antiacetylcholine receptor antibodies are not demonstrable in serum or muscle in congenital disease. There appears to be an absolute deficiency of acetylcholine receptors in the postsynaptic membrane.[132, 149]

Clinical signs, electrophysiologic findings, prognosis, and treatment of animals with acquired and congenital myasthenia gravis are similar.

A postanesthetic myasthenic syndrome is reported in three horses.[144] The syndrome was identical to botulism. However, all three horses recovered in a short period, and the possibility of a combination drug induced myasthenia was proposed.

Tick Paralysis

This is a flaccid, afebrile ascending motor paralysis that occurs in domestic and wild animals and humans and is produced by a neurotoxin generated by some but not all strains of certain species of ticks. Not all infested animals become paralyzed. The common wood tick, *Dermacentor variabilis*, and *Dermacentor andersonii* are incriminated most often in the United States, whereas in Australia, *Ixodes holocyclus* is usually responsible. Adult ticks, especially female, produce a salivary neurotoxin that circulates in the host animal and interferes with acetylcholine liberation at the neuromuscular junction.

Onset of clinical signs is gradual, paralysis first becoming evident as an incoordination in the pelvic limbs resulting in an unsteady gait. Altered voice, cough, and dysphagia may be early signs. Dogs become recumbent in 24 to 72 hours. Reflexes are lost, but sensation is preserved. Jaw muscle weakness and facial paresis may be present. Death may occur in several days from respiratory paralysis.

Electromyographic studies reveal absence of spontaneous potentials and lack of motor unit action potentials. No muscle response follows direct nerve stimulation. Nerve conduction velocity may be slower than normal.[39]

Prognosis is usually good, with recovery occurring in 1 to 3 days following tick removal or dipping the animal in an insecticide solution. In Australia, a hyperimmune serum is used to treat humans and dogs affected with paralysis caused by *Ixodes holocyclus*. The prognosis for this form of tick paralysis is guarded even with tick removal, insecticide application, and treatment with hyperimmune serum.

REFERENCES

1. Adams LG, Dolahite JW, Romane WM, et al: Cystitis and ataxia associated with sorghum ingestion by horses. JAVMA 155:518, 1969.
2. Adams OR: Lameness in Horses, 3rd ed. Philadelphia, Lea & Febiger, 1974, p. 320.
3. Alexander JW, deLahunta A, and Scott DW: A case of brachial plexus neuropathy in a dog. J Am Anim Hosp Assoc 10:515, 1974.
4. Averill DR: Diseases of the muscle. Vet Clin North Am 10:223, 1980.
5. Averill DR: The nervous system. In Holzworth J (ed): Diseases of the Cat. Philadelphia, WB Saunders Co, 1986.
6. Averill DR and deLahunta A: Toxoplasmosis of the canine nervous system: Clinicopathological findings in four cases. JAVMA 159:1134, 1971.
7. Bagshaw RJ, Cox RH, Knight DH, and Detweiler DK: Malignant hyperthermia in a greyhound. JAVMA 172:61, 1978.
8. Barsanti JA, Walser M, Hatheway CL, et al.: Type C botulism in American foxhounds. JAVMA 172:809, 1978.
9. Bartsch RC, McConnell EE, Imes GD, and Schmidt JM: A review of exertional rhabdomyolysis in wild and domestic animals and man. Vet Pathol 14:314, 1977.
10. Bennett D and Vaughan LC: The use of muscle relocation techniques in the treatment of peripheral nerve injuries in dogs and cats. J Small Anim Pract 17:99, 1976.
11. Bishop R: Fibrotic myopathy in the gracilis muscle of a horse. Vet Med Small Anim Clin 67:270, 1972.
12. Blakemore W: Personal communications, 1983.
13. Blakemore WF, Rees-Evans ET, and Wheeler PEG: Botulism in foxhounds. Vet Rec 100:57, 1977.
14. Blood DC, Henderson JA, and Radostits OM: Veterinary Medicine, 5th ed. Philadelphia, Lea & Febiger, 1979.
15. Blythe LL, Watrous BJ, Schmitz JA, and Kaneps AJ: Vestibular syndrome associated with temporohyoid joint fusion and temporal bone fracture in three horses. JAVMA 185:775, 1984.
16. Bowman KF, Vaughan JT, Quick CB, et al: Megaesophagus in a colt. JAVMA 172:334, 1978
17. Braund KG, Dillon AR, August JR, and Ganjam VK: Hypothyroid myopathy in two dogs. Vet Pathol 18:589, 1981.
18. Braund KG, Dillon AR, and Mikeal RL: Experimental investigation of glucocorticoid-induced myopathy in the dog. Exp Neurol 68:50, 1980.
19. Braund KG, Dillon AR, Mikeal RL, and August JR: Subclinical myopathy associated with hyperadrenocorticism in the dog. Vet Pathol 17:134, 1980.
20. Braund KG, Dillon AR, Pidgeon GL, and August JR:

Neuromuscular changes in dogs with spontaneous diabetes mellitus. Scientific Proceedings, Am Coll Vet Intern Med, 1981.

21. Braund KG, and Hoff MJ: Unpublished data, 1981.

22. Braund KG, Hoff EJ, and Richardson KEY: Histochemical identification of fiber types in canine skeletal muscle. Am J Vet Res 39:561, 1978.

23. Braund KG and Lincoln CE: Histochemical differentiation of fiber types in neonatal canine skeletal muscle. Am J Vet Res 42:407, 1981.

24. Braund KG, Luttgen PJ, Redding RW, and Rump RF: Distal symmetrical polyneuropathy in a dog. Vet Pathol 17:422, 1980.

25. Braund KG, Luttgen PJ, Sorjonen DC, and Redding RW: Idiopathic facial paralysis in the dog. Vet Rec 105:297, 1979.

26. Braund KG, Shires PK, and Mikeal RL: Type 1 fiber atrophy in the vastus lateralis muscle in dogs with femoral fractures treated by hyperextension. Vet Pathol 17:164, 1980.

27. Braund KG and Steiss JE: Distal neuropathy in spontaneous diabetes mellitus in the dog. Acta Neuropathol 57:263, 1982.

28. Braund KG, Walker TL, and Vandevelde M: Fascicular nerve biopsy in the dog. Am J Vet Res 40:1025, 1979.

29. Bright RM, Crabtree BJ, and Knecht CD: Brachial plexus neuropathy in the cat: A case report. J Am Anim Hosp Assoc 14:612, 1978.

30. Bryant SH: Altered membrane properties in myotonia. In Bolis L, Hoffman FJ, and Leaf A (ed): Membranes and Diseases. New York, Raven Press, 1976, p 197.

31. Bryant SH: Myotonia in the goat. Ann NY Acad Sci 317:314, 1979.

32. Buck WB: Physical and chemical disorders. In Howard JL (ed): Current Veterinary Therapy: Food Animal Practice. Philadelphia, WB Saunders Co, 1981.

33. Butler HC: An investigation into the relationship of an aortic embolus to posterior paralysis in the cat. J Small Anim Pract 12:141, 1971.

34. Cardinet GH, Fedde MR, and Tunell GL: Correlates of histochemical and physiologic properties in normal and hypertrophic pectineus muscles of the dog. Lab Invest 27:32, 1972.

35. Cardinet GH and Holliday TA: Neuromuscular diseases of domestic animals: A summary of muscle biopsies from 159 cases. Ann NY Acad Sci 317:290, 1979.

36. Cardinet GH, Wallace LJ, Fedde MR, et al: Developmental myopathy in the canine. Arch Neurol 21:620, 1969.

37. Carmichael S and Griffiths IR: Case of isolated sensory trigeminal neuropathy in a dog. Vet Rec 109:280, 1981.

38. Cheli R: Su di una particolare sindrome nervosa del suino (oto-encefalite). La Clinica Vet 92:76, 1969.

39. Chrisman CL: Differentiation of tick paralysis and acute idiopathic polyradiculoneuritis in the dog using electromyography. J Am Anim Hosp Assoc 11:455, 1975.

40. Clements RS: Diabetic neuropathy—new concepts of its etiology. Diabetes 28:604, 1979.

41. Clifford DH, Barboza PFT, and Pirsch JG: The motor nuclei of the vagus nerve in cats with and without congenital achalasia of the oesophagus. Br Vet J 136:74, 1980.

42. Clifford DH, Lee MO, Lee DC, and Ross JN: Clas-

sification of congenital neuromuscular dysfunction of the canine esophagus. J Am Vet Radiol Soc 17:98, 1976.

43. Clifford DH, Pirsch JG, and Mauldin ML: Comparison of motor nuclei of the vagus nerve in dogs with and without esophageal achalasia. Proc Soc Exp Biol Med 142:878, 1973.

44. Clifford DH, Soifer FK, Wilson MD, and Guillord GL: Congenital achalasia of the esophagus in 4 cats of common ancestry. JAVMA 158:1554, 1971.

45. Clifford DH, Waddell ED, Patterson DR, et al: Management of esophageal achalasia in miniature schnauzers. JAVMA 161:1012, 1972.

46. Cole CR: Changes in the equine larynx associated with laryngeal hemiplegia. Am J Vet Res 7:69, 1946.

47. Cook WR: The diagnosis of respiratory unsoundness in the horse. Vet Rec 77:516, 1965.

48. Cox VS: Understanding the downer cow syndrome. Comp Cont Ed Pract Vet 3:S472, 1981.

49. Cox VS, Breazile JE, and Hoover TR: Surgical and anatomic study of calving paralysis. Am J Vet Res 36:427, 1975.

50. Cox VS, McGrath CJ, and Jorgensen SE: The role of pressure damage in pathogenesis of the downer cow syndrome. Am J Vet Res 43:26, 1982.

51. Cox VS, Wallace LJ, Anderson VE, and Rushmer RA: Hereditary esophageal dysfunction in the miniature schnauzer dog. Am J Vet Res 41:326, 1980.

52. Cummings JF: Personal communications, 1983.

53. Cummings JF, Cooper BJ, deLahunta A, and van Winkle TJ: Canine inherited hypertrophic neuropathy. Acta Neuropathol 53:137, 1981.

54. Cummings JF and deLahunta A: Chronic relapsing polyradiculoneuritis in a dog. A clinical, light- and electron-microscopic study. Acta Neuropathol 28:191, 1974.

55. Cummings JF, de Lahunta A, Braund KG, and Mitchell WJ: Animal model of human disease: Hereditary sensory neuropathy: Nociceptive loss and acral mutilation in pointer dogs: Canine hereditary sensory neuropathy. Am J Pathol 112:136, 1983.

56. Cummings JF, de Lahunta A, Holmes DF, and Schultz RD: Coonhound paralysis. Further clinical studies and electron microscopic observations. Acta Neuropathol 56:167, 1982.

57. Cummings JF, deLahunta A, and Mitchell WJ: Ganglioradiculitis in the dog: A clinical, light- and electron-microscopic study. Acta Neuropathol 60:29, 1983.

58. Cummings JF, deLahunta A, and Timoney JF: Neuritis of the cauda equina, a chronic idiopathic polyradiculoneuritis in the horse. Acta Neuropathol 46:17, 1979.

59. Cummings JF, deLahunta A, and Winn SS: Acral mutilation and nociceptive loss in English pointer dogs. A canine sensory neuropathy. Acta Neuropathol 53:119, 1981.

60. Cummings JF and Haas DC: Coonhound paralysis. An acute idiopathic polyradiculoneuritis in dogs resembling the Landry-Guillain-Barré syndrome. J Neurol Sci 4:51, 1967.

61. Cummings JF, Lorenz MD, deLahunta A, and Washington LD: Canine brachial plexus neuritis: A syndrome resembling serum neuritis in man. Cornel Vet 63:589, 1973.

62. Dahme E, and Deutschlander N: Die neuritis der Cauda equina beim Pferde in electronmikroskopischen Bild. Beitrag zur weiteren Klarung der Pathogenese. Zentralbl Veterinarmed (A) 23:502, 1976.

63. Darke PGG, Roberts TA, Smart JL, and Bradshaw PR: Suspected botulism in foxhounds. Vet Rec 99:98, 1976.

64. Davis PE and Paris R: Azoturia in a greyhound: Clinical pathology aids to diagnosis. J Small Anim Pract 15:43, 1974.

65. Dawson JR: Myasthenia gravis in a cat. Vet Rec 86:562, 1970.

66. De Jong RH, Heavner JE, and Amory DM: Malignant hyperpyrexia in the cat. Anesthesiology 41:608, 1974.

67. deLahunta A: Veterinary Neuroanatomy and Clinical Neurology, 2nd ed. Philadelphia, WB Saunders Co, 1983.

68. Diamant N, Szczepanski M, and Mui H: Idiopathic megaesophagus in the dog: Reasons for spontaneous improvement and a possible method of medical therapy. Can Vet J 15:66, 1974.

69. Dillon AR and Braund KG: Distal polyneuropathy after canine heartworm disease therapy complicated by disseminated intravascular coagulation. JAVMA 181:239, 1982.

70. Dodd DC: Nutritional myopathy. In Mansmann RAB, McAllister ES, and Platt PW (ed): Equine Medicine and Surgery, 3rd ed. Santa Barbara, CA, American Veterinary Publications, 1982.

71. Drake JC and Hime JM: Two syndromes in young dogs caused by Toxoplasma gondii. J Small Anim Pract 8:621, 1967.

72. Duncan ID and Griffiths IR: Canine giant axonal neuropathy. Vet Rec 101:438, 1977.

73. Duncan ID and Griffiths IR: Peripheral nervous system in a case of canine giant axonal neuropathy. Neuropathol Appl Neurobiol 5:25, 1979.

74. Duncan ID and Griffiths IR: Canine giant axonal neuropathy; some aspects of its clinical, pathological and comparative features. J Small Anim Pract 22:491, 1981.

75. Duncan ID, Griffiths IR, Carmichael S, and Henderson S: Inherited canine giant axonal neuropathy. Muscle Nerve 4:223, 1981.

76. Duncan ID, Griffiths IR, and McQueen A: A myopathy associated with myotonia in the dog. Acta Neuropathol 31:297, 1975.

77. Duncan ID, Griffiths IR, McQueen A, and Baker GO: The pathology of equine laryngeal hemiplegia. Acta Neuropathol 27:337, 1974.

78. Duncan ID, Griffiths IR, and Munz M: The pathology of a sensory neuropathy affecting long haired dachshund dogs. Acta Neuropathol 58:141, 1982.

79. Duncan ID, Griffiths IR, and Nash AS: Myotonia in canine Cushing's disease. Vet Rec 100:30, 1977.

80. Eikelenboom G and Minkema D: Prediction of pale soft and exudative muscle with a non-lethal test for the halothane-induced porcine malignant hyperthermia syndrome. Neth J Vet Sci 99:421, 1974.

81. Fankhauser R, Gerber H, Cravero GC, and Straub R: Klinik und Pathologie der Neuritis caudae equinae (NCE) des Pferds. Schweiz Arch Tierheilkd 117:675, 1975.

82. Farnbach GC: Myositis in the dog. Comp Cont Ed Pract Vet 1:183, 1979.

83. Farrow BRH: Personal communications, 1982.

84. Farrow BRH and Malik R: Hereditary myotonia in the chow chow. J Small Anim Pract 22:451, 1981.

85. Feldman EC and Tyrrell JB: Hypoadrenocorticism. Vet Clin North Am 7:555, 1977.

86. Firth EC: Vestibular disease and its relationship to facial nerve paralysis in the horse: A clinical study of 7 cases. Aust Vet J 53:560, 1977.

87. Flecknell PA and Lucke VM: Chronic relapsing polyradiculoneuritis in a cat. Acta Neuropathol 41:81, 1978.

88. Freeman D and Donawick W: Occlusion of the internal carotid artery in the horse by means of a balloon-tipped catheter: Evaluation of a method designed to prevent epistaxis caused by guttural pouch mycosis. JAVMA 176:232, 1980.

89. Fregin GF: Aortoiliac occlusive disease. In Mansmann RA, MacAllister ES, and Pratt PW (ed): Equine Medicine and Surgery, 3rd ed. Santa Barbara, CA American Veterinary Publications, 1982, p 685.

90. Gannon JR: Exertional rhabdomyolysis (myoglobinuria) in the racing greyhound. In Kirk RW: Current Veterinary Therapy VIII. Philadelphia, WB Saunders Co, 1983.

91. Gray GW: Acute experiments on neuroeffector and function in canine esophageal achalasia. Am J Vet Res 35:1075, 1974.

92. Greene CE, Lorenz MD, Munnell JF, et al: Myopathy associated with hyperadrenocorticism in the dog. JAVMA 174:1310, 1979.

93. Greenwood AG, Barker J and McLeish I: Neuritis of the cauda equina in a horse. Equine Vet J 5:111, 1973.

94. Griffiths IR: Avulsion of the brachial plexus—1. Neuropathology of the spinal cord and peripheral nerves. J Small Anim Pract 15:165, 1974.

95. Griffiths IR and Duncan ID: Myotonia in the dog: A report of four cases. Vet Rec 93:184, 1973.

96. Griffiths IR and Duncan ID: The central nervous system in canine giant axonal neuropathy. Acta Neuropathol 46:169, 1979.

97. Griffiths IR and Duncan ID: Distal denervating disease: A degenerative neuropathy of the distal motor axon in dogs. J Small Anim Pract 20:579, 1979.

98. Griffiths IR and Duncan ID: Ischaemic neuromyopathy in cats. Vet Rec 104:518, 1979.

99. Griffiths IR, Duncan ID, and Barker J: A progressive axonopathy of boxer dogs affecting the central and peripheral nervous systems. J Small Anim Pract 21:29, 1980.

100. Griffiths IR, Duncan ID, and Lawson DD: Avulsion of the brachial plexus—2. Clinical aspects. J Small Anim Pract 15:177, 1974.

101. Griffiths IR, Duncan ID, McCulloch M, and Carmichael S: Further studies of the central nervous system in canine giant axonal neuropathy. Neuropathol Appl Neurobiol 6:421, 1980.

102. Griffiths IR, Duncan ID, and Swallow JS: Peripheral neuropathies in dogs: A study of five cases. J Small Anim Pract 18:101, 1977.

103. Griffiths IR, Nash AS, and Sharp NJH: The Key-Gaskell syndrome: The current situation. Vet Rec 111:532, 1982.

104. Gunn HM: Histochemical observations on laryngeal skeletal muscle in "normal" horses. Equine Vet J 4:144, 1972.

105. Gunn HM: Morphological aspects of the deep digital flexor muscle in horses having rigid flexion of their distal forelimb joints at birth. Irish Vet J 30:145, 1976.

106. Hartley WJ, Lindsay AB, and MacKinnon MM: Toxoplasma meningo-encephalomyelitis and myositis in a dog. NZ Vet J 6:124, 1958.

107. Harvey CE and O'Brien JA: Management of respira-

tory emergencies in small animals. Vet Clin North Am 2:243, 1972.

108. Harvey CE, O'Brien JA, Durie VR, et al.: Megaesophagus in the dog: A clinical survey of 79 cases. JAVMA 165:443, 1974.

109. Harvey CE and Venker-van Haagen AJ: Surgical management of pharyngeal and laryngeal airway obstruction in the dog. Vet Clin North Am 5:515, 1975.

110. Haynes PF: Surgery of the equine respiratory tract. In Jennings PB (ed): The Practice of Large Animal Surgery. Philadelphia, WB Saunders Co, 1984.

111. Higgs B, Kerr FWL, and Ellis FH: The experimental production of esophageal achalasia by electrolytic lesions in the medulla. J Thorac Cardiovasc Surg 50:613, 1965.

112. Holliday TA, Olander HJ, and Wind AP: Skeletal muscle atrophy associated with toxoplasmosis, a case report. Cornell Vet 53:288, 1963.

113. Holmes DF and deLahunta A: Experimental allergic neuritis in the dog and its comparison with the naturally occurring disease; coonhound paralysis. Acta Neuropathol 30:329, 1974.

114. Holmes DF, Schultz RD, Cummings JF, and deLahunta A: Experimental coonhound paralysis: Animal model of Guillain-Barré syndrome. Neurology 29:1186, 1979.

115. Hoskins JD, Nafe LA, and Cho DY: Myopathy associated with hyperadrenocorticism in a dog: A case report. Vet Med Small Anim Clin 77:760, 1982.

116. Hudson LC: The origins of innervation of the esophagus and the caudal pharyngeal muscles with histochemical and ultrastructural observations on the esophagus of the dog. Thesis (PhD), Cornell University, Ithaca, NY, 1982.

117. Innes JRM and Saunders LZ: Comparative Neuropathology. New York, Academic Press, 1962.

118. Jenkins WL, Van Dyk E, and McDonald CB: Myasthenia gravis in a fox terrier litter. J South Afr Vet Assoc 47:59, 1976.

119. Johnson RP, Watson ADJ, Smith J, and Cooper BJ: Myasthenia in springer spaniel littermates. J Small Anim Pract 16:641, 1975.

120. Jones BR, Anderson LJ, Barnes GRG, et al: Myotonia in related chow chow dogs. NZ Vet J 25:217, 1977.

121. Kao I, Drachman DB, and Price DL: Botulinum toxin: Mechanism of presynaptic blockade. Science 193:125, 1976.

122. Kaspar LV and Lombard LS: Nutritional myodegeneration in a litter of beagles. JAVMA 143:284, 1963.

123. Katherman AE and Braund KG: Polyneuropathy associated with diabetes mellitus in a dog. JAVMA 182:522, 1982.

124. Key TJA and Gaskell CJ: Puzzling syndrome in cats associated with pupillary dilation. Vet Rec 110:160, 1982.

125. Klein LV: Case report: A hot horse. Vet Anesth 2:41, 1975.

126. Kornegay JN, Gorgacz EJ, Dawe DL, et al: Polymyositis in dogs. JAVMA 176:431, 1980.

127. Kramer JW, Hegreberg GA, Bryan GM, et al: A muscle disorder of Labrador retrievers characterized by deficiency of type II muscle fibers. JAVMA 169:817, 1976.

128. Kramer JW, Hegreberg GA, and Hamilton MJ: Inheritance of a neuromuscular disorder of Labrador retriever dogs. JAVMA 179:380, 1981.

129. Krum SH, Cardinet GH, Anderson BC, and Holliday TA: Polymyositis and polyarthritis associated with systemic lupus erythematosus in a dog. JAVMA 170:61, 1977.

130. Kula RW: Neuromuscular disorders associated with systemic neoplastic diseases. In Vinken PJ and Bruyn GW (ed): Handbook of Clinical Neurology, vol 41. Amsterdam, North-Holland Publishing Co, 1979, p 317.

131. Langelier RM: Ischemic neuromyopathy associated with steel pellet BB aortic shot obstruction in a cat. Can Vet J 23:187, 1982.

132. Lennon VA, Palmer AC, Pflugfelder C, and Indrieri RJ: Myasthenia gravis in dogs: Acetylcholine receptor deficiency with and without anti-receptor antibodies. In Rose NR, Bigazzi PE, and Warner NL (ed): Genetic Control of Autoimmune Diseases. New York, Elsevier-North Holland, 1978, p 295.

133. Lesser AS: The use of a tendon transfer for the treatment of a traumatic sciatic nerve paralysis in the dog. Vet Surg 7:85, 1978.

134. Liu S-K: Acquired cardiac lesions leading to congestive heart failure in the cat. Am J Vet Res 31:2071, 1970.

135. Liu S-K and Dorfman HD: A condition resembling human localized myositis ossificans in two dogs. J Small Anim Pract 17:371, 1976.

136. Lorenz MD, de Lahunta A, and Alstrom DH: Neostigmine-responsive weakness in the dog, similar to myasthenia gravis. JAVMA 161:795, 1972.

137. Lucke JN, Hall GM, and Lister D: Malignant hyperthermia in the pig and the role of stress. Ann NY Acad Sci 317:326, 1979.

138. Lust G, Craig DH, Ross GE, and Geary JC: Studies on pectineus muscles in canine hip dysplasia. Cornell Vet 62:628, 1972.

139. Lyman R and Braund KG: Unpublished data, 1981.

140. MacLachlan NJ, Gribble DH, and East ME: Polyradiculoneuritis in a goat. JAVMA 180:166, 1982.

141. Maenhout D, Ducatelle R, Coussement W, et al: Space occupying lesions of cranial nerves in calves with facial paralysis. Vet Rec 15:407, 1984.

142. Manktelow BW: Myopathy of dogs resembling white muscle disease of sheep. NZ Vet J 11:52, 1963.

143. Mason KV: A case of myasthenia gravis in a cat. J Small Anim Pract 17:467, 1976.

144. Mayhew IG and MacKay RJ: The nervous system. In Mansmann RA, McAllister ES, and Pratt PW (ed): Equine Medicine and Surgery, 3rd ed, vol II. Santa Barbara, CA, American Veterinary Publications, 1982.

145. McKeran RO, Slavin G, Andrews TM, et al.: Muscle fiber type changes in hypothyroid myopathy. J Clin Pathol 28:659, 1975.

146. McKeran RO, Ward P, Slavin G, and Paul EA: Central nuclear counts in muscle fibers before and during treatment in hypothyroid myopathy. J Clin Pathol 32:229, 1979.

147. Meier H: Myopathies in the dog. Cornell Vet 48:313, 1958.

148. Mercer HD, Neal FC, Himes JA, and Edds GT: Cassia occidentalis toxicosis in cattle. JAVMA 151:735, 1967.

149. Miller LM, Lennon VA, Lambert EH, et al: Congenital myasthenia gravis in 13 smooth fox terriers. JAVMA 182:694, 1983.

150. Milne FJ and Carbonell PL: Neuritis of the cauda equina of horses. A case report. Equine Vet J 2:179, 1970.

151. Moore RW, Rouse GP, Piermattei DL, and Ferguson HR: Fibrotic myopathy of the semitendinosus muscle in four dogs. Vet Surg 10:169, 1981.

152. Nash AS, Griffiths IR, and Sharp NJH: The Key-Gaskell syndrome—an autonomic polyganglionopathy. Vet Rec 111:307, 1982.

153. Neal FC, and Ramsey FK: Cranial nerve injuries. *In* Catcott FJ and Smithcors JF (ed): Equine Medicine and Surgery. Wheaton, MD, American Veterinary Publications, 1972, p 470.

154. Nesbit JW, Lourens DC, and Williams MC: Spastic paresis in two littermate pups caused by *Toxoplasma gondii*. J South Afr Vet Assoc 52:243, 1981.

155. Nisbet DI and Ranwick CC: Congenital myopathy in lambs. J Comp Pathol 71:177, 1961.

156. Norris AM, Pallett L, and Wilcock B: Generalized myositis ossificans in a cat. J Am Anim Hosp Assoc 16:659, 1980.

157. Northington JW and Brown MJ: Acute canine idiopathic polyneuropathy. A Guillain-Barré-like syndrome in dogs. J Neurol Sci 56:259, 1982.

158. Northington JW, Brown MJ, Farnbach GC, and Steinberg SA: Acute idiopathic polyneuropathy in the dog. JAVMA 179:375, 1981.

159. O'Brien, JA, Harvey CE, Kelly AA, and Tucker JA: Neurogenic atrophy of the laryngeal muscles of the dog. J Small Anim Pract 14:521, 1973.

160. Oliver JE Jr and Lorenz MD: Handbook of Veterinary Neurologic Diagnosis. Philadelphia, WB Saunders Co, 1983.

161. Olmstead ML and Butler HC: Five-hydroxytryptamine antagonists and feline aortic embolism. J Small Anim Pract 18:247, 1977.

162. Orvis JS and Cardinet GH: Canine muscle fiber types and susceptibility of masticatory muscles to myositis. Muscle Nerve 4:354, 1981.

163. Osborne CA, Clifford DH, and Jessen C: Hereditary esophageal achalasia in dogs. JAVMA 151:572, 1967.

164. Palmer AC: Introduction to Animal Neurology, 2nd ed. London, Blackwell Scientific Publications, 1976.

165. Palmer AC: Myasthenia gravis. Vet Clin North Am 10:213, 1980.

166. Palmer AC and Barker J: Myasthenia in the dog. Vet Rec 95:452, 1974.

167. Palmer AC and Goodyear JV: Congenital myasthenia in the Jack Russell terrier. Vet Rec 103:433, 1978.

168. Palmer AC, Lennon VA, Beadle C, and Goodyear JV: Autoimmune form of myasthenia gravis in a juvenile Yorkshire terrier × Jack Russell terrier hybrid contrasted with congenital (non-autoimmune) myasthenia gravis of the Jack Russell. J Small Anim Pract 21:359, 1980.

169. Pemberton DH and Caple IW: Australian stringhalt in horses. Vet Ann 20:167, 1980.

170. Pflugfelder CM, Cardinet GH, Lutz H, et al.: Acquired canine myasthenia gravis: Immunocytochemical localization of immune complexes at neuromuscular junctions. Muscle Nerve 4:289, 1980.

171. Physick-Sheard PW and Maxie MG: Aortoiliofemoral arteriosclerosis. *In* Robinson NG (ed): Current Therapy in Equine Medicine. Philadelphia, WB Saunders Co, 1983, p 153.

172. Pilet C, Cazabat H, and Ardonceau R: Une nouvelle enzootie de botulisme chez le chien de meute. Bull Acad Vet Fr 32:297, 1959.

173. Pivnik L: Zur vergleichenden Problematic einiger akrodystrophischer Neuropathien bei Menschen und Hund. Schweiz Arch Neurol Neurochir Psychiatr 112:365, 1973.

174. Power HT, Watrous BJ, and deLahunta A: Facial and vestibulocochlear nerve disease in six horses. JAVMA 183:1076, 1983.

175. Reinke JD and Suter PF: Laryngeal paralysis in a dog. JAVMA 172:714, 1978.

176. Renegar WR: Auriculopalpebral nerve paralysis following prolonged anesthesia in a dog. JAVMA 174:1007, 1979.

177. Rogers WA, Fenner WR, and Sherding RG: Electromyographic and esophagomanometric findings in clinically normal dogs and in dogs with idiopathic megaesophagus. JAVMA 174:181, 1979.

178. Rolfe DL: Aortic thromboembolism in a calf. Can Vet J 18:321, 1977.

179. Rose RJ, Hartley WJ, and Baker W: Laryngeal paralysis in Arabian foals associated with oral Haloxon administration. Equine Vet J 13:171, 1981.

180. Sanda A and Pivnik L: Die Zehennekrose bei kurzhaarigen Vorstehhunden. Kleintierpraxis 9:76, 1964.

181. Scelsi R and Pinelli P: Subclinical myopathic findings in patients affected by malignant tumors. Acta Neuropathol 38:103, 1977.

182. Schunk KL and Averill DR: Peripheral vestibular syndrome in the dog: A review of 83 cases. JAVMA 182:1354, 1983.

183. Schutt I and Kersten U: Myasthenia gravis pseudoparalytica bei drei Deutschen Schaferhundinnen. Kleintierpraxis 22:45, 1977.

184. Schwartz A, Ravin CE, Greenspan RH, et al: Congenital neuromuscular esophageal disease in a litter of Newfoundland puppies. J Am Vet Radiol Soc 17:101, 1976.

185. Scott DW and deLahunta A: Eosinophilic polymyositis in a dog. Cornell Vet 64:47, 1974.

186. Shires PK, Braund KG, Milton JL, and Liu W: Effect of localized trauma and temporary splinting on immature skeletal muscle and mobility of the femorotibial joint in the dog. Am J Vet Res 43:454, 1982.

187. Shires PK, Nafe LA, and Hulse DA: Myotonia in a Staffordshire terrier. JAVMA 183:229, 1983.

188. Siebold HR and Davis CL: Generalized myositis ossificans (familial) in pigs. Pathol Vet 4:79, 1967.

189. Simpson ST, Braund KG, and Sorjonen DC: Muscular dystrophy of Labrador retrievers. Scientific Proceedings, Am Coll Vet Intern Med, 1982.

190. Sjolte IP: Polyneuritis equi. Maandsskr Dyrlaeger 56:357, 1944.

191. Sokolovsky V: Achalasia and paralysis of the canine esophagus. JAVMA 160:943, 1972.

192. Sorjonen DC, Braund KG, and Hoff EJ: Paraplegia and subclinical neuromyopathy associated with a primary lung tumor in the dog. JAVMA 180:1209, 1982.

193. Sova Z: Die Pfotennekrose (neurotrophische, erblich bedingte Osteopathie). Eine neue Erkrankung bei Welpen von Vorstehhunden. Tierarztl Prax 2:225, 1974.

194. Spangler WL and Muggli FM: Seizure-induced rhabdomyolysis accompanied by acute renal failure in a dog. JAVMA 172:1190, 1978.

195. Spencer PS, Sabri MI, Schaumburg HH, and Moore CL: Does a defect of energy metabolism in the nerve fiber underlie axonal degeneration in polyneuropathies? Ann Neurol 5:501, 1979.

196. Spencer PS and Schaumburg HH: Ultrastructural studies of the dying-back process. IV. Differential vulnerability of PNS and CNS fibers in experimental central-peripheral distal axonopathies. J Neuropathol Exp Neurol 36:300, 1977.

197. Spreull JSA: Treatment of otitis media in the dog. J Small Anim Pract 5:107, 1964.

198. Spreull JSA: Otitis media of the dog. *In* Kirk RW: Current Veterinary Therapy V. Philadelphia, WB Saunders Co, 1975.

199. Stead AC, Camburn MA, Gunn HM, and Kirk EJ: Congenital hindlimb rigidity in a dog. J Small Anim Pract 18:39, 1977.
200. Steinberg S and Botelho S: Myotonia in a horse. Science 137:979, 1962.
201. Steiss JE, Orsher AN, and Bowen JM: Electrodiagnostic analysis of peripheral neuropathy in dogs with diabetes mellitus. Am J Vet Res 42:2061, 1981.
202. Strombeck DR: Small Ánimal Gastroenterology. Davis, CA, Stonegate Publishing, 1979.
203. Swaim SF: Peripheral neuropathies. In Bojrab MJ (ed): Pathophysiology in Small Animal Surgery. Philadelphia, Lea & Febiger, 1981, p 233.
204. Sybesma W and Eikelenboom G: Malignant hyperthermia syndrome in pigs. Neth J Vet Sci 2:155, 1969.
205. Thomas PK: Metabolic neuropathies. In Aguayo AJ and Karpati G (ed): Current Topics in Nerve and Muscle Research. Amsterdam, Excerpta Medica, 1979, p 255.
206. Thomas PK and Eliasson SG: Diabetic neuropathy. In Dyck PJ, Thomas PK, and Lambert EH (ed): Peripheral Neuropathy. Philadelphia, WB Saunders Co, 1975, p 956.
207. Tilley LP and Liu S-K: Cardiomyopathy and thromboembolism in the cat. Feline Pract 5:32, 1975.
208. Tilley LP, Lord PF, and Wood A: Acquired heart disease and aortic thromboembolism in the cat. In Kirk RW: Current Veterinary Therapy V. Philadelphia, WB Saunders Co, 1974, p 305.
209. Tryphonas L, Hamilton GF, and Rhodes CS: Perinatal femoral nerve degeneration and neurogenic atrophy of quadriceps femoris muscle in calves. JAVMA 164:801, 1974.
210. Tyler HR: Paraneoplastic syndromes of nerve, muscle, and neuromuscular junction. Ann NY Acad Sci 230:348, 1974.
211. Vaughan LC: Muscle and tendon injuries in dogs. J Small Anim Pract 20:711, 1979.
212. Venker-van Haagen AJ,. Bouw J, and Hartman W: Hereditary transmission of laryngeal paralysis in Bouviers. J Am Anim Hosp Assoc 17:75, 1981.
213. Venker-van Haagen AJ, Hartman W, and Goedoge-buure SA: Spontaneous laryngeal paralysis in young Bouviers. J Am Anim Hosp Assoc 14:714, 1978.
214. Waldron-Mease E, Raker CW, and Hammel EP: The muscular system. In Mansmann RA, McAllister ES, and Pratt PW (ed): Equine Medicine and Surgery. Santa Barbara, CA, American Veterinary Publications, 1982.
215. Walker TL: Ischiadic nerve entrapment. JAVMA 178:1284, 1981.
216. Wentink GH, Hartman W, and Koeman JP: Three cases of myotonia in a family of chows. Tijdschr Diergeneeskd 14:729, 1974.
217. Wentink GH, van der Linde-Sipman JS, Meijer AEF, et al: Myopathy with a possible recessive X-linked inheritance in a litter of Irish terriers. Vet Pathol 9:328, 1972.
218. White NA: Postanesthesia myopathy-neuropathy. In Robinson NE (ed): Current Therapy in Equine Medicine. Philadelphia, WB Saunders Co, 1983.
219. Whitney JC: Eosinophilic myositis in dogs. Vet Rec 67:1140, 1955.
220. Whitney JC: Atrophic myositis in a dog: The differentiation of this disease from eosinophilic myositis. Vet Rec 69:130, 1957.
221. Whitney JC: A case of cranial myodegeneration (atrophic myositis) in a dog. J Small Anim Pract 11:735, 1970.
222. Wouda W, Vandevelde M, Oettli P, et al: Sensory neuronopathy in dogs: A study of four cases. J Comp Pathol 93:437, 1983.

Principles of Medical Therapy

As a tissue, the central nervous system (CNS) is anatomically and functionally unique in its response to both disease insults and therapeutic agents. To protect its delicate structures, the CNS is encased in a rigid framework of bony armor, making it more susceptible to compression injuries. Although it receives a proportionally higher blood flow than any other body tissue, the CNS has relatively few permanent cellular defense elements such as those of the mononuclear phagocytic and lymphocytic defense structures. Therefore, without adequate intrinsic defense mechanisms, the CNS must rely on physical barriers to protect itself from potential blood borne insults.[38]

Blood-Brain Barrier

The blood-brain barrier protects CNS structures by restricting passage of blood borne dyes, toxins, ions, metabolites, and drugs.[46] Historically, it had been observed that intravenously injected dyes stained all structures except the CNS. Similarly, animals with jaundice were found to have yellow staining of all body tissues with minimal staining of the brain. However, the CNS barrier could be overcome when substances were injected directly into the cerebrospinal fluid (CSF).

The anatomic nature of the blood-brain barrier has been primarily elucidated by ultrastructural examination. Unlike the capillary networks in other tissues, those in the CNS are lined by a continuous basement membrane. CNS endothelial cells are also connected by tight junctions, which exclude the passage of ionic or polar molecules or large molecules such as proteins in much the same manner as a continuous plasma membrane. In most tissues, transport of substances through capillary walls occurs primarily by pinocytosis. Pinocytosis is restricted across capillary barriers of the CNS presumably because of astrocytic foot processes on the capillary basement membrane, which are thought to inhibit the movement of compounds. The cerebral capillary endothelial cell also contains a large number of cellular enzymes responsible for selective transport of blood borne compounds into the CNS. Certain substances such as sugars, amino acids, and short chain fatty acids have facilitated transport across these cells.

The blood-brain barrier is present in all capillaries within the CNS, with exception of the hypophysis, tuber cinereum, area postrema, paraphysis, pineal gland, and preoptic recess.[5] It is thought that these areas are more permeable to compounds to enable the CNS to monitor blood borne elements. The area postrema is close to the emetic center and the chemoreceptor trigger zone of the medulla and is thought to be responsible for monitoring of blood borne toxins. The hypophyseal and pineal regions are important in assessing negative feedback of biologic hormones for homeostasis.

Blood–Cerebrospinal Fluid Barrier

The choroid plexus, unlike the rest of the CNS, readily stains following intravenous injection of dyes. However, the choroid plexus, the major site of CSF production, restricts the flow of these dye molecules into the CSF. Furthermore, capillary endothelium in the choroid plexus, as in the CNS, has been shown to prevent the passage of lipid insoluble compounds.

A CSF-brain barrier is relatively nonexistent; intraventricular or subarachnoid administration of compounds is known to provide more ready access of these substances into CNS tissues. Similarly, elimination of substances within CNS tissues is partly accomplished by their diffusion into the CSF and eventual removal by the arachnoid villi, which drain into the venous system. However, the arachnoid and other meningeal elements do restrict the diffusion of compounds out of the CSF into surrounding mesodermal tissues. These substances can only be eliminated from the CSF through normal drainage pathways.

Drug Penetration and Elimination in the Central Nervous System

Several properties determine whether or not substances will be able to cross the blood-brain and blood–cerebrospinal fluid barriers. The dissociation constant of the compound is important because substances cross primarily as undissociated molecules. Lipid solubility is also important in determining the ease with which substances can cross the endothelial lining of the blood-brain barrier. Measurements of plasma concentrations of various drugs can be misleading with respect to therapeutic efficacy in the CNS because they do not reflect the degree of protein binding of the compound. In the absence of inflammation or altered vascular permeability, blood proteins are excluded from entering CNS tissue.

The amount of blood flow to a given area in the CNS also affects the relative ease of entry and exit of blood borne compounds. In general, the brain has the potential to be exposed to large amounts of any circulating substances because, despite its small size, the brain receives 15 to 20% of cardiac output. The gray matter, containing a majority of neurons, receives a relatively high percentage (32%) of the blood flow to the CNS.

In addition to influences of blood-brain barrier and regional blood flow, the penetration and distribution of substances into the CNS is also determined by the affinity of different areas of the CNS for certain types of compounds. Drugs such as chlorpromazine, butyrophenones, and imipramine have an affinity for the caudate nucleus and hippocampus, whereas diazepam, diphenylhydantoin, and barbiturates

accumulate in the cerebral and cerebellar cortex, thalamus, and midbrain.

The rate of exit of compounds from the CNS is also important in determining their final concentration. In addition to venous removal, drugs in CNS tissue can leave via the CSF pathways. The brain and spinal cord have no lymphatic system. Drainage of extracellular fluid occurs through pericellular areas around neurons and glia; fluids cross the pial and ependymal linings and enter the CSF, where they are removed by the arachnoid villi. The arachnoid villi, responsible for the removal of CSF from the subarachnoid space, provide outgoing pathways to the venous circulation. The rate of CSF formation and drainage is, therefore, an important determinant for drug metabolism in the CNS. Not all drugs are eliminated by circulatory means, as many become locally inactivated by intrinsic metabolic processes in CNS tissue.

CONTROL OF CENTRAL NERVOUS SYSTEM EDEMA

Edema of any tissue is defined as an intra- or extracellular accumulation of excessive fluid. CNS edema is a common pathologic process that can result from a wide variety of abnormal influences on CNS tissue and CSF dynamics. Central nervous system edema has been classified according to its underlying cause, and some correlation has been made with the distribution pattern of edema fluid. Although not well documented, the composition of edematous fluid probably differs depending on its cause. *Cytotoxic edema* is thought to be caused by factors that directly injure neuronal and other cellular elements, thereby causing a breakdown in cellular osmoregulation and an intracellular shift in water. Brain volume is increased under such circumstances at the expense of a reduced extracellular space. Cytotoxic edema that primarily affects gray matter or neuronal regions is frequently caused by ischemia. *Vasogenic edema* is associated with diseases that increase cerebrovascular permeability, resulting in spread of edematous fluid from the vascular to the intra- and extracellular fluid spaces. Increased capillary endothelial permeability is also accompanied by increased CSF protein content. This form of edema has a predilection for white matter. *Interstitial edema* is associated with increased periventricular accumulation of CSF and occurs with diseases such as obstructive hydrocephalus.[18] In this condition, fluid is primarily found in the extracellular fluid space, but with increased intracranial pressure and reduced CSF absorption, more generalized parenchymal edema develops.

A number of therapeutic modalities have been attempted to control the process of CNS edema. Drug therapy has included the use of osmotic diuretics, glucocorticoids, dimethylsulfoxide, barbiturates, nonsteroid analgesics, antifibrinolytic agents, antibiogenic amine compounds, endorphin antagonists, and blood flow stimulants.[19, 58] Additional regimens have included hyperbaric oxygenation or hyperventilation and systemic or local hypothermia. (Decompressive surgery and medical therapy for spinal cord compression is considered in Chapters 11, 12, 16–18.)

Osmotic Diuretics

Hypertonic solutions have the advantage of rapidly reducing the swelling of CNS tissues. By producing relative blood hyperosmolality, osmotic diuretics cause movement of intra- and extracellular fluid into the intravascular space. The optimal osmotic agent has unrestricted glomerular filtration and restricted resorption at the renal tubule and behaves as a pharmacologically inert substance.

Osmotic agents must be used with caution in the presence of severe intracranial hemorrhage because they increase CNS blood flow and promote further bleeding as a result of arteriolar hypertension. A disadvantage of osmotic compounds is that they can only be used on a short-term basis because they interfere with fluid and electrolyte balance. Osmotic diuretics have the potential of producing rebound intracranial hypertension, which is associated with an influx of hypertonic solute in the brain following intravenous infusion. Rebound intracranial hypertension is more likely in the presence of a damaged blood-brain barrier because osmotic diuretics enter CNS tissue more readily.

Mannitol

This has been one of the most popular osmotic diuretics used for the treatment of cerebral edema. Its onset of action is slightly slower than that of urea or glucose, but it has fewer complications associated with the rebound phenomenon.

The dosage of mannitol used in dogs and cats ranges from 1 to 3 g/kg by intravenous infusion.[43] Given as a 20% solution it is infused over a 20 to 30 minute period to a maximum of 1.5 hours. A small initial dose of 1 g/kg should precede the infusion and is given over a 10 minute period. Mannitol, which begins to act within 1 hour, usually exerts its maximum antiedema effect within 2 to 4 hours. Synergistic effects have been found in treating cerebral edema in dogs when tubular diuretics have been concurrently administered.[59] Unfortunately, severe dehydration is a complication of this combined therapy.

Several precautions must be taken when administering mannitol to avoid serious side effects. Mannitol can crystallize in intravenous preparations kept at room temperature (22°C). Warming the solution to 37°C prior to infusion and using in-line filters are recommended to avoid any complications. Mannitol can be readministered every 6 to 8 hours for a maximum of 24 hours, but further administration results in electrolyte imbalance, arteriolar hypertension, and altered renal function. Mannitol given at a total dose of 3 g/kg has been shown to be safe and effective in reducing CSF pressure in normal dogs for 1.5 hours.[29] When a second dose of 3 g/kg was given 4 hours later, the effect was more prolonged; however, 50% of the dogs died. Mannitol is contraindicated in animals with severe hypovolemia because dogs with moderate blood loss have died immediately following infusion of 3 g/kg of mannitol.[42]

The cardiovascular response to hypertonic mannitol infusion in dogs is caused by a marked increase in vascular volume and is characterized by a dramatic increase in heart rate, blood pressure, and left ventricular end diastolic volume.[1] Mannitol must not be administered to animals with congestive heart failure because of its effect on increasing blood volume. Pulmonary edema has developed in dogs that received a high infusion rate of 2 g/kg mannitol over a 15 minute period during operative surgery with methoxyflurane anesthesia.[4]

Glycerol

Oral administration of glycerol has been effective in reducing CSF pressure in human patients with intracranial hypertension. Each dose of glycerol is accompanied by an increase in serum osmolality followed by a rapid decrease in intraventricular pressure. One disadvantage of glycerol in veterinary practice is the need for patient acceptance of orally administered liquids. Furthermore, oral therapy is often impossible in semicomatose or comatose patients with increased intracranial pressure. Glycerol is given at a dosage of 1 g/kg and, unlike mannitol, can be repeated as needed for more prolonged management. Repeated administration does not diminish the effectiveness of the drug, and rebound intracranial hypertension is not a problem if glycerol is not given more frequently than every 6 hours. However, if the drug is given too frequently (every 4 hours or more often), the CSF and serum osmolality will persistently increase because of incomplete metabolic removal. This rebound increased intracranial pressure can result in clinical deterioration.

Glucocorticoids

The benefit of glucocorticoids in treating CNS edema may relate to their effects on stabilization of plasma membranes.[13] Central nervous system edema from any cause is associated with disruption of the blood-brain barrier and altered cellular integrity. Membrane damage at the ultrastructural level results in alteration in the regular arrangement of the bimolecular layer of apposing phospholipid molecules in the membrane. It has been hypothesized that glucocorticoids fill the gaps in the lipid bilayer of the membrane, which has been disrupted by inflammatory processes and associated free radical peroxidation. Thus glucocorticoids are more effective in preventing than in correcting CNS edema. Additional proposed mechanisms for the protective effect of glucocorticoids include prevention of lysosomal breakdown by membrane stabilization, increasing energy supply to CNS tissue, and promotion of diuresis. It is known that glucocorticoids reach a high concentration in the choroid plexus, which may explain their effect on reducing CSF production and the resultant decrease in intracranial pressure.[60] Dexamethasone (0.15 mg/kg) has been shown to cause an immediate drop (by 50%) in CSF production in dogs within 1 hour of administration.[49] The effect of glucocorticoids is somewhat delayed as compared with osmotic diuretics, taking up to 12 to 24 hours before improvement is noted. Glucocorticoids are desirable, however, because they give a longer duration of action than osmotic agents.

Dexamethasone has been shown to be effective in reducing CNS edema in cats when administered at 0.25 to 2.5 mg/kg/day.[39] A threshold dosage of 1 mg/kg was effective in dogs in controlling experimentally induced cerebral edema[52] and spinal cord compression.[15]

Glucocorticoids, however, appear to be least effective in controlling CNS edema secondary to ischemic lesions.[12]

Studies on the treatment of acute experimental spinal cord trauma produced at L_2 in cats have shown a lack of efficacy of mannitol, dimethyl sulfoxide (DMSO), naloxone, thyrotropin releasing hormone, and dexamethasone given 45 minutes after spinal cord trauma.[20] Animals treated with these agents experienced no better results than untreated or saline treated controls. The highly soluble and fast acting glucocorticoid methylprednisolone sodium succinate produced a rapid sparing action on the spinal cord. The cats were ambulatory within a week after trauma, significantly better results than for those treated with other agents. Therefore, it is recommended that patients with acute CNS trauma be treated with a highly soluble glucocorticoid, such as methylprednisolone sodium succinate, as early as possible. Therapy can be maintained with dexamethasone as needed.

Side effects of glucocorticoid administration are usually, but not entirely, related to the use of increased dosages or long-term therapy. Severe gastrointestinal hemorrhage and ulceration are some of the most commonly observed side effects. Glucocorticoids should be used with caution if the patient has a history of erosive gastrointestinal disease or if concurrent drug therapy has such tendencies. Glucocorticoids are known to decrease gastric mucus production and decrease mucosal cell turnover, both of which increase the chance of bowel ulceration. Perforation of the proximal descending colon has been reported as a cause of death in dogs that received glucocorticoids as a supplement to surgical decompression for intervertebral disk disease.[56] The dosages in these cases ranged from 0.25 to 4.4 mg/kg of dexamethasone daily. In addition, surgical stress was thought to contribute to these fatal episodes.

High dosages of glucocorticoids have been shown to increase serum lipase activity without producing histologic lesions in the pancreas,[41] although acute pancreatitis has been associated with such therapy in dogs.[21] Glucocorticoids have also been incriminated as a precipitating factor of acute *Salmonella* gastroenteritis,[9] and many large animal clinicians are concerned about increasing the risk of laminitis in horses treated with glucocorticoids. A paradoxic case of cerebral edema associated with fluid and electrolyte retention in the CNS was reported in a dog that accidentally ingested 7.0 mg/kg prednisolone on two occasions.[26] The mineralocorticoid activity of prednisolone may have been responsible and, in addition to potency, is another reason that dexamethasone is more desirable for long-term treatment of CNS edema.

Barbiturates

Barbiturates were effective under experimental circumstances in protecting the brain against injuries caused by hypoxemia or ischemia and vasogenic cerebral edema.[32, 50] This effect may be mediated by the ability of barbiturates to reduce the energy requirements of CNS tissue. When given intravenously, thiopental and pentobarbital cause a significant decrease in intracranial pressure, especially when coupled with whole body hypothermia. A rapid and sustained reduction can be achieved when the blood level of barbiturate is maintained at 3 mg/dl.[48]

Hypothermia and Hyperventilation

Although it has been advocated alone and in conjunction with other forms of therapy to reduce cerebral edema, generalized or localized hypothermia has been recently abandoned because of increased risks due to the need for prolonged anesthesia to maintain hypothermia. A rebound and overshooting of the CNS pressure also frequently occurs when the animal's temperature is normalized. The benefits of localized hypothermic perfusion have not been well documented (see Chapter 16).

Hyperventilation or hyperbaric oxygenation has been proposed as a means of therapy for intracranial hypertension. High oxygen tension in CNS tissue is thought to cause relative vasoconstriction and reduced blood flow despite increased tissue oxygenation, which results in reduced CNS pressure. Unfortunately, prolonged vasoconstriction causes permanent ischemia of CNS tissue.

PAIN CONTROL AND SEDATION

Pain is probably the most common and least understood diagnostic dilemma presented to veterinary practitioners.[25, 61] Most pain originates from mechanical or inflammatory processes in the body that stimulate free nerve endings.[10] Pain impulses travel in the CNS in predetermined and sometimes diffuse pathways.[35] Specialized areas in the CNS around the periaqueductal gray matter in the midbrain are known to modulate these ascending impulses. When stimulated electrically or by local application of opiates, these pain suppressive areas blunt the response to painful stimulation. Neurotransmitters in these specialized regions consist of a heterogeneous group of polypeptides known as endorphins, enkephalins, or endogenous opiates.[33]

Two main classes of analgesic drugs for controlling pain in animals are available to the veterinarian.[22, 55] The opiates or narcotic analgesics are thought to produce analgesia by stimulating the receptors in the centrally located pain suppressive areas of the CNS by occupying the same receptors as the endogenous opiates. Narcotic antagonists occupy these same receptors by competitive binding but have reduced pharmacologic activities.[44]

Non-narcotic analgesics are thought to work by reducing inflammation at the peripheral pain receptors. Anti-inflammatory effects have also been associated with their ability to inhibit prostaglandin synthesis because prostaglandins are important biologic mediators of inflammation.

Narcotic Analgesics

Narcotic analgesics or opiates are a group of naturally occurring alkaloids derived from opium and its semisynthetic and synthetic derivatives. Narcotics have a wide variety of effects in addition to their modulating activity on impulses traveling in pain pathways. Structural differences among the narcotics determine the degree of agonist and antagonist activity at opiate receptors and the extraneural side effects that are produced. Opiates are potent cough suppressants and, when given in excessive dosages, can depress mental attitude to the point of general anesthesia. Excitatory effects can also result from overdosages or regular dosages in susceptible animals with low tolerance to these compounds. Horses and cats are prone to develop excitement, hallucinations, or convulsions. Autonomic side effects include bradycardia, hypotension, constipation, miosis, and spasms of biliary and pancreatic ducts. Antidiuresis results from stimulation of antidiuretic hormone release and from increased urinary bladder sphincter tone.

Narcotic drugs produce more pronounced effects when given intravenously, but the duration of action is relatively short. They should not be given in cases of cranial trauma because they cause a rise in intracranial pressure. Physical dependence and the potential for human drug abuse limit the widespread use of these compounds for controlling pain. Dosages recommended for use in various animal species are listed in Table 15–1.

Morphine, the naturally occurring opiate of the group, was the first narcotic analgesic to be used in veterinary practice. Parenteral administration is required because of poor oral absorption. Morphine is one of the most potent analgesics for clinical use in dogs and cats. As mentioned previously, cats and horses are most sensitive to the effects of morphine because they develop excitement; however, using one tenth the recommended canine dose in the cat gives effective analgesia with minimal side effects. Many of the undesirable autonomic side effects associated with morphine administration can be overcome by prior administration of atropine (0.05–0.1 mg/kg subcutaneously).

Meperidine (pethidine) is a synthetic narcotic used for analgesia in horses, dogs, and cats. Its use in cats is limited because of its rapid excre-

tion. Meperidine is commonly employed as a preanesthetic to reduce the amount of barbiturates or other drugs used as general anesthetics. Meperidine potentiates the effects of phenothiazines and can be combined with them for additive sedation.

Fentanyl is a narcotic analgesic that is up to 100 times more potent on a weight basis than morphine. In veterinary practice, it is combined with a phenothiazine, droperidol, in a fixed concentration for use in dogs. It is given primarily as a sedative for minor surgical procedures, although it may be used for short-term analgesia when other compounds are not readily available.

Codeine is a narcotic analgesic and antitussive compound that is absorbed orally. It is not metabolized to morphine in the liver of dogs as it is in humans. As a medium potency narcotic, it works well for low grade or visceral pain.

Butorphanol and nalbuphine are narcotic agonist-antagonist compounds that have lower abuse potential than other opiates. They have primarily been used experimentally to control

Table 15–1. DOSAGES OF COMMONLY USED NARCOTIC ANALGESICS

Drug	Formulations	Relative Potency Intramuscular	Oral	Species	Route	Dose (mg/kg)	Frequency (hours)
Narcotic Agonists							
Morphine, paregoric	Injectable, 2, 8, 10, 15 mg/ml; soluble tablets, 10, 15, 30 mg; oral tablets, 15, 30 mg	10	60	Dog	IM, SC	0.25–2.5	4–6
				Cat	IM, SC	0.1–0.2	4–6
				Horse	IM	0.4–0.66	8–12
Oxymorphone (Numorphan)	Injectable, 1–1.5 mg/ml	1	6	Dog	IM, SC	0.05–0.2*	12
				Cat	IM, SC	0.2–1.0 mg* (total)	≥ 24
Levorphanol (Levo-Dromoran)	Injectable, 2 mg/ml; tablets, 2 mg	2	4	Horse	SC, IM	0.01–0.033	4–6
Meperidine (pethidine, Demerol)	Injectable, 25, 50, 100 mg/ml; oral tablets, 50–100 mg; syrup, 50 mg/5 ml	75	300	Dog	IM, SC	10–15	2–8
				Cat	IM, SC	2–4	12–24
				Horse, cow	SC, IM	1–3	8–12
Fentanyl combined with droperidol (Innovar-Vet)	0.4 mg fentanyl and 20 mg droperidol/ml	0.1	—	Dog	IV	1 ml/11–27 kg (slow)	8–12†
					IM	1 ml/7–9 kg	
Codeine	Tablets, 15–60 mg; injectable, 30–60 mg/ml	130	200	Dog	PO	2–8	8–12
				Cat	PO	5–30 mg (total)	8–12
				Horse, cow	PO	200–2000 (total)	12
Dextropropoxyphene (Darvon)	Capsules, 32, 65 mg	—	130	Cat	PO	0.5–1	12
Narcotic Agonist-Antagonists							
Butorphanol (Torbugesil) Torbutrol	Injectable, 1 mg/ml	2–3 —	— —	Horse Dog	IV, IM IV, IM	0.01–0.04 0.5–2.0	2–4 2–4
Nalbuphine (Nubain)	Injectable 10 mg/ml	10	—	Dog	IV, IM	0.5–2.0	2–4
Pentazocine (Talwin)	Injectable, 30 mg/ml; tablets, 12.5, 25, 50 mg	30–60	166	Horse	IV, IM	0.33–0.44	4–6
				Dog, cat	IV, IM, SC	0.75–3.0‡	2–4

*Use lowest dosage for intravenous administration.
†Do not repeat product combined with droperidol. Repeat dose of fentanyl is 5–50 μg/kg.
‡Maximum of 6 mg/kg/day; use higher dosages orally.
IM, intramuscular; SC, subcutaneous; PO, oral.

Table 15–2. DOSAGES OF COMMONLY USED NON-NARCOTIC ANALGESICS

Drug	Species	Route	Dose (mg/kg)	Frequency (hours)
Acetylsalicylic acid (aspirin)	Dog	PO	25*	8–12
	Cat	PO	25	24
	Cow	PO	100	12
Sodium salicylate	Sheep, pig	PO	1–4 g†	24
	Horse, cow	PO	15–20 g†	24
	Dog	PO	0.3–1 g†	24
	Cat	PO	3–300 mg†	24
Phenylbutazone (Butazolidin)	Dog	PO, IV	15	6–8‖
	Cat	PO	6–12	12–24
	Horse	PO	4–8‡	12–24
		IV	3–6‡	12
Flunixin meglumine (Banamine)	Horse	IM, IV	1–2.2‡	24§
Meclofenamic acid (Arquel)	Horse	PO (feed granules)	2.2‡	24
Dipyrone (Novin)	Dog	IM, SC	100–500 mg†	4–6
	Cat	IM, IV, SC	125 mg†	6–12
	Horse, cow	IM, SC, IV	2.5–10 g†	24
	Sheep, pig	IM, SC	2.5 g†	24
Naproxen	Horse	PO (feed granules)	10	12
Orgotein (Palosein)	Horse	IM	5 mg†	24¶

*Analgesic dose has a high incidence of gastrointestinal ulceration; therefore, reduce to the lowest dosage that is effective.
†Total dosage.
‡After 5–7 days use lowest effective dosage.
§For up to 5 days.
‖Maximum of 800 mg/day.
¶This dose for 2 weeks, then 2–4 times weekly for 2–4 weeks.
PO, oral; IM, intramuscular; IV, intravenous; SC, subcutaneous.

visceral pain in horses.[23, 24] Levorphanol and propoxyphene are synthetic narcotics that are much more potent than morphine.[54]

Pentazocine is a synthetic benzomorphan derivative of weaker analgesic potency than morphine but approximately equivalent to codeine.[30] Being an agonist-antagonist it also has less potential for abuse. Pentazocine is well absorbed orally but undergoes substantial metabolism when entering the liver directly from the portal circulation, so that oral dosages have reduced effectiveness unless there is hepatic failure. The drug is often used for moderate pain or as an adjunct to surgical anesthesia. Side effects of ataxia and incoordination have been found in horses given high dosages.

A syndrome of tail chasing in dogs is thought to be caused by an imbalance in endogenous opiates within the CNS. Preliminary experience has shown that this aberrant behavior may be controlled by periodic administration of pentazocine or other narcotic antagonists.[6]

Non-narcotic Analgesics

Salicylates

The salicylates, acetylsalicylic acid (aspirin) and sodium salicylate, have been the most widely used drugs for control of pain in human medicine. Dosages of aspirin used for analgesia in animals are listed in Table 15–2. These dosages are much higher than those required for antiplatelet activity. Use of aspirin and other nonsteroidal antiinflammatory drugs has proceeded with caution because of the increased incidence of gastrointestinal toxicity. Aspirin is readily absorbed following oral administration. Acetylsalicylic acid and sodium salicylate both react with hydrochloric acid in the stomach to release the local irritant salicylic acid. Occult gastrointestinal hemorrhage is a common occurrence with the use of the drug. Toxicity is usually dose related, so that lower levels may be tolerable but unfortunately not effective in producing analgesia. Parenteral dosing should not be as irritating to the gastrointestinal mucosa as oral administration.

Phenylbutazone, a pyrazolone derivative with antipyretic and analgesic activity, has been used primarily as an analgesic for musculoskeletal pain in most domestic animals. It can be given orally or parenterally, and gastrointestinal irritation can occur with either route of administration.

Acetaminophen is a popular analgesic and antiinflammatory drug used in humans. It primarily has antipyretic activity and less peripheral antiinflammatory activity. The production of methemoglobinemia and Heinz body anemia in cats has deferred its use. Use of indomethacin has also been restricted in dogs and cats because of hepatotoxicity.

The fenamic acid group of analgesic and antiinflammatory drugs has been primarily marketed for use in horses. Flunixin meglumine, an antiprostaglandin derivative, can be administered orally or parenterally. Its efficacy as an analgesic has mainly been established in primates and in horses. On a dose per weight basis it was four times as potent as phenylbutazone as an analgesic in horses.[24] As with most prostaglandin synthesis inhibitors, flunixin's analgesic action is limited to pain caused by inflammatory, including traumatic, processes. Meclofenamic acid, a member of the fenamic acid group, has been marketed as a granulated compound, which can be mixed with feed. Toxic signs, including gastrointestinal blood loss, necessitate cessation of drug therapy.

Dipyrone is an antipyretic and analgesic drug that has commonly been used as an analgesic in veterinary practice, especially in the treatment of equine colic.

Naproxen is a relatively new antiinflammatory and analgesic drug that has been marketed for horses and has been formulated as granules for adding to feed.

Orgotein is a water soluble, low molecular weight compound that has been used as an antiinflammatory analgesic drug in horses. Its proposed mechanism of action is that it blocks the formation of free radicals in inflamed tissue, which are known to activate inflammatory processes.

Other Analgesics

Methocarbamol is a skeletal muscle relaxant derived from glyceryl guaiacolate. Its mode of action is unknown but is suspected to be a result of general CNS depression. Methocarbamol preferentially blocks polysynaptic reflex pathways in the CNS and, as such, functions as an anticonvulsant. Its effect as an analgesic for muscular spasm may stem from its tranquilizing effect rather than specific skeletal muscle relaxation. Its primary use in veterinary practice has been in horses, dogs, and cats to control pain associated with inflammatory, spinal, or musculoskeletal disorders or with muscular hypertonicity accompanying tetanus or strychnine intoxication. Oral and parenteral preparations are available, and the dosage is usually adjusted to the degree of relaxation desired (Table 15–3). Only the intravenous and intramuscular routes should be used parenterally because the solution is hypertonic and irritating and may produce sloughing when administered subcutaneously. The parenteral formulation should not be used in the presence of renal failure because polyethylene glycol is used as a vehicle for the drug. Additional side effects in dogs and cats include hypersalivation, vomiting, and paralysis.

Methotrimeprazine is a phenothiazine derivative that produces CNS depression. It works as an analgesic centrally by raising the pain threshold and peripherally by exerting antihistaminic and anticholinergic effects. This compound produces analgesia in humans comparable with that of morphine or meperidine but it produces greater sedation. Its nonhabit forming

Table 15–3. DOSAGES OF SEDATIVES AND MUSCLE RELAXANTS

Drug	Species	Route	Dose (mg/kg)	Frequency
Methocarbamol (Robaxin)	Dog, cat	PO	45 (MP)	8 hours*
		IV	45 (MP)	Once
			55–220 (SP)	Once
	Horse	IV (slow)	4.4–22 (MP)	Once
			22–55 (SP)	Once
Xylazine (Rompun)	Dog, cat	IM	8.4	Once
		IV	1	Once
	Horse	IM, IV	0.5–2.2	Once
	Cow	IM	0.1–0.2	Once
		IV	0.05–0.1	Once
Ketamine (Ketaset, Vetalar)	Dog	IV	10–50	≥ 24 hours
		IM	10–100	≥ 24 hours
	Cat	IV, IM	10–30	≥ 24 hours
	Horse	IV	2.2	≥ 24 hours

*For several days, then 25–45 mg/kg/day divided 2 to 3 times daily.
MP, Mild pain; SP, severe pain; PO, oral; IV, intravenous; IM, intramuscular.

Table 15–4. DOSAGES OF PHENOTHIAZINE TRANQUILIZERS

Drug	Species	Route	Dose (mg/kg)	Frequency (hours)
Acetylpromazine (Acepromazine)	Dog	IM, IV	0.05–0.5	8–12
		PO	0.55–3	8–12
	Cat	IM, IV	0.05–0.3	8–12
		PO	1.1–2.2	8–12
	Horse	IM, IV, SC	0.04–0.09	12
	Cow	Sublingual	0.04	12–24
		IM	0.08	12–24
Chlorpromazine (Thorazine)	Dog	IV	1–2	12
		IM	2	12
		PO	3–5	8
	Cat	IV, IM	1	12
		PO	2	12
	Cow, horse*	IV, IM	1–2	12–24
Promazine (Sparine, promazine granules)	Dog, cat	PO, IM, IV	2.5–6.5	4–12
	Cow, horse,† sheep, pig	IM, IV	0.4–1	8–12
	Horse	PO	0.45–0.9	12–24
	Cow	PO	0.6–1.2	12–24
Piperacetazine (Psymod)	Dog, cat	SC, IM	0.1	8–12
		PO	0.1	6–12
Perphenazine (Trilafon)	Dog, cat, cow, pig	IM	0.22	12–24
Trimeprazine	All	All routes	1–4	12–24

*Can cause imbalance and incoordination in horses.
†Use with caution, as some horses have allergic reaction.
IM, Intramuscular; IV, intravenous; PO, oral; SC, subcutaneous.

property makes it desirable. Because of irritation, it is usually given by deep intramuscular injection in large muscle masses. The sites are rotated to help alleviate the pain associated with the injection. The dosage in humans is 10 to 40 mg given every 4 to 6 hours.

Sedatives and Tranquilizers

Xylazine

Xylazine is a thiazine tranquilizer that produces sedation, analgesia, and muscle relaxation via its inhibition of intraneural impulses within the CNS. It has marked difference in potency for each species in which it is used (Table 15–3). Although licensed for administration in horses, dogs, and cats, it has been used extensively for sedation and analgesia in food animals. Relatively small dosages are needed to sedate cattle for surgical anesthesia. The drug produced marked analgesia when used for visceral pain in horses.[24] It has also been extensively used for sedation with minor surgery and endoscopic procedures in that species. Side effects in dogs include marked bradycardia from atrioventricular conduction blockade. Emesis also occurs in dogs and cats immediately after the drug is administered but prior to the onset of sedation.

Ketamine

Ketamine is a dissociative anesthetic that is thought to work by interrupting associative neural pathways to the CNS. It produces sedation and anesthesia without cardiorespiratory depression. The anesthetic state is better termed unconsciousness because, despite analgesia, normal pharyngeal and laryngeal reflexes are maintained. There are slight effects on muscle tone and only minimal cardiac and respiratory depression. The analgesia produced by ketamine is superficial and relaxation minimal, so that only minor surgical procedures can be performed unless adjunctive therapy is used. Convulsions or hallucinations that can occur following recovery from ketamine anesthesia can be controlled by ultrashort barbiturates, given to effect. Ketamine is detoxified by the liver and excreted by the kidneys, so that dosages must be reduced or its use avoided under circumstances of organ failure (Table 15–3).

Phenothiazines

A number of phenothiazine derivatives are effective tranquilizers; they produce CNS depression without interfering with consciousness, voluntary movement, or cardiorespiratory function (Table 15–4). These drugs act principally by suppressing the brain stem reticular activating system and its connections to the cerebral cortex. Acetylpromazine, chlorpromazine, piperacetazine, and promazine have been the most commonly used phenothiazine tranquilizers in veterinary practice. Phenothiazine tranquilizers also have antihistaminic activity and may produce α-adrenergic blockade, the latter causing a reduction in blood pressure. Phenothiazines have been used to facilitate general anesthesia, reduce fear and aggressive behavior, and decrease motion sickness. Some phenothiazines may potentiate the toxic effects of organophosphate compounds found in flea collars and anthelmintics. Phenothiazines also lower the seizure threshold and may precipitate convulsions in seizure prone animals.

Hydroxyzine is a piperazine antihistamine that may act by suppressing subcortical regions of the CNS. It has some properties of other antihistamines, including skeletal muscle relaxation, bronchodilation, antihistaminic and antiserotonin activity, and analgesia. It is rapidly absorbed from the gastrointestinal tract and is primarily metabolized and excreted by the liver. In veterinary medicine, its primary use has been as a sedative and analgesic to control pruritus in dogs.

Benzodiazepines

The benzodiazepines depress subcortical regions of the CNS, such as the limbic and reticular activating systems. They have antianxiety, hypnotic, anticonvulsant, and muscle relaxant properties. They have a wide margin of safety and produce depression in animals only at higher dosages. Oral or intravenous administration is desirable because of the pain they produce and erratic absorption with intramuscular usage. Benzodiazepines have relatively short duration of effectiveness because they are readily metabolized by the liver into inactive compounds that are excreted in the urine. Oxazepam (Serax) or lorazepam (Activan) is preferred in patients with hepatic insufficiency because they are most easily metabolized. There is little clinical evidence, however, that one benzodiazepine is more effective than another, because they are largely interconverted. Chlordiazepozide (Librium), oxazepam, and lorazepam have slower onset of action and reach a lower peak blood level compared with diazepam. Of the benzodiazepines, they are considered to be hypnotics and have been primarily used as appetite stimulants in dogs and cats. Clonazepam, chlorazepate, and diazepam have the best anticonvulsant activity. Because of their short duration of action they are primarily reserved for the treatment of status epilepticus. Diazepam has also been commonly employed as a muscle relaxant as an adjunct to the treatment of pain caused by muscle spasms. The use of these drugs in farm animals has been limited.

Barbiturates

The barbiturates are primarily discussed under anticonvulsant drugs (see Chapter 10). Some mention is also made of their use in the management of intracranial hypertension (see above).

TREATMENT OF CENTRAL NERVOUS SYSTEM INFECTIONS

Acute bacterial or fungal meningitis is the main type of infection of the CNS for which antimicrobial therapy is warranted.[27] Antiviral chemotherapy is still too limited and expensive to be of practical consideration in veterinary practice. Chronic bacterial or fungal infections of the CNS usually are associated with abscessation or granuloma formation.[17] Management of the latter conditions requires adjunctive treatment (such as surgical drainage), although this is usually difficult and impractical in the CNS.[36] Therapy for chronic infections, similar to that for meningitis (see below), requires an extended course.[11] Treatment for meningitis should be as expeditious as possible and usually involves immediate hospitalization. General nursing care for depressed, dehydrated, anorectic, or semicomatose animals may involve force-feeding or parenteral fluid therapy. Care must be taken not to overhydrate patients with CNS inflammation because of the risk of aggravating CNS edema.[2] Body temperature should be monitored closely in animals with meningitis. Hyperthermia commonly results from increased neuromuscular activity due to the irritative process or from convulsions. Fever may occur as a direct effect of the infectious process on hypothalamic thermoregulation. Cold water baths or other means of lowering body temperature may be required if the temperature becomes dangerously elevated or if the fever fails to respond to appropriate antimicrobial therapy alone.

Convulsions occur as the result of inflammation, which causes edema and irritation of forebrain structures. Status epilepticus is initially treated to effect with intravenous diazepam or an intermediate acting barbiturate such as pentobarbital. This should, however, be replaced by oral anticonvulsants as soon as the animal's condition stabilizes. Anticonvulsants should be administered for 1 to 2 months following clinical improvement, and the dose gradually reduced thereafter.

Antimicrobial Therapy

Oral and Parenteral Therapy

Antibiotics are the most important agents used to treat bacterial meningitis.[37] Because the CSF and nervous tissue spaces have reduced resistance to infection, antibiotic therapy has been responsible for decreases in meningitis associated mortality in recent years. Therapy usually begins before culture and sensitivity results are available. Antibiotics should be administered immediately after the CSF has been collected, with the understanding that appropriate changes will be made.[14] The initial choice of antibiotics should be based on the type of organisms suspected, as judged by the history, clinical findings, results of gram staining, and the knowledge of antibiotic pharmacodynamics within the CSF and CNS.[16] Antibiotics with high lipid solubility, low ionization, and low protein binding penetrate blood-brain and blood–cerebrospinal fluid barriers most effectively (Table 15–5). Penetration by many drugs, including penicillins and aminoglycosides, is increased with meningeal inflammation.[28] Except for chloramphenicol and isoniazid, the commonly used antibiotics do not enter the CSF or brain tissue in high concentration. Intravenous therapy using any antibiotic ensures the highest concentration possible. High dose oral or parenteral (other than intravenous) therapy should only be considered as a second choice if cost or other difficulties preclude intravenous therapy. Unlike other forms of therapy, intravenous administration of drugs requires that certain details, such as the stability of antimicrobials in solution, compatibilities when used in combined therapy, and the proper rate of administration, be considered.

The choice of appropriate antibiotic therapy can sometimes be difficult because in vivo response does not always correlate with in vitro testing. Furthermore, many cases of meningitis will respond to antibacterial therapy even when organisms cannot be cultured. Bactericidal antibiotics should be used in meningeal infections whenever possible to ensure complete destruction of the organisms.[51] Decreased bactericidal activity in the CNS relates to decreased opsonization and phagocytosis from decreased complement and immunoglobulin concentrations and decreased entry of phagocytic cells. It is also difficult for neutrophils to phagocytize encapsulated bacteria in the subarachnoid space because solid tissue support is lacking. Thus, therapy with bactericidal antibiotics should be continued for a minimum of 3 to 4 weeks after a good response is obtained.

Despite their ionized state and relatively poor passage through the blood-brain and blood–cerebrospinal fluid barriers, penicillin and its derivatives (especially ampicillin and amoxicillin) should be the drugs of first choice in treating acute bacterial meningitis.[34] Meningeal inflammation increases the antibiotic concentration in the meninges to 15% of serum concentration, which is adequate to kill many microorganisms. Inflammation elevates the concentration of antibiotics in the CNS by increasing permeability of blood-brain barrier to their entry and by preventing their removal by inhibiting the function of the arachnoid villi. As inflammation subsides, the drug concentration in CNS or CSF may fall to a level at which it is no longer effective. One cannot always correlate the degree of pleocytosis and increased protein concentration in the CSF with the degree of permeability to antibiotics. For this reason antimicrobials should be administered at high dosages for long periods even in the face of clinical improvement.[47] Penicillin is primarily reserved for gram-positive infections, and oxacillin can be used if resistant staphylococci are implicated. Ampicillin or amoxicillin and car-

Table 15–5. ANTIMICROBIAL DRUGS PENETRATING BLOOD-BRAIN AND BLOOD–CEREBROSPINAL FLUID BARRIERS

Good	Intermediate	Poor
Bactericidal		
Trimethoprim	Penicillin	Most cephalosporins
Metronidazole	Ampicillin	Aminoglycosides
Moxalactam	Methicillin	
	Oxacillin	
	Carbenicillin	
Bacteriostatic		
Chloramphenicol	Tetracyclines	Amphotericin B
Sulfonamides	Flucytosine	Erythromycin
Isoniazid		
Minocycline		
Rifampin		

Modified from Greene CE: Infections of the central nervous system. *In* Greene CE (ed): Clinical Microbiology and Infectious Diseases of the Dog and Cat. Philadelphia, WB Saunders Co, 1984, p 284.

benicillin, which have penetration abilities equivalent to those of penicillin, are used to treat gram-negative and anaerobic infections, respectively.[39] In the author's experience, ampicillin or amoxicillin should be the drug of first choice in small animals.

Chloramphenicol is one of the few antibiotics that reach higher concentrations in the brain tissue (nine times higher) than in serum. Although most other antibiotics fail to enter CSF, its concentration there, in the absence of inflammation, ranges from 33 to 76% of its concurrent serum concentration. Intravenous therapy is desirable but not essential because of the high concentration it attains by oral or other parenteral routes. Chloramphenicol sodium succinate, the available parenteral preparation, should only be given intravenously or subcutaneously because it is not well absorbed after intramuscular administration. Because of its toxicity and bacteriostatic properties, chloramphenicol would be the author's second choice of therapy under most circumstances. Its use, however, in treating gram-negative infections is associated with failures and relapses, presumably because it is bacteriostatic even at maximum dosages.

Despite adequate in vitro sensitivity, there are a number of reasons not to use aminoglycosides. Aminoglycosides are extremely ionic and diffuse poorly into the CNS tissue or CSF in the presence of inflammation. The lowered pH of infected CSF may actually inhibit aminoglycoside activity. High dosage therapy (2.2 mg/kg, given every 8 hours) or continuous intravenous infusion has been recommended for treating CNS infections, but use of aminoglycosides potentiates the development of renal toxicity. Although intrathecal administration has been advocated at 6 hour intervals, there is no justification for its use on a clinical or experimental basis. Aminoglycoside that enters the CSF diffuses poorly, which hinders its ability to spread to the entire nervous system. Resistant coliforms frequently are the cause of meningoencephalitis in immunodeficient large animals. Consequently, gentamicin or amikacin often are used, although the prognosis is poor.

Cephalosporins have relatively poor penetration into brain tissue and CSF. Only injectable and toxic cephaloridine has been shown to reach adequate concentrations in the presence of inflammation. Intrathecal therapy is an alternative possibility but not recommended. Some new cephalosporins, such as moxalactam, have been shown to penetrate the CSF in sufficient amounts to eradicate most encountered pathogens. These drugs may frequently fail in the clinical setting despite experimental success. Further, the cost of third generation cephalosporins may be prohibitive in most circumstances.

Sulfonamides and trimethoprim-sulfonamide combinations are extremely effective in penetrating blood-brain and blood–cerebrospinal fluid barriers and, in this regard, are similar to chloramphenicol. Trimethoprim-sulfonamide drugs have a relatively broad spectrum, are bactericidal, and can be used to treat a variety of infections within the CNS, including equine protozoal myeloencephalitis (see Chapter 7).

Metronidazole has been used to treat meningitis caused by anaerobic pathogens.[57] It is effective because it is bactericidal and diffuses in high concentration into all tissues, including the CNS and CSF. However, leukopenia may be a transient side effect following its administration.

Other antibiotics such as tetracycline and erythromycin have limited penetration into the CSF; they are rarely used because they are bacteriostatic, have a narrow spectrum of activity, and are frequently toxic at the doses employed. Lipid soluble tetracycline derivatives such as minocycline are more effective in treating CNS infections, although they have a relatively narrow spectrum of activity. Rifampin is a bacteriostatic antibiotic that penetrates CNS tissues and CSF and has been combined with isoniazid for the treatment of mycobacterial infections in the CNS.

An appropriate antibiotic choice and dosage regimen for treating various CNS infections are presented in Tables 15–5 and 15–6, respectively. Gram positive infections are initially treated with intravenous penicillin. Penicillinase-resistant organisms are treated with a resistant penicillin derivative or chloramphenicol. Gram-negative infections are treated with intravenous ampicillin or amoxicillin. Aminoglycosides can be used in combination. Chloramphenicol can be substituted if penicillin derivatives fail. Anaerobic infections should respond to penicillin, chloramphenicol, or metronidazole. Cephalosporins, other than moxalactam, should be used only as a last resort.

Bactericidal and bacteriostatic agents should not be combined. Studies with experimental meningitis demonstrated a marked reduction in the efficacy of penicillin when used in combination with tetracycline. Combination gentamicin-chloromycetin therapy has been recommended, even though chloromycetin is known to antagonize the bactericidal effect of genta-

Table 15–6. DOSAGES OF ANTIMICROBIAL DRUGS FOR CENTRAL NERVOUS SYSTEM INFECTIONS

Drug	Dose	Route	Frequency (hours)
Penicillin, aqueous	$10–20 \times 10^3$ U/kg	IV	4–6
Ampicillin	5–10 mg/kg	IV	6
Oxacillin	20 mg/kg	PO, IV	4–8
Gentamicin*	2 mg/kg	IV	8
Chloramphenicol	10–15 mg/kg	IV	4–6
Cephalexin*	20 mg/kg	PO	8
Cephapirin*	20 mg/kg	IV	8
Amphotericin B	0.15–0.25 mg/kg	IV	48
Flucytosine	50 mg/kg	PO	8
Rifampin	10–20 mg/kg	PO	8–12
Metronidazole	10–15 mg/kg	PO	8
Moxalactam	50 mg/kg	IV	8
Amikacin*	7.5 mg/kg	IV	8

*Poor penetration of CNS, but may be useful for treatment of primary infection.

IV, Intravenous; PO, oral.

Modified from Greene CE: Infections of the central nervous system. In Greene CE (ed): Clinical Microbiology and Infectious Diseases of the Dog and Cat. Philadelphia, WB Saunders Co, 1984, p 284.

micin in vivo. One justified combination is the use of two bactericidal agents such as penicillin and aminoglycosides. Because of their poor penetration, aminoglycosides should never be used alone in treatment of meningitis or intracranial abscessation.

Therapy for mycotic infection of the CNS or CSF most frequently involves amphotericin B. Because it is more practical and less toxic, intravenous therapy is primarily used, although intrathecal therapy has been recommended. Combinations of antimicrobial agents are relatively more effective than single drugs and have been frequently recommended in the treatment of fungal or bacterial meningitis or encephalitis. Flucytosine and amphotericin B have been combined to treat cryptococcosis. Greater efficacy of therapy and a lower incidence of relapse have been noted than with use of either drug alone. These two antifungal drugs have been combined with rifampin to treat histoplasmosis and aspergillosis. Rifampin is widely distributed in the body and reaches high concentration in the CSF. It also is effective against some bacteria. The use of ketoconazole is not recommended as a first choice because of its poor penetration of CNS tissue and CSF.

Intrathecal Therapy

Intrathecal therapy has been advocated in treating bacterial or fungal meningitis. In general, it should never be considered unless in-travenous antimicrobial therapy has failed. A major disadvantage of this therapy in animals is the frequent induction of anesthesia. Intrathecal gentamicin therapy has been recommended for treating meningitis, although the rationale has never been established. Experimental studies in dogs showed a high concentration for 12 to 18 hours with a wide individual range of concentrations.[45] Some bacteria were still cultured from the CSF after therapy was discontinued.

Additional Therapy

Glucocorticoids have been advocated for routine use in the therapy of meningitis in an attempt to minimize the inflammatory process.[7] Their use has been associated with increased morbidity, relapses, and mortality. They may minimize meningeal inflammation, but they also appear to impair host defense mechanisms.

Furthermore, although edema and swelling of the nervous tissue is associated with inflammation of the meninges, it is rarely of a magnitude to cause severe clinical signs. Affected animals usually improve with treatment of the primary infectious process. If they are considered, glucocorticoids should never be administered in the presence of bacterial or fungal meningitis without appropriate simultaneous antimicrobial therapy. In any event, bactericidal rather than bacteriostatic drugs should be used. Doses of glucocorticoids (2 mg/kg of dexamethasone) that have been required in experimental cases to reduce swelling in the nervous system are associated with immunosuppression. They may cause transient improvement in neurologic signs, but clinical deterioration eventually occurs because of spread of infection.

Edema or swelling of the CNS from bacterial or fungal infection is better controlled with osmotic agents than with glucocorticoids. Unfortunately, these cannot be administered on a long-term basis. Intravenous fluid therapy for symptomatic management of cases must be used with caution if cerebral edema is present. Neurologic deficits or permanent sequelae may occur following successful therapy of meningitis. Abscess formation may be the result of localization of a more disseminated infection and may be managed by combining antimicrobial therapy and surgical drainage. The latter requires extensive training in neurosurgery. Abscess formation usually involves anaerobes and as a result is treated with penicillin and chloramphenicol as first choices.

In large animals, meningitis is most often

seen in the neonatal period associated with failure of transfer of maternal immunoglobulin. Consequently, it is paramount in these cases to repair such immunodeficiency if therapy is to succeed.

Monitoring Therapy

Frequent monitoring of therapy for CNS infections has shown that CSF culture and gram stain results are negative and that glucose concentration is normal within 48 hours of initiation of therapy, if it has been successful. Improvement in cerebrospinal fluid protein levels and cytologic findings may lag by several days to weeks as the inflammatory process subsides. Repeated evaluation of the CSF is difficult in animal patients that require anesthesia. It may be possible if intrathecal administration of antibiotics is being performed. The inability to obtain frequent CSF samples means that clinical signs are primarily used to follow the course of therapy. Antimicrobial therapy should continue for at least 3 to 4 weeks following improvement. Some signs of neurologic disease may be permanent because of irreversible parenchymal destruction.

REFERENCES

1. Atkins JM, Wildenthal K, and Horwitz LD: Cardiovascular response to hyperosmotic mannitol in anesthetized and conscious dogs. Am J Physiol 225:132, 1973.
2. Bell WE: Treatment of bacterial infections of the central nervous system. Ann Neurol 9:313, 1981.
3. Brander GC, and Pugh DM: Veterinary Applied Pharmacology and Therapeutics. Philadelphia, Lea & Febiger, 1977.
4. Brock KA and Thurmon JC: Pulmonary edema associated with mannitol administration. Canine Pract 6:31, 1979.
5. Brodie BB, Kurz H, and Schanker LS: The importance of dissociation constant and lipid-solubility in influencing the passage of drugs into cerebrospinal fluid. J Pharmacol Exp Ther 130:20, 1960.
6. Brown S: Personal communication. University of Georgia, Athens, GA, 1984.
7. Bullmore CC and Sevedge JP: Canine meningoencephalitis. J Am Anim Hosp Assoc 14:387, 1978.
8. Calne DB: Therapeutics in Neurology. Oxford, Blackwell Scientific Publications, 1975.
9. Calvert CA and Leifer CE: Salmonellosis in dogs with lymphosarcoma. JAVMA 180:56, 1982.
10. Casey KL: The neurophysiologic basis of pain. Postgrad Med 53:58, 1973.
11. Ellner JJ: Chronic meningitis. In Mandell GL, Douglas, RG, and Bennett JE (ed): Principles and Practice of Infectious Disease. New York, John Wiley & Sons, 1979.
12. Fishman RA: Steroids in the treatment of brain edema. N Engl J Med 306:359, 1982.
13. Franklin RT: The use of glucocorticoids in treating cerebral edema. Comp Cont Ed Pract Vet 6:442, 1984.
14. Gotschlich EC: Bacterial meningitis: The beginning of the end. Am J Med 65:719, 1978.
15. Greene CE: An Experimental Model for Spinal Cord Compression Simulating Intervertebral Disc Protrusion in the Dog. Thesis (MS), Auburn University, Auburn, AL, 1976.
16. Greenlee JE: Anatomic considerations. In Mandell GL, Douglas RG, and Bennett JE (ed): Principles and Practice of Infectious Disease. New York, John Wiley & Sons, 1979.
17. Greenlee JE: Subdural empyema. In Mandell GL, Douglas RG, Bennett JE (ed): Principles and Practice of Infectious Disease. New York, John Wiley & Sons, 1979.
18. Higgins RJ, Vandevelde M, and Braund KG: Internal hydrocephalus and associated periventricular encephalitis in young dogs. Vet Pathol 14:236, 1977.
19. Hoerlein BF, Redding RW, Hoff EJ, and McGuire JA: Evaluation of dexamethasone, DMSO, mannitol, and solcoseryl in acute spinal trauma. J Am Anim Hosp Assoc 19:216, 1983.
20. Hoerlein BF, Redding RW, Hoff EJ, and McGuire JA: Evaluation of naloxone, crocetin, thyrotropin releasing hormone, methylprednisolone, partial myelotomy, and hemilaminectomy in the treatment of acute spinal cord trauma. J Am Anim Hosp Assoc, 21:67, 1985.
21. Hoerlein BF and Spano JS: Non-neurological complications following decompressive spinal cord surgery. Arch Am Coll Vet Surg 4:11, 1975.
22. Hughes HC and Lang CM: Control of pain in dogs and cats. In Kitchell RL and Erickson HH (ed): Animal Pain, Perception and Alleviation. Bethesda, MD, American Physiological Society, 1983.
23. Kalpravidh M, Lumb WV, Wright M, et al: Analgesic effects of butorphanol in horses; Dose response studies. Am J Vet Res 45:211, 1984.
24. Kalpravidh M, Lumb WV, Wright M, et al: Effects of butorphanol, flunixin, levorphanol, morphine, and xylazine in ponies. Am J Vet Res 45:217, 1984.
25. Kelly MJ: Pain. Proc 49th Annu Meet Am Anim Hosp Assoc, 155, 1982.
26. Knecht CD, Henderson B, and Richardson RC: Central nervous system depression associated with glucocorticoid ingestion in a dog. JAVMA 173:91, 1978.
27. Kornegay JN, Lorenz MD, and Zenoble RD: Bacterial meningoencephalitis in two dogs. JAVMA 173:1334, 1978.
28. Kramer PW, Griffith RS, and Campbell RL: Antibiotic penetration of the brain, a comparative study. J Neurosurg 31:295, 1969.
29. Leonard JL and Redding RW: Effects of hypertonic solutions on cerebrospinal fluid pressure in the lateral ventricle of the dog. Am J Vet Res 34:213, 1973.
30. Losacco CL and Miner WS: Pentazocine lactate for relief of pain in dogs. Vet Med Small Anim Clin 79:183, 1984.
31. Marshall LF, King J, and Langfitt TW: The complications of high-dose corticosteroid therapy in neurosurgical patients: A prospective study. Ann Neurol 1:201, 1977.
32. Marshall LF, Smith RW, and Shapiro HM: The outcome with aggressive treatment in severe head injuries. Part II: Acute and chronic barbiturate administration in the management of head injury. J Neurosurg 50:26, 1979.

33. Mayer DJ and Price DD: Central nervous mechanisms of analgesia. Pain 2:379, 1976.

34. McCracken GH: Dosage of ampicillin in the treatment of bacterial meningitis. J Pediatr 90:670, 1977.

35. Melzack R and Wall PD: Pain mechanisms: A new theory. Science 150:971, 1965.

36. Meyer RD: Brain abscess. *In* Mandell GL, Douglas RG, and Bennett JE (ed): Principles and Practice of Infectious Disease. New York, John Wiley & Sons, 1979.

37. Oliver JE Jr and Greene CE: Diseases of the brain. *In* Ettinger SJ: Textbook of Veterinary Internal Medicine, 2nd ed. Philadelphia, WB Saunders Co, 1983.

38. Oliver JE Jr and Lorenz MD: Handbook of Veterinary Neurologic Diagnosis. Philadelphia, WB Saunders Co, 1983.

39. Overturf GD, Steinberg EA, Underman AE, et al: Comparative trial of carbenicillin and ampicillin therapy for purulent meningitis. Antimicrob Agents Chemother 11:420, 1977.

40. Pappius HM and McCann WP: Effects of steroids on cerebral edema in cats. Arch Neurol 20:207, 1969.

41. Parent J: Effects of dexamethasone on pancreatic tissue and on serum amylase and lipase activities in dogs. JAVMA 180:743, 1982.

42. Parker AJ: Blood pressure changes and lethality of mannitol infusions in dogs. Am J Vet Res 34:1523, 1973.

43. Parker AJ, Park RD, and Stowater JL: Reduction of trauma-induced edema of spinal cord in dogs given mannitol. Am J Vet Res 34:1355, 1973.

44. Parkhouse J, Pleuvry BJ, and Rees, JMH: Analgesic Drugs. Oxford, Blackwell Scientific Publications, 1979.

45. Rahal JJ, Hyams PJ, Simberkoff MS, et al.: Combined intrathecal and intramuscular gentamicin for gram-negative meningitis. N Engl J Med 290:1394, 1974.

46. Sage MR: Review: Blood-brain barrier: Phenomenon of increasing importance to imaging. Am J Radiol 138:887, 1982.

47. Sande MA: Antibiotic therapy of bacterial meningitis: Lessons we've learned. Am J Med 71:507, 1981.

48. Saper JR and Yosselson S: Raised intracranial pressure. Postgrad Med 57:89, 1975.

49. Sato O, Hara M, Asai T, et al: The effect of dexamethasone phosphate on the production rate of cerebrospinal fluid in the spinal subarachnoid space of dogs. J Neurosurg 39:480, 1973.

50. Simeone FA, Frazer G, and Lawner P: Ischemic brain edema: Comparative effects of barbiturates and hypothermia. Stroke 10:8, 1979.

51. Sims MA: *Flavobacterium meningosepticum*: A probable cause of meningitis in a cat. Vet Rec 95:567, 1974.

52. Sims MH and Redding RW: The use of dexamethasone in the prevention of cerebral edema in dogs. J Am Anim Hosp Assoc 11:439, 1975.

53. Sorjonen DC, Dillon AR, Powers RD, et al: Effects of dexamethasone and surgical hypotension on the stomach of dogs: Clinical endoscopic and pathologic evaluations. Am J Vet Res 44:1233, 1983.

54. Spinelli JS and Enos LR: Drugs in Veterinary Practice. St Louis, CV Mosby Co, 1978.

55. Stowe CM: Analgesic drugs. JAVMA 158:789, 1971.

56. Toombs JP, Caywood DD, Lipowitz AJ, et al: Colonic perforation following neurosurgical procedures and corticosteroid therapy in four dogs. JAVMA 177:68, 1980.

57. Warner JF, Perkins RL, and Cordero L: Metronidazole therapy of anaerobic bacteremia, meningitis, and brain abscess. Arch Intern Med 139:167, 1979.

58. White RP, Hagen AA, and Robertson JT: Effect of nonsteroidal anti-inflammatory drugs on subarachnoid hemorrhage in dogs. J Neurosurg 51:164, 1979.

59. Wilkinson HA, Wepsic JG, and Austin G: Diuretic synergy in the treatment of acute experimental cerebral edema. J Neurosurg 34:203, 1971.

60. Withrow CD and Woodbury DM: Some aspects of the pharmacology of adrenal steroids and the central nervous system. *In* Reulen HJ and Scheerman K (ed): Steroids and Brain Edema. New York, Springer Verlag, 1972.

61. Yoxall AT: Pain in small animals, its recognition and control. ILAR News 25:16, 1981.

Chapter 16

CD Knecht, VMD, MS

Principles of Neurosurgery

The surgical treatment of disorders of the nervous system is within the province of the practicing veterinarian who is willing to learn the anatomic and physiologic peculiarities of the nervous system, to develop thorough techniques in neurologic and neuroradiographic examinations, to maintain strict asepsis in surgery, and to practice the surgical approaches.[18–20, 32] Some cases require special diagnostic tests, such as electroencephalography, electromyography, sensory or motor nerve conduction studies, and cerebrospinal fluid analysis, or require a surgical procedure so rarely done in practice as to prohibit competency. These should be handled at an approximate referral center.

The brain and spinal cord are soft, friable tissues supported by relatively weak connective tissue called neuroglia but surrounded by the meninges and by rigid osseous cranium and vertebrae, respectively.[10] The central nervous system has a good blood supply receiving 15% of total cardiac output, but is sensitive to oxygen deficiency. The oxygen consumption by the brain is estimated at 20 times that required for resting muscle per unit weight.[22]

Although the CNS is vascular, most neural tissue is protected from rapid alterations in environment by the blood-brain barrier. The barrier not only is protective but also may prevent chemotherapeutic agents from reaching the CNS in effective levels. Aseptic techniques are therefore essential in neurosurgery. If antibotics are needed, those that penetrate the blood-brain barrier should be used (see Chapter 15). The CNS is further protected by cerebrospinal fluid that acts as a cushion for the delicate tissues.

The CNS is sensitive to derangement of physiologic function, particularly as a result of edema and/or ischemia caused by accidental or iatrogenic trauma.[2] Severe or prolonged edema may result in herniation of parts of the brain or central necrosis of the spinal cord. Regrowth of CNS neurons, although demonstrated in experimental studies in neonates, is minimal in postneonates. Attempts to stimulate return of function using "deblocking" anticholinesterase drugs such as eserine and galanthamine, although reported favorably in the Russian literature, have not been effective for Western investigators.[24] Drugs used to facilitate neurotransmitter activity have improved recovery from behavior disorders.

Reactive synaptogenesis and silent synapses have also been suggested as factors in recovery of function following injury to the CNS, but the observed synaptogenesis has not been associated with marked improvement in function. Lastly, diaschisis, a relatively short-term suspension of function in neural tissue adjacent to, and in some instances distant from, the site of injury (likened to neural shock), may cause life threatening dysfunction of the CNS.[24, 41]

In view of the response of CNS tissue, unnecessary manipulation and resection should be avoided[25] and necessary procedures performed with a minimum of manipulation and distortion of the CNS. Even peripheral nerves, which do regrow, will be prevented from effective reinnervation by malalignment, interposition of adjacent tissues, and excessive trauma.

ANESTHESIA

The considerations for anesthesia in patients with lesions of the nervous system are similar to those for soft tissue or orthopedic surgery.

408

Total muscle relaxation, excluding the muscles of respiration; profound analgesia; and adequate oxygenation and ventilation are required. Local anesthetics are rarely indicated in neurosurgery.

Preanesthetic agents include anticholinergics, narcotics, and tranquilizers. The first are used to reduce parasympathetic stimulation and resultant- salivation, regurgitation, and bradycardia. Phenothiazine tranquilizers reduce the dose of barbiturate required for anesthesia induction and help prevent cardiac arrhythmia but are contraindicated for myelography or a history of seizures. Diazepam is the preferred drug for sedation or preanesthesia in these patients. Narcotics such as oxymorphone may be used in certain patients without detriment to the central nervous system. Neither tranquilizers nor narcotics should be administered while monitoring patients during diagnosis or therapy because they depress the central nervous system and mask neurologic signs.

Although pentobarbital appears to enhance cerebral cortical blood flow following prolonged cerebral bypass and resuscitation,[46] slow detoxification and elimination, and therefore prolonged depression of cardiopulmonary and neurologic function, prohibits its use for general anesthesia.[15] Short acting barbiturates are used for cerebrospinal fluid collection and for induction of general anesthesia, but the trachea should be intubated to ensure a patent airway.

Inhalant anesthetics such as methoxyflurane or halothane and nitrous oxide are appropriate for most other procedures.[11, 33] Increased intracranial (CSF) pressure results from halothane and possibly methoxyflurane. For this reason, some neurosurgeons avoid halogenated hydrocarbons in patients with cranial trauma or those being subjected to craniotomy. Nevertheless, use of these inhalant agents is generally considered appropriate in neurosurgery.[33, 37] Nitrous oxide facilitates anesthesia induction without barbiturates and enhances muscle relaxation and analgesia; however, it can increase intracranial pressure and is generally contraindicated in the patient with cranial trauma.[11] Nitrous oxide also reduces motor nerve conduction velocity and is contraindicated for electrodiagnostic testing.

A combination of narcotic analgesics, neuromuscular blocking agents, and controlled ventilation is preferred by some for craniotomy and for anesthesia following cranial trauma. Although such combinations provide benefits, control of the patient's status requires an anesthetist experienced in their use; thus they are best avoided for neurosurgery without a veterinary anesthesiologist. Cranial trauma is unique in that, as in encephalitis, the blood-brain barrier may be altered and permeability to barbiturates and other drugs increased. In general, it is not necessary to avoid short acting barbiturates for anesthesia induction and endotracheal intubation, but the intravenous injection should be given slowly and with careful observation of the depth of anesthesia.

The previous use of glucocorticosteroids in the treatment of intervertebral disk disease may affect liver function and elevate levels of serum enzymes, such as alanine aminotransferase (ALT, SGPT). Elevated levels of this enzyme, particularly when accompanied by neutrophilia, lymphopenia, and eosinopenia, indicates probable response to glucocorticosteroids in such patients. The functional capacity of the liver should be further tested if surgery can be delayed. If surgery cannot be delayed, induction of anesthesia without barbiturates using a mask or induction chamber is preferred.

Glucocorticosteroid treatment may also cause elevated serum lipase concentration, which is not necessarily indicative of pancreatitis.[39]

MONITORING THE PATIENT

Animals with spinal cord lesions are often subjected to a single, long anesthetic procedure for radiography, electromyography, myelography, and surgery to avoid repeated anesthesia and to effect early decompression. The duration of anesthesia is likely to encourage acidosis if ventilation is not assisted and the patient is not monitored carefully. Such prolonged anesthetic times may be intolerable for large animal patients. In tetraplegic animals, respiratory assistance is mandatory because of the effect of prolonged anesthesia on the thoracic musculature. Flaccidity of the abdominal musculature and pressures applied by the surgeon during decompression of the spinal cord may also decrease effective respiration. If the tests are available, blood gas tensions should be monitored every 30 to 60 minutes and adjusted by respiratory assistance and intravenous administration of sodium bicarbonate as indicated.

Respiratory assistance is no less important in cranial trauma, which is frequently accompanied by CNS depression, reduced respiratory minute volume, and increased acidosis. Sodium bicarbonate should not be used presumptively in such patients because the cerebral vasculature is responsive to carbon dioxide rather than to oxygen deficiency. An excess of sodium bicarbonate may reduce the apparent need to maintain increased vascular flow and result in secondary hypoxia and paradoxic acidosis. Hypoxia increases cerebral edema; hyperoxygenation reduces it. Similarly, intravenous calcium should be avoided because it tends to reduce effective cerebral cortical blood flow.[46]

It may be difficult to judge the depth of anesthesia by physical means in patients with brain disease or those undergoing surgical approach to the cranium or cervical vertebrae. Observation of pupillary and corneal responses, eye position, jaw tone, and swallowing may be difficult in the latter because of draping and be unreliable in diseases that reduce these signs. Electrocardiographic, electroencephalographic, blood pressure, and auditory monitors of the heart beat and respiration are particularly useful in these patients.

A discussion of the mechanisms and treatment of shock is not germane in this text. However, capillary refill, pulse rate, and pressure should be monitored carefully. Body temperature should be maintained within normal limits by water heating pads and effective table draping. Every animal undergoing major surgery should have the benefits of balanced fluid and crystalloid administration through an indwelling intravenous catheter but should not be overly hydrated.

PATIENT POSITIONING

The animal should be placed in a position that is convenient and comfortable for the surgeon and safe for the patient. In vertebral surgery, the animal should neither be stretched nor have the torso distorted or the limbs abducted strongly. Muscle fatigue results quickly in patients with the limbs firmly distracted in an attempt to maintain sternal or ventral recumbency.

Sandbags or towels may be placed lateral to the thorax with the patient in ventral or dorsal recumbency, or dorsal to the neck with the animal in dorsal recumbency. Ventral approaches to the cervical vertebrae are facilitated by extension of the neck. However, the amount of extension should be kept to a minimum in conditions in which extension causes increased pressure on the spinal cord. These include type II disk protrusions and most of the cervical vertebral malformation-malarticulation syndromes in both dogs and horses. Padding should not be placed under the abdomen to facilitate

the approach for laminectomy or hemilaminectomy with the animal in ventral recumbency.[8, 12, 27, 31, 35, 42] Abdominal padding combines with the pressure exerted by the surgeon to cause the following: reduced motion of the diaphragm; reduced venous return via the postcava; increased venous return via the vertebral venous plexus and, therefore, increased hemorrhage at the operative site; reduced urinary output because of pressure on the renal blood vessels and on the ureters; and increased likelihood of esophageal reflux. A heavy pad under the patient in lateral recumbency for prophylactic fenestration should be of minimal volume and exert minimal pressure on the dorsally placed lateral abdomen for the same reasons.

In recent years, trephination of the vertebral arches has been replaced by dissection and disarticulation of the articular processes in hemilaminectomy. Because the laminae are closely apposed at this point, the spinous process is elevated with towel clamps or forceps to open the articulation and the laminae are then dissected with rongeurs. Unfortunately, this maneuver also narrows the ventral intervertebral disk space, creating pressure ventrally to encourage extrusion of the remaining nucleus. Elevation should therefore be minimal, using only moderate tension and smooth motions. The procedure should never be used to approach a possible fracture or fracture luxation unless the cord and surrounding bone can be adequately visualized to be sure that spinal cord damage is not caused by the procedure.

In cranial surgery, the head should be slightly

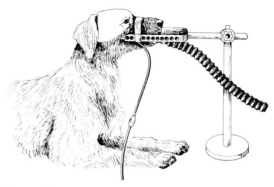

Figure 16–1. A device designed to stabilize the head in an elevated position for cranial surgery. The device allows for adjustments in height, as well as any oblique position of the head. This position inhibits cerebral venous congestion, edema, and subsequent brain swelling that could occur if the head were in a lower position. It also inhibits pressure on the jugular vein, which tends to raise venous pressure owing to impaired venous drainage.

elevated to reduce venous pressure, promote adequate drainage of fluids, provide easy access to the operative area, and allow the anesthetist access to the mouth. Figure 16–1 illustrates a simple device that can be used to accomplish adequate positioning of the patient. It is also useful for radiography of the head, especially ventriculography.[13]

INSTRUMENTS AND EQUIPMENT

The surgical packs used in neurosurgery are far from standard. The types of instruments differ for peripheral nerve anastomosis, hemilaminectomy and laminectomy, vertebral fusion, and craniotomy. Individual instruments among types differ because of the preference and experience of the surgeon. Many are depicted in standard surgical texts.[16, 20, 40] The surgical packs used by the neurosurgeon (Table 16–1) appear redundant and costly to the experienced practitioner who confines his or her neurosurgery to decompression of the thoracolumbar spinal cord and cervical fenestration. In this latter instance, the pack may include specialized rongeurs, a large bore hypodermic needle or claw dental scraper, self-retaining retractors (Gelpi), instruments for accomplishing adequate lavage and suction, and drapes and an optional trephine. Such a pack is relatively inexpensive but provides minimal latitude for complications or special techniques.

In addition to the standard surgical instruments an adequate method for lavage and controlled suction is mandatory to keep the neural tissue moist and to remove blood clots. The suction should be controllable so that excess negative pressure does not trap neural tissue and should not be applied to the brain or cord without interposed saline irrigated cotton flannel. An electrosurgical unit is also helpful to control the hemorrhage from small vessels. The unit should have a wide range of controls of output and should provide coagulation, as well as cutting currents.[9] Electrocoagulation of small vessels adjacent to nerves should be completed with minimal output and duration to prevent damage to the adjacent neural tissue. Bipolar coagulation is preferred around neural tissue.

Table 16–1. TYPICAL NEUROSURGERY INSTRUMENTS

General Soft Tissue Surgery	Hemilaminectomy
2 Scalpel handles (#3)	1 Stille-Ruskin double action rongeur
1 Adson thumb forceps	1 Lempert double action rongeur, very small
12 Backhaus towel clamp, 3¼″	2 Gelpi retractors
8 Halsted mosquito forceps	1 Periosteal elevator, thin
2 Allis tissue forceps	1 Curet, size 000
1 Metzenbaum scissors	2 Frazier suction tips, #80 Fr, #10 Fr
1 Mayo scissors	2 Claw-type tartar scrapers
1 Suture cutting scissors	1 14 gauge needle, straight with stylet
1 Saline bowl	1 14 gauge needle, curved with stylet
1 Senn hand retractor	Bulb syringe
1 Needle holder	2 Cloth towels
4 Disposable drapes	
	Optional
	1 Michele trephine
	1 Love-Kerrison bone forceps
	1 Stryker or Hall air drill
	1 Micrometer trephine—for toy dogs and cats
	Equine instruments (see Chapter 17)
Peripheral Nerve Surgery	**Craniotomy**
1 Small ophthalmic needle holder	1 Craniotome, Stryker, or 3 M drill
1 Jeweler's forceps	2 Handles for wire saw
1 Adson forceps, 1 × 2 teeth	1 Wire saw
1 Small, blunt pointed, curved scissors	1 Groove director
Razor blades	1 Dural scissors
Wooden tongue depressors	2 Dural hooks
Surgical sponges, lint free	1 Ophthalmic needle holder
	1 Iris scissors
	1 Iris forceps
	1 Frazier suction tip
	Cotton flannel (Cottonoid)
	Bone wax
	Silver or stainless steel vessel clips

Hemorrhage is not unique to neurosurgery, but the methods of hemostasis are. Although large vessels should be avoided, small vessels and venous sinuses may be damaged during dissection or manipulation. Meningeal vessels may be ligated with 6–0 silk ligatures or other nonreactive suture material, or with small silver or stainless steel clips carefully applied. Capillary hemorrhage from the brain parenchyma, muscles, and other tissues may be controlled with bipolar electrocoagulation. Cotton flannel is used with copious saline irrigation to control surface hemorrhage and to promote clotting. Similarly, methylcellulose gel is used for venous sinus bleeding and is removed after clotting occurs. Bone wax may be pressed into bone marrow after craniotomy, laminectomy, or vertebral body slotting to stop medullary hemorrhage. All hemorrhage adjacent to the nervous system should be controlled before the tissues are closed.

A large number of towel clamps are necessary for adequate towelling-in and to fix the electroscalpel and surgical suction to drapes. Gelpi retractors are frequently used in lieu of laminectomy retractors because they provide adequate exposure with the moderate length of incision made in small animals. A ball stop on the tines of the retractor will reduce penetration, but care is needed to prevent accidental damage to vessels, nerves, and, in the cervical region, viscera. A Frazier laminectomy retractor is useful in ventral cervical approaches in the dog. (For more details on instruments for large animal procedures, see Chapter 17 and reference 40.

The type of rongeur used varies with the surgeon. The small Lempert rongeurs are excellent for small dogs and cats but are easily damaged by use on thick or dense bone. In larger breeds and in ventral cervical decompression, Love-Kerrison bone cutting forceps of appropriate large (6–8 mm) and small (2–3 mm) sizes, respectively, are beneficial. The latter should have the thinnest foot available. Double action Stille-Ruskin or Beyer rongeurs are the most versatile instruments for vertebral surgery.

Several companies supply air drills.* The equipment should be high speed and air or nitrogen driven. Conversions are available for craniotomy and for orthopedic use. Available burs should include a 3 to 4 mm pineapple and a 1.5 to 2 mm round and should not be reused

---

*Stryker, Zimmer Co, Warsaw, IN; 3M, Santa Barbara, CA.

or overused because of the heat created by a dull bur.

CEREBRAL EDEMA

Heat is only one form of iatrogenic trauma that result in edema of the CNS. Direct trauma during manipulation and ischemia are common causes. The effects of edema of the CNS are frequently profound. The brain is enclosed in a nonyielding bony vault, which limits expansion. Increases in the parenchymal compartment must be compensated by reduction in the vascular, subarachnoid, and ventricular compartments. Any increase beyond the limits of compensation is likely to result in ischemia and in herniation of the occipital cortex ventral to the tentorium cerebelli and the cerebellum through the foramen magnum. Edema is best prevented by minimizing trauma and hypoxia. Edema is treated by hyperventilation, particularly hyperoxygenation, by administration of glucocorticosteroids and hyperosmolar agents, and by positioning.[5, 10, 13, 26, 28, 29, 34, 35]

Hyperventilation is used to prevent and treat cerebral edema during and following craniotomy. The procedure involves an increase of 25 to 50% in total minute volume by artificial respiration and increased inspiratory volume at approximately 15 breaths per minute with an inhalant high in oxygen concentration. The arterial blood pressure remains within normal limits during hyperventilation, provided sufficient time is permitted for expiration.

Aspiration from the basal cisterns or through cottonoid applied to the external brain parenchyma will facilitate the removal of fluid during craniotomy. Maintenance of slight end expiratory positive pressure until the endotracheal tube is removed and a high oxygen environment following removal of the tube will also help prevent cerebral edema and may help avert pulmonary edema.

Glucocorticoids, hyperosmolar agents, and other methods of treating edema of the CNS are discussed in Chapter 15.

Lavage of the spinal cord with ice slush made from lactated Ringer's solution has been advocated[1, 3, 4, 23, 44, 45, 49] in prolonged and routine decompressive procedures. The purpose is to reduce the blood flow and metabolic needs of the traumatized tissue and to reduce the postsurgical inflammation through local hypothermia. Nevertheless, Tator and Deecke,[43] using Elliott's B solution, concluded that normothermic and hypothermic solutions were equally efficacious in treating moderately traumatized spinal cords and normothermic lavage was more effective in treating severely traumatized spinal cords. The explanation for this remains unknown, but the studies suggest that normothermic lavage is beneficial and, more important, that copious lavage with physiologic solutions is an important part of surgery to decompress the spinal cord.

Regional and total body hypothermia are used in selected neurosurgical procedures in humans but require a trained team and intensive monitoring and are fraught with complications.

POSTOPERATIVE CARE

Vertebral immobilization is rarely needed after fenestration or decompression of the vertebral column in small animals. A firm bandage should be applied for 2 to 3 days to lessen discomfort and edema and reduce unnecessary and possibly traumatic movements. Effective immobilization is indicated for 7 to 14 days after internal fixation of fractures and luxations of the vertebral column and for longer times when internal fixation is not required or not possible. An external cast or splint may also be applied[20] if any combination of two of the three joint surfaces of one intervertebral articulation (articular processes and vertebral body) are removed or weakened during surgery. Internal fixation usually should also be applied.

The primary postoperative concerns include care of urinary function and physical therapy. Urine retention and secondary urinary tract infection are common in paraplegic animals. The urinary bladder should be emptied at least three times daily by manual expression, catheterization, and, in the case of large animals, promotion to rise and void urine. Cystocentesis has been advocated, but the use of repeated cystocentesis alternating with attempts at manual expression of the urinary bladder increases the possibility of urinary bladder rupture. Leakage may occur from cystocentesis punctures in the neurogenic bladder.

Some paraplegic patients develop reflex bladder function in 5 to 7 days. In these patients, a volume of urine may be expelled in response to bladder expansion with urine or to manual pressure. The false impression of effective voluntary urination can be dispelled by determination of bladder volume by palpation at the end of urination. In dogs, if more than 10 ml of urine is retained, then the urination is not adequate and manual expression should be continued.

Pulsed urine flow may also be misinterpreted as voluntary urination. The combination of overflow incontinence and "spurts" of urine, particularly during manual expression of the bladder, is common 7 to 14 days after the occurrence of lesions in the sacrum or pelvic plexus. The spurts result from bladder wall contraction without central enhancement or inhibition. The volume of urine expelled is always small, and the volume retained is excessive. More commonly, pulsatile flow is caused by uninhibited contractions of the urethra in upper motor neuron (UMN) lesions, especially in male dogs.

It may be difficult to express the bladder in some paraplegic animals. This form of dyssynergia results from centrally or peripherally mediated parasympathetic deficit and persistent urethral tone. The latter appears to be the result of α-adrenergic stimulation of the urethral continence zone and somatic innervation of the striated muscle, which is released from UMN control.[6, 17] Excessive urethral tone can be reduced with α-adrenergic blocking agents such as phenoxybenzamine[17, 27] (see Chapter 13).

Frequent and thorough emptying of the urinary bladder should be combined with frequent bathing to prevent urine scalding and systemic antibiotics to prevent or treat urinary tract infections. Should bladder function be adequate in the paretic patient, antibiotic therapy is not indicated.

Enemas or physical rectal evacuation should be used as needed to treat fecal retention.

Physical therapy should include passive manipulation of the paretic limbs in a full range of motion and encouragement of volitional activity. Active and passive motions should be encouraged in a water bath, whirlpool, or sling support until the animal takes a few steps. Whirlpool therapy is particularly useful because it facilitates passive movement, encourages active movement by reducing weightbearing on paretic limbs, reduces muscle spasticity, and cleanses the skin, reducing urine scalding and the tendency to decubital ulcers. Physical therapy should be given for 5 to 10 minutes at least two or three times daily. Whirlpool therapy should be delayed for 2 to 3 days after surgery, and the incision should be covered with collodion. Urination and defecation should be encouraged before the animal is placed in the bath. An effective and safe germicide, such as povidone-iodine or chlorhexidine, should be used routinely in the whirlpool.

Mock walking with the pelvic limbs and trunk supported by a towel placed under the abdomen, or the caudal body supported by the tail, helps to encourage walking. This should not replace hydrotherapy in small animals but can be an effective adjunct to therapy. Encouraging free exercise on grass or other nontraumatic surface is also valuable. Some clinicians use a paraplegic cart* during recovery.[38] The mobility achieved without use of the paretic limbs may be counterproductive by reducing the desire of some patients to walk normally.

Other forms of physical therapy include diathermy, heating pads, warm towels applied to the incision area, and ultrasound. None is curative, but the proper use of each may add to the physical comfort of the patient.

Every effort should be made to prevent decubital ulcers. These are common on bony prominences, such as the shoulder, hip, elbow, stifle, and hock, in paralyzed animals. Healing with any treatment is slow and rarely complete until the animal can stand and walk. All paraplegic animals should be placed on soft clean bedding, such as deep straw or synthetic sheepskin,† placed on an elevated grating, if possible. With or without grating, soiled bedding should be replaced promptly and the skin kept scrupulously clean. Quadriplegic animals may be placed in a sling for 2 to 4 hours daily to reduce ulceration and encourage motor activity. Bandaging techniques using combination circumferential, ring, and stint bandages, and foam rubber padding, have been described[18, 40] and should be used on the pressure points of all large paralyzed patients.

Lastly, patients should be observed for signs of gastrointestinal distress and laminitis (horses), particularly if glucocorticosteroids have been used. Vomiting and diarrhea should be treated promptly and vigorously and a normal state of hydration maintained.

---

*K-9 Cart Company, Berwyn, PA.

†Decub-a-rest Pads, American Hospital Supply, McGaw Park, IL.

REFERENCES

1. Albin MS, White RJ, Acosta-Rua G, and Yashon D: Study of functional recovery produced by delayed localized cooling after spinal cord injury in primates. J Neurosurg 29:113, 1968.
2. Anderson DK, et al: Susceptibility of feline spinal cord energy metabolism to severe, incomplete ischemia. Neurology 33:722, 1983.
3. Bouzarth WF, Kazi KH, Bubelin J, and Shenki HA: Effect of temperature upon craniocerebral trauma. JAMA 199:567, 1967.
4. Brasmer TH and Lumb WV: Lumbar vertebral prosthesis in the dog. Am J Vet Res 33:493, 1973.
5. Chasen RA, Cooke PM, Pandolfi S, et al: Hypertonic urea in experimental cerebral edema. Arch Neurol 12:424, 1965.
6. Elbadawi A and Schenk E: New theory of innervation of bladder musculature. IV. Innervation of vesicourethral junction and external urethral sphincter. J Urol 111:613, 1974.
7. Faden AI, Jacob TP, Smith MT, and Holaday TW: Comparison of thyrotropin releasing factor (TRH), naloxone, and dexamethasone treatment in experimental spinal surgery. Neurology 33:673, 1983.
8. Gage ED: Modification in dorsolateral hemilaminectomy and disc fenestration in the dog. J Am Anim Hosp Assoc 11:407, 1975.
9. Greene JA and Knecht CD: Electrosurgery. A review. J Vet Surg 9:27, 1980.
10. Guyton AC: Textbook of Medical Physiology, 7th ed. Philadelphia, WB Saunders Co, 1985.
11. Henriksen HT and Jorgensen PB: Effect of nitrous oxide on intracranial pressure in patients with intracranial disorders. In Yearbook of Anesthesia. Chicago, Year Book Medical Publishers, 1974.
12. Hoerlein BF: The treatment of intervertebral disc protrusions in the dog. Proc Am Vet Med Assoc 206, 1952.
13. Hoerlein BF: Canine Neurology, 3rd ed. Philadelphia WB Saunders Co, 1978.
14. Hoerlein BF, Redding RW, Hoff EJ, and McGuire JA: Evaluation of dexamethasone, DMSO, mannitol and solcoseryl in acute spinal cord trauma. J Am Anim Hosp Assoc 19:216, 1983.
15. Homburger F, Himwich WA, Etstein B, et al: Effect of Pentothal anesthesia on canine cerebral cortex. Am J Physiol 147:343, 1946.
16. Hurov L: Handbook of Veterinary Surgical Instruments and Glossary of Surgical Terms. Philadelphia, WB Saunders Co, 1978.
17. Khanna OP, Heber D, and Gonick P: Cholinergic and adrenergic neuroreceptors in urinary tract of female dogs. J Urol 5:616, 1975.
18. Knecht CD: Results of delayed hemilaminectomy in intervertebral disc protrusion. J Am Anim Hosp Assoc 7:346, 1971.
19. Knecht CD: Results of surgical treatment for thoracolumbar disc protrusion. J Small Anim Pract 13:449, 1972.
20. Knecht CD, Allen AR, William DJ, and Johnson JH: Fundamental Techniques in Veterinary Surgery, 2nd ed. Philadelphia, WB Saunders Co, 1981.
21. Long DM, Hartman JF, and French DA: The response of human cerebral edema to glucosteroid administration. Neurology 16:521, 1966.
22. Luhan JA: Neurology, A Concise Clinical Textbook. Baltimore, Williams & Wilkins Co, 1968.
23. Lumb WV and Brasmer TH: Improved spinal plates and hypothermia as adjuncts to spinal surgery. JAVMA 157:338, 1970.
24. Luria AR, Nayden VL, Tretkova LS, and Vinarskaya EN: Restoration of higher cortical function following local brain damage. In Vinken PJ and Bryn GW: Handbook of Clinical Neurology 3. Amsterdam, Holland, Elsevier, 1969, p 368–443.
25. Martin JG: The feasibility of delayed surgery in intervertebral disc protrusion causing paraplegia and paresis. 36th Annu Sci Proc Am Anim Hosp Assoc 423, 1969.

26. Matson DD: Treatment of cerebral swelling. N Engl J Med 272:626, 1965.
27. Moreau PM: Neurogenic disorders of micturition in the dog and cat. Comp Cont Ed Pract Vet 4:12, 1982.
28. Oliver JE Jr: Canine Cranial Surgery. Thesis, Auburn University, Auburn, AL, 1966.
29. Oliver JE Jr: Surgical approaches to the canine brain. Am J Vet Res 29:353, 1978.
30. Parker AJ: Blood pressure changes and lethality of mannitol infusions in dogs. Am J Vet Res 34:1523, 1973.
31. Prata RG: Neurosurgical treatment of thoracolumbar disks: The rationale and value of laminectomy with concomitant disk removal. J Am Anim Hosp Assoc 17:17, 1981.
32. Redding RW: Laminectomy in the dog. Am J Vet Res 12:123, 1951.
33. Sawyer DC: The Practice of Small Animal Anesthesia. Philadelphia, WB Saunders Co, 1982.
34. Sims MH and Redding RW: The use of dexamethasone in prevention of cerebral edema in dogs. J Am Anim Hosp Assoc 1975.
35. Shenkin HA, Goluboff B, and Hoft H: The use of mannitol for the reduction of intracranial pressure in intracranial surgery. J Neurosurg 19:897, 1962.
36. Shores A: Intervertebral disc syndrome in the dog. Part III. Thoracolumbar surgery. Comp Cont Ed Pract Vet 4:1, 1983.
37. Short CE: Clinical Veterinary Anesthesia. St Louis, CV Mosby Co, 1974.
38. Short TR: Experiences with a mobile support for paraplegic dogs. JAVMA 152:973, 1968.
39. Sorjonen DC, Dillon RA, Powers RD, and Spano, JJ: Effects of dexamethasone and surgical hypotension on the stomach of dogs: Clinical, endoscopic, and pathologic evaluations Am J Vet Res 44:1233, 1983.
40. Stashak TS and Mayhew IG: Neurosurgical procedures. In Jennings PB (ed): The Practice of Large Animal Surgery. Philadelphia, WB Saunders Co, 1984.
41. Stricker E and Zigmond M: Recovery of fundamental damage to control catecholamine containing neurons. In Sprague JM and Epstein AN (ed): Progress in Psychobiology and Physiological Psychology. New York, Academic Press, 1976, p 121.
42. Swaim SF: Ventral decompression of the cervical spinal cord in the dog. JAVMA 162:276, 1973.
43. Tator CH and Deecke L: Value of normothermic perfusion and durotomy in the treatment of experimental acute spinal cord trauma. J Neurosurg 39:52, 1973.
44. Trotter EJ: Modified dorsal laminectomy and selective regional spinal cord hypothermia in the treatment of thoracolumbar disk disease. In Bojrab MJ (ed): Current Techniques in Small Animal Surgery I. Philadelphia, Lea & Febiger, 1975.
45. Trotter EJ, Brasmer TH, and deLahunta A: Modified deep dorsal laminectomy in the dog. Cornell Vet 65:402, 1975.
46. White BC, et al.: Effects of flunarizine on canine cerebral cortical blood flow and vascular resistance post cardiac arrest. Ann Emerg Med 11:119, 1982.
47. Wise BL and Chater N: Use of hypertonic mannitol solutions to lower cerebrospinal fluid pressure and decrease brain bulk in man. Surg Forum 12:398, 1961.
48. Wise BL and Chater N: The value of hypertonic solution in decreasing brain mass and lowering cerebrospinal fluid pressure. J Neurosurg 19:1038, 1962.
49. Yturraspe DJ and Lumb WV: Second lumbar spondylectomy and shortening of the spinal column of the dog. Am J Vet Res 34:521, 1973.

Chapter 17

Vertebral and Spinal Cord Surgery

Section 1   SF Swaim, DVM, MS

SMALL ANIMAL THORACOLUMBAR, LUMBOSACRAL, AND SACROCAUDAL SURGERY

Vertebral and spinal cord surgery in small animals is based on three procedures: decompression, fixation, and exploration. Decompression relieves pressure on the spinal cord. This is accomplished by removal of part of the vertebral arch and removal of space occupying material (ie, disk material or neoplastic tissue) from the vertebral canal. In instances of vertebral fracture or luxation, decompression can also be accomplished by realignment of the two vertebral segments. Fractures and/or luxations require stabilization to prevent further trauma to the spinal cord. This is achieved with various internal and external fixation devices. Exploratory surgery is performed to determine the source of spinal cord abnormality if other diagnostic measures (eg, neurologic examination, radiographs, electrodiagnostic testing) have not fully explained the nature of the abnormality. Exploratory surgery can be performed to obtain biopsy and culture samples.

INDICATIONS

The indications for vertebral and spinal cord surgery include diseases of traumatic, congenital, neoplastic, infectious, and degenerative origins. Herniated intervertebral disks, fractures, and luxations are examples of traumatic diseases necessitating surgery. Congenital conditions requiring surgery include atlantoaxial luxation and subluxation, malformations of the vertebrae, and multiple cartilaginous exostoses. Neoplasia can be vertebral, extramedullary, or intramedullary; each can result in damage to the spinal cord and the necessity for exploratory, decompressive, and possibly fixation surgery. Osteomyelitis and diskospondylitis are examples of infectious conditions that can cause spinal cord pressure or pain, thereby requiring exploratory and possibly decompressive and/or fixation surgery. Degenerative disorders such as lumbosacral malformation or malarticulation can result in spondylosis deformans and impingement on neural tissue, thus necessitating decompressive surgery.[8, 28, 39, 56]

Surgical management of diseases involving the spinal cord is indicated for animals showing severe motor involvement, deteriorating neurologic status, and lack of response to conservative therapy. For herniated thoracolumbar disks, spinal fractures, and spinal luxations at all levels, surgery is generally performed within the first 24 hours.

PREOPERATIVE PROCEDURES

An accurate and complete history should be obtained on the animal; thorough physical and neurologic examinations should also be performed before arriving at a diagnosis. When vertebral instability is suspected, only those reactions and reflexes necessary for lesion localization should be carefully performed (ie, evaluations that can be done with the animal in lateral recumbency). Client education should include an assessment of the animal's condition and a basic explanation of the pathophysiology involved, information about therapeutic methods available, the approximate cost, the advantages and disadvantages of each procedure, and the complications of the various treatment modalities.[47]

A minimum data base should be obtained on the animal (including urinalysis, BUN, CBC, and SGPT). Radiographs are imperative. With suspected intervertebral disk herniation, the dog should be anesthetized prior to radiography. Anesthesia should include tracheal intubation and maintenance with an inhalation anesthetic agent. Intravenous fluid therapy should be administered during surgery, and the patient should be closely monitored during the procedures.[47]

DORSOLATERAL THORACIC AND LUMBAR SURGERY

Hemilaminectomy and Fenestration

Hemilaminectomy is indicated when there is diagnostic evidence (from neurologic examination, radiographs, or myelogram) of spinal cord compression. Compression could be related to many factors (see Indications above). Decompression is indicated when an animal demonstrates conscious proprioceptive deficits and paresis. If a dog still has sensory function in the pelvic limbs, it is a candidate for decompressive surgery.[9] The most important factor determining recovery rate from decompressive surgery is the presence of preoperative sensory perception.[25] If an animal has complete pelvic limb paralysis with loss of deep pain perception and motor function, it may still benefit from surgery if these signs are of less than 24 hours' duration.[9, 27] However, a guarded prognosis should accompany such surgery.

Disk fenestration is indicated primarily as a prophylactic measure to prevent future disk herniation. It is performed at the time of hemi-laminectomy on dogs that demonstrate recurrent back pain due to disk disease, or on dogs showing pain with minimal neurologic deficits.[9, 29, 61] A fenestration alone should be considered in dogs under 8 years of age with signs that vary from lumbar pain to caudal paresis.[10] A survey has shown that disk fenestration combined with hemilaminectomy is the most frequently used technique for treating spinal cord compression resulting from disk herniation.[29]

The dorsal area of the animal is prepared for aseptic surgery from the level of the scapulae to the level of the tuber coxae for approximately 5 cm on either side of the dorsal midline. An intravenous catheter is placed in the jugular vein and secured with tape around the animal's neck. The animal is placed on the surgery table in ventral recumbency and is draped for aseptic surgery.

A skin incision is made parallel to, but just off, the dorsal midline between the spinous processes of T9 and L6. After palpating the spinous processes to locate the midline, the subcutaneous fat and fascia are incised longitudinally *right next to* the tips of these processes for the length of the skin incision. This exposes the underlying dense thoracolumbar fascia, which is incised in like manner to expose the epaxial musculature (Fig. 17–1). All dissection of muscle from the bone should be done as close to the bone as possible to obtain adequate exposure and hemostasis.

Dissection and retraction of the muscles to expose the dorsolateral surface of the vertebrae are done by a three step method to coincide with the three distinct muscle layers and attachments to the vertebrae. Each muscle layer is removed separately, always proceeding in a caudal to cranial direction. The first step involves retraction and dissection of the muscles from the spinous processes. A periosteal elevator or the blunt end of a scalpel handle is inserted between the muscle and bone at the tip of the spinous processes and is pushed ventrally while pulling laterally. With lateral retraction of the muscles, the tendinous attachments of the multifidus muscles are incised from caudal to cranial[23, 24, 47] (Fig. 17–2).

The second step separates the muscle attachments to the articular processes. The scalpel handle or periosteal elevator is placed on the bone between the two most caudally exposed articular processes. While lateral traction is applied, the tendinous attachments of the muscles to the articular processes are cut by closely encircling the articular processes with a scalpel blade. The same procedure is repeated on each

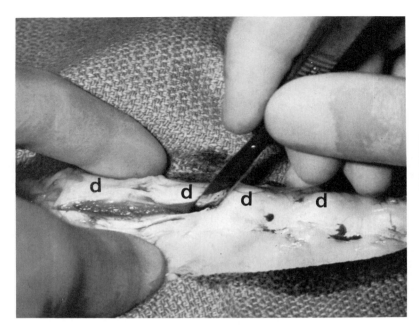

Figure 17–1. Incising the thoraco-lumbar fascia right next to the tips of the spinous processes (d) to expose the underlying epaxial musculature.

successive pair of articular processes, working from caudal to cranial[23, 24] (Fig. 17–3).

The third step involves incision of the muscle attachments to the accessory processes. Care must be taken to prevent damage to the spinal nerves and vessels emerging from the intervertebral foramina. Working from caudal to cranial, a finger is inserted between the last two articular processes to the level of the lateral vertebral process. With lateral retraction of the mus-

cle, the tight band of tendinous insertion to the accessory process is identified. With this tendon stretched tightly, a scalpel blade is used to sever the tendon about 0.5 cm lateral to its insertion. This avoids possible damage to the

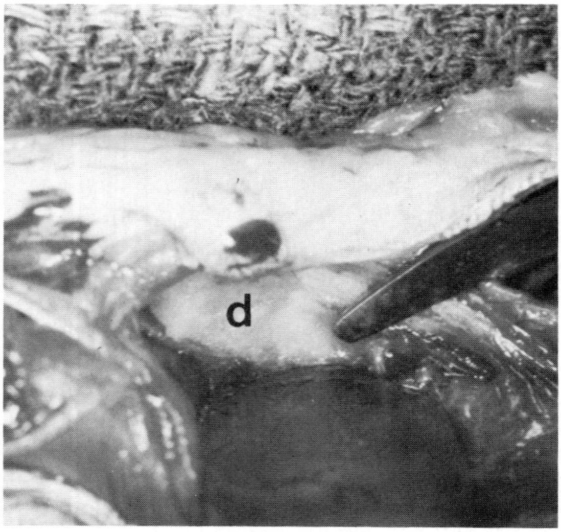

Figure 17–2. With the lateral retraction of the epaxial musculature from the spinous process (d), scissors are used to cut the ligamentous attachments of the muscles to the process.

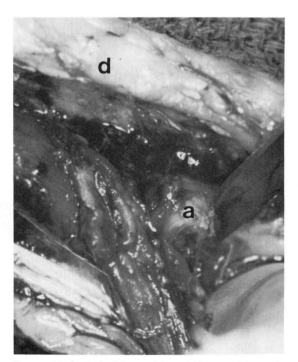

Figure 17–3. Scalpel is used to cut the epaxial muscle attachments from the articular process (a). d, Tip of spinous process.

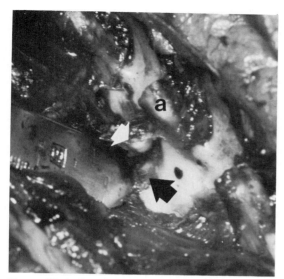

Figure 17–4. Just below the articular process (a), the ligamentous attachment of the epaxial muscles to the accessory process (white arrow) has been cut, and the muscle is retracted cranially to expose the lateral aspect of the disk (black arrow).

The thirteenth rib is palpated to its articulation with the thirteenth thoracic vertebra. Using this vertebra as a landmark, the vertebrae can be counted caudally or cranially to identify the area for hemilaminectomy as determined radiographically.[23, 24, 28]

A pair of bone rongeurs* and a 5/16 inch diameter laminectomy trephine† can be used to begin the hemilaminectomy procedure. The rongeurs are used to remove the articular processes between the two involved vertebrae as flush with the surface of the vertebral arches as possible (Fig. 17–6). The trephine is centered over this area at about a 45° angle from the dorsal midline (Fig. 17–7). Trephination is started by turning the trephine on the bone with slight pressure. Periodic removal of the trephine to check for looseness of the bone plug or periodic rocking of the trephine helps determine when the plug is loose enough to be removed.[23, 24, 28] A micrometer trephine,‡ on which the depth of trephination can be set, may also be used for entering the vertebral canal.[35]

Once the plug of bone has been removed from the vertebral arches, rongeurs*§ are used to create the hemilaminectomy defect cranially and caudally from the trephine opening (Fig. 17–8). Care should be exercised when using the rongeurs so that no pressure is ever exerted toward the spinal cord.[28] Generally, the cranial and caudal extent of the defect should be the bases of the adjacent articular processes, and

spinal nerves and vessels emerging from the intervertebral foramen just ventral to the accessory process.[23, 24] No attempt should be made to dissect the muscle ventral to the accessory process. This is left as a pad to protect the nerves and vessels as the muscle is retracted cranially to expose the lateral aspect of the disk for fenestration (Fig. 17–4).

By dissecting close to the bone and cutting muscles at their insertion to the bone, muscle trauma and hemorrhage are minimized. If there is some hemorrhaging from the muscle, the area between the retracted muscle and vertebral column can be packed with a surgical sponge for a few minutes to achieve hemostasis[23, 24] (Fig. 17–5).

---

*Blumenthal rongeurs, available through various distributors.

†Michelle laminectomy trephine, available through various distributors.

‡Micrometer trephine, CL Lippincott, Pacific Palisades, CA.

§Lempert rongeurs, available through various distributors.

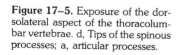

Figure 17–5. Exposure of the dorsolateral aspect of the thoracolumbar vertebrae. d, Tips of the spinous processes; a, articular processes.

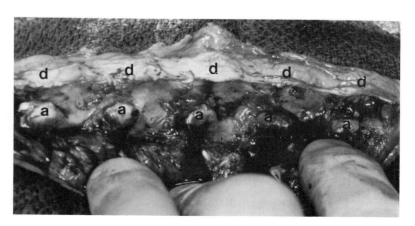

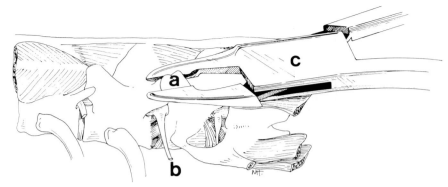

Figure 17–6. In the dorsolateral hemilaminectomy the articular processes (a) are being removed to produce a flat surface for trephination or burring. b, The intervertebral nerves and vessels; c, rongeurs.

Figure 17–7. A Michelle laminectomy trephine is used to expose the epidural space and spinal cord.

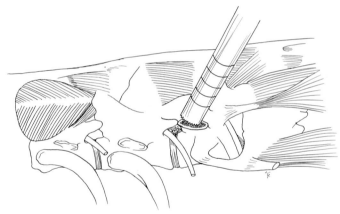

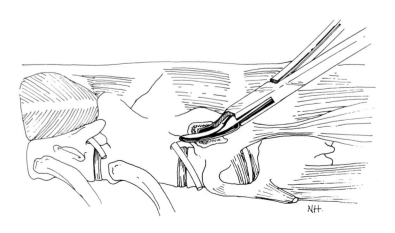

Figure 17–8. Lempert rongeurs are used to create the hemilaminectomy defect cranially and caudally from the trephination opening.

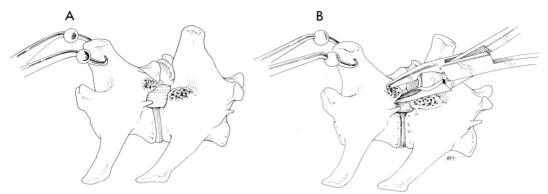

Figure 17–9. Towel forceps and rongeurs can be used to enter the vertebral canal. A, After the articular processes are removed, towel forceps are placed on the spinous process of the cranialmost involved vertebra and elevated to open the interarcual and articular spaces. B, Small rongeurs are inserted at the opening to begin the hemilaminectomy.[54]

the dorsal and ventral extent should be from the bases of the spinous processes to the floor of the vertebral canal. The defect can be extended over four to five vertebrae in cases of severe spinal cord compression without postoperative problems.[23,24]

A second method for entering the vertebral canal utilizes towel forceps and rongeurs.[54] The technique is best suited to the lumbar vertebrae of small to medium-sized dogs; however, it can be used on the thoracic vertebrae and in large dogs. The articular processes are removed as previously described, then a pair of towel forceps is placed on the spinous process of the cranialmost involved vertebra. By lifting on the two forceps the interarcual and articular spaces are opened enough to allow a small pair of rongeurs to remove enough bone to gain a starting point for the rongeurs to create the previously described hemilaminectomy defect (Fig. 17–9).

A third method of creating a hemilaminectomy defect employs electric hobby* or pneumatic† drills and burs.[51, 62] After removing the articular processes in the area, the drill, with a sharp unused bur, is used to brush away the bone within the limits of the hemilaminectomy (Fig. 17–10). A brushing action is used to remove outer cortical and cancellous bone down to a thin crust of inner cortical bone, which is removed with rongeurs or a tartar scraper to expose the vertebral canal.[28, 51, 62] The electric hobby drill is less expensive than the pneumatic drill; however, it requires gas sterilization and cannot be immersed for cleaning. The possibility of electric shock is always present when using an electric appliance. This hazard can be minimized by using an appropriate electric ground.[62]

---

*Moto-flex tool, Dremel Mfg, Racine, WI.
†Airdrill 100, Hall International, Inc, Santa Barbara, CA.

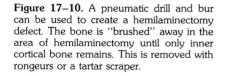

Figure 17–10. A pneumatic drill and bur can be used to create a hemilaminectomy defect. The bone is "brushed" away in the area of hemilaminectomy until only inner cortical bone remains. This is removed with rongeurs or a tartar scraper.

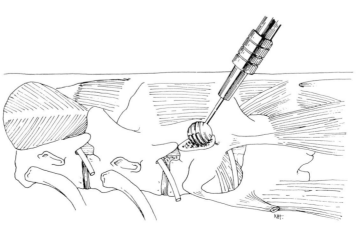

A 12 mm skull trephine equipped with an automatic clutch and depth gauge, which is powered by an air driven orthopedic drill, has also been used for performing hemilaminectomies in dogs.[11]

If hemilaminectomy was performed as treatment for intervertebral disk herniation, the degenerated disk material can be carefully removed from the vertebral canal using a tartar scraper, small curet, or similar instrument. Care must be taken to avoid excessive spinal cord manipulation during this procedure[24, 28] (Fig. 17–11).

If maximum decompression of the spinal cord is necessary, a bilateral hemilaminectomy can be performed over the length of two vertebrae, leaving the articular processes at either end of the hemilaminectomy defects intact to support the spinous processes. Irreducible vertebral luxations and fractures, as well as severe disk herniations, are examples of conditions in which this might be indicated. When articular processes are removed bilaterally, the vertebral column is weakened at the point of removal. If, in addition, a disk has herniated, the disk is weakened also; therefore, some form of vertebral fixation (eg, plates or pins) may be necessary.[55]

Thoracolumbar intervertebral disks may be fenestrated via the hemilaminectomy approach. Working from caudal to cranial to approach each disk, the musculature in the area of the accessory process is retracted cranially with a periosteal elevator or scalpel handle until the lateral aspect of the intervertebral disk is exposed (Fig. 17–4). The disk lies just cranial to the attachment of the lateral process with the vertebrae; in the thoracic area the disk is located slightly more cranial to the junction of the rib with the vertebral body. A sharp pointed, claw-type tartar scraper is moved from the cranial border of the lateral process and is inserted through the lateral aspect of the anulus fibrosus. With a downward and outward motion, the disk is fenestrated[23, 24] (Fig. 17–12).

An alternative technique for disk fenestration is to insert a 2 to 2.5 inch, 12 to 14 gauge needle through the lateral aspect of the disk and direct it transversely toward the opposite side of the disk. Using a boring action, several plugs of nuclear material are removed, and the bevel of the needle is used to scrape disk material out of the disk using a downward and outward motion.[28]

Regardless of where the hemilaminectomy was performed for spinal cord decompression, the disks from T11–T12 to L3–L4 should be fenestrated. Fenestration not only removes a large amount of disk material, but it also produces an inflammatory tissue response that transforms the progressive degenerative process into a stabilized fibrosis.[9, 28, 29]

A dorsolateral approach can be used for lateral disk fenestration from T9–10 to L5–6. A dorsolateral approach is made to the vertebrae and disks, and the disks are fenestrated by passing a 2 to 3 mm diameter Steinmann pin horizontally through the longissimus dorsi muscle to locate the disk. A curet is passed similarly to remove the disk material.[19]

The advantages of hemilaminectomy are that it allows spinal cord decompression and thus a more rapid reduction of cord ischemia than by medical therapy in the presence of protrusions; it allows removal of disk material from the vertebral canal with minimal spinal cord manipulation; it leaves a cosmetically acceptable appearance to the dog's back because the spinous processes are left intact; and it allows removal of disk material still present in the affected disk space, as well as prophylactic fenestration of other high risk disks.[9, 52] However, there is the

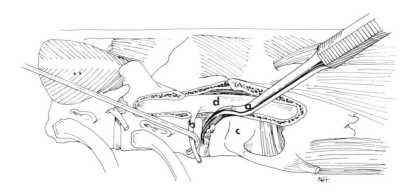

Figure 17–11. The tartar scraper (a) is used to remove the protrusion and remainder of the disk, care being employed not to injure the spinal cord during the manipulations. (b), Spinal nerve; c, lateral process; d, spinal cord.

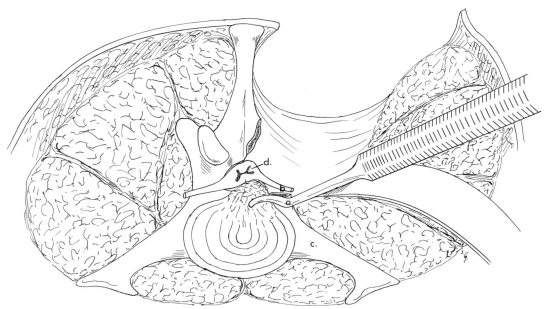

Figure 17–12. Cross section through the vertebral column at the level of hemilaminectomy. After removing protruded disk material from under the spinal cord, the tartar scraper (a) can be moved from the cranial border of the lateral process (c) and be inserted through the lateral aspect of the anulus fibrosus. Downward and outward motion of the tartar scraper removes remaining nucleus pulposus from the disc. b, Spinal nerve; d, spinal cord.

potential for rupture of the venous sinus on the floor of the vertebral canal as the defect is carried ventrally.[52, 61] This is not a major problem and application of crushed muscle or gelatin sponge usually stops the hemorrhage.

The advantage of disk fenestration is its value in preventing future disk protrusions.[9, 10, 19, 28, 47] It will also stop further protrusion of disk material into the vertebral canal when a protruding disk is fenestrated.[9, 10, 61]

Durotomy and Cord Perfusion

Durotomy by means of a longitudinal incision in the dura mater has been described for decompression. It was believed that this incision would lessen the compressive action of the dura on the swollen cord and help to at least partially restore the blood supply to the cord and reduce hypoxia.[1] Durotomy can serve a prognostic function when the neurologic examination reveals questionable results with regard to an animal's ability to recover neurologically, and there is the possibility of spinal cord malacia.[28, 41] Durotomy can be performed through a hemilaminectomy defect (Fig. 17–13).

Clinically, the advantage of durotomy is its

prognostic value. If the spinal cord is malacic and flows from the durotomy site, the prognosis is grave. The surgeon can observe the cord for thrombosis and disappearance or rupture of spinal cord vasculature, as well as absence of normal spinal cord pulsations.[28, 41, 61] Durotomies performed immediately after trauma are beneficial to neurologic recovery in dogs; however, if there is a 2 hour delay in durotomy after trauma there is no benefit.[28, 41–43]

Normothermic saline perfusion of the spinal cord has been beneficial in improving the functional recovery of dogs subjected to spinal cord trauma.[41] This perfusion has been shown to be as effective as hypothermic perfusion, perhaps because of dialysis of noxious substances from the cord tissue.[58] Research has shown that 120 minutes of exposure to hypothermic perfusion causes significantly more severe clinical and histopathologic cord change in normal spinal cords than does 30 minutes of hypothermic perfusion, 30 minutes of normothermic perfusion, or 120 minutes of normothermic perfusion.[56] The use of hypothermic cord perfusion for 20 minutes following spinal cord surgery of dogs has been advocated to reduce inflammation and the ischemia caused by edema and vasospasm. In addition, there may be a reduction of the noxious substances within the cord.[61]

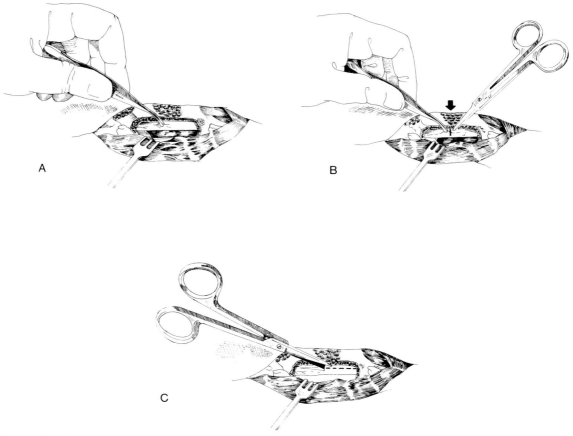

Figure 17–13. A, Elevating the dura from the cord with iris forceps. B, Incising the dura with iris scissors. C, Opening the dura longitudinally from central slit.

Closure

Placement of absorbable gelatin sponge (Gelfoam) or a piece of crushed muscle tissue over the hemilaminectomy site has been described as a means of attaining hemostasis.[28] The author prefers to take a piece of fresh subcutaneous fat that has not been exposed to the air and surgical lights and place it over the hemilaminectomy defect just prior to closure. Such fat grafts have been effective in preventing adhesions of the paravertebral muscles to the dura.[31, 32, 44] The epaxial musculature is replaced alongside the vertebral column, and simple interrupted absorbable 2–0 or 3–0 sutures are used to close the thoracolumbar fascia. The subcutaneous tissue is closed using the same suture material in a continuous pattern, and the skin is fastened with 3–0 or 4–0 nonabsorbable suture in a simple interrupted or continuous lock stitch pattern.

Vertebral Stabilization with Hemilaminectomies

When vertebral fractures or luxation is present, stabilization of the vertebral segments must be performed in conjunction with decompression. Stabilization devices can be affixed to the spinous processes, the transverse processes, or the vertebral bodies.

Spinous Processes

The approach to the vertebrae is the same as described for a hemilaminectomy. However, the spinous processes will have to be dissected out on both sides.

Metal Plates. These plates* are available in various lengths and thicknesses with attachment

---

*Auburn spinal plates, Richards Mfg Co, Memphis, TN.

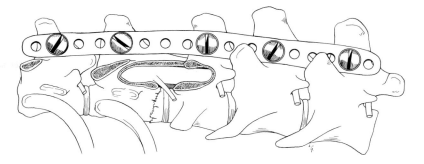

Figure 17–14. The drill holes are made in the spinous processes after one plate has been positioned. A bolt is inserted through each hole as it is drilled to keep the spines and plates in position as all the holes are drilled. Bolts are placed to afford the greatest stability and immobilization.

bolts, washers, and nuts. Based on the dog's size and the vertebral size and conformation as observed on radiographs, the proper sized spinal plates are selected by the surgeon. They should be long enough to include at least one normal vertebra on each side of the fractured one. With larger dogs, at least two vertebrae should be included on each side of the fracture.[28] Inclusion of three normal vertebrae has also been advocated.[26, 63] One plate is positioned on each side of the dorsal spinous processes. It is important that the bolts be placed in the heaviest and most central part of the process, and that the plates be placed as close to the dorsal lamina as possible. This may necessitate the removal of articular processes and/or grooving the bone of the dorsal arch with rongeurs or pneumatic drill and bur. Proper positioning prevents friction or rubbing of plates against the dorsal fascia and skin and affords stability of the spine.[26, 28, 36, 52]

Decompression via hemilaminectomy and/or manipulation of the fracture segments into alignment should be performed. With one plate

in place, holes are drilled in the processes with a drill bit or intramedullary pin with a diameter slightly larger than that of the bolt to be used for fixation. Bolts are inserted as holes are drilled to keep the processes and plate in position during the remaining drilling procedure (Fig. 17–14). After the holes are drilled and the bolts are in place, the second plate is applied to the other side of the spinous processes, and washers and nuts are secured (Fig. 17–15). Excessive tightening of these should be avoided. Excess bolt is cut with side-cutting pin cutters as close to the nut as possible.[26, 28, 36, 53] If the vertebral segments can be manipulated, it would be best to affix the plates to one segment, realign the vertebral column, and then affix the plates to the remaining segment.[63]

Closure of the surgical site is as described for hemilaminectomy.

Auburn spinal plates allow rapid easy immobilization, with the degree of immobilization being dependent on the type of fracture or luxation and the degree of instability. The technique can also be used with vertebral body

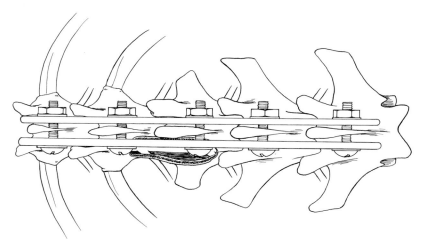

Figure 17–15. The second plate is applied to the other side of the spinous processes and washers and nuts are secured.

plating or cross pinning.[28, 36] Metal plates have the following disadvantages: excessive tightening of the nuts and bolts may result in ischemic bone necrosis or fracture of the spinous processes. Conversely, insufficient tightening can result in plate slippage;[28, 36, 52] a long segment of the vertebral column is immobilized, and excessive spinal flexion or torsion may cause fracture of the spinous processes;[36] vertebral body fractures with structural loss or shortening are difficult to stabilize adequately with a stabilization device affixed to the spinous processes;[36] it is difficult to apply plates to the caudal thoracic region because of the smaller, weaker spinous processes, especially in small dogs;[36, 52] the technique cannot be used if the spinous processes or laminae are fractured.[26, 36, 52]

Vinylidene Plates. The design of these plates* is basically the same as that of the metal plates. However, the surface of the plate applied to the spinous processes is crosshatched with grooves to provide a friction grip-type surface.[53, 63] The surgical preparation and application of these plates are basically the same as that described for metal plates.

When applying these plates, 3.175 mm diameter Wilson vitallium bolts are used. The bolts are directed between the spines rather than through them as with metal plates. Because of their flexibility, the plates tend to wrap themselves around the spines when the nuts and bolts are tightened[28, 53, 63] (Fig. 17–16).

The advantages of these plates are basically the same as for metal plates. In addition, the spinous processes are not weakened by passing bolts through them, and the plates can be cut and molded to the spine using a scalpel, rongeur, or pneumatic drill and bur at the time of surgery.[15, 36, 52, 53] The disadvantages of these plates are the same as those stated for metal plates.

Spinal Staples and Modifications. This form of stabilization is indicated for small dogs and cats. A small flexible stainless steel intramedullary pin (0.045–0.062 cm in diameter) is fashioned into a staple configuration as it is attached to the spinous processes.[22, 28, 36, 53]

Following a hemilaminectomy at the fracture site, *small* holes are drilled at the center of the bases of the spinous processes of the involved vertebra and two on each side of it, using a stainless steel pin. The intramedullary pin to be used for fixation is bent at a right angle 2 to 3 cm from one end. The bent portion is inserted through the drill hole at the base of the spinous process of the second vertebra cranial to the fracture or luxation.[22, 28, 36, 53]

The pin is laid parallel to the bases of the spinous processes, and a second 90° angle bend is made in the pin at the level of the hole in the spinous process of the caudalmost vertebra to be stabilized. The bent end of the pin is cut 2 to 3 cm from the angle. After inserting the bent ends of the pin through their corresponding holes, the ends are bent in toward the fracture or luxation until they press tightly against the spinous processes. Segments of 22 to 24 gauge stainless steel orthopedic wire are passed through the holes at the bases of the intervening spinous processes. The wires are bent to encircle the pin and are twisted tightly to affix the pin to the spinous processes[22, 28, 36, 53] (Fig. 17–17).

Long Staple. A modification of this technique entails leaving one arm of the staple long. It is doubled back the entire length of the immobilized segment, and all aspects of the pin are wired to the intervening spines to afford double strength immobilization[28] (Fig. 17–18A).

U Pin. The intramedullary pin is bent in half to form an exaggerated U shape. The ends of the pin are cut off so that the pin is just long enough for stabilizing the five vertebrae. It may be necessary to bend the pin slightly so that it will conform to the dorsoventral curvature of the vertebral column. One arm of the U pin is inserted through the hole in the spinous process of the caudalmost vertebra until the base of the U is situated in the hole. The pin is stood upright so it can be pivoted downward at the hole and laid so that one arm of the U is on each side of the bases of the spinous processes. Segments of 22 or 24 gauge wire are passed

*Lubra plates, Lubra Co, 1905 Mohawk, Ft Collins, CO.

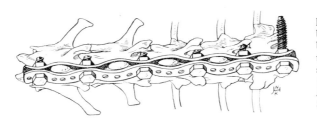

Figure 17–16. The spinous processes are sandwiched between the friction grip surfaces of the plastic plates. The bolts pass between the spines; when the nuts are tightened the plates are almost pulled into apposition between the spines. This tends to wrap the plates around the spines. (From Swaim SF: Thoracolumbar and sacral spine trauma. *In* Bojrab MJ (ed): Current Techniques in Small Animal Surgery I. Philadelphia, Lea & Febiger, 1975.)

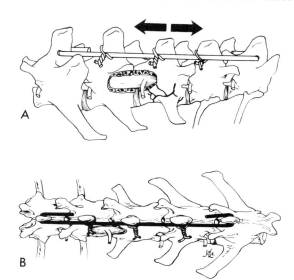

Figure 17–17. Gage's spinal staple used on small breed dogs. Small holes are drilled at the bases of the spines of the vertebrae to be fixed. A small stainless steel intramedullary pin is bent at right angles at the appropriate length. The bent arms are inserted through the holes at the ends of the spinal segment to be fixed and are bent back along the spines to form a staple. Intervening spines are wired to the pin. A, Lateral view; B, dorsoventral view. (From Swaim SF: Thoracolumbar and sacral spine trauma. *In* Bojrab MJ (ed): Current Techniques in Small Animal Surgery I. Philadelphia, Lea & Febiger, 1975.)

through the holes in the remaining four spinous processes and are bent to encircle the pin on both sides of the spine before they are twisted to attain spinal stabilization[28, 52, 53] (Fig. 17–18B).

U Pin Wired to Lateral Processes. The procedure is basically the same as that for U pin fixation; however, no holes are drilled in the spinous processes. The pin is affixed to each vertebra by a loop of orthopedic wire that has been passed under the pin and under the lateral process (rib on thoracic vertebra). The ends of the wire are twisted together behind the articular processes. This is performed bilaterally on each vertebra. For additional support, two U pins can be placed, one based at each end of the vertebral segment to be immobilized.[26, 36] With this procedure, it is necessary to dissect both sides of the vertebrae, including the bases of the lateral processes.

The advantages of staples are that they are economical, are easily applied, and can be used on small dogs and cats. The long staple, U pin, and U pin with lateral process wiring have the same advantages. In addition, these techniques have an added advantage of supplying a length of pin on both sides of the spinuous processes that can be utilized in the wire stabilization process.[26, 36, 52]

A disadvantage of these techniques is that they immobilize long segments of the vertebral column.[26, 52] With the exception of U pins wired to the lateral processes, these techniques are all dependent on the spinous processes being intact.[52] Compression and wedge vertebral body fractures with structural bone loss or shortening cannot be completely immobilized. Because the spinal staple acts as a tension band constraint to flexion, ventral body defects will exaggerate flexional and torsional forces placed on the

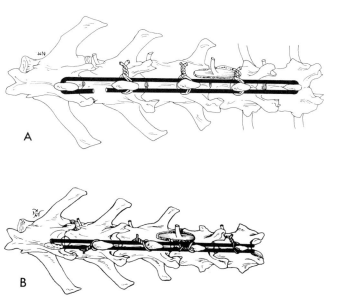

Figure 17–18. Modifications of the spinal staple. A, Hoerlein's modification leaves one arm of the staple long to provide double strength. B, Swaim's U pin modification has an arm of the pin on either side of the spines for added stability. There is an open end to the bent pin at the cranialmost vertebrae. (From Swaim SF: Thoracolumbar and sacral spine trauma. *In* Bojrab MJ (ed): Current Techniques in Small Animal Surgery I. Philadelphia, Lea & Febiger, 1975.)

dorsal spines and the fixation device. The result is pin bending, wires tearing, or breakage.[36] Fractures of the dorsal spinous processes during manipulation occurs easily because these structures are more delicate in the smaller animals on which these procedures would be used.

Vertebral Bodies

The approach to the vertebral bodies is the same as described for hemilaminectomies. However, application of methylmethacrylate and pins requires bilateral dissection of the vertebral column to expose both sides of the dorsal aspect of the vertebral bodies.

Cross Pins. Intramedullary pins are used to stabilize the vertebral bodies. When the vertebral bodies are intact (ie, luxation) two vertebrae are pinned together. One pin is inserted into the middle of the lateral aspect of the cranialmost vertebral body and is angled slightly ventrally and diagonally as it is advanced through the bone and across the intervertebral disk to be seated in the caudalmost vertebral body. The second pin is inserted in like manner cranially from the vertebra just caudal to the lesion. The pins are cut as close to the vertebral bodies as possible (Fig. 17–19).

Using the same technique, three vertebral bodies and two disks are involved when cross pinning a particularly unstable fracture, such as a compression-type fracture.[21, 26, 28, 36, 53] To keep pins parallel to the dorsal plane they may be inserted laterally through the paravertebral muscles into the vertebral body. In the caudal lumbar area, the ilial wings may interfere with placement of the caudal pin; therefore, both pins can be passed from cranial to caudal with one pin being passed from each side of the vertebral body. Similar placement from caudal to cranial can be performed in the thoracic area.[26]

Crossed pin fixation is not dependent on the spinous processes, it takes advantage of the increased osseous tissue of the vertebral bodies for fixation, and it does not immobilize long segments of the vertebral column.[36, 53] Crossed pins have some disadvantages: It is technically difficult to place the pins accurately, and it may be difficult to maintain reduction while pins are being placed. If placed improperly, the pins can damage the aorta, vena cava, vertebral sinuses, or spinal cord. It may be difficult to cut the pins off because of surrounding musculature. It is difficult to stabilize comminuted vertebral body fractures effectively.[36]

Methylmethacrylate and Pins. This technique is described for use with a laminectomy; however, it will be covered in this section on vertebral fixation. The approach to the vertebrae is bilateral. After a laminectomy is performed, two Steinmann pins are placed into the vertebral body cranial to the area of instability. Two more pins are placed in like manner in the vertebra just caudal to the area of instability. The pins are cut at the height of the articular processes[45] (Fig. 17–20A).

Gelfoam that has been soaked in cold lactated Ringer's solution is placed over the exposed spinal cord, and a dry surgical field is obtained. The fracture is reduced, and the liquid and powder of the methylmethacrylate are mixed to a doughy consistency. The methylmethacrylate is preformed into a 1 to 2 cm diameter strand for about 4 minutes and is then carefully laid around the laminectomy defect, pins, and articular processes (Fig. 17–20 B and C). The area should be irrigated with iced lactated Ringer's solution.[36, 45]

The technique has the advantages of requiring less soft tissue dissection than with other vertebral body fixation techniques. Rib insertion on the vertebrae and interference with nerve roots in the caudal lumbar area are not problems with the technique. A short segment of vertebral column is immobilized.[36, 45] Disadvantages of the technique include the potential for implant associated infection and possible

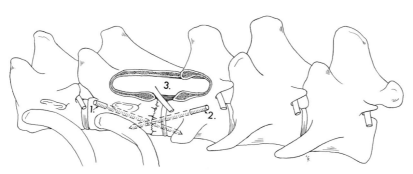

Figure 17–19. Stabilization across a single intervertebral space by cross-pinning the involved vertebral bodies. 1, Pin directed caudally; 2, pin directed cranially; 3, area of hemilaminectomy and decompression. (After Gage ED: A new method of spinal fixation in the dog. Vet Med/Small Anim Clin 64:295, 1969.)

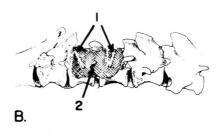

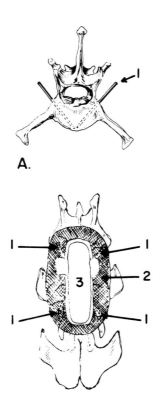

Figure 17–20. Methyl methacrylate and pins for vertebral fixation. A, Cross section showing pin placement in vertebral bodies. B, Lateral view. C, Dorsoventral view. 1, Pins; 2, methyl methacrylate; 3, dorsal laminectomy site.

rejection. It may be difficult to stabilize the vertebrae if the vertebral body fracture involves loss or shortening of the bone. Closure of the dorsal thoracolumbar fascia over the implant may be difficult.[36]

Vertebral Body Plates. Small bone plates may be applied to the dorsolateral surface of the vertebral bodies for fixation of luxations, subluxations, epiphyseal body fractures, and transverse fractures with the majority of the vertebral body intact. They can be used on both large and small dogs. Plates can be applied to vertebrae from T12 to L5. Generally, two vertebral bodies are stabilized when repairing a luxation, subluxation, or fracture near the intervertebral disk. A longer plate may be used to span three vertebral bodies if a midbody transverse or compressive fracture exists.[28, 36, 50, 53]

The approach to the vertebrae is as previously described; however, the artery, vein, and nerve are isolated as they emerge from the intervertebral foramen. The vessels are double ligated with 3–0 absorbable suture material and severed between ligatures. The spinal nerve is severed.[26, 36, 50, 53]

The proper length of small bone plate* is selected and laid on the dorsolateral surface of the vertebral body just below the hemilaminectomy defect. When two vertebrae are to be stabilized, the plate is placed with two holes over each vertebral body. If three vertebrae are involved, a longer plate† with multiple holes is laid over the vertebrae. A 5/64 inch diameter drill bit is used to drill a hole through the cranialmost hole in the plate, directing the bit slightly ventrally toward the opposite side of the vertebral body (Fig. 17–21). A 7/64 inch diameter drill bit is used to enlarge the lateral aspect of the holes to make insertion of the bone screws easier.[26, 28, 36, 50, 53]

A bone depth gauge is used to measure the depth of the hole in the vertebral body. The proper length screw‡ is selected and secured in the hole.[50, 53] When stabilizing two vertebrae,

---

*Swaim vertebral body plates, Richards Mfg Co, Memphis, TN.

†Auburn spinal plates.

‡Bechtol radial fluted point and buttress threads, Richards Mfg Co, Memphis, TN.

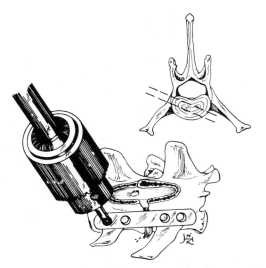

Figure 17–21. Vertebral body plating. After decompression by hemilaminectomy, a vertebral body plate is placed on the dorsolateral aspect of the vertebral body. A drill bit is used to drill a hole in the cranialmost hole of the plate, directing the bit slightly ventral toward the opposite side of the vertebral body. (From Swaim SF: Thoracolumbar and sacral spine trauma. *In* Bojrab MJ (ed): Current Techniques in Small Animal Surgery I. Philadelphia, Lea & Febiger, 1975.)

a screw is placed in the remaining plate hole over the cranialmost vertebral body, the fracture segments are realigned if possible, and screws are placed in the two plate holes over the caudalmost vertebra (Fig. 17–22). With a midbody transverse or compression fracture, the plate is affixed to the vertebrae cranial and caudal to the fractured vertebra, providing a buttress effect.[28, 36, 50, 53] If there is sufficient solid bone in the fractured vertebra, one or two screws can be placed in it.

When applying vertebral body plates to the thoracic vertebrae, the vertebrae and rib heads are exposed and a small intramedullary pin is used to drill a dorsoventral hole in the head of each involved rib. The ribs are separated from the vertebra at the costovertebral junction using bone forceps. As the ribs retract ventrally, the dorsolateral surface of the vertebral bodies is exposed. After smoothing the surfaces, a vertebral body plate is applied as previously described.[28, 50, 53]

A piece of stainless steel wire is threaded through each of the predrilled holes in the rib heads. These wires are then threaded through holes drilled in the spinous processes of the plated vertebrae. The rib heads are elevated to their original level.[28, 36, 50, 53]

Vertebral body plates have several advan-

tages. They are not dependent on intact spinous processes; however, the processes can be plated also for additional support in large dogs. The plates utilize the increased osseous tissue of the vertebral bodies to stabilize a short segment of the vertebral column, thus reducing the chance of implant failure. Compressive forces can be withstood by this type of fixation, even when fractures have caused vertebral body collapse and shortening.[28, 36, 52]

Disadvantages of vertebral body plates include difficulty in applying the plates to the thoracic vertebrae because of the costovertebral articulations and the potential for creating pneumothorax, difficulty in obtaining access to the vertebral bodies cranial to T12, and potential damage to some of the spinal nerves supplying the lumbosacral plexus if applied caudal to L4.[26, 36, 50, 52, 53]

EXTERNAL VERTEBRAL STABILIZATION

External vertebral stabilization is not necessary following intervertebral disk surgery. However, the use of a body bandage is sometimes advocated to protect the wound and to help prevent seromas. External stabilization is generally indicated as an adjunct to internal fixa-

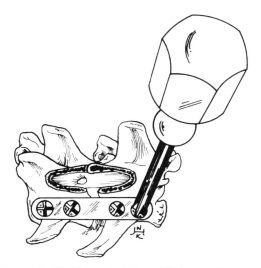

Figure 17–22. After each hole is drilled, a depth gauge is used to select the correct length for the screw. The screws should have Bechtol radial-fluted points with buttress threads (Richards). They are applied firmly so there will be no movement of the plate. (From Swaim SF: Thoracolumbar and sacral spine trauma. *In* Bojrab MJ (ed): Current Techniques in Small Animal Surgery I. Philadelphia, Lea & Febiger, 1975.)

tion, especially in larger animals. External stabilization alone is occasionally used when there are minor vertebral fractures and luxations or when there is minimal if any displacement of the vertebral segments. However, the radiographic position of the spinal segments only indicates their position at the time of radiography. Vertebral segments may have been maximally displaced at the time of injury, causing severe spinal cord damage, and yet they may have returned to a near normal position at the time of radiography. Thus, it is important to correlate the neurologic and radiographic examinations. If any animal demonstrates minimal neurologic abnormalities and a minor fracture or luxation, and the owner does not wish to undertake the expense of surgery, external fixation may be considered. However, the pet owner should be warned that external fixation alone is not as effective as internal and external fixation.

Several criteria must be met for a cast to be functional and comfortable. The dog should be anesthetized or strongly sedated (cast is usually

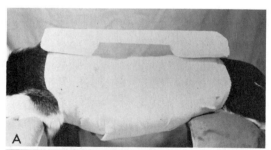

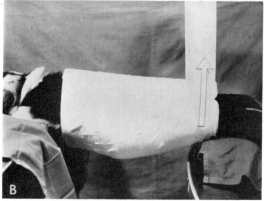

Figure 17–23. Body splint and cast. A, After applying a bandage from the axillary region to the folds of the flanks, a premeasured dorsal splint that is well padded at the ends is placed over the top of the bandage. B, The splint is taped in place with special tension in the caudal areas so it does not fit too loosely. (From Swaim SF: Body casts. Vet Med/Small Anim Clin 65:1179, 1970.)

placed immediately after surgery). The thin plywood, basswood, or aluminum splint that is to be used for dorsal support should be cut to the appropriate length (ie, dorsal scapulae to tuber coxae) and be well padded on its ends to prevent it from pressing on the incision. After placing dressing sponges over the incision line, the animal is wrapped from the axillae to the folds of the flanks with three or four layers of soft absorbent bandage wrap.* Two inch wide adhesive tape is used to cover this wrap. The dorsal splint is then taped in place over the dorsal midline using circumferential body wrapping. A snug fit is important; however, the bandage should not be so tight that it impairs respiration. Cranially, it should be anchored slightly to the hair or "suspenders" of tape should be crisscrossed between the thoracic limbs to keep the bandage from slipping caudally. In the flank area the bandage should be applied with special tension so it does not fit too loosely (Fig. 17–23). This may require placing the bandage over the prepuce in males, followed by cutting an aperture for it after bandaging is complete.[28, 49]

If internal stabilization has supplied strong fixation of the appliance to adequate amounts of bone (eg, vertebral body plates) or if the animal is a quiet, small dog or cat, the bandage and splint are usually sufficient for external support. However, if the appliances have been applied to lesser amounts of bone (eg, spinous process fixation), if the animal is large or fractious, or if the surgeon believes that additional support is necessary, a light, strong casting material† may be applied over the bandage splint. Casting is also indicated if no internal fixation is applied.

An assortment of removable and reuseable neck and body braces are currently available.‡ These could be used on dogs with vertebral trauma.

Bandages and casts should be kept in place for 10 to 14 days and possibly longer if no internal fixation was used. During this time the base of the prepuce, folds of the flanks, axillary folds, dorsal scapular areas, and flexion surfaces of the elbows (if tape suspenders were used), should be observed for friction and pressure sores.

---

*Sheet wadding, American Hospital Supply, Evanston, IL.

†Delta-lite, fiberglass casting tape, Johnson & Johnson, New Brunswick, NJ.

‡Canine Orthopedics, 107 7th St, Broadmoor, Colorado Springs, CO.

DORSAL THORACIC, LUMBAR, SACRAL, AND CAUDAL SURGERY

Thoracolumbar Laminectomy

The indications for performing a dorsal laminectomy are the same as those for hemilaminectomy, with the end result being decompression of the spinal cord. The positioning of the dog and preparation for aseptic surgery are the same as for a hemilaminectomy. The approach to the vertebrae is basically the same as for a hemilaminectomy; however, the dissection is carried out on both sides of the vertebrae in the affected area down to the articular processes. [17, 20, 28]

After removing the supraspinous and interspinous ligaments, the spinous processes of two to six vertebrae are removed with bone cutting forceps. To perform a Funkquist type B laminectomy, a pneumatic drill and bur are used to brush away the bone on the dorsolateral portions of the arches, removing outer compact bone, cancellous bone, and inner compact bone. [17, 18, 20, 28] When the inner compact bone is burred to a thin shell, rongeurs may be used to remove the remaining bone. The outer articular processes are left intact, as is the outer compact bone of the dorsolateral portion of the vertebral arch (Fig. 17–24). This keeps bone above the level of the top of the spinal cord to help prevent dorsoventral cord compression by secondary fibrosis. The laminectomy defect is extended cranially and caudally until normal epidural fat is seen at each end. No attempt is made to remove disk material from around the cord unless it is above or lateral to the cord. [17, 18, 20, 28, 51, 61]

This technique provides good dorsal decompression of the spinal cord. However, it leaves a palpable and sometimes a visible defect over the surgical site owing to removal of the spinous processes. [28, 52] Prata[44] reports that this can be prevented by passing a loop of 20 or 22 gauge orthopedic wire through the cranial and caudal spinous processes and suturing the thoracolumbar fascia and muscle over the wire with 2–0 or 3–0 nylon. The technique does not lend itself to removal of disk material from the floor of the vertebral canal or removal of remaining disk material from the involved disk. [52, 61]

Thoracolumbar Modified Dorsal Laminectomy

Following bilateral subperiosteal exposure of the dorsal aspect of the vertebrae down to the level of the accessory processes, the spinous processes of the vertebrae cranial and caudal to the involved disk space are removed with rongeurs. Using a pneumatic drill and bur, the lamina of the vertebral arches are removed as far lateral as the joint spaces of the articular processes, which entails removing the caudal articular process while leaving the cranial process on each vertebra. Bone is removed from the lamina down to the inner cortical bone over the spinal cord. A small bur is used to remove

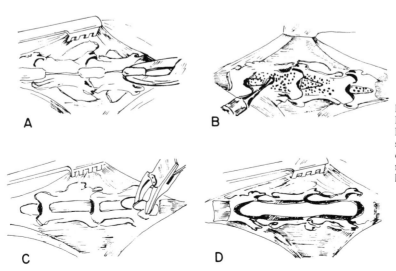

Figure 17–24. Dorsal laminectomy. A, Removal of spinous processes. B, Pneumatic drill and bur removing dorsal laminae between articular processes. C, Rongeurs removing the last remnants of the laminae. D, Complete Funkquist type B dorsal laminectomy.

A

B

C

D

cancellous bone along the sides of the vertebral arch between the two cortical layers. The shell of inner cortical bone is cut through with the small bur at the level of the lateral aspect of the spinal cord bilaterally (Fig. 17–25) and is lifted to expose the full width of the vertebral canal. The laminectomy defect usually extends for two or three vertebrae; however, it may be lengthened until normal epidural fat is observed at each end of the defect.[61]

Disk material can be removed from under the spinal cord with minimal cord manipulation. However, radiculotomy or rhizotomy are beneficial in removing disk material. "Sling sutures" of 5–0 silk placed in the dura also allow gentle retraction of the spinal cord for removal of disk material.[61]

This modification has the advantage of providing a more spacious decompression of the spinal cord than a hemilaminectomy or Funkquist type B laminectomy, and disk material can be removed from the vertebral canal. The technique is primarily used along with durotomy in cases of sudden onset of paraplegia with loss of sensory function. Disadvantages of this technique are that it requires delicate use of the pneumatic drill and burs, there is more instability of the vertebral column resulting from the bilateral removal of articular processes, and a palpable and visible defect remains over the surgical area.[28, 29, 52, 61]

Thoracolumbar Deep Dorsal Laminectomy

Deep dorsal laminectomy involves the removal of the entire vertebral arch (pedicles and lamina) of the vertebra so that the spinal cord rests on the vertebral body with no arch covering it.[30, 55] The technique should be considered when radical decompression of one vertebral length is indicated. Such indications would include a severely comminuted fracture of a vertebral arch or a tumor or infectious process confined to one vertebral arch. The technique should not be used over more than one vertebral length, and this vertebral segment should be stabilized by means of vertebral body fixation or spinous process fixation to stabilize the vertebrae on each side of the defect.

Thoracolumbar Midline Myelotomy

Dorsal midline myelotomies have been described in conjunction with dorsal laminectomy and durotomy procedures as a means of early radical spinal cord decompression.[28, 37, 46] Careful myelotomy on the precise midline in the dorsal median sulcus down to the central canal using a sharp instrument such as a razor blade will cause minimal to moderate neurologic signs

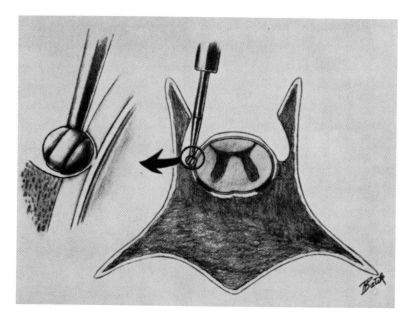

Figure 17–25. Modified dorsal laminectomy. A pneumatic drill and bur bilaterally remove the lamina down to the inner cortical bone as far as the lateral aspect of the cord, where the inner cortical bone is cut through. (From Trotter EJ: Thoracolumbar spine: Thoracolumbar disk disease. *In* Bojrab MJ (ed): Current Techniques in Small Animal Surgery, 2nd ed. Philadelphia, Lea & Febiger, 1983.)

in normal dogs.[3] The technique has been reported to reduce norepinephrine levels at the injury site and thus reduce cord hemorrhage and necrosis.[40, 46] Myelotomy has also been claimed to release increased intramedullary pressure and increase the oxygen interface with exposed surface area.[46] It has been found that, if not performed carefully, varying degrees and permanence of proprioceptive deficits may result, especially if the incision is off the midline.[3, 28] A study on normal dogs has revealed that a full thickness midline myelotomy causes severe necrosis of the spinal gray matter as the result of damage to its blood supply via the ventral sulcal artery.[60] Clinically, the procedure has not been used for cervical spinal injuries and is rarely used for thoracolumbar spinal injuries.[29]

Lumbosacral Laminectomy

Dorsal laminectomy at the lumbosacral junction is indicated as an exploratory diagnostic or therapeutic procedure of the cauda equina syndrome, which is caused by compression, displacement, or destruction of nerve roots or the vasculature of the cauda equina (ie, L7–Cd5).[4, 34] (For information about the pathologic changes associated with the cauda equina syndrome, see Chapters 6 and 12.)

To decompress the cauda equina, the animal is placed in sternal recumbency with the pelvic limbs extended forward on each side of the body to slightly flex the lumbosacral area.[33, 39] Others recommend extending the limbs caudally and placing a sandbag under the caudal abdomen.[13]

A dorsal midline skin incision is made from L6 to the midline sacral area. The subcutaneous fat is bluntly dissected to the lumbosacral fascia. This fascia is incised parallel and adjacent to the spinous processes of L6–S3. After bilaterally severing their ligamentous attachments to the spinous processes of L6–S3, the multifidus lumborum, sacrocaudalis dorsalis lateralis, and medialis muscles are bluntly dissected and reflected bilaterally from the vertebrae to the level of the articular processes. The attachments of the sacrocaudalis dorsalis lateralis are incised from the articular processes, and the lateral surface of the pedicle of L7 is stripped of muscle if a foraminotomy is planned.[13, 33, 38]

The interarcuate ligament is removed between L7 and S1, and the spinous processes of L7 and S1 are removed. Using rongeurs or a pneumatic drill, the laminae of L7 and S1 are

removed, leaving the articular processes intact. The components of the cauda equina can be retracted laterally in the canal via this opening, thus exposing the dorsal aspect of the disk for fenestration (Fig. 17–26). If either or both of the seventh lumbar nerves are compressed in their respective intervertebral foramina, the articular processes and pedicles may be removed to provide adequate nerve decompression. Laminectomies can be extended either cranially or caudally for further decompression in instances of more severe canal stenosis or neoplasia. Prior to closure, a fat graft from the subcutaneous area is placed over the laminectomy site. The musculature is returned to the midline, and the lumbosacral fascia is closed with simple interrupted absorbable sutures. Subcutaneous tissues and skin are closed in routine fashion.[4, 13, 33, 38, 39, 57]

If, by clinical examination and ancillary tests, the area of cauda equina compression can be relatively localized to the vertebral canal or intervertebral foramen, surgical decompression should be concentrated to that area as much as possible. This helps avoid the possible sequelae

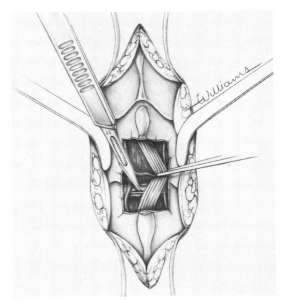

Figure 17–26. The dorsal laminae have been removed with a rongeur or air drill. Epidural fat normally fills the vertebral canal but is not illustrated. The cauda equina is retracted with umbilical tape, exposing the dorsal anulus of the intervertebral disk. The prominent venous sinuses should be avoided. (From Oliver JE Jr and Selcer RR: Decompression of the lumbosacral spinal cord and nerve roots. *In* Bojrab MJ (ed): Current Techniques in Small Animal Surgery I. Philadelphia, Lea & Febiger, 1975.)

of cicatrix formation and instability with future exacerbation of clinical signs.[34]

Postoperative complications include seroma formation and cystitis. Seromas are frequent but easily resolved. Cystitis is often present when the animal is initially examined, and it requires care and treatment for about 2 to 4 weeks until bladder function returns.[39]

Thoracolumbar Stabilization with Dorsal Laminectomy

The fixation devices that are affixed to the vertebral bodies and lateral processes of the vertebrae (see above) can be used in conjunction with a dorsal laminectomy without any problem. However, fixation devices that are applied to the spinous processes must be applied to spinous processes on each side of the laminectomy defect so that the device bridges the laminectomy defect. If the defect is long, it is important for adequate numbers of spinous processes to be affixed to the device on each end of the defect. In such instances the surgeon should also consider the use of vertebral body fixation in the area of decompression to ensure adequate vertebral stabilization.

Dorsal Lumbosacral Stabilization

Transilial Pin. With fractures at the lumbosacral junction, it is not uncommon to have the fracture line extend cranioventrally from the lumbosacral intervertebral foramina across the vertebral body of L7. The caudal segment luxates ventrally and cranially either minimally or with complete overriding of the vertebral body

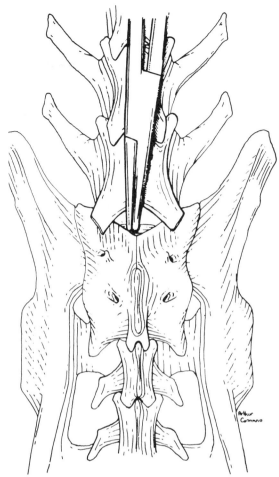

Figure 17–28. Leverage to reduce a displaced lumbosacral fracture. With traction on the head and tail, forceps are used to lever segments into position. Tip of the lever is just ventral to the dorsal sacral arch. The fulcrum of the lever is dorsal to the arch of the seventh lumbar vertebra. The end of the lever is cranial to the seventh lumbar vertebra. (From Slocum B and Rudy RL: Fractures of the seventh lumbar vertebra in the dog. J Am Anim Hosp Assoc 11:167, 1975.)

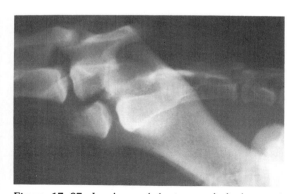

Figure 17–27. Lumbosacral fracture and displacement. Caudodorsal displacement of cranial segment and cranioventral displacement of the caudal segment.

fragments (Fig. 17–27). The objective of the surgery is to elevate this segment back into place and stabilize it with a pin affixed in the ilial wings.[26, 48]

Exposure of the lumbosacral area is as previously described for decompression of this area. Fracture reduction is accomplished with traction on the head and tail of the dog to move the sacrum caudally while a lever is used to elevate the sacrum. The tip of the lever is just ventral to the sacral arch, the fulcrum of the lever is at the arch of L7, and the free end of the lever is cranial to L7. Ventral depression of the free end of the lever raises the sacrum dorsally into anatomic reduction of the articular processes[26, 48] (Fig. 17–28).

Reduction is maintained by a transilial pin, which is placed between the ilial wings dorsocaudal to the base of the spine of L7. To place the pin, the skin is retracted laterally over the middle gluteal muscle. A Steinmann pin is inserted through the middle gluteal muscle and the ilium and emerges just dorsal to the articular facet of L7. It is advanced to the opposite ilium and inserted through it. The nerves of the cauda equina can be explored by removing the remains of the interarcuate ligament between L7 and S1. The pin is cut flush with the gluteal muscles, and closure is routine[26, 48] (Fig. 17–29).

The technique relieves pressure on the spinal nerves, gives stability to the fracture site, and decreases pain and osteophytic response. However, a disadvantage is that a smooth Steinmann pin may migrate if it becomes loose in the ilium. Application of Kirschner clamps external to the skin may prevent pin migration. Deep bacterial infection may occur around the pin, and the dorsal spine of L7 may fracture.[26, 48]

Vinylidene Plates and Pins. A modification of transilial pinning incorporates polyvinylidene plates in the fixation. The plates are applied to the spinous processes of three lumbar vertebrae cranial to the fracture site, leaving portions of the plates extending over the caudal spinal segment. After the fracture is reduced, an intramedullary pin ranging in size from $3/32$ to $1/8$ inch in diameter, depending on the size of the dog, is placed through the gluteal muscle and through the lateral aspect of the ilial wing about 1 cm from the dorsal margin of the iliac crest and 1 cm from its cranial margin. The pin is advanced through holes in the plates and placed through the opposite ilial wing and gluteal muscle. In like manner, a second pin is placed just caudal to the first pin. The pins are bent upward at 90° angles just lateral to the gluteal muscles and are cut, leaving 5 mm protruding lateral to each ilial wing. Closure is routine[14] (Fig. 17–30).

The technique has the advantage of increased stability owing to the many contact points between the plates and the spinous processes. Two pins give greater stability than one pin, because rotation may occur around one pin. Potential disadvantages of the technique are fractures of the spinous processes, pin migra-

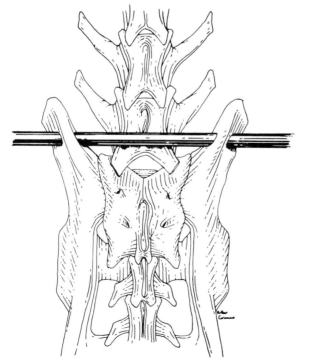

Figure 17–29. Transilial stabilization of a fracture of the body of the seventh lumbar vertebra. The pin passes between the wings of the ilia dorsocaudal to the base of the spine of the seventh lumbar vertebra. (From Slocum B and Rudy RL: Fractures of the seventh lumbar vertebra in the dog. J Am Anim Hosp Assoc 11:167, 1975.)

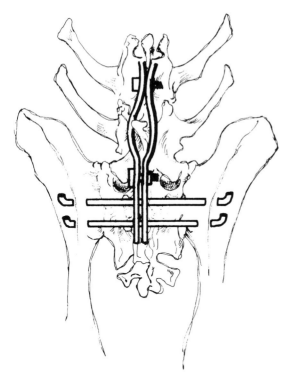

Figure 17–30. Stabilization of lower lumbar fractures with plastic plates and transilial pins. Two transilial pins pass through holes in the plastic plates, which extend over the caudal vertebrae. (After Dulisch ML and Nichols JB: A surgical technique for management of lower lumbar fractures: Case report. Vet Surg 10:90, 1981.)

tion, and postoperative swelling and irritation of the subcutaneous tissues near the pin ends.[14]

Ventral Lumbosacral Stabilization

Ventral stabilization of traumatic lumbosacral spondylolisthesis has been described.[5] With the dog in dorsal recumbency, a routine midline approach is made to the caudal abdominal area. Following abdominal viscera retraction, large vessel identification, and muscle retraction, the ventral lumbosacral area is exposed. A malleolar screw is placed from cranial to caudal across the L7–S1 intervertebral disk space into the body of S1.

The technique has the potential disadvantage of creating a dorsoventral shearing of the vertebral canal at the L7–S1 level as the screw is tightened. In addition, the tip of the screw may traverse the sacral vertebral canal.[5]

Sacrocaudal Decompression, Stabilization, or Amputation

Repair of sacrocaudal fractures and luxations is indicated whenever moderate displacement or neurologic dysfunction is present. Amputation of the tail is indicated when there is lack of deep pain sensation, there is caudal vertebral displacement that may cause traction on nerves of the cauda equina, and it is necessary to relieve pain, especially when rigid internal fixation of small fragments and articular processes is impossible. Amputation prevents self mutilation and fecal soiling of the tail.[26, 59] Even with tail amputation, repair of moderately displaced caudal vertebrae, along with internal stabilization, is indicated because of potential or evident trauma to the sacral nerves. Likewise, repair of greatly displaced sacral fractures is recommended because neurologic complications may accompany large callus formation at the healed fracture site. It is important to remember that not all of the caudal vertebrae may be removed without involvement of the structures of the perineum, especially the external anal sphincter muscles.[26]

Minor displacement of sacral or caudal vertebrae in a small dog may require only wires through the articular processes for fixation. When surgical exposure reveals the need for decompression, a Funkquist type B dorsal laminectomy may be performed to relieve cauda equina compression. This serves as a diagnostic measure to visualize the affected nerves. If the nerve tissue appears salvageable, rigid fixation of the unstable vertebrae is employed. Such fixation may be difficult because of the small size of the bones and the associated trauma.[59]

Sacral fractures may be more adequately stabilized using a U shaped intramedullary pin and wires. The base of the U pin rests in a hole in the dorsal spinous process of L6 or L7 with the legs of the U extending caudally on the vertebral laminae, medial to the articular processes. Segments of orthopedic wire are used to affix the caudal vertebrae to the U pin by passing the wires under the transverse processes ventrally and twisting them together over the legs of the pin dorsally. The articular processes should also be wired to prevent distraction[26] (Fig. 17–31).

Surgical exploration and laminectomy allow direct visualization of the area, which is important because if nerve fibers are completely severed a less favorable prognosis is rendered. Rigid internal fixation can be difficult because

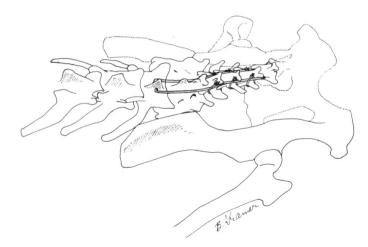

Figure 17–31. Caudal vertebral stabilization with U pin and wires. A U-shaped intramedullary pin is placed through the spinous process of L7 and is contoured to the lamina of the sacral and caudal vertebrae. Orthopedic wire is used to secure the transverse processes to the pin laterally. (From Helphrey M: Spinal trauma. *In* Bojrab MJ (ed): Current Techniques in Small Animal Surgery, 2nd ed. Philadelphia, Lea & Febiger, 1983.)

of the small size of the bones and difficulty in achieving arthrodesis of the articular surfaces.[59]

LATERAL THORACIC AND LUMBAR SURGERY

Fenestration

Thoracolumbar disk fenestrations are generally indicated as a prophylactic measure when dogs show signs of initial or recurrent thoracolumbar pain or paresis.[6, 10, 12, 16, 28, 29, 47] However, some have stated that fenestrations have also been used to successfully treat paraplegic animals.[12, 16]

Similar lateral approaches for fenestrating thoracolumbar disks have been described.[12, 16] One technique for lateral disk fenestration requires that the dog be placed in lateral recumbency over a 4 inch diameter sandbag. A paramedian skin incision is made from the lateral aspect of the dorsal spine of T9 toward the ventral aspect of the ilial wing, stopping at L5. The subcutaneous fat, lumbar fascia, and underlying fat are incised along this same plane to expose the iliocostalis lumborum muscle. The tip of each lateral process is palpated through this muscle. The muscle is separated just dorsal to this tip, elevated, and retracted medially, exposing the lateral aspect of the disk. The fascia lying over the disk is carefully retracted and held cranially with a blunt instrument while a rectangular window is cut in the anulus fibrosus from the 2 to 4 o'clock position. An alligator forceps and blunt probe are then used to remove the nucleus pulposus[16, 47] (Fig. 17–32).

Thoracic disks are exposed similarly, except the iliocostalis lumborum insertion is on the rib. After elevating this muscle, the levator costae muscle, which attaches to the cranial surface of the rib neck, is separated and retracted ventrally to give limited exposure to the disk.[16, 47]

After fenestrating all of the disks from T10 to L4 the vertebral column is flexed and the disks are reexplored for loose disk material. The surgical area is then closed in layers, and a bandage is applied.[16]

The advantages of the technique over laminectomy or hemilaminectomy with fenestration are that there is less hemorrhage and tissue trauma,[12, 16] there is less likelihood of iatrogenic cord damage, no expensive equipment is needed, and exact identification of the offending disk by myelography is not mandatory.[16] The approach does not require entering the thoracic or abdominal cavity, and it can be used in conjunction with a hemilaminectomy for decompression.[47] The disadvantages of the procedure are the need for an assistant to hold the retractors, more difficult muscle retraction in the caudal lumbar area, difficult exposure and fenestration of the thoracic disks,[16] the possibility of creating pneumothorax while working on the thoracic disks,[12, 16] and a temporary mild worsening of clinical signs for 1 to 2 days after surgery, especially if the dog has been treated with antiinflammatory drugs prior to, but not after, surgery.[16]

A dorsolateral muscle separating approach to the thoracolumbar disk has also been described. A dorsal midline or paramedian incision is made from the level of T9 to L6. The subcutaneous tissue and cutaneous trunci muscle are incised along the same plane as the skin. The lumbodorsal fascia, aponeurosis of the longissimus

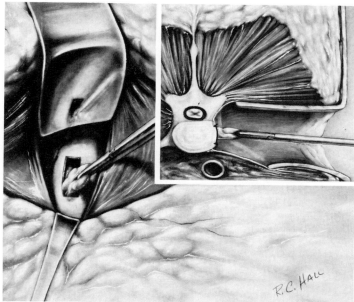

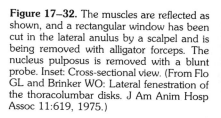

Figure 17–32. The muscles are reflected as shown, and a rectangular window has been cut in the lateral anulus by a scalpel and is being removed with alligator forceps. The nucleus pulposus is removed with a blunt probe. Inset: Cross-sectional view. (From Flo GL and Brinker WO: Lateral fenestration of the thoracolumbar disks. J Am Anim Hosp Assoc 11:619, 1975.)

thoracis and lumborum muscle and the caudal edge of the spinalis and semispinalis muscles are incised from a point 5 cm lateral to the spinous process of T9 to a point 1 to 2 cm lateral to the spinous process of L6. The lateral aspects of the disks are exposed by opening the intramuscular septum between the multifidus muscle group medially and the longissimus muscle group laterally. This septum is the first one lateral to the spinous processes. The surgeon should completely separate muscles to get complete exposure and prevent damage to the dorsal branches of spinal nerves. The disk is incised, and nuclear material is removed with a modified dental tartar scraper. Caution should be used to keep fenestration below the intervertebral foramen and yet not so low on the disk that the ventral branches of the spinal nerves are damaged as they cross the ventrolateral aspect of each disk.[10, 28, 64]

Following fenestration, closure is routine and a light pressure bandage is applied.[10]

The dorsolateral muscle separating approach for disk fenestration has the advantages of permitting decompression by hemilaminectomy, inflicting minimal trauma, and allowing relatively easy access to nine intervertebral disks.[10] Potential surgical complications and disadvantages of the technique include trauma to the multifidus muscle if decompression is used with the technique, failure to fenestrate a disk, pneumothorax, cutting of spinal arteries, damage to the spinal cord, and spinal nerve injury.[2, 10]

Trauma to the spinal nerves may result in scoliosis, ventral abdominal muscle paralysis, and femoral nerve deficits.[2] Some of these complications and disadvantages may also be encountered with other techniques of spinal surgery.

Decompression

The lateral approach can also be utilized for spinal cord decompression. The initial approach to the tips of the lateral processes is basically the same as for the lateral fenestration technique previously described.[16] The epaxial musculature is dissected and retracted dorsally from the lateral processes and intertransverse ligaments to expose the vertebral bodies and adjacent disk. Continued dorsal dissection and retraction exposes the intervertebral foramen with its nerves and vessels. Muscles are separated from the accessory process, and rongeurs or a high speed drill are used to remove the pedicle, beginning at the intervertebral foramen[7] (Fig. 17–33). The caudal thoracic vertebrae and disks are exposed in a manner similar to that for decompression and fenestration. The musculature is returned to its original position, followed by routine closure of the tissues and application of an abdominal bandage.[7]

Lateral decompression has the advantage of being a simple and quick approach to the vertebral column. There is minimal muscle trauma,

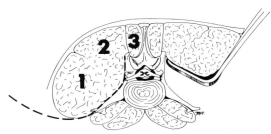

Figure 17–33. This cross-sectional illustration demonstrates the route for the proposed periosteal elevation (on the left). The dorsal retraction of the epaxial muscle mass is shown on the right. 1, 2, 3, Epaxial muscles. (From Braund KG, Taylor TKF, Ghosh P, and Sherwood AA: Lateral spinal decompression in the dog. J Small Anim Pract 17:583, 1976.)

and it does not require further disruption of vertebral stability by removal of dorsal vertebral elements. The cord is decompressed from its ventral aspect without excessive bone resection.[7] Exposure is limited, however.

VENTRAL THORACIC AND LUMBAR SURGERY

Fenestration

The ventral approach for fenestration is also indicated as a prophylactic measure. With the dog in right lateral recumbency, a skin incision is made from the dorsal to the ventral midline along the thirteenth rib. The incision is slid caudally to allow a paracostal incision into the abdomen. After reflecting the left kidney ventrally, Frazier laminectomy retractors are positioned, and the abdominal viscera are packed off. The iliopsoas muscle is retracted from the ventral midline. The crus of the diaphragm, aorta, and sympathetic trunk are also depressed from the surgical site. After palpating and numbering the lateral processes, the area medial to the first lateral process is identified as the T13–L1 intervertebral disk. This area is used as a starting point to count lumbar disks caudally for fenestration from L1–L2 to L5–L6 using a modified tartar scraper. After fenestration, structures are allowed to return to their normal position, and the abdominal muscle layers are sutured.[6, 47]

The skin incision is slid forward, and an entry is made into the thoracic cavity between the tenth and eleventh ribs. Frazier laminectomy retractors hold the ribs apart while positive pressure respiration is administered. While carefully avoiding the sympathetic trunk and intercostal vessels, the pleura is dissected free

from the T9–T10 to the T13–L1 disks, and they are fenestrated. The retractors are removed, followed by routine closure of the thorax, latissimus dorsi muscle, and skin.[6, 47]

Ventral fenestration has the advantage of allowing access to all the potentially offending disks with a minimum of surgical trauma and hemorrhage, as well as avoiding the spinal nerve roots.[6, 47] However, the technique requires a laparotomy, thoracotomy, positive pressure respiration, and reestablishment of a negative thoracic pressure after thoracic closure. In addition, major structures must be handled and retracted to avoid damage to them, decompression of the spinal cord is not possible, and there is risk of pushing nucleus pulposus into the vertebral canal.[47, 52] The animal must be monitored closely during the anesthetic recovery period.[6]

REFERENCES

1. Albin MS, White RJ, Yashon D, and Harris LS: Effects of localized cooling on spinal cord trauma. J Trauma 9:1000, 1969.
2. Bartels KE, Creed JE, and Yturraspe DJ: Complications associated with the dorsolateral muscle-separating approach for thoracolumbar disc fenestration in the dog. JAVMA 183:1081, 1983.
3. Belcher WR: Evaluation of the lumbar myelotomy and durotomy in the dog. Senior Seminar Report, School of Veterinary Medicine, Auburn University 1:217, 1974.
4. Berzon JL and Dueland R: Cauda equina syndrome: Pathophysiology and report of seven cases. J Am Anim Hosp Assoc 15:635, 1979.
5. Betts CW, Kneller SK, and Skelton JA: An unusual case of traumatic spondylolisthesis in a red bone hound; diagnosis and therapy. J Am Anim Hosp Assoc 12:470, 1976.
6. Bojrab MJ: Thoracolumbar spine: Prophylactic thoracolumbar disk fenestration. In Bojrab MJ (ed): Current Techniques in Small Animal Surgery, 2nd ed. Philadelphia, Lea & Febiger, 1983.
7. Braund KG, Taylor TKF, Ghosh P, and Sherwood AA: Lateral spinal decompression in the dog. J Small Anim Pract 17:583, 1976.
8. Chrisman CL: Problems in Small Animal Neurology. Philadelphia, Lea & Febiger, 1982.
9. Coulter SB: Fenestration, decompression, or both? Vet Clin North Am 8:379, 1978.
10. Creed JE and Yturraspe DJ: Thoracolumbar spine: Intervertebral disk fenestration. In Bojrab MJ (ed): Current Techniques in Small Animal Surgery, 2nd ed. Philadelphia, Lea & Febiger, 1983.
11. David T: Thoracolumbar hemilaminectomy in the dog using a power skull trephine. Vet Med Small Anim Clin 71:477, 1976.
12. Denny HR: The lateral fenestration of canine thoracolumbar disc protrusions: A review of 30 cases. J Small Anim Pract 19:259, 1978.
13. Denny HR, Gibbs C, and Holt PE: The diagnosis and treatment of cauda equina lesions in the dog. J Small Anim Pract 23:245, 1982.
14. Dulisch ML and Nichols JB: A surgical technique for

management of lower lumbar fractures: A case report. Vet Surg 10:90, 1981.

15. Dulisch ML and Withrow SJ: The use of plastic plates for fixation of spinal fractures in the dog. Can Vet J 20:326, 1979.

16. Flo GL and Brinker WO: Lateral fenestration of thoracolumbar discs. J Am Anim Hosp Assoc 11:619, 1975.

17. Funkquist B: Decompressive laminectomy for cervical disk protrusion in the dog. Acta Vet Scand 3:88, 1962.

18. Funkquist B: Thoracolumbar disk protrusion with severe cord compression in the dog. I. Clinical and pathoanatomic observations with special reference to the rate of development of the symptoms of motor loss. II. Clinical observations with special reference to the prognosis in conservative treatment. III. Treatment by decompressive laminectomy. Acta Vet Scand 3:256, 1962.

19. Funkquist B: Investigations of the therapeutic and prophylactic effects of disc evacuation in cases of thoracolumbar herniated discs in dogs. Acta Vet Scand 19:441, 1978.

20. Funkquist B and Schantz B: Influence of extensive laminectomy on the shape of the spinal canal. Acta Orthop Scand (Suppl) 56:1, 1962.

21. Gage ED: A new method of spinal fixation in the dog (a preliminary report). Vet Med Small Anim Clin 64:295, 1969.

22. Gage ED: Surgical repairs of spinal fractures in small breed dogs. Vet Med Small Anim Clin 66:1095, 1971.

23. Gage ED: Spinal disc surgery the dog: Part 3— Thoracolumbar hemilaminectomy and disc fenestration. Southwest Vet 25:209, 1972.

24. Gage ED: Modifications in dorsolateral hemilaminectomy and disc fenestration in the dog. J Am Anim Hosp Assoc 11:407, 1975.

25. Gambardella PC: Dorsal decompressive laminectomy for treatment of thoracolumbar disc disease in dogs: A retrospective study of 98 cases. Vet Surg 9:24, 1980.

26. Helphrey M: Spinal trauma. In Bojrab MJ (ed): Current Techniques in Small Animal Surgery, 2nd ed. Philadelphia, Lea & Febiger, 1983.

27. Henry WB Jr: Dorsal decompressive laminectomy in the treatment of thoraco-lumbar disc disease. J Am Anim Hosp Assoc 11:627, 1975.

28. Hoerlein BF: Canine Neurology, 3rd ed. Philadelphia, WB Saunders Co, 1978.

29. Hoerlein BF: The status of the various intervertebral disc surgeries for the dog in 1978. J Am Anim Hosp Assoc 14:563, 1978.

30. Horne TR, Powers RD, and Swaim SF: Dorsal laminectomy techniques in the dog. JAVMA 171:742, 1977.

31. Keller JT, Dunsker SB, McWhorter JM, et al: The fate of autogenous grafts to the spinal dura. J Neurosurg 49:412, 1978.

32. Kiviluoto O: Use of free fat transplants to prevent epidural scar formation: An experimental study. Acta Orthop Scand (Suppl) 164:3, 1976.

33. Leighton RL: Surgical treatment of canine lumbosacral spondylopathy. Vet Med Small Anim Clin 78:1853, 1983.

34. Lenehan TM: Canine cauda equina syndrome. Comp Cont Ed Pract Vet 5:941, 1983.

35. Lippincott CL: Use of the micrometer trephine in surgical treatment of the intervertebral disc syndrome. Vet Med Small Anim Clin 67:643, 1972.

36. Matthiesen DT: Thoracolumbar spinal fractures/luxations: Surgical management. Comp Cont Ed Pract Vet 5:867, 1983.

37. Mendenhall HV, Litwak P, Yturraspe DJ, et al: Aggressive pharmacologic and surgical treatment of spinal cord injuries in dogs and cats. JAVMA 168:1026, 1976.

38. Oliver JE Jr and Selcer RR: Decompression of the lumbosacral spinal cord and nerve roots. In Bojrab MJ (ed): Current Techniques in Small Animal Surgery I. Philadelphia, Lea & Febiger, 1975.

39. Oliver JE Jr, Selcer RR, and Simpson S: Cauda equina compression from lumbosacral malarticulation and malformation in the dog. JAVMA 173:207, 1978.

40. Osterholm JL: The pathophysiological response to spinal cord injury: The current status of related research. J Neurosurg 40:5, 1974.

41. Parker AJ: Durotomy and saline perfusion in spinal cord trauma. J Am Anim Hosp Assoc 11:412, 1975.

42. Parker AJ and Smith CW: Functional recovery from spinal cord trauma following incision of spinal meninges in dogs. Res Vet Sci 16:276, 1974.

43. Parker AJ and Smith CW: Functional recovery from spinal cord trauma following delayed incision of spinal meninges in dogs. Res Vet Sci 18:110, 1975.

44. Prata RG: Neurosurgical treatment of thoracolumbar disks: The rationale and value of laminectomy with concomitant disk removal. J Am Anim Hosp Assoc 17:17, 1981.

45. Rouse GP and Miller JI: The use of methylmethacrylate for spinal stabilization. J Am Anim Hosp Assoc 11:418, 1975.

46. Rucker NC, Lumb WV, and Scott RJ: Combined pharmacologic and surgical treatments for acute spinal cord trauma. Am J Vet Res 42:1138, 1981.

47. Shores A: Intervertebral disk syndrome in the dog. Part III. Thoracolumbar disk surgery. Comp Cont Ed Pract Vet 4:24, 1982.

48. Slocum B and Rudy RL: Fractures of the seventh lumbar vertebra in the dog. J Am Anim Hosp Assoc 11:167, 1975.

49. Swaim SF: Body casts: Technics of application to the dog. Vet Med Small Anim Clin 65:1179, 1970.

50. Swaim SF: Vertebral body plating for spinal immobilization. JAVMA 158:1683, 1971.

51. Swaim SF: Use of pneumatic surgical instruments in neurosurgery. Part I. Spinal surgery. Vet Med Small Anim Clin 68:1275, 1973.

52. Swaim SF: Surgical approaches to spinal cord disease of small animals. Sci Proc Am Anim Hosp Assoc Meet 1:311, 1975.

53. Swaim SF: Thoracolumbar and sacral spine trauma. In Bojrab MJ (ed): Current Techniques in Small Animal Surgery I. Philadelphia, Lea & Febiger, 1975.

54. Swaim SF: A rongeuring technique for performing thoracolumbar hemilaminectomies. Vet Med Small Anim Clin 71:172, 1976.

55. Swaim SF and Vandevelde M: Clinical and histologic evaluation of bilateral hemilaminectomy and deep dorsal laminectomy for extensive spinal cord decompression in the dog. JAVMA 170:407, 1977.

56. Swaim SF, Vandevelde M, Sammons WC, et al: Comparison of hypothermic and normothermic spinal cord perfusion in the dog. Vet Surg 8:119, 1979.

57. Tarvin G and Prata RG: Lumbosacral stenosis in dogs. JAVMA 177:154, 1980.

58. Tator CH and Deecke L: Value of normothermic perfusion, hypothermic perfusion, and durotomy in the treatment of experimental acute spinal cord trauma. J Neurosurg 39:52, 1973.

59. Taylor RA: Treatment of fractures of the sacrum and sacrococcygeal region. Vet Surg 10:119, 1981.

60. Teague HD and Brasmer TH: Midline myelotomy of the clinically normal canine spinal cord. Am J Vet Res 39:1584, 1978.

61. Trotter EJ: Thoracolumbar spine: Thoracolumbar disc disease. In Bojrab MJ (ed): Current Techniques in

Small Animal Surgery, 2nd ed. Philadelphia, Lea & Febiger, 1983.

62. Walker TL, Roberts RE, Kincaid SA, and Bratton GR: The use of electric drills as an alternative to pneumatic equipment in spinal surgery. J Am Anim Hosp Assoc 17:605, 1981.

63. Yturraspe DJ and Lumb WV: The use of plastic spinal plates for internal fixation of the canine spine. JAVMA 161:1651, 1972.

64. Yturraspe DJ and Lumb WV: A dorsolateral muscle separating approach for thoraco-lumbar intervertebral disc fenestration in the dog. JAVMA 162:1037, 1973.

Section 2   DC Sorjonen, DVM, MS

SMALL ANIMAL CERVICAL SURGERY

PREOPERATIVE PROCEDURES

The indications for cervical surgery are generally the same as those for thoracolumbar, lumbosacral, and sacrocaudal surgery. Tracheal intubation and patient positioning require special consideration when performing cervical surgery, however. The endotracheal tube must be of sufficient length to prevent tracheal collapse when the patient is positioned for surgery (dorsal approach) or tracheal manipulation (ventral approach). Precaution in patient positioning to prevent hyperflexion or hyperextension of the injured area is critical when vertebral instability is present.

DORSAL TECHNIQUES

Cranial Cervical Vertebral Exposure and Decompression

The dorsal cranial cervical approach is most commonly employed to correct atlantoaxial instability or fracture (Fig. 17–34). The approach can also be used to explore the cranial cervical vertebral column for other conditions (eg, neoplasia). The caudal cephalic and cranial cervical area is prepared for aseptic surgery, and the patient is positioned in ventral recumbency with the head slightly flexed. Compression of the external jugular veins is avoided because occlusion may cause exaggerated hemorrhage if the ventral vertebral venous plexus is entered. The skin is incised on the dorsal midline from the external occipital protuberance to the level of the fourth cervical vertebra. Using the spinous process of C2 as a landmark, the incision is continued ventrally by sharp incision on the median plane to gently remove the paravertebral muscles from the spinous process of C2 and from the arches of C1 and C2. Paravertebral muscle dissection is repeated on the opposite side if bilateral exposure is required. The spinal cord can be exposed cranial and caudal to C1 by dissecting the overlying atlantooccipital and interarcuate ligaments, respectively, along with adjacent fibrous tissue. The dura is usually attached to the cranial edge of the atlas. It may be separated without penetration by careful subperiosteal dissection over the cranial border of the atlas. The vertebral and cerebrospinal arteries, the anastomotic veins, and the first and second cervical nerves are usually located lateral to the area of exposure, but must be isolated and preserved if dissection is extended laterally (Fig. 17–35).

Hemilaminectomy is not needed in most luxations, as reduction accomplishes the decompression.[21] If additional decompression is necessary, a hemilaminectomy is performed using a 2 mm rongeur* to include one side of the caudal half of C1 and one side of the cranial half of the arch of C2.

Cranial Cervical Stabilization

Nearly 90% of all cervical fractures in dogs occur cranial to C3.[31] Fractures of the bodies of C1 and C2 or their end plates can be repaired through the dorsal approach, provided dorsal structures can support fixation devices.

Longitudinal Atlas Fixation

Vertebral stabilization can be achieved by using a double strand of 20 or 22 gauge orthopedic stainless steel wire.[7, 21] A wire loop with the caudal strands on opposite sides of C2 is advanced from the dorsal atlantoaxial space cranially under the arch of C1 (Fig. 17–36). Head flexion, removal of a caudal portion of the occipital bone, or caudal traction with an ovariohysterectomy hook on the cranial brim of the arch of C1 will facilitate passage of the wire. Continuous downward pressure on the axis re-

---

*Lempert rongeurs, Codman and Shurtleff Inc, Randolph, MA.

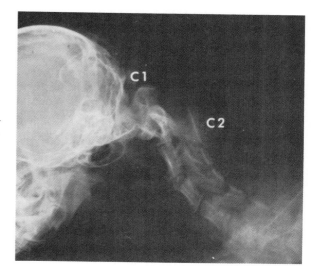

Figure 17–34. Lateral radiograph of an atlantoaxial subluxation showing dorsal displacement of the axis (C2). C1 = atlas.

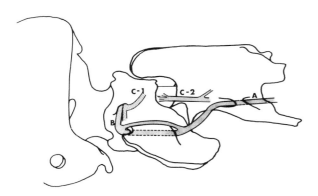

Figure 17–35. Lateral view of atlantoaxial area demonstrating major arteries and nerves. A, Vertebral artery; B, cerebrospinal artery; C–1, first cervical nerve; C–2, second cervical nerve. (From Oliver JE Jr and Lewis RE: Lesions of the atlas and axis in dogs. J Am Anim Hosp Assoc 9:304, 1973.)

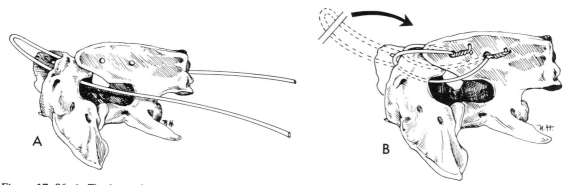

Figure 17–36. A, The loop of wire is passed under the atlas with the caudal strands on opposite sides of the axis. B, The cranial and caudal pairs of strands are tied together in their respective predrilled holes. (From Swaim SF: Surgical approaches to spinal cord disease of small animals. Proc Am Anim Hosp Assoc 1:311, 1975).

duces the luxation, relieving the compression and facilitating passage of the wire. Careful passage of the wire will prevent trauma to the spinal cord. After retrieval of the loop from the atlantooccipital space, the wire loop is cut and the strands are folded back over C1. The atlantoaxial subluxation is gently held in reduction by ventral depression of C2 using hemostatic forceps. The two strands of wire from the atlantoaxial space are twisted together through the most caudal of two predrilled holes in the spine of C2, while the two other ends of the strands of wire exiting from the atlantooccipital space are twisted together through the cranial hole (Fig. 17–36).

When the epidural space is too small to safely manipulate a loop of heavy orthopedic wire under the arch of C1, nonmetallic suture material (0–2 nylon or impregnated silk* or Dacron†) can be used. The nonmetallic suture material is threaded through a loop of small stainless steel wire (32–36 gauge) that has been passed under the arch at C1 from caudal to cranial. The nonmetallic suture material is then pulled from cranial to caudal under the arch of C1, transected, and tied to the dorsal spine of C2 as described for the wiring technique.[4]

Anatomic alignment and adequate stabilization of C1 and C2 can be achieved with the dorsal wiring technique (Fig. 17–37). However, trauma to the cord during wire passage, wire breakage, slippage, or dislodgement from bone, and inadequate space to safely pass the fixation wire are reported disadvantages.[20] The nonmetallic suture fixation can overcome the problem of lack of space to pass the wire; however,

---

*Silky, Polydek, Deknatel, Inc, Queens Village, NY.
†Tevdek, Deknatel, Inc, Queens Village, NY.

breakage of the suture material and inadequate bone mass (in toy breeds) to allow concurrent decompressive hemilaminectomy (which is rarely needed) are reported disadvantages.[4] When original wiring techniques have failed, methylmethacrylate bone cement has been packed around the dorsal aspects of C1 and C2 to create stability.[25]

Transverse Atlas Fixation

To avoid passage of the fixation wire beneath the arch of C1, small holes can be drilled on opposite sides of the arch.[15] After transverse passage of a double wire loop through the holes, the wire loop is cut and the individual strands are tightened through holes predrilled in the spine of C2. Trauma to the cord is reduced with this technique; however, the bony support provided by C1 may not be as great as that of longitudinal wire passage under the arch of C1.

Atlantooccipital Fixation

An atlantooccipital instability has been repaired by wiring a wing of the atlas to the ipsilateral occipital condyle.[8] A hemilaminectomy was performed over the area of greatest cord compression. Bone fragments and blood clots were gently removed from the surgical area, and the area was flushed with an isotonic solution.

Caudal Cervical Vertebral Exposure and Decompression (C3–T1)

The dorsal caudal cervical approach can be used for the cervical vertebral malformation-

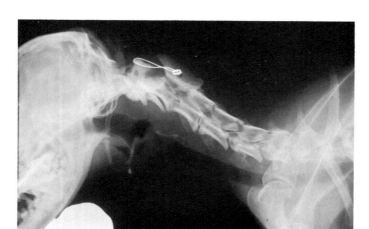

Figure 17–37. An atlantoaxial subluxation after decompression and dorsal wire fixation.

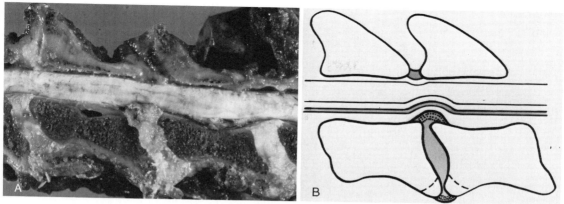

Figure 17–38. A, Sagittal section of the cervical spine. B, The ligamentous changes and subsequent spinal cord compression that can occur with cervical vertebral malformation-malarticulation. (From Seim HB and Withrow SJ: Pathophysiology and diagnosis of caudal-cervical spondylo-myelopathy with emphasis on the Doberman pinscher. J Am Anim Hosp Assoc 18:241, 1982.)

malarticulation (CVMM) syndrome, fractures and luxations of the cervical vertebrae, spinal cord or vertebral neoplasia, and, less commonly, intervertebral disk prolapse.

In cervical vertebral malformation-malarticulation, cord compression can occur dorsally as a result of interarcuate ligament hypertrophy and stenosis of the cranial orifice of a vertebral foramen, or ventrally as a result of hypertrophy of the dorsal longitudinal ligament, hypertrophy of the dorsal anulus fibrosus, and herniation of the nucleus pulposus[3, 5, 24, 28, 38] (Fig. 17–38). Cord compression from disk prolapse, neoplasia, and vertebral fractures can occur from any direction. Because of the variety of disease conditions possible in the caudal cervical area, a single surgical decompression technique cannot be recommended for all cases. In general, a dorsal laminectomy can be used in dogs with dorsal cord compression. If ventral cord compression exists, or damage to dorsal structures prevents their use in stabilization, ventral decompression and/or stabilization may be indicated (see below).

The patient is positioned in ventral recumbency with the head down and the caudal cervical vertebrae elevated with sandbags. A skin incision is made on the dorsal midline from the external occipital protuberance to the first thoracic vertebra to expose the almost transparent platysma muscle. The dorsal midline can be identified by noting the emergence of cutaneous branches of the cervical nerves through the median fibrous raphe and by palpating the spinous process of C2. A sharp incision through the median raphe is deepened to expose the nuchal ligament. This incision is extended to expose the caudal aspect of the spine of C2 and the spinous process of T1 (the cranial and caudal attachments of the nuchal ligament, respectively), which serve as landmarks. The nuchal ligament and dorsolateral cervical muscles are retracted laterally, and the spinous processes from C3 to C7 can be palpated between the straplike spinalis cervicis muscles. The spinous process of C3 may be difficult to perceive because the spinous process of C2 overhangs the dorsum of C3 and the dorsal spine of C3 is often small. The spinalis cervicis muscles over the spinous processes are incised on the midline and dissected from the vertebral laminae with a periosteal elevator. A surgical sponge on the blunt end of a scalpel handle is also helpful in removing muscle from the dorsal laminae. A large, self-retaining retractor* is helpful in maintaining vertebral exposure. Large branches of the vertebral artery course through muscles near the articular processes. Hemorrhage may be reduced by separating muscles close to bone; however, all vessels encountered should be ligated[17] (Figs. 17–39 and 17–40).

To expose the C2–C3 interspace, a uni- or bilateral incision and retraction of the muscles from the spinous process of C2 is required. Removal of the multifidus cervicis muscle from the dorsolateral aspect of C2 will expose the C2–C3 interspace (Fig. 17–41). Extreme care should be taken to avoid the vertebral artery as it courses through the transverse foramen and the cervical vessels and nerves at the intervertebral foramen.

---

*Downing laminectomy retractor, Zimmer USA, Warsaw, IN.

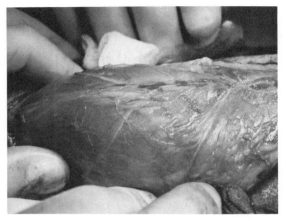

Figure 17–39. The dorsal midline is identified by emergence of cutaneous branches of the cranial nerves. (From Hurov L: Dorsal decompressive cervical laminectomy in the dog: Surgical considerations and clinical cases. J Am Anim Hosp Assoc 15:301, 1979.)

To decompress the spinal cord over C2, the caudal articular process of C2–C3 on the side with the most neurologic involvement is removed with a rongeur. A hemilaminectomy can then be started at the caudal aspect of C2 and extended from caudal to cranial, lateral to the spinous process of C2. Generally, the hemilaminectomy can be performed with a rongeur on smaller animals; however, a high speed pneu-

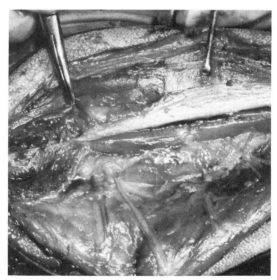

Figure 17–40. The nuchal ligament attaches cranially to the spinous process of the axis and caudally to the tip of the T1 spinous process. (From Hurov L: Dorsal decompressive cervical laminectomy in the dog: Surgical considerations and clinical cases. J Am Anim Hosp Assoc 15:301, 1979.)

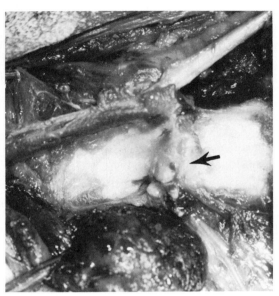

Figure 17–41. Exposure of the C2–C3 interspace (arrow). (From Hurov L: Dorsal decompressive cervical laminectomy in the dog: Surgical considerations and clinical cases. J Am Anim Hosp Assoc 15:301, 1979.)

matic drill* equipped with a bur may be required in larger animals[35, 38] (Fig. 17–42).

Cervical vertebral decompression caudal to C2 is usually by laminectomy. Removal of the spinous processes and interarcuate ligament overlying each interspace to be decompressed will enhance exposure of the bony laminae. The laminectomy is usually performed with a rongeur, starting on the caudal border of the cranial vertebra of each pair composing an interspace. In larger animals, duck bill rongeurs† will facilitate bone removal. The laminectomy is continued cranially and caudally until the cord is no longer compressed. The presence of epidural fat usually indicates adequate cord decompression. Laterally, the laminectomy should not involve the articular processes, which may be needed for vertebral stabilization.[17, 18, 34, 38]

When hypertrophy of the cranial articular processes produces stenosis of the vertebral canal (CVMM), undercutting of the inner cortical and middle cancellous bone of the involved laminae by means of a high speed pneumatic drill and bur can be performed[38] (Fig. 17–43).

To facilitate undercutting of the laminectomy edges or removal of a spinal cord tumor or prolapsed disk, 5–0 or 6–0 silk sling sutures

*Airdrill 100, Hall International, Inc, Santa Barbara, CA.
†Echlin laminectomy rongeurs, double action, Codman and Shurtleff Inc, Randolph, MA.

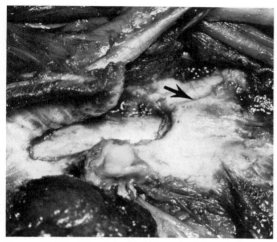

Figure 17–42. Dorsal cervical decompression at C2–C3. The C2 hemilaminectomy is performed laterally to spare the spinous process. Incomplete C3 laminectomy illustrates location of the bony opening and partial removal of the C3 spinous process (arrow). (From Hurov L: Dorsal decompressive cervical laminectomy in the dog: Surgical considerations and clinical cases. J Am Anim Hosp Assoc 15:301, 1979.)

may be placed in the dura mater to elevate and retract the cord laterally; however, excess spinal cord manipulation should be avoided. Extramedullary neoplasia can be gently dissected

from the cord using ophthalmic scissors and forceps. To expose intradural-extramedullary neoplasia, a durotomy is performed over the lesion.[39]

Hemilaminectomy may be performed on the cervical vertebrae caudal to C3. Exposure is similar to that described above, but the bone removal only involves one side of the vertebral arch to include the laminae, pedicles, and articular processes. The vertebral artery in the transverse foramen must be preserved.

Although generally not indicated in the cervical area, additional procedures, such as myelotomy or spinal cord perfusion, may be performed. Adipose tissue is applied to the bony defect prior to closure. Secure closure of all separated muscle layers is performed to help prevent seroma formation.

The advantages of the dorsal approaches to the cervical vertebrae are the potential for extensive decompression and exposure allowing for the inspection of osseous, ligamentous, and neural lesions; however, soft tissue dissection diverging from the dorsal midline can result in muscle trauma and excessive hemorrhage.[38] The decompressive techniques described can be used alone or in combination. The dorsolateral hemilaminectomy is advantageous for decompression of C2 and whenever cord compres-

Figure 17–43. In cervical vertebral malarticulation-malformation, undercutting of the inner cortical and middle cancellous bone with a high speed air drill and bur will provide more spacious decompression. (From Trotter EJ, deLahunta A, Geary JC, and Brasmer TH: Caudal cervical vertebral malformation-malarticulation in Great Danes and Doberman pinschers. JAVMA 168:917, 1976.)

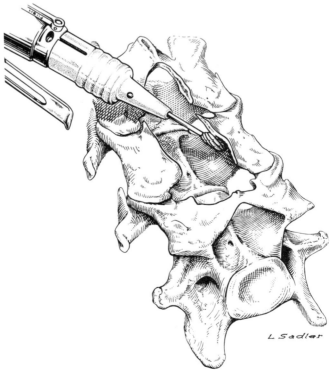

sion (disk, tumor) is lateralized; however, the potential for vertebral stabilization is reduced with removal of articular processes.[35] The laminectomy, which is most commonly used caudal to C2 or when dorsal structures compress the cord, provides maximum cord decompression and exposure while allowing vertebral stabilization; however, constrictive fibrosis with subsequent cord compression may occur.[15]

Caudal Cervical Stabilization

Stabilization of the caudal cervical vertebrae from the dorsal approach is indicated to manage vertebral instability. When cord compression coexists with instability, stabilization can be combined with decompressive techniques.

The dorsal approach for vertebral stabilization is contraindicated if vertebral instability coexists with fractures of the articular processes of the involved vertebrae. Detailed ventrodorsal and oblique radiographs of the vertebral fractures will aid in determining the status of the articular processes before surgery. Additionally, fractures that produce dorsal displacement of the vertebral body may be difficult to reduce from a dorsal approach.[31] In these instances, ventral decompression and stabilization may be indicated.

Articular Process Screws

Stabilization of the caudal cervical vertebrae is most commonly performed in treating cervical vertebral malformation-malarticulation and vertebral fractures. In CVMM, vertebral stabilization can be achieved by placing screws bilaterally through the articular processes. Vertebral exposure is similar to that described for caudal cervical decompressive techniques. Using a 5/64 inch diameter drill bit in a small hand drill,* a hole is drilled caudoventrally and slightly laterally through the center of the overlapping articular processes of the unstable vertebrae. The drilling is stopped as the drill bit penetrates the cortical bone on the ventral surface of the cranial articular process, thus preventing damage to the vertebral artery and cervical vessels and nerves as they emerge from the intervertebral foramen. The hole is enlarged with a 7/64 inch diameter drill bit, and the depth of the hole measured.† A 9/64 inch

diameter Bechtol radial fluted point bone screw with buttress threads* is advanced into the hole. The procedure is repeated on the opposite articular process[34] (Fig. 17–44). The screw is tightened slowly to avoid fracture of the articular processes. Near the end of tightening, the surgeon should observe the cervical musculature for fasciculations as the screw is turned. This could indicate that the tip of the screw is irritating a cervical nerve as it emerges from the intervertebral foramen. The surgeon should remove the screw and use a shorter one.

Articular Process Arthrodesis

Arthrodesis of unstable articulations using cancellous bone grafts or corticocancellous bone grafts has been described.[38] Preparation for the cancellous graft is by removal of the joint capsules and hyaline cartilage from the articular surfaces of the unstable vertebrae. The spinous processes of the unstable vertebrae are removed and cancellous bone harvested from them is packed into the prepared articulation.[38] Eighteen gauge orthopedic wire is passed through 1 mm diameter holes predrilled through the center of the articular processes. The wire is twisted tightly to immobilize and compress the articulation.

In addition, a thoracic spinous process can be wired to the denuded articular surface of unstable cervical vertebra.[9]

Long-term evaluation is lacking for any of the dorsal decompressive and stabilizing techniques discussed. In general, the best results are obtained when the cord is decompressed at the site of maximum compression (dorsal or ventral) and stabilization is provided when needed.[3, 18, 38]

Fractures of the caudal cervical vertebrae that produce dorsal cord compression are repaired best from the dorsal approach.[31] The laminectomy is performed over the area of greatest cord compression.[21] Any bone fragments or blood clots are gently removed, and the area is flushed with an isotonic solution. The fracture is gently reduced and stabilization can be performed utilizing the techniques described for CVMM repair.[18, 31]

If articular processes fracture, screws loosen, or wires break, exacerbation of clinical signs may develop.[3, 18, 28] Recurrences may also occur in animals with multiple vertebral involvement. Stabilization of one vertebral segment may act

---

*Richards pistol grip drill, Richards Mfg Co, Memphis, TN.

†Calibrated depth gauge, Richards Mfg Co, Memphis, TN.

*Richards bone screw, Richards Mfg Co, Memphis, TN.

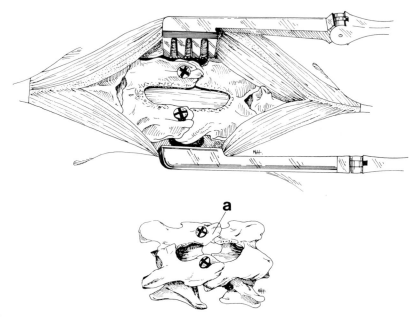

Figure 17–44. In cervical vertebral malarticulation-malformation, a dorsal laminectomy is performed to relieve the fibrous and osseous constriction of the cord. Immobilization is obtained by bilateral placement of Bechtol radial-fluted point, buttress-threaded screws in the heaviest portion of the overlapping articular processes (a) of the involved vertebrae. Notice the angulation of the screws in the lower drawing. (Courtesy of Dr SF Swaim).

as a fulcrum to increase instability of another segment. In one report, 25 of 36 (70%) cases of cervical vertebral malformation-malarticulation involved multiple vertebrae.[23]

VENTRAL TECHNIQUES

Cranial Cervical Vertebral Exposure and Decompression (C1–C2)

The cranial cervical vertebrae should be approached ventrally when ventral spinal cord compression is present or when vertebral instability exists and dorsal structures cannot support fixation devices.[30, 31] Fractures of the dens, abnormally angulated dens, fractures involving the body of C1 or C2, and atlantoaxial or atlantooccipital subluxation can be repaired through the ventral approach.

The patient is positioned in dorsal recumbency with the head and neck extended over a sandbag and thoracic limbs pulled caudally. Tracheal intubation to the level of the manubrium is imperative because of tracheal manipulation during surgery. The ventral cervical area is prepared for aseptic surgery from the caudal intermandibular area to the manubrium of the sternum. A ventral midline skin incision is made from the level of the larynx to the level of the fourth cervical vertebra. The sternohyoid muscles are divided along the midline and retracted laterally. The trachea and esophagus are isolated and retracted away from the surgeon. The carotid sheath nearest the surgeon is isolated and protected from damage during soft tissue retraction. Craniolateral retraction of the larynx, cranial portion of the trachea, and esophagus and thyroid glands exposes the longus colli muscles. The atlas is located by palpating the pointed ventral tubercle that marks the midline. The longus colli muscles are separated on the midline using a periosteal elevator and scissors to expose the underlying bone from the occipital condyles to C4. Vertebral exposure is maintained with self-retaining retractors positioned on opposite ends of the incision through the longus colli muscles.[33, 36]

Odontoidectomy is indicated to treat congenital angulation of the dens producing spinal cord compression.[36] Initially, a defect is created in the caudal one half of the ventral arch of C1 using rongeurs. The dens is removed at its junction with C2 using rongeurs or a high speed pneumatic drill equipped with an oblong bur. The dens is reflected cranially and removed by incising any ligamentous structures attached to the apex (Fig. 17–45).

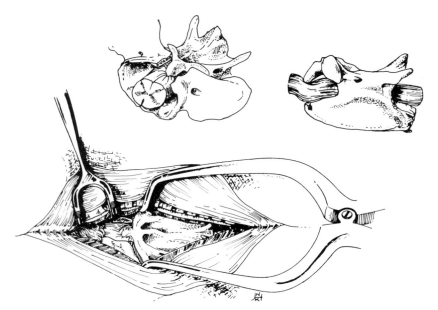

Figure 17–45. Angulation of the dens. The dog is in the dorsal recumbent position. The upper right view shows the dens angulated against the spinal cord. In the ventral approach, the ventral arch of the atlas is burred off by means of a pneumatic drill and bur, and the dens is removed. (From Swaim SF and Greene CE: Odontoidectomy in the dog. J Am Anim Hosp Assoc 11:663, 1975.)

Cranial Cervical Stabilization

Atlantoaxial Pin Fixation

Atlantoaxial subluxation can coexist with fractures, or congenital defects of the dens can occur with a normal, intact dens. The ventral approach to atlantoaxial subluxation repair utilizes odontoidectomy for cord decompression along with vertebral fixation by orthopedic pins or screws and joint arthrodesis.[30] In atlantoaxial subluxation, ventral exposure will reveal a step deformity of the atlantoaxial interface, with C2 displaced dorsocranially. The atlantoaxial articulations are exposed bilaterally by complete removal of their joint capsules. By placing a periosteal elevator or dental tartar scraper in the atlantoaxial joint, the luxated vertebrae can be levered back into alignment. If the dens is present an odontoidectomy (see above) should be performed. Articular cartilage is removed from the surface of C1 and C2 using a number 15 scalpel blade and dental tartar scraper. If a bone graft is used, the right proximal humerus is surgically exposed and cancellous bone is obtained. This bone is transferred to the scarified atlantoaxial joint spaces. The atlas and axis are held in alignment with small reduction forceps.*

_____

*Bone fragment forceps, Synthesis Limited, Wayne, PA.

In smaller animals, a premeasured 0.45 inch or 0.625 inch nonthreaded Kirschner pin is used to establish joint stability. The pin is drilled into the caudoventral body of C2 near the midline and is directed craniolaterally nearly parallel to the ventral surface of C2 toward the alar notch that lies on the cranial edge of C1. The pin crosses the atlantoaxial joint and is seated in C1 (Fig. 17–46). A hand drill or pneumatic drill* can be used for pin placement. By laying the pin across the ventral surface of the atlantoaxial joint over the proposed placement route, exact pin length can be determined. A second pin is placed through the opposite atlantoaxial joint in like fashion. The pins are cut close to their entrance into the body of C2. The tissues are approximated in individual layers for closure.[30]

Atlantooccipital Pin Fixation

Repair of atlantooccipital subluxation can be performed through the ventral approach. The atlantooccipital articulation is exposed, scarified, reduced, and held in alignment in a similar manner to that described for atlantoaxial subluxation. Gentle traction on the head will aid

_____

*Airdrill 200-S, 3M, Surgical Products Division, Costa Mesa, CA.

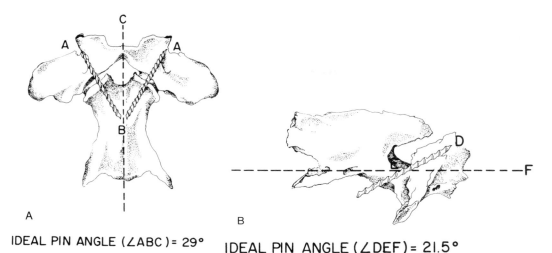

IDEAL PIN ANGLE (∠ABC)= 29°   IDEAL PIN ANGLE (∠DEF)= 21.5°

Figure 17–46. A, ventrodorsal view of atlantoaxial joint showing the ideal pin placement. BC designates the midline. A is the medial border of the alar notch of the atlas. ABC is the ideal angle for pin placement. B, Lateral view of atlantoaxial joint showing ideal pin placement. F is a line along the floor of the canal. D indicates the most craniolateral point of the cranial articular surface of the atlas. DEF is the ideal for pin placement. (From Sorjonen DC and Shires PK: Atlantoaxial instability: A ventral surgical technique for decompression, fixation and fusion. Vet Surg 10:22, 1981.)

in reduction. A premeasured nonthreaded Kirschner pin is positioned nearly parallel to the ventral surface of C1 and drilled into the caudoventral body of C1 just medial to the alar notch. The pin is directed craniomedially through the atlantooccipital joint into the occipital condyle. Measurement of the proposed pin route taken from radiographs of the atlantooccipital joint can aid in determining the pin length necessary. The fixation is performed bilaterally. The remainder of the procedure is similar to that described for atlantoaxial subluxation.

In larger animals, screws can be used to maintain atlantoaxial or atlantooccipital joint stability. In place of pins, 9/64 inch diameter self-tapping screws placed in 7/64 inch diameter tunnels are used. Additional aspects of the screw technique are similar to those described for repair of subluxation using Kirschner pins. Atlantooccipital subluxation in a pygmy goat[29] and combined atlantoaxial and atlantooccipital subluxation in a 4 month old Doberman pinscher have been successfully repaired by the author with screw fixation via the ventral approach (Fig. 17–47).

Advantages of the ventral approach not provided by dorsal approach include odontoidectomy if the dens is abnormal or has remained intact, ease of reduction and alignment of dorsally displaced vertebral body fractures or subluxations, and joint arthrodesis to prevent

clinical recurrence if long-range orthopedic appliance failure should occur. Joint arthrodesis is considered the treatment of choice for atlantoaxial instability in humans.[30] With the ventral approach improper angulation of the pins or screws may lead to pin or screw migration and joint instability or may result in entrance into the vertebral canal or puncturing the vertebral artery.[30]

Axial Plate Fixation

Fractures involving the body of C2 can be repaired with bone plates via a ventral approach.[1] The fracture segments are identified and the fracture reduced with a periosteal elevator. Gentle traction on the head will aid in the reduction. One or two small utility plates* are molded to fit the body of C2. After the median ridge of the axis has been removed flush with the vertebral body, the plate is applied on the midline so that two screws can be placed on each side of the fracture line. When two plates are used, they are applied on each side of the median ridge of the axis. The plates are held in place with a hemostat until all screws are placed. Screws should engage inner cortical bone but not enter the vertebral canal. Preop-

---

*Finger plates, Richards Mfg Co, Memphis, TN.

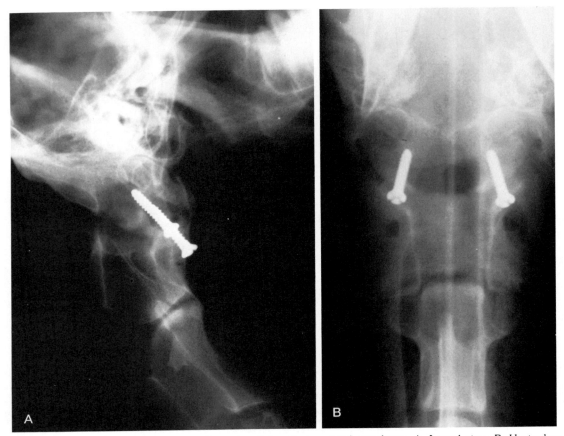

Figure 17–47. Immediate postoperative radiographs of the atlantooccipital articulation. A, Lateral view. B, Ventrodorsal view. (From Sorjonen DC, Powe TA, West M, and Edmonds S: Ventral surgical fixation and fusion for atlantooccipital subluxation in a goat. Vet Surg 12:127, 1983.)

erative radiographs may be used to ensure proper screw length.

Axial Methylmethacrylate and Pin Fixation

Axial fractures have been repaired using orthopedic pins and methylmethacrylate*.[26] Stabilization of the cervical vertebrae with methylmethacrylate obviates the use of bone plates and the inherent risk of spinal cord injury due to screw penetration of the vertebral canal; however, osteomyelitis is always a potential complication when using methylmethacrylate. Additionally, hypotension and fat emboli, sometimes followed by complete cardiovascular collapse, have occurred following methylmethacrylate use during total hip arthroplasty.[26]

---

*Methylmethacrylate, Howmedia, Inc, Medical Division, Rutherford, NJ.

Caudal Cervical Vertebral Exposure with Fenestration and Decompression (C3–C7)

The ventral approach to the caudal cervical vertebral column is indicated when ventral cord compression is present or when vertebral instability exists and dorsal structures cannot support fixation devices.

Dogs demonstrating only cervical pain as the result of a Hansen's type I disk herniation are candidates for disk fenestration unless there is clear herniation into the vertebral canal seen radiographically.[6, 16, 27]

Ventral cord decompression is performed for Hansen's type I disk protrusion, for Hansen's type II disk protrusion, and for dorsal subluxation of the craniodorsal aspect of the vertebral body common in nonchondrodystrophoid breeds (CVMM). Dogs are considered candidates for ventral decompressive surgery when severe cervical pain or motor dysfunction is present or when disk material is radiographically present in the vertebral canal.[5, 6, 16]

The patient positioning and surgical approach are identical to the ventral approach to the cranial cervical vertebrae. To improve exposure to vertebrae C4 to C7, the incision in the skin and sternohyoid muscles is extended to the manubrium. The landmarks used for identification of the disk spaces include the sharp ventral process of C1 marking the C1–C2 articulation cranially, and the large transverse processes of C6, caudally. Beginning with the C1 process, each successive ventral process is palpated and enumerated. When localization is correct, transverse processes can be palpated on each side of the ventral process to confirm that the surgeon is still on the midline. The disks are located just caudal to the ventral processes (Fig. 17–48). The large transverse processes of C6 can be palpated just caudolateral to the C5 ventral process.[15]

To fenestrate the cervical disk, the tips of a small, curved hemostatic forceps are placed over the disk space and used to gently separate the longus colli muscle fibers, thus exposing the ventral anulus. The hemostatic forceps is held in place, and a window is cut in the ventral anulus with a number 11 scalpel blade.[2] The depth of the disk space can be measured from a radiographic view of the lateral cervical vertebrae. The nucleus pulposus can be removed using a thin bladed tartar scraper or small bone curet. The C2–C3, C3–C4, C4–5, C5–C6, and C6–C7 disk spaces are routinely fenestrated.[2, 6] To facilitate evacuation of the last two cervical disks, the sandbag support is repositioned under the withers and a small curet bent to form a 60° angle can be used.[10]

When cord decompression is indicated, the longus colli muscles are separated from the vertebral bodies cranial and caudal to the affected disk. Exposure is maintained with self-retaining retractors. The tip of the ventral process just cranial to the disk is removed by bone rongeurs. Using a pneumatic drill with an oblong bur, a slot defect is created in the involved vertebrae that extends from the caudal one half of the cranial vertebra to the cranial one half of the caudal vertebra. In cases of Hansen's type I disk disease, the width of the slot should not exceed one half the width of the disk space.[13, 33] In Hansen's type II disk disease associated with cervical vertebral malformation-malarticulation, the slot should be one half to three fourths the width of the disk space.[22, 38]

Knowledge of the bone layers that compose the vertebral body is essential when the slot is created by drill and bur. Removal of the thin layered white outer cortical bone exposes the thick layered and red medullary bone. With further drilling, the appearance of white bone identifies the thin layered inner cortical bone. Careful use of the drill will allow all but a thin layer of inner cortical bone to be removed. The drilling is frequently stopped to irrigate the surgical site and evaluate the depth of the slot.

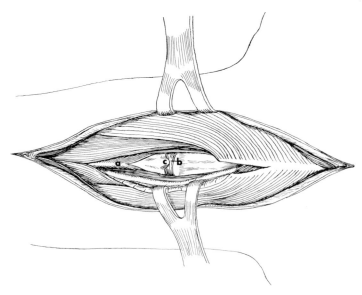

Figure 17–48. The fibers of the deep subvertebral musculature join in the midline (a), which should be identified to locate the midline ventral processes. The disk (b) is located immediately caudal to the prominent ventral protuberance (c) on the caudal end of each vertebra.

The remaining inner cortical bone can be removed with a bone rongeur or fine upbiting laminectomy rongeur.*

Disk material can be removed from the vertebral canal with a blunt claw-type tartar scraper or ear curet. Remnants of the anulus fibrosus and dorsal longitudinal ligament should be excised to allow removal of any disk material ventral and ventrolateral to the spinal cord.[38] In cervical malformation-malarticulation, spinal cord compression created by subluxation of the craniodorsal tip of the caudalmost involved vertebral body can be carefully removed with an upbiting laminectomy rongeur. The vertebral venous plexus, located just lateral to the slotted area, should not be damaged. However, if the plexus is invaded, hemorrhage is evacuated with suction and controlled with an absorbable gelatin sponge (Gelfoam) packed into the slot. Bone wax applied to the cut edges of the slot will stop hemorrhage from cancellous bone.

In chondrodystrophoid breeds, routine disk fenestration as previously described is performed as a prophylactic measure on remaining disks in addition to cord decompression.

A micrometer trephine† can be used in place of a pneumatic drill.[33] Dorsoventral measurements of the involved vertebral bodies taken from a lateral radiographic view of the cervical vertebrae are used to set the stop limits on the micrometer, thus preventing excessive trephination and spinal cord damage. A hole is tre-

phined in the vertebral body on the midline just cranial to the involved disk. A second hole is similarly made just caudal to the involved disk. A slot is created by removing the intervening bone and disk with bone rongeurs (Fig. 17–49). Disk material and ligamentous tissue are removed as previously described.

The choice of surgical approach to the cervical vertebrae is based primarily on the site of maximum cord compression; however, the ventral approach has several advantages over the dorsal techniques. The ventral approach is less traumatic and requires less operating time.[38] Ventral fenestration is a simple technique for relief of cervical pain associated with herniated disks; however, it does not provide cord decompression and does not allow removal of disk material within the vertebral canal.[6, 15, 16] The ventral slot can relieve ventral cord compression arising from disk, ligament, or bone and can be combined with prophylactic fenestration of adjacent cervical disks.[15, 38] The principal disadvantage of spinal cord decompression by the ventral slot technique includes potential rupture of the vertebral venous plexuses during disk removal and difficulty in decompressing the cord at the last two disk spaces owing to limited exposure. In addition, with expansive lesions there is the inability to adequately decompress and visualize the spinal cord.[10, 33, 38]

The primary indication for utilization of the ventral approach to stabilize the caudal cervical vertebrae is a case of malformation-malarticulation that demonstrates vertebral instability coexistent with ventral spinal cord compression and vertebral body fractures.[5, 16, 38]

---

*Kerrison laminectomy rongeur, Codman and Shurtleff Inc, Randolph, MA.

†Micrometer trephine, CL Lippincott, Pacific Palisades, CA.

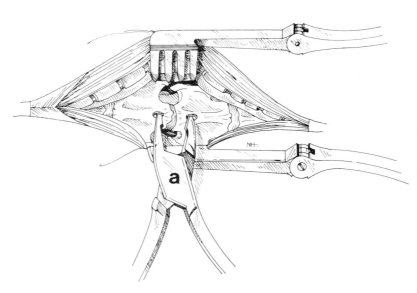

Figure 17–49. A rongeur (a) is used to remove the bone between the drill holes down to the mass and the vertebral canal. (From Swaim SF: Ventral decompression of the cervical spinal cord in the dog. JAVMA 164:491, 1974.)

Caudal Cervical Stabilization

In cervical malformation-malarticulation, vertebral stabilization can be performed alone and in combination with spinal cord decompression. The patient positioning, surgical approach, and spinal cord decompression are similar to those previously described for the ventral approach to the caudal cervical vertebrae (see above). A bone graft taken from the wing of the ilium can be placed in the decompression defect to achieve stabilization.[22, 38]

To harvest the bone graft, the skin, subcutis, and deep gluteal fascia are incised in a straight line from the crest of the ilium to the greater trochanter. The middle gluteal muscle is freed from the ilium by an incision from the iliac crest to the superficial gluteal muscle along the dorsal edge of the body of the ilium. Lateral retraction of the middle gluteal muscle and medial retraction of the iliocostal and longissi-mus muscles will expose the entire dorsal aspect of the ilium. An osteotome and mallet are used to remove a full thickness rectangular graft.

The graft is shaped to be approximately 1 mm wider, 2 mm longer, and 2 mm less than the depth of the decompressive defect. The bone graft is tapped into place with a bone tamp* and mallet (Fig. 17–50). Traction applied to the head and pelvis will aid in graft placement. Bone wax applied to the cut edges of the vertebral body defect must be completely removed prior to placement of the graft. The head and neck are splinted in a neutral position for 1 month.

A technique utilizing a corticocancellous bone graft and ventral plating of the involved interspace has recently been reported.[40] After exposure of the involved vertebrae, a partial thickness slot is created that extends three fourths

---

*Kiene bone tamp, Zimmer USA, Warsaw, IN.

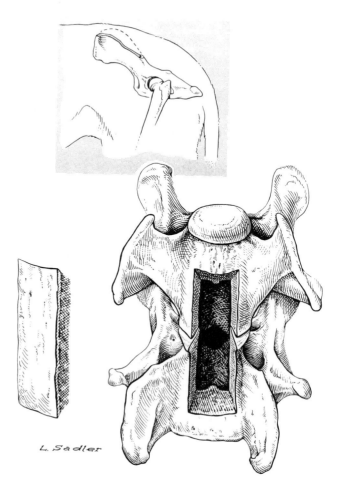

Figure 17–50. Extent of defect in the vertebral bodies in ventral decompression prior to placement of the iliac graft for arthrodesis of the symphyseal joint. (From Trotter EJ, deLahunta A, Geary JC, and Brasmer TH: Caudal cervical vertebral malformation-malarticulation in Great Danes and Doberman pinschers. JAVMA 168:917, 1976.)

L. Sadler

the distance to the vertebral canal, two thirds the width of the vertebral body, and approximately 1 cm long.

The patient's head is grasped behind the base of the skull, and longitudinal traction is applied until the slot is approximately doubled in length. A bone graft is shaped to fit the distracted slot. Pelvic autografts, tibial allografts from a frozen bone bank, and bovine heterografts* have been used. If tibial grafts are used, they should be packed into the medullary defect with fresh autogenous cancellous bone.

A medium-sized plastic plate† is cut to fit across the interspace such that two cortical 3.5 mm diameter screws can be placed into 2.0 mm diameter holes drilled into each vertebral body. The drill holes are angled away from the vertebral canal. Screws are inserted without tapping the drilled holes (Figs. 17–51 and 17–52). The head and neck are placed in a collar for 3 months.

Although fractures of the caudal cervical vertebrae occur rarely, a dorsally displaced vertebral body fracture is best reduced from the ventral approach.[31] After reduction, vertebral body fractures can be stabilized by techniques (bone plates and methylmethacrylate) similar to those described for stabilization of cranial cervical vertebrae through the ventral approach.

In addition to the previously stated advantages and disadvantages of the ventral approach for spinal cord decompression, vertebral stabilization through the ventral approach provides excellent sites for bone grafts and bony mass for orthopedic fixation.[38] In cases of CVMM with multiple sites involved, disk fenestration may prevent disk prolapse subsequent to fixation of the primary site of instability. The principal disadvantages of ventral stabilization are the additional surgical time required to harvest the bone graft,[38] partial crushing of the bone graft, and collapse of the disk space.[40] Loss of spinal cord decompression can occur if collapse follows the partial thickness decompression technique.[40]

EXTERNAL STABILIZATION

External support bandages are needed occasionally to promote immobilization of vertebral fractures when internal fixation is not indicated or to provide additional support for internal

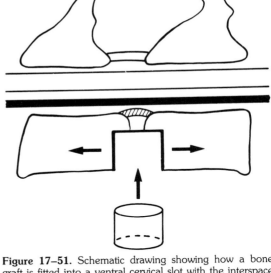

Figure 17–51. Schematic drawing showing how a bone graft is fitted into a ventral cervical slot with the interspace distracted. (From Withrow SJ and Seim HB: Caudal cervical spondylopathy and myelopathy in large breed dogs. *In* Bojrab MJ (ed): Current Techniques in Small Animal Surgery, 2nd ed. Philadelphia, Lea & Febiger, 1983.)

fixation. Nonsurgical management of traumatic injury to the cervical vertebral column has been reported.[1, 12, 14, 19, 37] Atlantooccipital subluxation can be reduced by applying traction to the atlantooccipital joint while the head is rotated into proper alignment. The head and neck are immobilized in a flexed position with an external support bandage.[14, 19] Atlantoaxial subluxation can be reduced by applying traction to the atlantoaxial joint while pressing the atlas dorsally and the axis ventrally. The atlantoaxial joint is immobilized in a neutral or slightly hyperextended position.[12] Similarly, dislocations of the caudal cervical vertebrae can be reduced and maintained in a neutral or slightly hyperextended position. External support bandages should be maintained for 8 weeks. Following internal fixation, support bandages should complement the surgical alignment and be maintained for 2 or 3 weeks.[26, 30, 31]

The principles for applying external support in the cervical area are the same as those for the thoracolumbar area. The support material should be applied so that the bandage fits snugly and is anchored slightly to the hair at each end of the bandage. Cranially, the bandage should extend to the lateral canthus of the eyes and caudally to the midthoracic area. Adequate aperture size for the ears and thoracic limbs should be provided. All pressure points and

---

*Kiel surgibones, Unilab, Inc, Hillside, NJ.

†Lubra plate, Lubra Co, 1905 Mohawk, Fort Collins, CO.

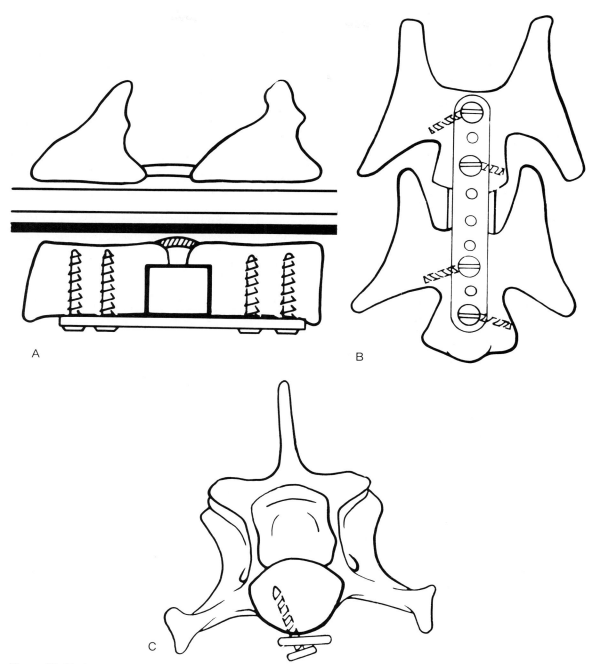

Figure 17–52. A, Postoperative view with plastic plate, screws, and bone graft in place. B, Plate and screws as seen from ventral aspect. Note that screws diverge away from the canal. C. Cross-sectional view showing appropriate angulation of screws to avoid injury to the spinal cord. (From Withrow SJ and Seim HB: Caudal cervical spondylopathy and myelopathy in large breed dogs. *In* Bojrab MJ (ed): Current Techniques in Small Animal Surgery, 2nd ed. Philadelphia, Lea & Febiger, 1983.)

areas of possible friction must be observed and relieved appropriately before friction and pressure lesions occur.[32]

REFERENCES

1. Archibald J, Pennock PW, and Cawley AJ: Trauma of the vertebral column in dogs. Vet Med 54:518, 1959.
2. Cechner PE: Ventral cervical disc fenestration in the dog: A modified technique. J Am Anim Hosp Assoc 16:647, 1980.
3. Chambers JN and Betts CW: Caudal cervical spondylopathy in the dog: A review of 20 clinical cases and the literature. J Am Anim Hosp Assoc 13:571, 1977.
4. Chambers JN, Betts CW, and Oliver JE Jr: The use of nonmetallic suture material for stabilization of atlantoaxial subluxation. J Am Anim Hosp Assoc 13:603, 1977.
5. Chambers JN, Oliver JE Jr, Kornegay JE, and Malnati GA: Ventral decompression for caudal cervical disk herniation in large and giant-breed dogs. JAVMA 180:410, 1982.
6. Colter SB: Fenestration, decompression, or both? Vet Clin North Am 8:379, 1978.
7. Cook JP and Oliver JE Jr: Atlantoaxial luxation in the dog. Comp Cont Ed Pract Vet 3:242, 1981.
8. Crane SW: Surgical management of traumatic atlantooccipital instability in a dog. Vet Surg 7:39, 1978.
9. Deuland R, Furneaux RW, and Kaye MM: Spinal fusion and dorsal laminectomy for midcervical spondylolisthesis in a dog. JAVMA 162:366, 1973.
10. Funkquist B and Svalastoga E: A simplified surgical approach to the last two cervical discs of the dog. J Small Anim Pract 20:593, 1979.
11. Gage ED: Surgical repair of a fractured cervical spine in the dog. JAVMA 153:1407, 1968.
12. Gilmore DR: Nonsurgical management of four cases of atlantoaxial subluxation in the dog. J Am Anim Hosp Assoc 20:93, 1984.
13. Gilpin GN: Evaluation of three techniques of ventral decompression of the cervical spinal cord in the dog. JAVMA 168:325, 1976.
14. Greenwood KM and Oliver JE Jr: Traumatic atlantooccipital dislocation in two dogs. JAVMA 173:1324, 1978.
15. Hoerlein BF: Canine Neurology, 3rd ed. Philadelphia, WB Saunders Co, 1978.
16. Hoerlein BF: The status of the various intervertebral disc surgeries for the dog in 1978. J Am Anim Hosp Assoc 14:563, 1978.
17. Hurov LI: Dorsal decompressive cervical laminectomy in the dog: Surgical considerations and clinical cases. J Am Anim Hosp Assoc 15:301, 1979.
18. Hurov LI: Treatment of cervical vertebral instability in the dog. JAVMA 175:278, 1979.
19. Lappin MR and Dow S: Traumatic atlantooccipital luxation in a cat. Vet Surg 12:30, 1983.
20. LeCouteur RA, McKeown D, Johnson J, and Eger CE: Stabilization of atlantoaxial subluxation in the dog, using the nuchal ligament. JAVMA 177:1011, 1980.
21. Oliver JE Jr and Lewis RE: Lesions of the atlas and axis in dogs. J Am Anim Hosp Assoc 9:304, 1973.
22. Prata RG and Stoll SG: Ventral decompression and fusion for the treatment of cervical disc disease in the dog. J Am Anim Hosp Assoc 9:462, 1973.
23. Rafee MR and Knecht CD: Cervical vertebral malformation: A review of 36 cases. J Am Anim Hosp Assoc 16:881, 1980.
24. Rendano UT Jr and Smith LL: Cervical vertebral malformation-malarticulation (wobbler syndrome)—the value of the ventrodorsal view in defining lateral spinal cord compression in the dog. J Am Anim Hosp Assoc 17:627, 1981.
25. Renegar WR and Stoll SG: The use of methyl methacrylate bone cement in the repair of atlantoaxial subluxation stabilization failures—case report and discussion. J Am Anim Hosp Assoc 15:313, 1979.
26. Rouse GP: Cervical spine stabilization with methyl methacrylate. Vet Surg 8:1, 1979.
27. Seim HB and Prata RG: Ventral decompression for the treatment of cervical disk disease in the dog: A review of 54 cases. J Am Anim Hosp Assoc 18:233,1982.
28. Seim HB and Withrow SJ: Pathophysiology and diagnosis of caudal cervical spondylo-myelopathy with emphasis on the Doberman pinscher. J Am Anim Hosp Assoc 18:241, 1982.
29. Sorjonen DC, Powe TA, West M, and Edmonds S: Ventral surgical fixation and fusion for atlanto-occipital subluxation in a goat. Vet Surg 12:127, 1983.
30. Sorjonen DC and Shires PK: Atlantoaxial instability: A ventral surgical technique for decompression, fixation, and fusion. Vet Surg 10:22, 1981.
31. Stone EA, Betts CW, and Chambers JN: Cervical fractures in the dog: A literature and case review. J Am Anim Hosp Assoc 15:463, 1979.
32. Swaim SF: Bodycasts: Technics of application to the dog. Vet Med Small Anim Clin 65:1179, 1970.
33. Swaim SF: Ventral decompression of the cervical spinal cord in the dog. JAVMA 164:491, 1974.
34. Swaim SF: Evaluation of four techniques of cervical spinal fixation in dogs. JAVMA 166:1080, 1975.
35. Swaim SF: Cervical laminectomy for the treatment of cervical discs: Indications and surgical technique. Am Coll Vet Surg Forum V, 1977.
36. Swaim SF and Greene CE: Odontoidectomy in a dog. J Am Anim Hosp Assoc 11:663, 1975.
37. Trotter EJ: Surgical repair of fractured axis in a dog. JAVMA 161:303, 1972.
38. Trotter EJ, deLahunta A, Geary JC, and Brasmer TH: Caudal cervical vertebral malformation-malarticulation in Great Danes and Doberman pinschers. JAVMA 168:917, 1976.
39. Troy GC, Hurov LI, and King GK: Successful surgical removal of a cervical subdural neurofibrosarcoma. J Am Anim Hosp Assoc 15:997, 1979.
40. Withrow SJ and Seim HB: Caudal cervical spondylopathy and myelopathy in large breed dogs. In Bojrab MJ (ed): Current Techniques in Small Animal Surgery, 2nd ed. Philadelphia, Lea & Febiger, 1983, p 541.

Section 3   *PC Wagner, DVM, MS*

LARGE ANIMAL VERTEBRAL AND SPINAL CORD SURGERY

INDICATIONS

Compressive lesions of the spinal cord in large animals carry a grave prognosis for recovery and, until recently, conservative treatment or humane destruction were the only alternatives. Several surgical techniques have been reported that substantially improve the prognosis in selected spinal cord compressive lesions in horses.[10, 15, 24–27]

The prognosis for return to function of neural tissue in cases of spinal cord or nerve root compression decreases with the duration of the signs and the degree of compression. The importance of relieving pressure on the neural tissue as rapidly as possible cannot be overemphasized. With increased client education, and the improvement in therapy and prognosis for compressive lesions, owners of large animals have been seeking treatment earlier.

The physical bulk of large animals and the difficulty of surgical access to many portions of the vertebral column limit corrective surgical techniques to the cervical and caudal vertebral canal and the dorsal spinous processes of the thoracic vertebrae. Surgery of these areas will be discussed, with emphasis on the horse.

CERVICAL SURGERY

Spinal cord compression in the cervical area is usually due to fractures or cervical vertebral malformations. Osteomyelitis, spina bifida, hemivertebrae, and neoplasia have been reported to cause compression; however, these are rare.[6, 7, 24]

There are basically three indications for surgery of the cervical vertebrae in large animals: signs of cervical cord compression such as ataxia, dysmetria, spasticity, and paresis of all four limbs,[17] with demonstration of a cervical cord compressive lesion by radiography. Plain radiographs may indicate the area of involvement (fractures of the body or articular processes); however, myelography is necessary to define the extent of most lesions[14, 16]; lack of response or deterioration of signs with conservative therapy; and retention of some degree of pain perception in the limbs in the presence of paresis or paralysis. Loss of all pain perception indicates such a grave prognosis that surgery is not indicated.

Surgical correction of cervical vertebral fractures may involve internal or external stabilization in the acute stage, or decompression if callus formation impinges on the vertebral canal later following fracture healing.

Ventral Approach for Decompression and Stabilization

Bone Dowel or Basket Fixation

The ventral approach has been described to relieve ventral cervical cord compression or to stabilize subluxations and fractures.[10, 25, 27] The ventral surface of the neck is clipped from the mandible to the thoracic inlet prior to anesthetic induction. After induction, the horse is placed in dorsal recumbency with the head extended over a brace placed at the approximate operative level (Fig. 17–53). Lateral radiographs are

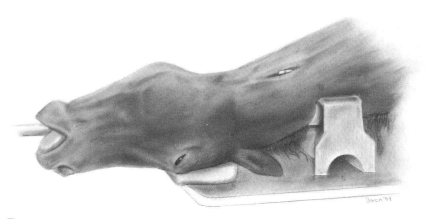

Figure 17–53. The approach to the ventral cervical vertebral column is performed with the horse in dorsal recumbency with the neck extended over a firm brace.

made with radiopaque markers in place in the lateral skin of the neck at the approximate surgical level. This is a simple, safe way to ensure that the approach is at the correct level because the ventral processes of C2–C6 cannot be readily differentiated by palpation during surgery.

After preparation of the ventral cervical area for aseptic surgery, the site is draped, and a 30 cm ventral midline skin incision is made over the selected site. Subcutaneous tissues and the cutaneous colli muscles are incised to expose the paired sternothyrohyoid muscles. These are separated, and the underlying trachea is retracted to the left. The right carotid sheath and vagosympathetic trunk are carefully retracted to the left and protected by moistened gauze under large, hand held retractors. This exposure allows the surgeon to palpate the ventral crest of the vertebrae through the overlying longus colli muscles (Fig. 17–54). Using this landmark in conjunction with the previously placed skin markers, the surgeon locates the vertebrae to be stabilized. The longus colli muscles are incised and elevated from the bone with a periosteal elevator or osteotome. Self-retaining retractors* are used to expose the surgical site.

Cervical vertebral fusion in the horse is a modification of anterior cervical fusion in humans as described by Cloward.[1] The technique consists of drilling a large hole in the vertebral bodies at the intervertebral disk space that removes portions of two vertebral epiphyses and a majority of the intervertebral disk. An autogenous or homologous bone graft, slightly larger than the hole, is tamped into the hole. This provides immediate stabilization and even-

*Inge lamina spreaders, Jarit Instrument, Elmsford, NY.

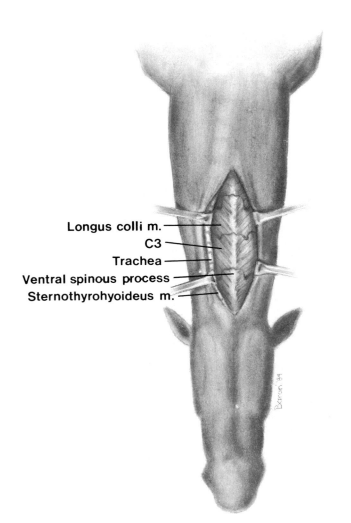

Longus colli m.
C3
Trachea
Ventral spinous process
Sternothyrohyoideus m.

Figure 17–54. After incision of the skin, subcutaneous tissues, and ventral cervical muscles, the trachea is drawn to the left and the ventral spinous processes may be palpated through the longus colli muscles.

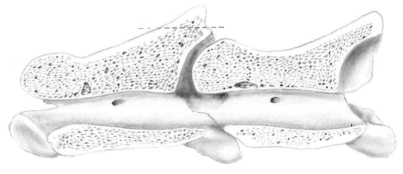

Figure 17–55. The ventral crest of the cranial vertebrae is rongeured to provide a level surface for seating of the drill guide. (Ventral is up).

tual arthrodesis of the intervertebral space.[26] Recently, a metal basket implant has been substituted for the bone dowel.[2] Collapse of the graft is less frequent using the metal implant.

After the ventral crest of the cranialmost of the two vertebrae to be fused is exposed, it is removed with rongeurs to provide a level surface for the seating of the drill guides and drills used to create the hole (Fig. 17–55).

The depth of the hole to be drilled is measured on lateral radiographs. The hole between the vertebrae is created in two steps. First, a small guide hole is created with an 18 mm twist drill on a Hudson cranial drill* brace (Fig. 17–56). The cone shaped equine intervertebral disk points cranially, and this must be taken into account when drilling the guide hole. The physeal scar on the caudal portion of the ventral crest of the cranialmost vertebra acts as a reference point for drilling the guide hole. The drill is positioned just cranial to this scar and directed in a craniodorsal direction.

Disk material will appear at the caudal edge of the hole as drilling begins and then at the cranial edge as the hole is deepened owing to the cranial curvature of the intervertebral disk

---

*Hudson cranial drills, Jarit Instrument, Elmsford, NY.

space. Drilling is continued to three quarters of the depth of the vertebrae. This leaves a shelf of bone and disk between the drill and the vertebral canal. The depth is measured with a depth gauge periodically during drilling. If ventral decompression is necessary, drilling continues to the vertebral canal. When the desired depth is reached, the hole is enlarged using a 25 mm core saw (Fig. 17–57). If the guide hole has been placed too far caudally or cranially, corrections can be made by angling the core saw appropriately. The core produced is removed using rongeurs, and the hole is completed using a depth finisher to provide an even base for the implant site. When the surgeon views the completed hole, the disk should lie in the center to allow contact of the bone dowel or metal basket with maximum surface area of the cranial and caudal vertebrae.

If a bone dowel is used for stabilization, it is obtained aseptically from an equine cadaver ilium.[25, 27] A trephine 26 mm in diameter is used to cut a dowel from the wing of the ilium. By using the entire thickness, a dowel with cortical bone at both ends and cancellous bone in the center is obtained. It may be frozen at −20°C prior to use.

If a bone dowel is used, it is now tamped

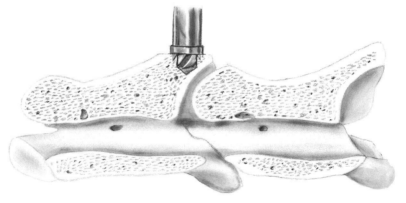

Figure 17–56. A small guide hole is created with an 18 mm twist drill.

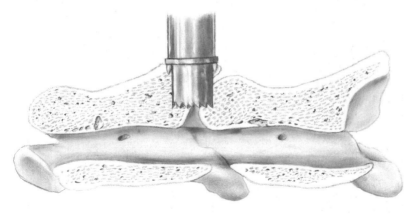

Figure 17–57. The hole is enlarged to 25 mm in diameter using a core saw.

into place (Fig. 17–58). If a metal basket is used, it is packed with portions of cancellous bone that have been removed from the vertebral bodies during drilling. The metal basket (total diameter, 26 mm) is then tamped into place. Both the bone dowel and metal basket are approximately 1 mm larger than the hole to ensure a secure fit. The hole should be 2 to 4 mm deeper than the implant to allow countersinking without fracture of the plate of bone still adjacent to the vertebral canal.

After copious flushing with cold sterile saline, the longus colli, sternothyrohyoid muscles, and cutaneous colli muscles are closed with absorbable suture using a continuous pattern. The skin is apposed with nonabsorbable suture or skin staples. Lateral radiographs after closure are necessary to evaluate implant positioning (Fig. 17–59).

Postsurgical care includes covering the surgical site with a light dressing and confining the horse to a stall to limit activity. Antibiotics may be indicated if there was a protracted surgical time. Antiinflammatory or analgesic agents are not given, thereby discouraging the patient from overactive use of the neck. In uneventful recoveries, supervised walking may be started 2 to 3 weeks postoperatively. Fusion, in young horses, may be complete in 3 months[25]; however, postoperative radiographs are needed to confirm this.

Dynamic Compression Plate Fixation

One instance of successful compression plating of a fractured dens in a young filly has been reported.[9] After exposure of the ventrum of the first and second vertebrae, these two vertebrae were gently manipulated to realign the odontoid process with C2. The alignment was temporarily stabilized using small bone holding forceps across the lateral articulation of C1 with C2. The ventral tubercle of C1 was flattened, using bone rongeurs. Two, 6 hole, broad dynamic compression plates stabilized C1 and C2, by placing one plate on each side of the ventral

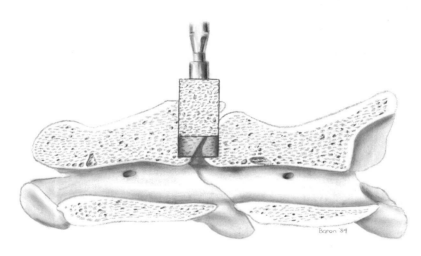

Figure 17–58. If a bone dowel is used, it is tamped into place.

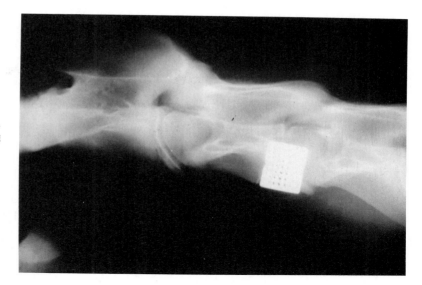

Figure 17–59. Postsurgical radiograph shows correct positioning when a metal basket is used.

midline of the vertebrae (Fig. 17–60). Cortical bone screws anchored the plates, angling the screws laterally to avoid the vertebral canal and the atlantooccipital joint. Recovery was complete.

Stabilization of vertebrae prevents further trauma to the spinal cord and reduces pressure from venous congestion and cord edema. Improvement of clinical signs may be expected as early as 2 to 3 weeks postoperatively, and may continue for up to 1 year after surgery. Insufficient data are available to predict which horses will regain full function and which will not,[12] although the severity and duration of neurologic signs are undoubtedly important.

Complications of the ventral approach to the cervical vertebrae for decompression or stabilization are related to surgical technique and, for the most part, are avoidable.[27] Hemorrhage and spinal cord trauma are possible if the surgeon overestimates the desired depth of drilling and enters the vertebral canal. The large venous plexus ventral to the spinal cord may be perforated, resulting in severe, usually fatal, hemorrhage. Spinal cord trauma from the drill may produce immediate respiratory arrest and death or may cause permanent quadriplegia or paresis. Retraction of the right recurrent laryngeal nerve as it runs in the carotid sheath has resulted in right laryngeal hemiplegia ("roaring") in several cases. This complication can be avoided by protecting the nerve with damp sponges to eliminate the pressure of the retractors. Collapse of the bone dowel, dislodgment of the metal implant, lack of complete fusion, or reestablishment of a functional joint space are infrequent complications. If the implant dislodges or fails, surgical correction is necessary. Lack of fusion, partial fusion, or reestablishment of a functional joint space may or may not require correction, depending on the clinical signs. Seroma formation and postoperative swelling have been seen in some instances but usually resolve uneventfully. In one case, postoperative sepsis with migration of infection along the fascial planes of the neck resulted in death of the horse.

Strict attention to detail in placement of the implant, proper handling of equipment and tissues, and effective confinement of the horse after surgery reduce the incidence of complications.

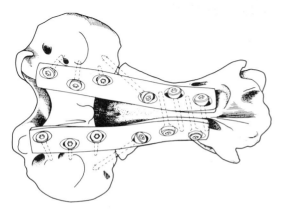

Figure 17–60. Ventrodorsal view of skull showing stabilization of the first and second cervical vertebrae. Six hole, broad dynamic compression plates are used. The cortical bone screws must be angled to avoid the vertebral canal.

Ventral Atlantooccipital Fixation and Fusion

Successful ventral fixation of traumatically induced atlantooccipital subluxation in a pygmy goat has been described[22] (see Cranial Cervical Stabilization, Section 2, above and Fig. 17–47).

Dorsal Approach for Decompression or Stabilization

Dorsal Laminectomy

A dorsal approach to the equine cervical vertebrae is used when a compressive lesion of the spinal cord cannot be alleviated by extension of the neck. This type of lesion can occur at any level of the spinal cord but is most commonly seen at the level of the fifth, sixth, and seventh cervical vertebrae.[11, 16] Degenerative joint disease with bony proliferation of the dorsal articular processes, soft tissue hypertrophy, and synovial and epidural cysts contribute to this static compression.[29] Confirmation of this lesion is via myelography with the neck in extension and flexion.

The mane and dorsal cervical area are clipped and the mane area treated with a depilatory agent from poll to withers prior to anesthetic induction.[26] Dorsal decompressive laminectomy may be performed with the horse in sternal or lateral recumbency or suspended in a sling.[4, 11, 16, 24, 27] If a sling is used, the head and neck are supported on a surgical table after anesthesia induction. If lateral recumbency is elected, the neck is flexed to allow easier access to the dorsal portion of the vertebrae.[4] Sternal recumbency with the legs positioned under the horse is avoided in all but the lightest patient because of the danger of postanesthetic neuromyopathy.

After positioning and aseptic surgical preparation, the horse is draped. A 30 to 40 cm skin incision is made on the dorsal cervical midline over the lesion. A generous incision makes retraction for exposure of the vertebrae easier. The incision is carried through the subcutaneous fat to the funicular portion of the ligamentum nuchae. Hemorrhage is profuse but easily controlled by ligation or electrocautery. The funicular portion of the nuchal ligament is incised longitudinally on the midline. This allows blunt dissection between the lamellar portions of the nuchal ligament to the dorsal spinous processes of the cervical vertebrae, which are easily palpated (Fig. 17–61). The dorsal spinous process of the seventh cervical vertebrae is approximately 2 cm high and that of T1 is up to 5 cm high.[16] This allows orientation by using T1 as a point of reference, and the correct

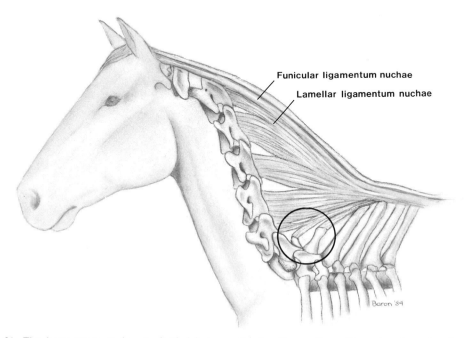

Funicular ligamentum nuchae

Lamellar ligamentum nuchae

Figure 17–61. The ligamentum nuchae is divided between the lamellar portions. These insert on the dorsal spinous processes. The seventh cervical vertebral spinous process is about 2 cm high and the first thoracic is up to 5 cm (circled). This height discrepancy allows orientation by the surgeon without use of intraoperative radiographs.

site for decompression can be located by counting cranially.

The attachments of the lamellar nuchal ligament and multifidus muscles are elevated from the dorsal arches of the two involved vertebrae using a rongeur or osteotome, and the dorsal spinous processes are removed from these vertebrae. Large self-retaining retractors* are used to retract the musculature. The caudal half of the arch of the cranial vertebra and the cranial half of the arch of the caudal vertebra are removed. However, the distance to be decompressed may vary among animals and is estimated from the myelogram. In some patients the interarcual space is encased in heavy fibrous or osseous material that makes localization difficult. After the soft tissue is removed from the interarcual space, a pneumatic instrument and bur† are used to remove the majority of the bone of the laminae. Caution in burring is imperative because sudden trauma to the cord is possible. A 20 mm diameter cranial drill bit in a Hudson drill brace has been used for initial openings. Cranial drill bits are designed to allow penetration of the bone without trauma to the underlying nervous tissue. The depth of the bone varies with the animal and is difficult to estimate from lateral radiographs. In lesions with extensive proliferation of bone, the drilling can be a tedious procedure.

When the lamina has been perforated in one area with the cranial drill bit and thinned by the use of the pneumatic instrument and bur in other areas, the final shelf of bone can be removed using reverse biting laminectomy rongeurs.* The spinal cord is completely exposed over the area of compression (Fig. 17–62). The presence of epidural fat at the cranial and caudal limits of the laminectomy usually indicates a satisfactory extent of decompression. The nature of these lesions is usually that of chronic compression, and a durotomy to reduce pressure from edema or hemorrhage is not necessary.

Hemorrhage from the cancellous bone may be controlled by applying bone wax or thrombin soaked sponges. Removal of redundant interarcuate ligament or other soft tissue structures is done at this time. The decompression site should bracket the area of myelographic compression. After smoothing of the bony edges and control of blood seepage, a thin sheet of fat from the subcutaneous fat pad of the mane is placed over the laminectomy site. A continuous suction drain is anchored with fine absorbable suture near the decompression site with exits through the lateral cervical musculature. This is used to withdraw fluid that accumulates in the first 24 to 36 hours.

Closure is with absorbable suture using a continuous pattern in the funicular portion of the nuchal ligament; the subcutaneous tissue is apposed using absorbable continuous suture and the skin closed with interrupted nonabsorbable suture or staples. A stent-type bandage is applied and the continuous drain affixed.

---

*Finochietto rib spreader, Jarit Instrument, Elmsford, NY.

†Max-driver, 3M, Surgical Products Division, Eagan, MN.

---

*Kerrison laminectomy rongeur, Codman and Shurtleff Inc, Randolph, MA.

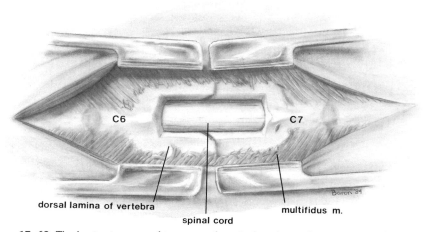

dorsal lamina of vertebra

spinal cord

multifidus m.

C6   C7

Baron '84

Figure 17–62. The lamina is removed to expose the spinal cord over the entire area of compression.

Recovery from anesthesia is often prolonged, and the horse may require constant attention to prevent self-inflicted trauma during this period. The drain should be evacuated frequently to prevent pressure from fluid accumulation around the spinal cord. Postoperative care should include bandaging and administration of antibiotic and antiinflammatory agents.

Complications of this surgery include hemorrhage, vertebral fracture, spinal cord trauma, insufficient decompression, seroma formation, and sepsis. Seepage of blood from the cervical muscles into the surgical area is unavoidable after closure. Lavage of the cervical muscles with heparinized saline during closure prevents clotting of the blood and allows removal of the initial hemorrhage through the continuous suction drain. The drain is removed 48 hours after surgery. If further seepage occurs a seroma may develop. The seroma can be drained by needle aspiration or left to resolve on its own. Accumulation of fluid or blood clots over the spinal cord may lead to compression with increased neurologic deficits. Formation of a restrictive membrane at the laminectomy site during healing has not been noted.[27]

Laminectomy in an area of cord compression may result in spinal cord trauma, and proper instrumentation is necessary to avoid this. Even mild trauma can produce severe weakness and proprioceptive deficits in the limbs after recovery. Laminectomy should extend the entire length of cord compression, as determined by myelogram, if surgery is to be successful. Removal of bone too far laterally may cause weakening of the pedicles of the vertebral arch and the articular processes. This can lead to fractures with resultant cervical instability, especially if the recovery is prolonged or violent.[12, 13]

If sepsis and dehiscence occur, they usually involve the tissue dorsal to the nuchal ligament. Purulent discharge may be substantial, but in the one such case treated by the author sepsis did resolve following nursing care and antibiotic therapy.

Response to surgical decompression may be rapid in acute compressive lesions or may be prolonged with clinical improvement occurring over a year's time.

THORACOLUMBAR SURGERY

Fractures of thoracolumbar vertebrae resulting in spinal cord compression in heavy (500 kg) patients are usually not amenable to surgical stabilization. Spinal cord decompression and possible vertebral débridement and stabilization of thoracolumbar osteomyelitis or fractures are possible in smaller animals and has been achieved in a 1 month old Simmental heifer. Collapse of L3 in the calf was believed to be due to osteomyelitis. Laminectomy of L1–L5 relieved the spinal cord compression. The calf was recumbent prior to surgery and apparently made a full recovery by a year of age.[21]

SACROCAUDAL SURGERY

Fractures of the sacral and caudal vertebrae are relatively uncommon in the horse, accounting for 4 of 42 fractures of the vertebrae in one study[5] and 0 of 125 in another.[23] Trauma to the sacral and caudal vertebrae occurs when the horse goes over backward and lands on its hindquarters. Surgical decompression of the caudal vertebral nerves has been successful.[28] Surgical repair of sacral fractures has not been reported.

Indications for caudal vertebral surgery are evidence of a fracture compressing nerves or nerve roots, inability to move the tail due to nerve root or nerve compression causing soiling during defecation and during urination in the mare, and lack of response to antiinflammatory therapy.

Dorsal Approach for Decompression

The dorsal approach is indicated for decompression and fracture fragment removal when the lamina of Cd1–Cd4 have been shattered. The horse is positioned in lateral recumbency with the base of the tail close to the edge of the surgical table for easier access. The hair around the base of the tail and the proximal one third of the tail is removed. The rest of the tail is wrapped to prevent contamination of the surgical site. Prior to surgical preparation a temporary pursestring suture is placed in the anus to prevent fecal contamination, and a catheter is introduced into the bladder in mares for controlled drainage during surgery.

An incision is made on the dorsal midline over the fracture fragments to be removed. The dorsal sacrocaudal muscles are divided and the lateral sacrocaudal muscles undermined and retracted to expose the fracture fragments. The traumatized soft tissue around the fracture obliterates normal landmarks, and caution is advised to avoid further damage to nerves that cannot be visualized. Once exposed, the fragments

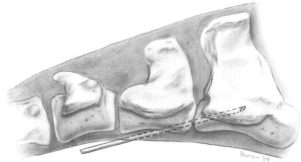

Figure 17–63. A Steinmann pin engages the fractured caudal vertebra and anchors it onto the vertebra cranial to the fracture.

should be removed with as little manipulation of the soft tissues as possible.

The incision is closed by reapposition of the dorsal sacrocaudal muscles, subcutaneous tissues, and skin. A stent-type bandage may be sutured in place to prevent soiling of the incision.

Ventral Approach for Decompression

The ventral approach is indicated when fracture of a vertebral body has allowed luxation and impingement of the vertebra on nerve roots or nerves, or when vertebral luxation alone renders the horse unable to move the distal part of the tail. In such cases use of Steinmann pins to affix the body of the fractured vertebra to the next cranial vertebra may return function to the tail.

The horse is placed in lateral recumbency and is prepared as for the dorsal approach; in some cases both ventral and dorsal approaches may be made. A small stab incision is made to one side of the midline on the ventral aspect of the tail at the caudal margin of the last affected vertebra, avoiding the middle coccygeal artery and paired veins. A 0.25 inch diameter trocar tip Steinmann pin can be introduced to engage the fractured or luxated vertebral body and then directed forward to engage the vertebral body just craniad (Fig. 17–63). After correct alignment is ascertained by radiographs, a second pin is placed similarly to maintain the reduction. The stab incisions are closed with a single mattress suture of nonabsorbable suture material.

Complications of this surgery include possible perforation of the caudal artery on entry into the ventral tail and possible perforation of the rectal mucosa as the pin is advanced to engage the cranial vertebra. In most cases surgical resection of fragments or reduction of fractures is made more difficult because of the time lapse between diagnosis and surgery. Conservative therapy may allow return of function to the tail. However, after several weeks with no improvement, the chances of surgical correction are minimal; therefore, the decision to perform surgery should be made within several days of injury.

In one instance of decompression and stabilization, movement of the tail was noticed 48 hours after surgery. Pins were removed 6 weeks after surgery and the horse was used successfully as a broodmare the next season.

THORACIC SURGERY

Indications for surgery on the dorsal spinous processes of the thoracic vertebrae include fracture and displacement of tips of the dorsal spinous processes causing pain and/or drainage, osteomyelitis of the dorsal spinous processes secondary to fracture or supraspinous bursitis ("fistulous withers"), and overlapping of the dorsal spinous processes causing lameness and back pain.[18] These conditions do not result in neurologic signs unless the vertebral body or arch becomes involved. The horse is usually presented for evaluation because of swelling, pain, drainage from a tract, or reluctance to perform at a previous level. Diagnosis may be based on history and physical examination but in most cases requires radiography for confirmation.[3, 4, 5]

Dorsal Approach

Surgical removal of the summits of fractured, infected, or overriding dorsal spinous processes is done to relieve pain and promote healing.

The surgical approach is similar in all situations.[18, 24] The horse is placed in lateral recumbency with the affected area of the spine near the edge of the table for better access. In instances of fracture, the loosened fragments will move laterally and their location should be ascertained prior to positioning the animal. The loosened fragments should be uppermost in position to facilitate removal.

The area over affected spinous processes is clipped and prepared for aseptic surgery. A longitudinal paramedian incision is made in the skin approximately 2 cm lateral to the dorsal midline. The supraspinous ligament is located. This ligament runs from the head to the sacrum, and its function is to assist in extension of the head and neck. Complete transection may result in inability of the horse to raise its head. In the cervical region it is well defined as the nuchal ligament. It broadens at the withers to measure 4 to 5 inches in width with thin edges overlying the trapezius and rhomboid muscles. Caudal to T6 it narrows to 1.5 inches to form the lumbodorsal segment of the supraspinous ligament, and the edges are clearly defined. Identification of the ligament, therefore, may be more difficult when fractures or osteomyelitis of the withers is being treated. By keeping the incision lateral to the midline to remove the summits of spinous processes, transection of the ligament may be avoided. In surgery of overriding dorsal spinous processes, which commonly occurs between T12–T17, this ligament is more easily defined.

The spinous processes are dissected from the ligament and removed using bone rongeurs. A bone saw may be required when removing an overriding process. Infected processes are easily identified by their soft consistency and purple-blue color. Copious flushing and reapposition of soft tissues is advised prior to skin closure. Large drainage holes may be left lateral and ventral to the incison if infection was the reason for surgery.

Stall rest is advised for 2 months after surgery, and signs of clinical improvement may not be evident for several months after that. If the wound is left open, flushing, protecting skin beneath the wound from the scalding, and antibiotic therapy are advised.

Complications of this surgery include continued or recurring drainage, sinking in of the area as the wound heals, interruption of the nuchal ligament or supraspinous ligament resulting in the inability of the horse to raise its head, and dissection of drainage medial to the scapula causing pockets of exudate to develop between the scapula and body wall. Careful surgical technique and complete excision of affected material can reduce complications.

EXTERNAL STABILIZATION

Because of the physical strength of the horse, external stabilization has not been frequently employed in injury to the vertebral column. Few reports in the equine literature refer to external stabilization.[8, 15, 19] The reports concern cast and pin fixation applicable to cervical vertebral fractures. When contemplating use of external fixation, one should bear in mind that the horse makes extensive use of the weight of the head and flexibility of the neck for rising from recumbency. Although this may not be a problem in the young foal that can be manually placed on its feet, it might be a considerable deterrent with a full grown horse. For this reason, the adult horse should be standing when external stabilization is applied.

Application of a cervical cast is a modification of the human halo vest technique.[19] The materials required are large stockinette material, cast padding or roll cotton padding, and a lightweight casting material.*

The horse is restrained with a minimal dosage of tranquilizer (xylazine,† 0.5 mg/kg; acetylpromazine,‡ 0.04 mg/kg) intravenously to avoid movement. Larger doses will cause the horse to lower its head, making cast placement more difficult. The head is extended slightly and 6 inch stockinette or other protective material is applied. A layer of cotton under the casting material reduces pressure sores and facilitates removal with a cast saw. The casting material is applied from behind the ears to the shoulders; care should be taken that padding covers the ends of the cast cranially and caudally. (When using 3M casting, two layers should suffice, whereas with the Cutter cast three or four layers are usually required.) The cast is set in 20 minutes; however, continued monitoring of the animal is required to ascertain whether it will tolerate the cast. Fractures of C1, C2, and C3 have been successfully handled by this method.[19]

After application of the cast, the horse should be confined to a stall and food and water provided at an elevated level. If the horse lies

---

*3M cast, Animal Care Products, 3M, St Paul, MN; Cutter cast, Biomedical Division of Cutter Laboratories, San Diego, CA.

†Rompun, Haver-Lockhart, Shawnee, KS.

‡Acepromazine, Med-Tech, Inc, Elwood, KS.

down, assistance to stand will be needed. The cast may be left in place for 3 to 4 weeks, at which time radiographic evaluation and clinical signs are used to assess the advisability of replacing the cast.

REFERENCES

1. Cloward RB: The anterior approach for removal of ruptured cervical discs. J Neurosurg 5:602, 1958.
2. DeBowes RM, Grant BD, Bagby GW, et al: Cervical vertebral interbody fusion in the horse: A comparative study of bovine xenografts and autografts supported by stainless steel baskets. Am J Vet Res 45:191, 1984.
3. Jeffcott LB: The diagnosis of disease of the horse's back. Equine Vet J 7:69, 1975.
4. Jeffcott LB: Disorders of the equine thoracolumbar spine—a review. J Equine Med Surg 2:9, 1978.
5. Jeffcott LB and Whitewell KE: Fractures of the thoracolumbar spine of the horse. Proc 22nd Annu Conv Am Assoc Equine Pract 91, 1976.
6. Klaassen JK and Wagner PC: Congenital vertebral abnormalities in a foal. Equine Pract 3:11, 1981.
7. Leathers CW, Wagner PC, and Milleson BD: A case report: Cervical spina bifida with meningocele in an appaloosa foal. J Vet Orthop 1:55, 1979.
8. Mayhew IG and MacKay RJ: The nervous system. *In* Mansmann RA, McAllister ES, and Pratt PW (ed): Equine Medicine and Surgery, 3rd ed. Santa Barbara, CA, American Veterinary Publications, 1982.
9. McCoy DJ, Shires PK, and Beadle R: A ventral approach for stabilization of atlantoaxial subluxation secondary to an odontoid fracture in a foal. JAVMA 185:545, 1984.
10. Nixon AJ and Stashak TS: Surgical management of cervical vertebral malformation in the horse. Proc Am Assoc Equine Pract 267, 1982.
11. Nixon AJ, Stashak TS, and Ingram JT: Diagnosis of cervical vertebral malformation in the horse. Proc Am Assoc Equine Pract 253, 1982.
12. Nixon AJ, Stashak TS, Ingram JT, et al: Dorsal laminectomy in the horse—II. Evaluation in the normal horse. Vet Surg 12:177, 1983.
13. Nixon AJ, Stashak TS, and Ingram JT: Dorsal laminectomy in the horse—III. Results in horses with cervical vertebral malformation. Vet Surg 12:184, 1983.
14. Nyland HG, Blythe LL, Pool RR, et al: Metrizamide myelography in the horse: Clinical, radiographic and pathologic changes. Am J Vet Res 41:204, 1980.
15. Owen R and Smith Maxie LL: Repair of fractured dens of the axis in a foal. JAVMA 173:854, 1978.
16. Rantanen NW, Gavin PR, Barbee DD, and Sande RD: Ataxia and paresis in horses. Part 2. Radiographic and myelographic examination of the cervical vertebral column. Comp Cont Ed Pract Vet 3:S161, 1981.
17. Reed SM, Bayly WM, Traub JL, et al: Ataxia and paresis in horses. Part 1. Differential diagnosis. Comp Cont Ed Pract Vet 3:S88, 1981.
18. Roberts EJ: Resection of the thoracic or lumbar spinous processes for the relief of pain responsible for lameness and some other locomotor disorders of the horse. Proc Am Assoc Equine Pract 13, 1968.
19. Schneider JE: Immobilizing cervical vertebral fractures. Proc Am Assoc Equine Pract 253, 1981.
20. Slone DE, Bergfeld WA, and Walker TL: Surgical decompression for traumatic atlantoaxial subluxation in a weanling filly. JAVMA 174:1234, 1979.
21. Smith KD and Miller CW: Dorsal laminectomy in a calf. JAVMA 184:1508, 1984.
22. Sorjonen DC, Powe TA, West M, and Edmonds S: Ventral surgical fixation and fusion for atlanto-occipital subluxation in a goat. Vet Surg 12:127, 1983.
23. Vaughan JT and Mason BJE: A clinico-pathological study of racing accidents in horses. A report of a study on equine fatal accidents on race courses, financed by the Horserace Betting Levy Board. Royal Veterinary College, Hatfield, Herts, England, 1976.
24. Wagner PC: Diseases of the spine. *In* Mansmann RA, McAllister ES, and Pratt PW (ed): Equine Medicine and Surgery, 3rd ed. Santa Barbara, CA, American Veterinary Publications, 1982.
25. Wagner PC, Bagby GW, Grant BD, et al: Surgical stabilization of the equine cervical spine. Vet Surg 8:7, 1979.
26. Wagner PC, Grant BD, Bagby GW, et al: Evaluation of cervical spine fusion as a treatment in the equine "wobbler" syndrome. Vet Surg 8:88, 1979.
27. Wagner PC, Grant BD, Gallina AM, and Bagby GW: Ataxia and paresis in horses. Part III. Surgical treatment of cervical spinal cord compression. Comp Cont Ed Pract Vet 3:S192, 1981.
28. Wagner PC, Long GG, Chatburn CC and Grant BD: Traumatic injury of the cauda equina in the horse: A case report. J Equine Med Surg 1:282, 1977.
29. Whitewell KE: Causes of ataxia in horses. In Practice 2:17, 1980.

Chapter 18

JE Oliver, Jr, DVM, PhD
BF Hoerlein, DVM, PhD

Cranial Surgery

INDICATIONS

Brain surgery is indicated for elevation of depressed fractures,[25, 56] brain biopsy,[85] or removal of hematoma,[34] neoplasms,[46] or epileptic foci.[57, 63] Behavior disorders may be treated by prefrontal lobotomy.[70, 71] Ventriculoatrial and ventriculoperitoneal shunts are used to treat hydrocephalus.[11, 20, 21] Surgical decompression of traumatic lesions has been the most common use of brain surgery in veterinary medicine, but removal of brain tumors is becoming more frequent.

Elevation of fracture fragments is relatively easy and the location of the fracture can be determined on survey radiographs.[16, 61] Other problems, such as neoplasia, require precise localization of the lesion, usually involving special radiographic procedures.

Brain surgery in large animals is rarely reported.[72, 83, 88, 91] A number of procedures are described for research involving pinealectomy[8, 73] or hypophysectomy.[44] The removal of parasitic cysts from the brains of sheep has been reported.[6, 78] A brain abscess in a cow has been treated successfully using surgical drainage.[77]

SURGICAL APPROACHES TO THE BRAIN

The cranial vault is divided anatomically into two compartments, the rostral and caudal fossae, which are separated by the tentorium cerebelli. These areas are often referred to as rostrotentorial (supratentorial in humans) and caudotentorial (infratentorial in humans). The caudal fossa or compartment contains the cerebellum, the brain stem, and the fourth ventricle; the rostral compartment contains the cerebral hemispheres; and the midbrain is located at the junction of the two compartments. The surgical approaches developed to expose these areas are the lateral (lateral rostrotentorial), the bilateral (rostrotentorial), the suboccipital (caudotentorial), and the ventral.[34, 35, 58, 60]

Lateral (Lateral Rostrotentorial) Craniotomy

This approach involves an opening into the cranial cavity through portions of the frontal, parietal, temporal, or sphenoid bones, depending on the amount of exposure desired. This approach can expose the frontal, parietal, temporal, and occipital lobes. The pituitary gland, the rostral aspect of the cerebellum, and the lateral ventricles may also be approached via this route. The craniotomy can be extended caudally to expose the tentorium cerebelli and the midbrain. By surgically splitting the tentorium, the rostral aspect of the cerebellum can be explored. The craniotomy defect can be extended ventrally to expose the arterial circle, the pituitary gland, and other ventral structures. The lateral ventricle can be explored through a cortical incision in the suprasylvian gyrus.

Technique

The animal is positioned with the head elevated as described in Chapter 16.

The skin incision can be made on the dorsal midline, but to afford a more spacious approach it is generally made in the shape of a horseshoe, extending from the lateral canthus of the eye to the dorsal midline and carried caudally to curve behind the ear. The skin should be carefully draped around the edges and folded back with some compression to inhibit bleeding. Ligation of major vessels and coagulation cautery of minor ones are always indicated.

The superficial muscles are severed slightly lateral to the external sagittal crest. The dissection is continued along the nuchal crest, and the muscles are reflected ventrolaterally. In preparing the isolated bone flap, the temporal muscle is incised slightly lateral to its dorsal attachment and is elevated from the entire lateral aspect of the cranium by means of a periosteal elevator. If maximum exposure is required, the superficial temporal artery and palpebral nerve can be ligated and severed at the rostral portion of the zygomatic arch near the lateral canthus of the eye. The caudal deep temporal artery and nerve are located at the dorsocaudal margin of the zygomatic arch. For greater exposure, it is possible to transect the zygomatic arch at its rostral attachment and caudally just lateral to the mandibular articulation (Fig. 18–1).

Bone Flap

The bone over the lateral calvaria should generally be preserved by means of a bone flap. When the defect is covered with the bone flap, it is part of a craniotomy procedure. If the bone is not preserved and a permanent defect results, the procedure is termed a craniectomy.[4] The bone flap can be of two types, the isolated bone flap or the combined muscle-bone (hinged) flap. The advantage of the latter procedure is that less muscle is transected and that the blood supply to the bone is better maintained by the attached muscle. In dolichocephalic canine breeds, exposure is a problem with this technique because the ventral aspects of the temporal muscle are so thick. In the brachiocephalic breeds, such as the Chihuahua, the combined flap is a satisfactory technique. However, the isolated bone flap, if kept warm and moist during the isolation period, is a satisfactory method and gives better exposure.

The technique of making the flap involves four bur, drill, or trephine holes placed in the extreme corners of the desired exposure area. If hand equipment is used, the bur technique is preferable, starting with a pointed bur and finishing with a round one until the endosteal layer of dura is exposed. Making bur holes with the ultra high speed drill (Hall or Stryker air drill) is faster, easier, and safer.[84] The time involved is a fraction of that needed with hand equipment, which is also more traumatic. If a craniotome attachment is used with the air driven drill, only one drill hole is needed and the flap is promptly cut from it. The outermost boundaries of the bone flap are located 0.5 cm rostral to the nuchal crest, to avoid the transverse sinus; 1.0 cm lateral to the dorsal midline, to avoid the dorsal sagittal sinus; at the orbit and frontal sinus rostrally; and at the temporal musculature, coronoid process of the mandible, and zygomatic arch ventrally (Figs. 18–2 and 18–3).

If a craniotome attachment is not used, the dura mater must be separated from the skull by means of a curved, grooved director or a flat probe passed between the dorsal and lateral holes. The bur holes generally need additional shaping by means of a rongeur forceps to facilitate passing the director. Using high speed equipment, the flap between the drill holes is cut with a fine pointed drill bit on the dorsal, caudal, and cranial sides of the proposed flap (Fig. 18–4). Without the power equipment, a wire saw is then passed between the holes, and the grooved director is passed ventral to the wire to protect the dura during the sawing procedure (Fig. 18–5). The bone is sawed or burred in as diagonal a direction as possible,

Figure 18–1. The incision in the temporal fascia is made approximately 3 to 4 mm from its attachment to facilitate later suturing.

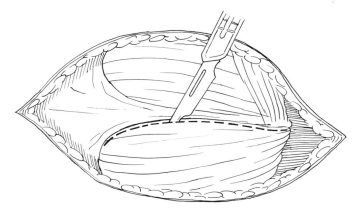

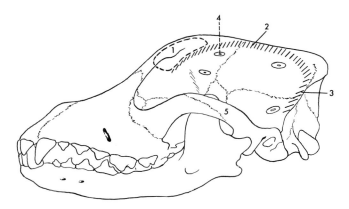

Figure 18–2. Position of bur holes for a lateral rostrotentorial craniotomy. 1, Frontal sinus; 2, sagittal sinus (on midline in dura); 3, transverse sinus (under nuchal crest in dura and partially in bone); 4, bur holes; 5, zygomatic arch.

Figure 18–3. A, Using the hand-powered drill or bit, bur holes can be started more easily with a pointed bur and finished with a spheric bur. The burring should stop when the endosteum is exposed and should be finished with a rongeur. B, Using the air-powered drill, only the spheric bur is needed. 1, Pointed bur; 2, spheric bur; 3, air drill.

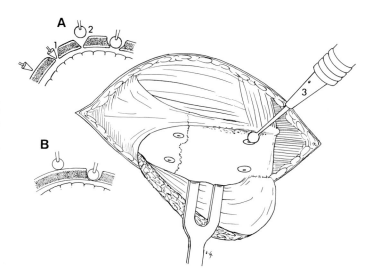

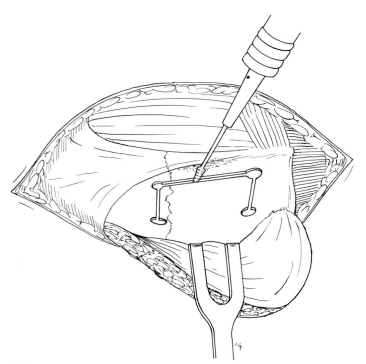

Figure 18–4. The bur holes are joined by grooving and carefully penetrating the bone with a small pointed bur. The ventral side of the flap is broken rather than risk cutting the middle meningeal artery.

472

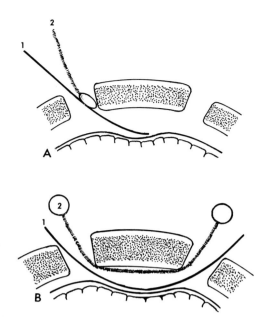

Figure 18–5. If an air drill is not available, the bur holes can be joined by using a wire saw guide or grooved director to separate the dura from the bone and to protect the dura from the wire saw that is used to cut the bone. 1, Saw guide; 2, wire saw.

producing a beveled edge, so that the flap will sit firmly when replaced. After the dorsal, rostral, and caudal sides are sawed, the ventral border is broken by means of prying the dorsal border (Fig. 18–6). The act of sawing the ventral border increases the chance of lacerating the

middle meningeal artery close to its origin. The ventral aspect of the craniotomy is enlarged by rongeurs as needed (Figs. 18–7 and 18–8).

The air driven equipment is the least traumatic and least time consuming means of performing a craniotomy. In larger canine skulls, the craniotome attachment may be used, assuring even greater reduction in operating time. The craniotome end is inserted in a suitably placed bur hole; the attachment works best when a curved rather than a straight rectangular cut is made. The blunt rounded guard pushes the dura away from the calvarium as the bur cuts the bone (Fig. 18–9). In addition, the procedure of making holes in the flap and adjacent skull needed for wiring the flap in place is facilitated with the power equipment. This power equipment is now also used widely in veterinary hospitals in which orthopedic surgery is performed.[84]

The diploic hemorrhage is controlled by rubbing bone wax over the cut bone edges. The isolated bone flap is kept warm and moist in saline soaked sponges. Generally, greater exposure is needed ventrally, and this is obtained by careful use of the rongeur, which leaves a permanent defect in this area. The thick temporal muscle and zygomatic arch protect the brain underlying this defect from injury.

Handling the Dura Mater

The dura mater must be preserved from laceration during the burring, sawing, and ron-

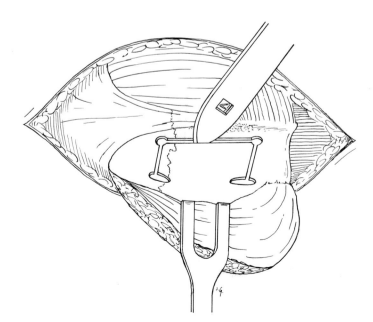

Figure 18–6. The bone flap is carefully pried open. The ventral border of the flap breaks straight because the lower bur bones are notched inward with the rongeur.

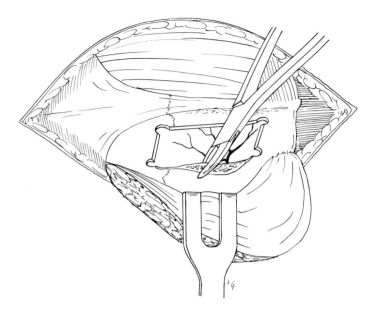

Figure 18–7. For exposure of the ventral portion of the cranial cavity, the rongeur is used to enlarge the craniotomy opening. The ventral defect is well protected by temporal muscle. (Courtesy of ED Gage.)

geuring procedures. It is emphasized that the dura mater is one of the chief barriers to infection and that once it is invaded, asepsis must be strictly maintained. The dura can be retracted from the calvarium in young dogs, but occasionally it adheres so closely to the calvarial bone in old patients that separation is difficult. One must be extremely careful not to lacerate or damage the cerebral cortex in such patients.

In preparing the dural flap, the dura mater is incised 2 to 4 mm inward from the margin of the craniotomy defect. A dural hook, a small, sharp suture needle placed in a needle holder, or a 23 to 25 gauge injection needle with the point bent into a hook, can be used to elevate the dura mater to facilitate making a small incision with a scalpel. The incision is enlarged in a rectangular fashion with small dural scissors, taking care not to incise the soft, fragile brain tissue. The middle meningeal artery is ligated by means of 6–0 silk or silver clips near its origin at the ventral incision of the craniotomy (Fig. 18–8). The flap can be reflected dorsally or ventrally to suit the surgeon's need.

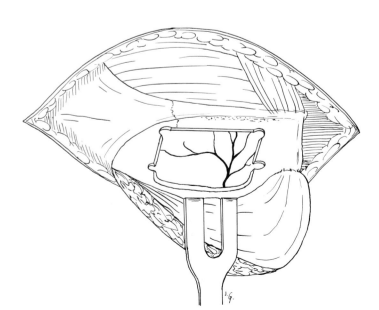

Figure 18–8. The craniotomy is completed.

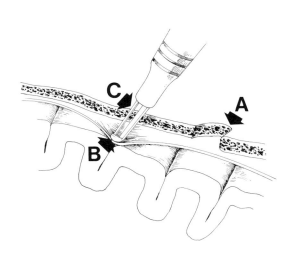

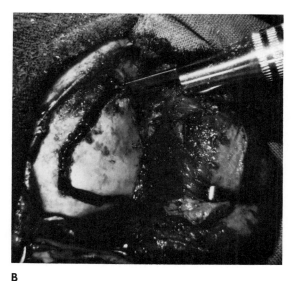

A   **B**

Figure 18–9. The use of the craniotome. A, A cross section of the skull and brain with the craniotome in place. Bur hole in skull (A) with dural guard (B) protecting the underlying dura and brain from the rotating cutting blade (C). B, The craniotome is shown cutting the bone flap from a standard bur hole. (From Swaim SF: Use of pneumatic surgical instruments in neurosurgery, Part 2. Cranial and paracranial surgery. Vet Med/Small Anim Clin 68:1404, 1973.)

The flap may be easier to suture when it is reflected ventrally (Fig. 18–10).

The dura is a tough but still a delicate membrane that will shrink if it is not kept moist and under stretching tension during the procedure. If such care is not taken, the flap will not be large enough to close the dural defect at the time of closure. Therefore, 5–0 to 6–0 silk sutures are placed in the extreme corners of the flap, and the atraumatic needles are allowed to remain attached so that they can be used later to suture the flap. The reflected flap is sandwiched between cotton flannel strips that are kept moist with saline, and forceps are attached to the corner stay sutures. The forceps are allowed to hang over the edge of the surgical area and provide tension to the flap, and it is constantly bathed in saline. This care of the dural flap will facilitate later closure of the dural defect.

The dura and brain tissue must be kept moist and warm and must not be exposed excessively to air. A collagen sponge material (Biocol) has been used in over 300 patients in operations lasting from 1 to 13 hours. The material is soft, white, and pliable and has excellent wet strength; it absorbs 100 times its weight in water compared with an absorbing power of 30 times for most available gelatin sponges (Gelfoam). It reportedly protects the brain tissue from the trauma of contact retraction by instru-

mentation. It is nonabsorbable and should be removed after use.[45]

The usual surgical sponge materials may leave lint on central nervous system tissues that is said to promote connective tissue reactions. Therefore, use of lint free sponges should be considered, especially when controlling hemorrhage on neural tissue. Cotton flannel (Cottonoid) is lint free and smooth.

The question that arises is whether the dural flap is important. Most neurosurgeons feel that is is essential to maintain a watertight dura mater even if a graft or substitute material has to be used. If there is no major damage to the pia arachnoid a neodura will form with no apparent adhesions in approximately 2 weeks.[40, 66, 74] This is particularly true in the absence of a bone flap.[39] However, in the neurosurgical procedure, at least minimal injury to the pia arachnoid will occur, and a dural and bone flap should be preserved if at all possible.

The method of suturing the dura mater will be discussed later (see Closure). Fat tissue sutured on the inside of a small dural tear will promote a watertight seal and is quickly invaded by connective tissue.[50] If the dura cannot be closed, the craniotomy should be left open. Autogenous transplants from temporal fascia or fascia lata have proved successful as a substitute.[24, 58, 59] Homologous dura mater is sterilized and stored in Hank's solution for 8 to 10 weeks

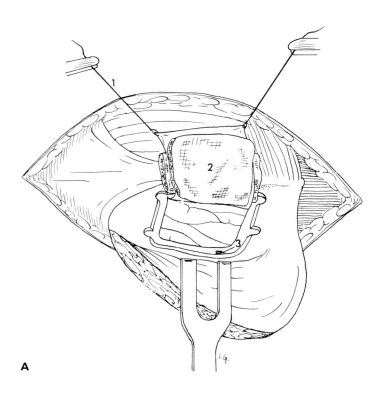

A

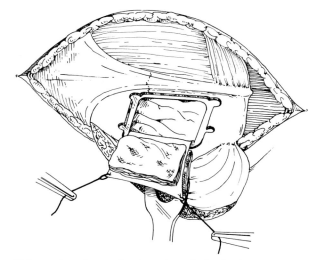

B

Figure 18–10. A, After the middle meningeal artery has been ligated, the dural flap is carefully protected from the calvarial edge by cotton flannel moistened with warm saline. 1, Tension sutures; 2, cotton flannel applied to both sides of the dural flap; 3, middle meningeal artery ligation. Dural flap is hinged toward the midline to facilitate surgery in this area. B, Usually, the dural flap is hinged downward to facilitate surgery in areas that are not near the midline. This facilitates resuturing of the dura. To preserve the integrity of the dural flap for subsequent closure, continuous tension is applied to the stay sutures in each corner of the flap. Warm saline is applied periodically to the dural flap to prevent shrinkage.

or lyophilized and stored for 2 to 3 years.[49] Plastic adhesives have been proposed for non-suture sealing of the dura but have proved to be irritating to neural tissues.[42] Plastic materials such as polythene film,[9] polyvinyl sponges,[14] Vinyon "N,"[86] Orlon,[37] Teflon,[2] and Silastic rubber dural replacement have been used. Cargile membrane* has been used as dural substitute in cats.[46] Silicone reinforced with Dacron mesh is commercially available.† Charged gold leaf has been used to help seal dural lacerations and defects.[23] The authors have found temporal fascia available and satisfactory when a graft is necessary to complete the closure.

Examination of the Brain Cavity

Reduction of the brain volume is necessary when the cranial cavity needs examining or exploration or if edema and brain swelling exist. If a gaseous anesthetic and oxygen mixture is employed, the simplest and most effective means of performing such a reduction is hyperventilation. Hyperventilation in conjunction with the elevated position of the head, administration of glucocorticosteroids prior to surgery, and hypertonic mannitol prior to, during, and even after surgery will generally be highly effective in controlling brain swelling.[26, 27, 30] However, mannitol has been incriminated in promoting occasional intracranial hemorrhage during surgery. The addition of regional or systemic hypothermia to these procedures should make them even more efficacious.[22]

Controlled ventilation is generally started at

*Ethicon, Somerville, NJ.
†Heyer-Schultz Corp, Goleta, CA.

the time of skin incision in an exploratory craniotomy. Because it requires 30 to 40 minutes of hyperventilation to produce maximal reduction in brain volume, the brain is already shrinking at the time of exposure. An increased rate of hyperventilation is started at this point (one and a half times the normal rate and in sufficient volume to visibly expand the chest). If the surgeon retracts the brain toward the midline and carefully aspirates the cerebrospinal fluid from the ventral cisterns, the brain rapidly recedes from the cranial walls, and surgical examination with a lighted brain retractor is facilitated. Hyperventilation for long periods of time will result in a lowering of blood carbon dioxide levels, systemic alkalosis, and cerebral vascular constriction (producing cellular hypoxia). These effects have not generally been a problem[59] (see Chapter 16).

The brain should be bathed almost continuously in warm saline. Moist cotton flannel sponges overlying its surface will help prevent inflammation resulting from retraction and aspiration. One should never aspirate directly against nervous tissue, but only against cotton, absorbable, or lint free sponges overlying the tissue. The use of gelatin sponge pledgets pressed in place with cotton flannel, combined with saline irrigations and patience, will prove to be an effective means of controlling surface hemorrhage[59] (Fig. 18–11).

Incisions into the cortex should be made through a gyrus, because relatively large vessels are located in a sulcus. Hemorrhage from the pia mater can be controlled by use of low intensity bipolar electrocautery, and the invasion of brain tissue should be as delicate as possible.[10, 89] Occasional cautery with separation

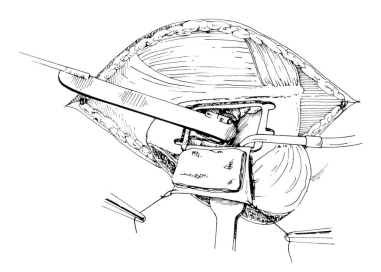

Figure 18–11. Exploration of the ventral cerebral areas is facilitated by moderate hyperventilation, gentle retraction of the brain with a padded retractor, and continuous aspiration of cerebrospinal fluid from basal cisterns.

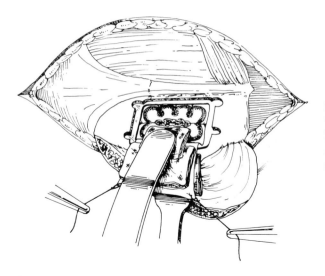

Figure 18–12. To explore deep lesions, the pia is cauterized with bipolar cautery and incised, and the cortex separated with a thin spatula or the catheter balloon (see text). Incised tissue should be protected from instruments by cotton flannel soaked in warm saline.

of tissues rather than flagrant incision could be tried. Separated surfaces should be protected with gelatin sponge material (Fig. 18–12).

A new technique for making cortical incisions has been tried experimentally on dogs.[76] A ventricular needle was inserted through a gyrus to make a tract for a balloon catheter. The catheter was a 5 Fr feeding tube with multiple holes cut in the side. The catheter was inserted into a finger cot and tied with 4–0 silk at its proximal end. The catheter was placed in the needle tract, and small amounts of saline were injected and withdrawn over a 5 to 6 minute period. The tissues were gently separated along cleavage planes produced by the balloon. Histologic and functional studies confirmed that this method was superior to conventional dissection.

Many lesions will have undergone necrosis and liquefaction; this tissue can frequently be removed by aspiration. Hemorrhage in any cavity in the brain after removal of pathologic tissue must be controlled before closure. It is also best not to leave excessive gelatin sponge material in the area, because the clot formation in its substance makes an excellent cultural medium for any bacterial contamination.

Closure

After the surgical procedure in the brain, the dura is closed with interrupted or continuous sutures of 5–0 or 6–0 nonabsorbable material. The stay sutures in the flap corners are secured initially. The same material can be used for the rest of the closure. If the flap has been well cared for during surgery, the closure is routine

(Fig. 18–13). The bone flap is secured by means of orthopedic stainless steel wire through appropriate drill holes in the cranium and flap. Either a high speed drill or a small Steinmann pin in a hand drill will suffice. One must be careful not to damage the dura or underlying brain when drilling these holes. The human drill guides and protectors are too large for most dogs; however, a scalpel handle or brain retractor placed beneath the cranial edges will afford the desired protection (Fig. 18–14).

In cases of cranial fractures, cranial bone lesions, or severe traumatic brain damage, a craniectomy defect may be indicated. A myoplastic flap can be cosmetically satisfactory and in some cases may even afford ample protection against future injury, especially if the defect is in a ventrolateral area and the dog is dolichocephalic. However, a prosthetic bone flap can be fashioned from acrylic, plastic, or metal.[28]

Stainless steel screen material is satisfactory for maintaining a cosmetic appearance, as well as affording more protection to the area. Such a cranioplasty can be performed at the time of the initial surgery or at a later time to give protection to the brain. Caution is again advised in making certain that the dura or dural substitute completely shields the cerebral cortex from the skull flap or prosthesis to prevent cortical adhesions and future seizure episodes.

The temporal muscle, superficial muscles, subcutis, and skin are closed routinely. Careful suturing of layers of tissue, maintaining proper hemostasis, and obliterating all dead space will reduce the possibility of formation of a subcutaneous hematoma or seroma. A snug but loose bandage of elastic adhesive will also aid in

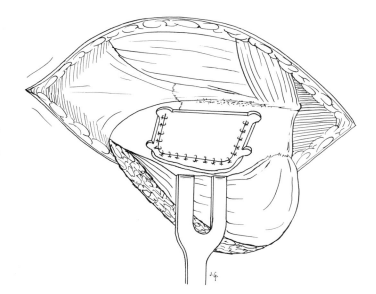

Figure 18–13. The dura should be securely closed with 5–0 or 6–0 nonabsorbable suture; either interrupted or continuous pattern may be used.

preventing a seroma. Maintaining a patent airway, preventing postsurgical delirium and self mutilation, good nursing care, and other immediate postsurgical considerations are discussed in detail in Chapters 15 and 16.

Modifications of Lateral Craniotomy

Transfrontal Craniotomy

In the lateral craniotomy, lesions of the prefrontal cerebrum, which is adjacent to the frontal sinus and olfactory areas, are difficult to expose. If there is a small focal lesion in this area, an isolated approach through the frontal sinus may be large enough to correct it. A combination of the transfrontal and lateral craniotomies will be necessary for adequate exposure of most lesions in this area.[13, 64]

The skin incision is a modified horseshoe, extending from the lateral canthus of the eye and curving rostrodorsally about 2 cm behind the dorsal palpebral margin to the midline between the eyes. The incision is continued caudally along the midline to the external occipital protuberance and then ventrally along the nuchal crest. The skin, subcutis, muscula-

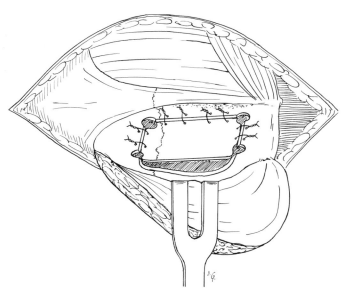

Figure 18–14. The bone flap is replaced and secured with stainless steel orthopedic wire. The ventral craniectomy will be protected by the temporal muscle.

ture (where present), and periosteum are removed from the area of the frontal sinus and the part of the calvarium involved in the exposure. The limits of the frontal sinus in the patient's particular type of skull are determined, and a triangular flap of outer frontal bone is removed by means of the smallest available drill bur for the air powered drill (a small saw blade or hand saw may be used instead). The flap is wrapped in warm saline soaked sponges or towel and preserved for final replacement. The exposed frontal sinus is thoroughly flushed with sterile saline, and the mucosal lining is removed. The rostral opening of the frontal sinus is packed with bone wax and covered with cotton flannel.[33] At this point, all previously used pieces of equipment are removed from the surgical area, surgical gloves are replaced with sterile ones, and drapes are replaced. Every effort is made to alleviate the chances of introducing infection from the sinus area into the cranial cavity.

The cranial cavity is entered at least 0.5 cm from the midline and as far distal to the caudal limit of the frontal sinus as deemed necessary for proper exposure. If a complete unilateral cerebral and transfrontal approach is desired, there should be three bur holes (two caudal holes and the ventrocranial one) for the lateral flap previously described, and the dorsal bone incision should be extended to remove the inner

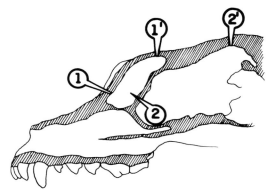

Figure 18–15. In transfrontal craniotomy (lateral view), access to the frontal lobe of the brain is made through the frontal sinus. An initial bone flap is made through the frontal sinus (1 to 1'). The craniotomy flap is between 2 and 2'.

or ventral (frontal bone) plate of the frontal sinus. The smallest air driven bur drill should be used if at all possible. If the inner frontal bone plate in the sinus is diseased and cannot be removed for a flap, it should be carefully removed with rongeurs; the bone defect will then remain. If the small frontal sinus approach is sufficient, only the ventral flap of bone in the sinus is cut with the drill bit. Great care is needed to avoid lacerating the dura (Figs. 18–15 and 18–16).

Osteotomy of the zygomatic arch caudal to the orbital ligament and rostral to the tempo-

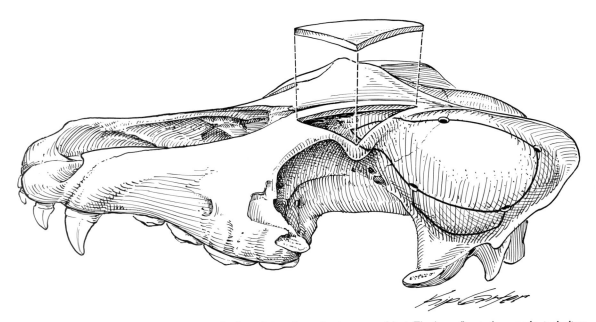

Figure 18–16. In a transfrontal craniotomy, the frontal sinus bone flap is removed first. The large flap is then made, including the area inside the frontal sinus. Notice the increased area of the flap rostrally, as compared with that in Figure 18–2. Additional exposure can be obtained ventrally by removal of bone with rongeurs to the level of the zygomatic process.

romandibular joint allows slightly greater exposure ventrally.[58] The craniotomy flap can be extended ventrally and rostrally to expose most of the frontal lobe (Fig. 18–16). DeWet et al[13] have described the development of a bone flap providing maximal exposure in this region. In many instances, a smaller flap can be made and the opening enlarged as needed with rongeurs. The defects that remain are well protected by the temporal muscle. Preservation and replacement of the dorsal portions of the flap, including the frontal sinus, are necessary for a good cosmetic effect.

The dural flap is cut at least 1 to 2 mm smaller than the bone flap so that it can be securely sutured after correction of the lesion. If the dura cannot be securely closed, temporal muscle fascia is removed and grafted over the dural defect to ensure a watertight closure. Autogenous fat can be packed in the frontal sinus to help obliterate the cavity.[87] All bone flaps are securely wired in place to prevent secondary compression of brain tissue from loose flaps. If necessary, a small tube into the frontal sinus can be left exposed for postoperative antibiotic infusions.

The dangers of the surgery are the chance of recurring infection because of the invasion of the frontal sinus, and the possibility that dural defects will promote leakage of cerebrospinal fluid into the sinus. However, this approach should be utilized when exposure of a cranial frontal lesion is expected to be difficult.[13, 64]

The prefrontal lobotomy may be performed using this approach. Prefrontal lobotomy, as described by Redding,[70, 71] has been recommended as a treatment for aggressiveness, de-

structive behavior, fear biting, and self mutilation in dogs. Results have been variable, and it is rarely used.[3] A simplified approach provided little exposure.[71] Complications of the procedure may be attributable to improper placement of the lesion or disruption of other structures such as the caudate nucleus or its blood supply[13] (Fig. 18–17).

Bilateral Craniotomy

This approach can be used for midline lesions or for massive cerebral decompressions in trauma. The authors prefer to use lateral craniotomies involving both sides separately rather than disturbing the dorsal sagittal sinus and possibly injuring it in a single dorsal bone flap.[54, 60] Of course, midline pathologic lesions, such as lacerations of the sagittal sinus and tumors of the falx cerebri, demand the midline approach.[28, 54] The anatomic considerations already described are appropriate for this approach. The sagittal sinus is the primary problem. Ligation of the sagittal sinus caudal to the dorsal cerebral veins results in severe congestion and edema of the cerebral hemisphere.[58]

TECHNIQUE

The incision can be midline or an **H** incision. The **H** incision consists of a dorsal midline incision with transverse incisions at its extremities; it unquestionably gives the best exposure. The skin and musculature are retracted as in the lateral approach. The amount of temporal muscle reflected per side depends on the need for exposure. Perhaps one side will need com-

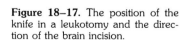
Figure 18–17. The position of the knife in a leukotomy and the direction of the brain incision.

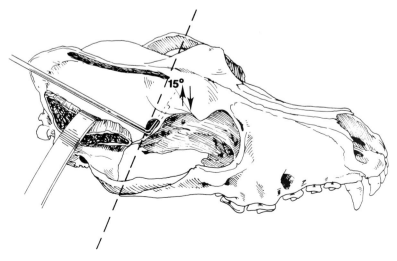

plete reflection but the other will need to extend only 2 to 3 cm from the midline.

The bone flap differs somewhat from that in the unilateral approach. Bur holes are made at the extreme corners of the proposed area on the side of largest exposure, but the dorsal holes are closer to the midline (0.5 cm instead of 1.0 cm). Two more dorsal bur holes are made in like fashion on the opposite side, for a total of six bur holes. If a larger dorsal exposure is desired, a total of eight holes can be made, four on each side. On the side with the four holes, the rostral and caudal pairs are joined by sawing. The two dorsal holes on this side are enlarged with a rongeur forceps so that the endosteal layer of the dura can be separated from the bone over the sagittal sinus. This will provide for less damage to the sinus when the bone flap is lifted. The bur holes on the opposite side of the midline are united by a rostrocaudal cut. The sagittal sinus must be protected while the rostral pair of dorsal bur holes (one on each side of the midline) are joined across the midline by sawing or rongeuring. The caudal dorsal pair of holes are likewise joined across the midline. Finally, the bone flap is carefully lifted upward from the side with the two bur holes; any remaining dura is separated from bone, and the ventral border of the flap is broken on the side with four holes (Fig. 18–18). Use of an air drill or craniotome is preferred. It is not necessary to make all of the bur holes when using power equipment, but the midline holes are used to elevate the dura and sagittal sinus from the bone.

Bleeding emissary veins that have been ruptured between the skull and the sagittal sinus are covered with pieces of crushed muscle or gelatin sponge and held in place by cotton flannel moistened with saline. Bone wax is used on cut bone edges to control diploic hemorrhage. The dural flap is prepared on the larger side of the opening. It is reflected dorsally to the midline. If a complete exposure of the midline and the longitudinal fissure is needed, it may be necessary to ligate and sever one or more of the dorsal cerebral veins that enter the sagittal sinus in the frontal area. Cauterization or application of gelatin sponge may be necessary to stop bleeding from some of these small vessels.

The continuity of the sagittal sinus must be preserved caudal to the largest dorsal cerebral veins. Occlusion of these veins or the sagittal sinus causes severe cerebral congestion and brain swelling. The sagittal sinus can be occluded rostral to the dorsal cerebral veins with little problem.

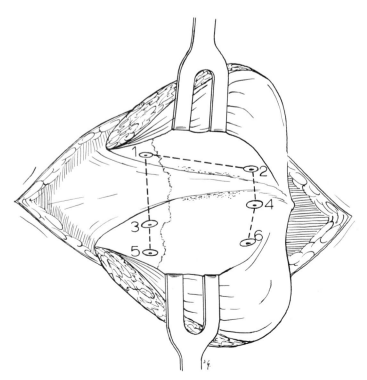

Figure 18–18. The bur holes for a bilateral craniotomy. Holes 3 and 4 are enlarged so that the dura and sagittal sinus can be carefully separated from the skull. Cuts between holes 1 and 3 and holes 2 and 4 are carefully performed to avoid lacerating the sagittal sinus. After all cuts are made, the flap is lifted from line 1–2 toward holes 5 and 6 until it breaks at this point, separating the dura from the bone during the procedure. Dotted lines indicate saw lines.

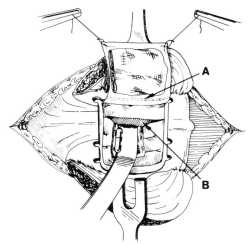

Figure 18–19. Retracting the cerebral hemisphere to examine the area for a midline lesion. A, The dural flap containing the sagittal sinus (dotted line), which must not be occluded; B, the longitudinal fissure between the hemispheres.

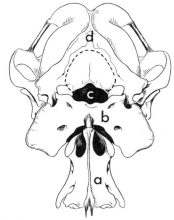

Figure 18–20. Caudal view of the skull. The dotted line indicates the maximum extent of the usual craniectomy for an approach to the cerebellum. a, Axis: b, atlas; c, foramen magnum; d, occipital protuberance. (After Miller ME: Guide to the Dissection of the Dog, 3rd ed. Ann Arbor, MI, Edwards Bros, 1952, © Dr Malcolm E Miller.)

In this manner, even such deep midline structures as the cingulate gyrus, the corpus callosum, the third ventricle, and, caudally, the tentorium cerebelli can be exposed (Fig. 18–19). The dura, bone, muscle, and skin can be closed as described above.

Caudal Suboccipital or Caudotentorial Craniectomy

The suboccipital approach to the brain is used to expose the caudal aspect of the cerebellum, the dorsal aspect of the medulla, the fourth ventricle, and the rostral portions of the spinal cord, if necessary. Because the bone is irregularly thin and the musculature is extremely heavy, one does not generally attempt to preserve a bone flap (Fig. 18–20).

Technique

The head should be flexed nearly at a right angle to the cervical vertebrae. The skin incision may be either a midline or a crossbow incision (midline and curved over the nuchal crest). The superficial fascia is severed on the midline to expose the dorsal cervical muscles, which are removed from the caudal aspect of the occiput about 0.5 cm from their tendinous attachments. These stumps of insertion will facilitate suturing at the time of closure. The caudal aspect of the occipital bone is cleaned of all muscle by elevation. Greater exposure can be obtained by splitting the dorsal musculature

on the midline at least to the level of the atlas. Electrocautery coagulation will control bleeding from the small vessels in the muscle.

One or more bur holes can be made in the base of the skull lateral to the midline. The rongeur is used to expand the craniectomy defect carefully up to the transverse sinuses laterally, the occipital protuberance dorsally, and the foramen magnum ventrally (Fig. 18–21). Because the bone is irregular and the dura adheres tightly to it, the dura is frequently torn

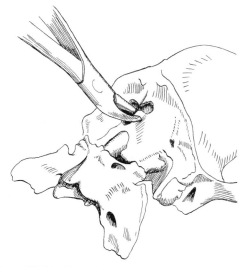

Figure 18–21. After a bur hole is made, the rongeur is used to enlarge the craniectomy to the extent illustrated in Figure 18–20.

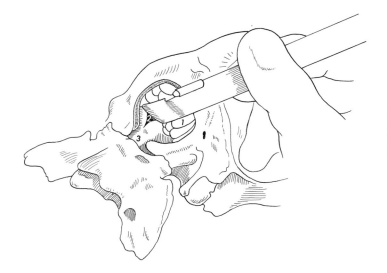

Figure 18–22. The cerebellum can be elevated gently to examine the fourth ventricle. Lateral exposure is limited. 1, Cerebellum; 2, fourth ventricle; 3, medulla oblongata.

and a flap is not possible. The cerebellum is exposed and examined, and the procedure is accomplished as necessary. The dorsal aspect of the medulla and the area of the fourth ventricle can be exposed by lifting the vermis of the cerebellum (Fig. 18–22).

The dura is sutured, if possible, or a graft can be furnished, if necessary. Because a bone flap is not preserved, the dural closure is not critical to prevent adhesions. The musculature is securely sutured, and the remainder of the closure is routine. An appropriate external brace placed either ventrally or dorsally will promote healing of the supporting muscles.

When the cerebellar exposure was inadequate, the authors tried three different procedures to solve the problem. Removal of the nuchal crest resulted in invasion of the transverse sinus, which had to be ligated. Even though good exposure of the lateral aspects of the cerebellum was achieved, the patient rarely survived. Exposure of the tentorium through a lateral craniotomy, splitting it to expose the anterior portions of the cerebellum, is possible, but time consuming. An approach made by separate suboccipital and lateral rostrotentorial openings affords good exposure of the cerebellum and tentorium. A cerebellar lesion could be exposed initially with a suboccipital approach and then, if necessary, the lateral flap could be made, leaving the nuchal crest and its transverse sinus intact.[60]

Ventral Craniectomy

The ventral approach seems to have limited clinical value, as only the pituitary gland, the ventral surfaces of the medulla, and the pons can be exposed.

Technique

The usual approach to this area of the brain is through either the mouth[31, 47, 48, 52] or the ventral midline.[90, 92] For the oral approach, the dog is placed in a dorsal recumbent position with its mouth wide open. An endotracheal or tracheotomy tube is essential. The pharynx is packed with gauze sponges to prevent aspiration of fluid, and the oral cavity is swabbed with antiseptic solution. The incision is made with an electrocautery knife, through the mucosa and soft palate and down to the base of the skull. A palpable landmark is the pterygoid process, which is located directly even with the intersphenoid suture. The periosteum and mucosa are removed caudally over the basisphenoid bone until the occipitosphenoid suture is exposed. The pituitary gland lies directly dorsal to the middle of the basisphenoid bone. The available craniectomy area is limited, in most cases, to a section about 0.5 cm wide and 0.7 cm long because of the ventral petrosal sinuses caudally and the cavernous sinuses laterally and rostrally.

The bur is used directly over the pituitary, and the hole is enlarged appropriately with curets. Lesions of the pituitary gland can frequently be removed by aspiration, as can the pituitary gland itself. A large tumor of the gland would be difficult to remove via this approach.

More exposure can be achieved by splitting the symphysis of the mandible, elevating the digastric and mylohyoid muscles from one mandible laterally.[31] The additional exposure is generally not worth the extra time and trauma to the patient.

In closure, the dura is left open. Fat may be left as a dural substitute. The mucosa is securely sutured with 3–0 medium monofilament nylon.

This approach is difficult and has the disadvantage that asepsis is nearly impossible.

In the neck approach, the dog is placed in the dorsal recumbent position with the head extended and firmly immobilized. An endotracheal catheter is essential. A midline incision is made from the body of the mandible to the level of the third and fourth cervical vertebrae. The trachea and sternohyoid and the sternothyroid muscles are retracted from the carotid sheath to allow for dissection through fascial planes. The larynx can be palpated at the level of the occipital condyles. Blunt dissection is extended to the base of the skull, where the bodies of the atlas and axis can be palpated. A self retaining retractor is applied and the rectus capitis ventralis and longus capitis muscles are elevated from their insertions on the basioccipital bone.

The bur hole is made directly over the pituitary gland or started just rostral to the rim of the foramen magnum and enlarged rostrally up to the pituitary gland. The total lateral dimension can be only about 1 cm because of large venous sinuses. To expose the pituitary gland adequately, the pharyngeal mucosa must be elevated, but one must be careful not to enter the oral cavity and permit contamination. The dura is opened, and the area is examined as

necessary. Fat may be left as a dural substitute. The closure is made routinely. The large basilar artery would make surgical corrections in this area difficult.

INTRACRANIAL MANIPULATION

Intracranial structures must be handled carefully and gently. Distinction between normal and abnormal tissues can be difficult. As small hemorrhages occur, the distinction is even less clear. Blunt dissection with a smooth, flat spatula is preferred. Most lesions and all normal brain tissue can be removed by suction. In removing a tumor, suction is used as much as possible once a piece has been obtained for histopathologic examination. Normal cleavage lines are followed if possible. Intravenous fluorescein dye has been recommended to help delineate the boundaries of brain tumors.[55] Bipolar coagulation is used on small arteries.[10, 89] Venous hemorrhage is best controlled with gelatin sponge and gentle compression.[59] Almost constant irrigation of the tissues with warm saline is essential to prevent drying.

Biopsy of the brain may be indicated to establish a diagnosis.[85] This technique is especially valuable in making an antemortem diagnosis in animals with inheritable diseases, such as the storage diseases. Biopsy may be important in the future if specific antiviral drugs become available. Either the cerebral cortex or the cerebellum can be exposed using the tech-

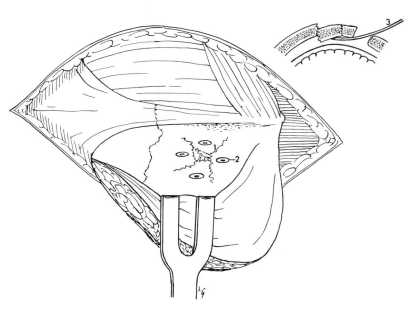

Figure 18–23. Depressed fracture fragments must be carefully elevated in an effort to alleviate injury. Appropriately placed bur holes allow examination for subdural hemorrhage, as well as providing access to these fragments. 1, Fracture; 2, bur holes; 3, elevating fragments through a bur hole.

niques described. The biopsy is obtained by using a number 11 scalpel blade to make four stab incisions into a gyrus to remove a pyramid of tissue including both gray and white matter.[85] This tissue must be handled carefully as it is friable.

Elevation of depressed fracture fragments is a common application of brain surgery in animals. If the fragments are loose, they are easily removed. If they are depressed, but attached on one or more sides, simple elevation may cause depression of the opposite side resulting in additional injury. To safely elevate such a fragment, a bur hole is made adjacent to the fracture site, a probe is carefully passed through the bur hole and under the fragment, and the fragment pushed up (Fig. 18–23).

The major branches of the middle cerebral artery must be preserved. Occlusion of the rostral or caudal cerebral arteries is less critical because there are anastomotic branches, but the middle cerebral artery is an end artery.[32, 69]

SURGICAL TREATMENT OF HYDROCEPHALUS

The diagnosis and medical management of hydrocephalus was discussed in Chapter 6. Medical management is effective in many animals with hydrocephalus, but some are unresponsive.[17, 21] Surgical shunting of the excess fluid is the only alternative. It is not used frequently because of the risk, cost, and complications. Revision of the shunt because of growth of the animal is frequently necessary. Occlusion of the system is also common, necessitating replacement of portions of the shunt system. In spite of these problems, the procedure can be effective and result in a relatively normal animal for many years.[34] The procedure has been described only in dogs.

Surgical shunts are used to drain the fluid from the ventricular system to some other portion of the body. Ideally, the shunt should be established where it will remain patent, be free from infection, maintain normal intraventricular pressure, and provide for reabsorption of the fluid. The fluid has been diverted to numerous sites in the body,[67] but only two are recommended for animals, the ventriculoatrial and ventriculoperitoneal shunts.[11, 17, 18, 20, 21, 43]

Ventriculoatrial Shunt

Several systems are available, including the Holter, Denver, Pudenz, and various modifi-

cations of these.[34, 67] All systems include a fenestrated Silastic ventricular catheter, a Silastic tube to pass through the jugular vein into the right atrium, various connecting devices, and a valve to restrict flow to one direction and to maintain appropriate pressure. The type of valve is the main difference in the systems. Most valves are placed between the ventricular tubing and the venous tubing. The Pudenz system has a slit valve in the atrial tube[68] (Fig. 18–24).

Installation of the shunt is simple but requires strict attention to detail to be successful.[34] Careful anesthesia, strict asepsis, and avoidance of introducing air into the system, which might cause air embolism, are essential.

The patient is positioned in lateral recum-

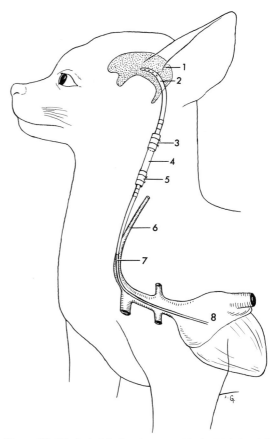

Figure 18–24. A sketch showing a ventriculoatrial shunt. 1, Lateral ventricle; 2, ventricular catheter made of siliconized rubber; 3, proximal Holter one way valve; 4, intermediate silicone tube that can be manipulated by hand to stimulate CSF flow in case of temporary occlusion of the system; 5, distal Holter one way valve; 6, jugular vein; 7, venous catheter ligated in place in jugular vein over a connector apparatus so as not to diminish lumen of tube; 8, right atrium.

bency with the head slightly elevated. The skin incision varies depending on the conformation of the animal. If the skull is dome shaped, the ventricular catheter can be inserted from caudal to cranial through a bur hole dorsal to the nuchal crest. If the skull is not dome shaped, the catheter must be inserted from the lateral side. The caudal approach is preferred, because the catheter can extend the full length of the lateral ventricle.

The incision can be extended from the head to the proximal cervical area over the jugular groove.[20, 21] Preferably, two small incisions are made, one at the location of the ventricular catheter and one at the jugular vein. Subcutaneous tissues are undermined between the two sites to place the valve and connecting tubes. The placement of the tube is caudal to the ear when the caudal site is used, and rostral to the ear when the lateral site is used.

A bur hole is made at the selected site after muscles are elevated from the skull. The dura mater is incised and a spinal needle is inserted to estimate the thickness of the cerebral cortex and to establish a path for the ventricular tube. The ventricular tube is inserted, establishing a free flow of fluid. It is clamped to prevent excessive loss of fluid, which can cause subdural hematoma. The valve is attached, which prevents excessive fluid loss, and the clamp can be removed. The valve is tied securely to the ventricular catheter and placed in the subcutaneous tunnel. The previously exposed jugular vein is mobilized below the bifurcation of the internal and external maxillary branches. An incision is made in the vein, and the atrial tube is inserted. The length of the atrial tube may be estimated from radiographs and measurements of the dog prior to surgery. If difficulty is encountered passing the tubing into the vein, the opening may be stabilized by three 6–0 stay sutures. The atrial catheter must be clamped to stop back flow of blood. A radiograph should be made at this time to verify proper location of the distal tip of the catheter in the atrium (Fig. 18–25). Improper placement will invariably result in early occlusion of the system.[41]

After proper placement is verified, the atrial catheter is connected to the valve with appropriate connectors and tubes. A metal adaptor must be inserted at all cut segments to support ligatures without occluding the tubes. The jugular vein is ligated. During all manipulations, the atrial catheter is periodically flushed with saline-heparin solution to prevent clot formation.

Muscle and skin incisions are closed in a

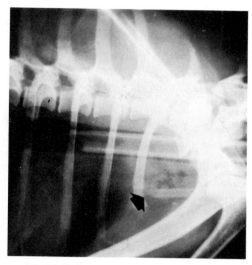

Figure 18–25. Radiograph taken during surgery indicating that the atrial catheter (arrow) needs to be inserted farther to reach the right atrium. (From Gage ED and Hoerlein BF: Surgical treatment of canine hydrocephalus by ventriculoatrial shunting. JAVMA 153:1423, 1968.)

routine fashion. The valve should be situated in a position for easy manipulation under the skin. When the system is thought to be occluded, the valve can be pumped by squeezing it, which often clears the obstruction. Patency of the system can also be assessed, because the middle segment of the valve will not refill if the ventricular catheter is plugged, and it will not empty if the distal catheter is plugged.

Ventriculoperitoneal Shunt

In the ventriculoperitoneal shunt, the ventricular catheter is placed as in the ventriculoatrial shunt.[11, 43] An incision is made in the paralumbar skin and the shunt tubing routed through a subcutaneous channel to the paralumbar incision. A small incision is made in the paralumbar region through the abdominal muscles into the peritoneal cavity, leaving 4 to 6 inches of extra tubing loosely coiled to allow for movement and growth (Fig. 18–26).

Several special catheters are made to place in the peritoneal cavity. Some have slit valves and others have modifications to prevent kinking.[43] Clemmons[11] suggests using plain Silastic tubing, fenestrated when necessary, for the entire assembly. This is considerably cheaper, but there is some risk of excessive fluid flow and collapse of the cerebral cortex in severe

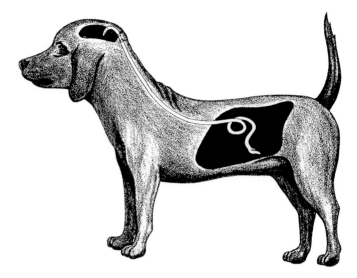

Figure 18–26. Ventriculoperitoneal shunt. Any extra length of tubing is coiled at the distal end to allow for movement and growth. (From Knecht CD: Ventriculoperitoneal shunt for hydrocephalus. *In* Bojrab MJ (ed): Current Techniques in Small Animal Surgery I. Philadelphia, Lea & Febiger, 1975.)

hydrocephalus when there is no valve to regulate flow.

Comparison of Shunting Methods

The ventriculoatrial shunt is more difficult to install. Precise placement of the atrial catheter necessitates a radiograph during surgery. A jugular vein must be sacrificed for insertion of the atrial catheter. The ventriculoperitoneal shunt requires extensive subcutaneous dissection and entry into the peritoneal cavity. Revisions for growth may be less frequent. There are no long-term studies comparing the two systems in animals, but frequency of revision is similar in humans.[38, 41, 75] Hoerlein[34] summarized results of shunting on 52 hydrocephalic dogs with good results (1 year survival) in 29 (55%).

Failures in surgical shunting may be related to irreversible neurologic disease, anesthetic and surgical problems, and postoperative problems associated with the shunt. Postoperative complications are usually caused by occlusion of the system. Growth of the animal may displace the catheters, requiring revision. Hemorrhage or inflammation in the ventricle may plug the catheter or valve. Clots may form on the distal atrial tube. Adhesions may occlude the peritoneal tubing. Many of these problems can be corrected by replacement of malfunctioning tubing.

Harrison[29] has reported successful use of the Ommaya reservoir without a complete shunt system. A ventricular tube with the reservoir attached is placed in the lateral ventricle. Small amounts of fluid can be removed to manage the animal in the acute stages of increased pressure. The theory is that the increased volume afforded by the reservoir reduces the effect of pulsatile pressure in the ventricles, which has been considered a factor in ventricular enlargement.

Surgical shunting should be reserved for animals that cannot be managed medically. It is more satisfactory in the more mature animal. Animals with severe neurologic deficits prior to shunting are unlikely to return to normal after surgery.

BULLA OSTEOTOMY

Inflammatory disorders of the middle and inner ear (otitis media and interna) were discussed in Chapter 7. Most middle ear infections can be resolved by drainage through the tympanic membrane (myringotomy, tympanotomy) and administration of topical and systemic antibiotics.[34, 65, 82] Occasionally the process is so advanced that surgical drainage and débridement is necessary.[12]

Technique

The ventral bulla osteotomy is performed with the animal in a dorsal recumbent position with the head extended.[1, 7, 36, 53] A 7 to 8 cm longitudinal incision is made directly over the bulla, medial to the digastric muscle. The digastric muscle, laterally, is separated from the styloglossus and hyoglossus muscles medially

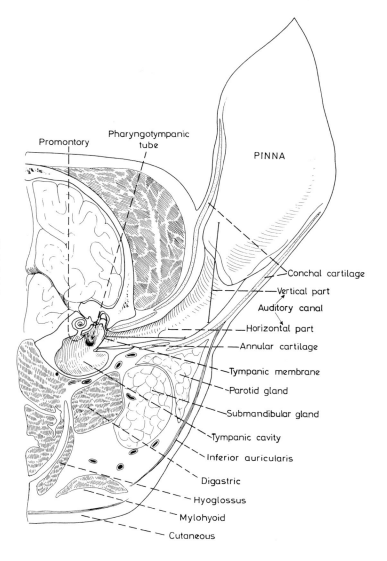

Figure 18–27. The anatomic structure of the outer, middle, and inner ear and their surrounding tissues. (From Spruell JSA: Ablation of ear canal. *In* Bojrab MJ (ed): Current Techniques in Small Animal Surgery I. Philadelphia, Lea & Febiger, 1975).

Promontory

Pharyngotympanic tube

PINNA

Conchal cartilage
Vertical part
Auditory canal
Horizontal part
Annular cartilage
Tympanic membrane
Parotid gland
Submandibular gland
Tympanic cavity
Inferior auricularis
Digastric
Hyoglossus
Mylohyoid
Cutaneous

(Fig. 18–27). The bulla can be palpated directly. Care must be exercised to retract the hypoglossal nerve, which is on the lateral surface of the hyoglossus muscle.[15] The external carotid artery may be directly over or just medial to the bulla.[34] It should be identified and retracted if necessary (Fig. 18–28). Soft tissue is elevated from the bulla. The bulla is opened with a rongeur, a small chisel or gouge, or a Steinmann pin. The opening is enlarged with rongeurs.

Swabs for culture and sensitivity testing and tissue for histopathologic examination are obtained. Curettage and flushing of the bulla is used to remove all pathologic material. If severe inner ear disease is present, the medial wall of the promontory is opened with an air drill or a small chisel[82] (Fig. 18–29).

A drain is sutured to adjacent soft tissue with absorbable suture. The drain may be single or double tubing or a small rubber tube inside a Penrose drain.[19, 36, 80] A second tube may be inserted in the external ear canal through the tympanic membrane to provide more thorough irrigation.

The drain tubes are incorporated in the closure to prevent displacement. Administration of systemic antibiotics and twice daily irrigation of the bulla are continued for a varying time depending on the problem. Drains are usually removed within 1 week, but systemic antibiotics are continued for 2 to 3 weeks. Culture and sensitivity testing results dictate the choice of antibiotics.

Animals with otitis media often improve

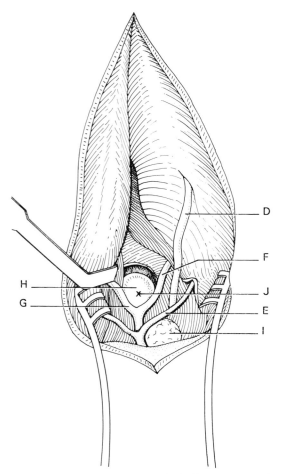

Figure 18–28. Ventral approach for bulla osteotomy—the dissection between the digastric muscle laterally and the styloglossus and hyoglossus muscles medially. D, Hypoglossal nerve; E, lingual vein; F, lingual artery; G, external carotid artery; H, tympanic bulla; I, submandibular salivary gland; J, the point to open the bulla. (From Denny HR: The results of surgical treatment of otitis media and interna in the dog. J Small Anim Pract 14:585, 1973.)

markedly in the first week. Significant improvement is not expected in animals with otitis interna in less than 3 weeks.[79, 81]

An alternative procedure is to establish drainage of the middle ear into the pharynx. An intramedullary pin is inserted through the external ear canal, rupturing the tympanic membrane, and then drilled medially through the wall of the bulla into the pharynx.[36, 51, 62] A lateral approach to the bulla, made immediately below the external ear canal, can also be used to enter the bulla.[5] A drain tube is placed and sutured in the pharynx and externally. Flushing is accomplished as previously described. The authors have not used this method in recent years, preferring the ventral approach.

REFERENCES

1. Adler PL and Boothe HW: Ventral bulla osteotomy in the cat. J Am Anim Hosp Assoc 15:757, 1979.
2. Albin MS, D'Agostino AN, White RJ, and Grindlay JH: Nonsuture sealing of a dural substitute utilizing a plastic adhesive, methyl-2-cyanoacrylate. J Neurosurg 19:545, 1962.
3. Allen DB, Cummings JF, and deLahunta A: Effects of lobotomy on aggressive behavior. Cornell Vet 64:201, 1974.
4. Asenjo A: Neurosurgical Techniques. Springfield, IL, Charles C Thomas, 1963.
5. Barrett RE and Rathfon BL: Lateral approach to a bulla osteotomy. J Am Anim Hosp Assoc 11:203, 1975.
6. Berge E and Westhues M: Veterinary Operative Surgery. Copenhagen, Medical Book Co, 1977.
7. Bojrab MJ and Robertson JJ: Surgical treatment for middle and inner ear infections. In Bojrab MJ: Current Techniques in Small Animal Surgery, 2nd ed. Philadelphia, Lea & Febiger, 1983.
8. Braun RK, Gideon LA, Riebold TW, and Peters RR: Surgical approach for pinealectomy in the calf. Am J Vet Res 12:1973, 1977.
9. Brown MH: Use of polythene film as a dural substitute. Surg Gynecol Obstet 86:663, 1948.

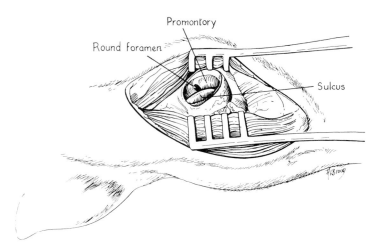

Figure 18–29. Landmarks for a vestibular osteotomy. The medial wall of the promontory is chipped away to open the vestibule of the inner ear. (From Spruell JSA: Tympanotomy, bulla osteotomy, and vestibular osteotomy. In Bojrab MJ (ed): Current Techniques in Small Animal Surgery I. Philadelphia, Lea & Febiger, 1975.)

10. Cherzai B and Collins WF: A comparison of effects of bipolar and monopolar electrocoagulation in brain. J Neurosurg 54:197, 1981.

11. Clemmons RM: Ventriculoperitoneal shunt for hydrocephalus. *In* Bojrab MJ: Current Techniques in Small Animal Surgery, 2nd ed. Philadelphia, Lea & Febiger, 1983.

12. Denny HR: The results of surgical treatment of otitis media and interna in the dog. J Small Anim Pract 14:585, 1973.

13. DeWet PD, Ali II, and Peters DN: Surgical approach to the rostral cranial fossa by radical transfrontal craniotomy in the dog. J South Afr Vet Assoc 53:40, 1982.

14. Dodge HW Jr, Grindlay JH, Craid W McK, and Ross PJ: Use of polyvinyl sponge in neurosurgery. J Neurosurg 11:258, 1954.

15. Evans HE and Christensen GC: Miller's Anatomy of the Dog, 2nd ed. Philadelphia, WB Saunders Co, 1979.

16. Fenner WE: Head trauma and nervous system injury. *In* Kirk RW: Current Veterinary Therapy VIII. Philadelphia, WB Saunders Co, 1983.

17. Few AB: The diagnosis and surgical treatment of canine hydrocephalus. JAVMA 149:286, 1966.

18. Few AB: Ventriculoatrial shunt for internal hydrocephalus. *In* Bojrab MJ: Current Techniques in Small Animal Surgery I. Philadelphia, Lea & Febiger, 1975.

19. Fraser G, Gregar WW, Mackenzie CP, et al: Canine ear disease. J Small Anim Pract 10:725, 1970.

20. Gage ED: Surgical treatment of canine hydrocephalus. JAVMA 157:1729, 1970.

21. Gage ED and Hoerlein BF: Surgical treatment of canine hydrocephalus by ventriculoatrial shunting. JAVMA 153:1418, 1968.

22. Galbraith JG: Hypothermia in the management of brain injuries. J Med Assoc 30:197, 1960.

23. Gallagher JP and Geschickter CF: The use of charged gold leaf in surgery. JAMA 189:928, 1964.

24. Glaser MA and Thienes CH: Dural defects: How important is their surgical repair? An experimental and clinical study on heteroplastic autoplastic dural grafts. Calif West Med 48:163, 1938.

25. Gleeson LN and Larkin HA: Fracture of the occipital bone with cerebellar compression in a dog. JAVMA 161:111, 1972.

26. Goluboff B, Shenkin HA, and Haft H: The effects of mannitol and urea on cerebral hemodynamics and cerebrospinal fluid pressure. Neurology 14:891, 1964.

27. Gunn CG, Williams GR, and Parker IT: Edema of the brain following circulatory arrest. J Surg Res 2:141, 1962.

28. Gurdjian ES: Operative Neurosurgery, 2nd ed. Baltimore, Williams & Wilkins Co, 1964.

29. Harrison EO: The use of the Ommaya reservoir in hydrocephalic dogs. Proc Am Vet Neurol Assoc, San Antonio, 1983.

30. Hayes GJ and Slocum HC: The achievement of optimal brain relaxation by hyperventilation technic of anesthesia. J Neurosurg 19:65, 1962.

31. Henry RW, Hulse DA, Archbald LF, and Barta M: Transoral hypophysectomy with mandibular symphysiotomy in the dog. Am J Vet Res 43:1825, 1982.

32. Himwich WA, Costa E, Canham RG, and Goldstein SL: Isolation and injection of selected arterial areas in the brain. J Appl Physiol 15:303, 1960.

33. Hoerlein BF: Nasal sinus surgery. *In* Kirk RW (ed): Current Veterinary Therapy III. Philadelphia, WB Saunders Co, 1968.

34. Hoerlein BF: Canine Neurology, 3rd ed. Philadelphia, WB Saunders Co, 1978.

35. Hoerlein BF, Few AB, and Petty MF: Brain surgery in the dog—preliminary studies. JAVMA 143:21, 1963.

36. Howard PE, Neer TM, and Miller JS: Otitis media. Part II. Surgical considerations. Comp Cont Ed Pract Vet 5:18, 1983.

37. Huertas J: The use of Orlon for dural replacement. J Neurosurg 12:550, 1955.

38. Ignelzi RJ and Kirsch WM: Follow-up analysis of ventriculoperitoneal and ventriculoatrial shunts for hydrocephalus. J Neurosurg 42:679, 1975.

39. Keener EB: An experimental study of reactions of the dura mater to wounding and loss of substance. J Neurosurg 16:424, 1959.

40. Keener EB: Regeneration of dural defects, a review. J Neurosurg 16:415, 1959.

41. Keucher TR and Mealey J: Long-term results after ventriculoatrial and ventriculoperitoneal shunting for infantile hydrocephalus. J Neurosurg 50:179, 1979.

42. Kline DB and Hayes GJ: Experimental evaluation of the effect of a plastic adhesive, methyl-2-cyanoacrylate, on neural tissue. J Neurosurg 20:647, 1963.

43. Knecht CD: Ventriculoperitoneal shunt for hydrocephalus. *In* Bojrab MJ (ed): Current Techniques in Small Animal Surgery I. Philadelphia, Lea & Febiger, 1975.

44. Kraeling RR: A modified supraorbital approach to hypophysectomy in the pig. Am J Vet Res. 34:283, 1973.

45. Kurze T, Apuzo ML, Wess M, and Keiden JS: Collagen sponge for surface brain protection. J Neurosurg 43:637, 1975.

46. Lawson DC, Burk RL, and Prata RG: Cerebral meningioma in the cat: Diagnosis and surgical treatment of ten cases. J Am Anim Hosp Assoc 20:333, 1974.

47. Lubberink AAME: Therapy for spontaneous hyperadrenocorticism. *In* Kirk RW: Current Veterinary Therapy VII. Philadelphia, WB Saunders Co, 1980.

48. Markowitz J, Archibald J, and Downie HG: Central nervous system. *In* Experimental Surgery, 5th ed. Baltimore, Williams & Wilkins Co, 1960.

49. Mason MS and Reaf J: Homologous dura mater grafts. Ann Surg 153:423, 1961.

50. Mayfield FH, and Kurokawa K: Watertight closure of spinal dura mater. J Neurosurg 43:639, 1975.

51. McBride NC: Persistent otorrhea in the dog. 90th Annu Meet Am Vet Med Assoc, 1953.

52. McLean AJ: Transbuccal approach to encephalon in experimental operations upon carnivoral pituitary, pons and ventral medulla. Ann Surg 88:985, 1928.

53. McNutt GW and McCoy JE: Bulla-osteotomy in the dog. JAVMA 77:617, 1930.

54. Meirowsky AM: Wounds of dural sinuses. J Neurosurg 5:496, 1953.

55. Murray KJ: Improved surgical resection of human brain tumors: Part I. A preliminary study. Surg Neurol 17:316, 1982.

56. Oliver JE Jr: Surgical decompression in a cranial fracture. Auburn Vet 20:78, 1964.

57. Oliver JE Jr: Surgical relief of epileptiform seizures in a dog. Vet Med Small Anim Clin 60:367, 1965.

58. Oliver JE Jr: Canine, Cranial Surgery. Thesis, Auburn University, Auburn, AL, 1966.

59. Oliver JE Jr: Principles of canine brain surgery. Anim Hosp 2:73, 1966.

60. Oliver JE Jr: Surgical approaches to the canine brain. Am J Vet Res 29:353, 1968.

61. Oliver JE Jr: Management of the patient with acute head injury. The newer knowledge about dogs. Gaines Dog Research Center, October, 1969.

62. Ott RL: Ears. *In* Archibald J (ed): Canine Surgery, 2nd ed. Santa Barbara, CA, American Veterinary Publications, 1974.

63. Parker AJ and Cunningham JG: Successful surgical removal of an epileptogenic focus in a dog. J Small Anim Pract 12:513, 1971.
64. Parker AJ and Cunningham JG: Transfrontal craniotomy in the dog. Vet Rec 90:622, 1972.
65. Parker AJ, Schiller AG, and Cusick PK: Bulla curettage for chronic otitis media and interna in dogs. JAVMA 168:193, 1976.
66. Penfield WG: Meningocerebral adhesions. Surg Gynecol Obstet 39:803, 1924.
67. Pudenz RH: The surgical treatment of hydrocephalus—a historical review. Surg Neurol 15:15, 1981.
68. Pudenz RH, Russell FE, Hurd A, and Shelden CH: Ventriculo-auriculostomy. A technique for shunting cerebrospinal fluid into the right auricle; preliminary report. J Neurosurg 14:771, 1947.
69. Rasmussen, TB: Experimental Ligation of the Cerebral Arteries of the Dog. Thesis, University of Minnesota, St Paul, MN, 1938.
70. Redding RW: Prefrontal lobotomy of the dog. Scientific Presentations, Am Anim Hosp Assoc 374, 1972.
71. Redding RW: Prefrontal lobotomy. In Bojrab MJ (ed): Current Techniques in Small Animal Surgery I. Philadelphia, Lea & Febiger, 1975.
72. Reed SM: Head trauma. In Robinson NE: Current Therapy in Equine Medicine. Philadelphia, WB Saunders Co, 1983.
73. Roche JF and Dzuik CJ: A technique for pinealectomy of the ewe. Am J Vet Res 30:2031, 1969.
74. Sayad WY and Harvey SC: The regeneration of the meninges. The dura mater. Ann Surg 77:129, 1923.
75. Sekhar LN, Moossy J, and Guthkelch AN: Malfunctioning ventriculoperitoneal shunts. J Neurosurg 56:411, 1982.
76. Shahbabian S, Keller JT, Gould HJ, et al: A new technique for making cortical incisions with minimal damage to cerebral tissue. Surg Neurol 20:310, 1983.
77. Sharma HN, Nigam JM, and Ramkumar: Successful surgical treatment of the brain abscess in a cow. Indian Vet J 52:398, 1975.
78. Skerritt GC and Stalbaumer MF: Diagnosis and treatment of coenuriasis (gid) in sheep. Vet Rec 115:399, 1984.
79. Spreull JSA: Treatment of otitis media in the dog. J Small Anim Pract 5:107, 1964.
80. Spreull JSA: Otitis media. Anim Hosp 2:80, 1966.
81. Spreull JSA: Otitis media of the dog. In Kirk RW (ed): Current Veterinary Therapy III. Philadelphia, WB Saunders Co, 1968, p 482.
82. Spreull JSA: Tympanotomy, bulla osteotomy, and vestibular osteotomy. In Bojrab MJ (ed): Current Techniques in Small Animal Surgery I. Philadelphia, Lea & Febiger, 1975.
83. Stashak TS and Mayhew IG: Neurosurgical procedures. In Jennings PB (ed): The Practice of Large Animal Surgery. Philadelphia, WB Saunders Co, 1984.
84. Swaim SF: Use of pneumatic surgical instruments in neurosurgery, part 2: Cranial and paracranial surgery. Vet Med Small Anim Clin 68:1404, 1973.
85. Swaim SF, Vandevelde M, and Faircloth, JC: Evaluation of brain biopsy techniques in the dog. J Am Anim Hosp Assoc 15:627, 1979.
86. Teng P and Feigin I: Vinyon "N" as a dural substitute. J Neurosurg 12:591, 1955.
87. Tomlinson MJ and Schenck NL: Autogenous fat implantation as a treatment for chronic frontal sinusitis in a cat. JAVMA 167:927, 1975.
88. Turner AS: Surgical management of depression fractures of the equine skull. Vet Surg 8:29, 1979.
89. Vallfors B and Erlandson BE: Damage to nervous tissue from monopolar and bipolar electrocoagulation. J Surg Res 29:371, 1980.
90. Verdura J, White RJ, and Albin M: New technique for aseptic hypophysectomy in the dog. J Surg Res 3:174, 1963.
91. White ME: Central nervous system trauma. In Howard JL: Current Veterinary Therapy: Food Animal Practice. Philadelphia, WB Saunders Co, 1981.
92. White RJ and Donald DE: Basilar artery ligation and cerebral ischemia in dogs. Arch Surg 84:108, 1962.

Chapter 19

SF Swaim, DVM, MS

Peripheral Nerve Surgery

INDICATIONS

Trauma is a common cause of peripheral nerve damage. Most injuries due to violent external pressure, traction, laceration, or gunshots can cause severe damage or severance of the nerve. Neglected fractures can injure a nerve owing to the internal movement of fragments and jagged ends of bone. In some instances, medical personnel may induce injury by injecting a chemical or therapeutic agent in or around a nerve. Other sources of peripheral nerve damage or defect include prolonged x-ray administration, peripheral nerve tumors, and passage of large electric currents through nerve tissue.[38, 42, 70] Based on history, physical examination, neurologic examination, and electrodiagnostic testing, the surgeon must determine the location and extent of the injury to recommend the best mode of repair.

ANATOMY

To fully understand the principles of peripheral nerve surgery, it is necessary to know the anatomy of peripheral nerves. Likewise, knowledge of anatomy is necessary to appreciate the nerve degeneration and regeneration processes that occur.

The neuron is the primary unit of a peripheral nerve. It is composed of dendrites (dendritic zone), a nerve cell body, an axon, and a terminal sensory end organ or motor end plate. The relative proportions of these structures are expressed in the following analogy: if the cell body were the height of a man, the axon would be 1 to 2 inches in diameter and extend for more than 2 miles.[16, 17, 69]

The axon is the basic component of a peripheral nerve. In mixed nerves, sensory neuron dendrites are structurally like axons and are referred to as axons. Axons may or may not have a coating of myelin, which is composed of lamellar wrapping of the Schwann cell plasma membrane. The myelin circumferentially covers the axon in laminated layers, similar to an onion peel.[61] The Schwann cells form the Schwann sheath, also known as the Schwann membrane, Schwann tube, Schwann tubule, or neurilemma. Nodes of Ranvier, junctional areas between Schwann cells, are found at discrete intervals along the entire length of the myelinated nerve. Outside the axon and its covering is the connective tissue known as the endoneurium, composed of collagen fibrils, fibroblasts, and vascular tissue. From the endoneurium come intrafunicular septa that divide nerve fibers and carry a blood supply. Large bundles of axons and their associated structures are surrounded by the multilayered perineurium, composed of collagen and elastic fibers. This gives the nerve bundles most of their tensile strength and elasticity, in addition to serving as a diffusion barrier to keep out various substances. The connective tissue around the entire nerve is called the epineurium. It is composed of areolar connective tissue and collagen fibrils[22, 24, 45, 49, 59, 61, 69] (Fig. 19–1).

The blood supply to a nerve enters via a mesoneurium similar to the intestinal mesentery. Within the nerve the blood supply has well-developed collaterals between layers and different segments of the nerve, and thus a

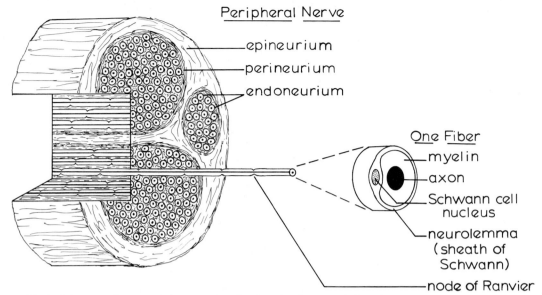

Figure 19–1. Schematic drawing of the structure of a peripheral nerve. (Adapted from Ham AW: Histology, 5th ed. Philadelphia, JB Lippincott Co, 1965.)

considerable margin of safety exists if the vascular supply is compromised.[22, 24, 59, 61] It has also been stated that the blood supply to a nerve comes from adjacent tissues and vessels and not via a mesoneurium.[37, 73] An entire peripheral nerve has the consistency of a piece of cooked spaghetti.[24, 59, 61]

PATHOPHYSIOLOGY

Classification of Nerve Damage

The most common classification of peripheral nerve damage utilizes the terms neurotmesis, axonotmesis, and neurapraxia.[1, 7, 9, 42, 45, 49, 52, 69, 73, 75] Neurotmesis is complete severance of all nerve structures with wallerian degeneration of the distal stump. This includes severance of all essential structures despite the apparent maintenance of anatomic continuity. Axonotmesis is damage to the nerve fibers of such severity that wallerian degeneration of the distal stump follows. However, the internal architecture of the nerve, including the endoneurium and Schwann sheath, is fairly well preserved. Recovery is spontaneous and of good quality. Neurapraxia is an interruption in the function and conduction of a nerve. There is paralysis without structural change. Additionally, in closed injury to peripheral nerves functional loss (neurapraxia) or axonal loss (axonotmesis) is

difficult to distinguish clinically from nerve severance (neurotmesis), which has a poorer prognosis. Electrodiagnostic testing can be useful in determining the type of damage (see Chapter 5).

Lesions in Continuity

Lesions in continuity are lesions of peripheral nerves in which the nerve is damaged but not severed.[75] The important factor about such lesions is the ability of the nerve to regenerate. The regenerative ability is directly proportional to the amount and continuity of the nerve's connective tissue structures. With neurapraxic and axonotmesic lesions in which the endoneurial connective tissue and Schwann sheaths remain intact, axonal regeneration is comparatively better than with a neurotmesic lesion in which some axons never regenerate successfully because of blockage of their growth by scar tissue at the site of severance and resultant neuroma formation.[69] It has been shown in crushing nerve injuries in cats that regenerating axons use intact endoneurial tubules as they regenerate.[27]

Causes of lesions in continuity include intraneural injections, intraneural hemorrhage, gunshot wounds, contusions, fractures near nerves, crushing, and compression by casts and splints.[7, 34] A major source of peripheral nerve injury, which can result in severe damage, is nerve traction. Traction can produce damage that extends for some distance along the nerve in the form of root avulsion from the cord, axonal division, rupture of neural connective tissues, rupture of blood vessels with intraneural hemorrhage, and intraneural scarring.[24, 42, 69, 75] Studies on cats have shown that their peroneal nerves may be stretched 100% of their length, yet functional recovery was complete 14 days later.[8] Rabbit nerves have been found to tolerate lengthening of 69% above control measurements before epineurial rupture occurred.[25, 28]

Lesions in continuity may be noted at the time of surgery to correct other problems (eg, fractures) or they may be seen accompanying open wounds. Such lesions may be suspected when an animal demonstrates peripheral neurologic deficits following trauma, such as crushing, contusing, or stretching injuries, or suspected intraneural injections. Electrodiagnostic examination may aid in evaluating recovery or lack of recovery of nerve function. However, the question arises as to when exploratory surgery should be undertaken. The recommended practice is to delay exploration for 8 to 10 weeks. By this time, neurapraxic lesions will have reversed; in addition, the surgeon will be able to accurately evaluate the injury at the time of surgery.[32] Neuroma inspection and direct electrodiagnostic testing could be done at the time of exploratory surgery.

Nerve Degeneration

Following nerve severance or damage, nerve degeneration and regeneration occur simultaneously; however, for ease of presentation these will be considered separately. The most accepted theory of degeneration is that proposed by Waller. He suggested that the portion of the nerve that has been severed and completely separated from the central trophic area degenerates. Regeneration begins from the undegenerated proximal stump, which remains connected to the trophic center. Many factors influence the potential for recovery following transection. These include the site of the lesion, the age of the individual, the length of the nerve destroyed, the width of the severance gap, the alignment of the cut ends, and the amount of damage and hemorrhage in adjacent tissues.[1]

Immediately after severance there is hemorrhage and projection of a clot from the severed nerve ends. Within 1 hour there is marked swelling about 0.5 to 1 cm on either side of the point of severance owing to the accumulation of acid mucopolysaccharides, which have an affinity for water. The accumulation of blood serum and plasma in the area also contributes to the swelling. This swelling persists for about 1 week, then slowly subsides.[15–17, 22, 24]

Degeneration occurs in the proximal nerve stump, but it is not as extensive as that in the distal nerve stump. It has been called traumatic degeneration, and it extends no farther than the second or third node of Ranvier from the point of severance.[4, 9, 10, 22, 24, 35] However, it has also been stated that axons many inches above an interrupted nerve trunk show a break in continuity.[28] With extensive trauma (eg, from a high-speed missile), axon, myelin, and sheath connective tissue damage may extend several centimeters proximal and distal from the point of severance.[22, 24] There may also be some loss of motor neurons following nerve transection, with survival of neurons being proportional to the distance from the cell body at which axonal severance occurs.[28]

Wallerian degeneration occurs in the entire distal nerve stump, with the axons and their myelin coatings undergoing degeneration. However, the axons at the proximal end of the distal stump tend to enlarge and isolate themselves from the rest of the distal stump as a unit that survives for approximately 2 weeks.[4, 15–17, 22, 24] The remaining portions of the distal axons break down more rapidly, and at 48 hours after severance axon and myelin degeneration is evident all along the distal stump. Myelin loses its layered appearance and becomes homogeneous, breaking into ovoids and ellipsoids surrounding axonal fragments.[1, 4, 30] Neurofibrils in the axoplasm degenerate and disappear, as the axoplasm increases in optical density and forms clumps.[30]

The degeneration products of axons and myelin are removed, leaving only the connective tissue framework of the distal nerve stump. Macrophages appear from intra- and extraneural sources to begin this process. In addition to these, Schwann cells play a role in phagocytizing axonal and myelin breakdown products.[10, 16, 17, 21, 28, 30] One study has shown that there may be two different types of Schwann cells: those associated with cleaning up axon and myelin debris, and those involved with protecting and remyelinating regenerating axons.[12] The macrophages appear about 7 days after injury and reach the peak of their invasiveness during the third week after injury.[24] The process of debris removal takes place for as long as 21 to 56 days after injury, during which time the nerve stump becomes less swollen, phagocytic activity subsides, an orderly realignment of neurilemmal sheaths occurs, and endoneurial sheaths shrink or disappear. If regenerating axons do not penetrate the distal nerve stump, it becomes increasingly contracted and replaced by connective tissue.[1, 16, 17, 24]

The neuromuscular junctions also are involved in the degenerative process. However, studies in dogs have shown that their neuromuscular junctions remain functional for approximately 5 days following nerve severance[56] (Fig. 19–2A).

Nerve Regeneration

Regeneration of a peripheral nerve is based on the peripheral growth of new axons from the central nondegenerated portion of the nerve. The process requires the nerve cell body to expend considerable energy. The process begins within the cell body of the severed axon and is the same for both sensory and motor nerves. The cell body undergoes chromatolysis and becomes progressively larger for approximately 10 to 20 days. It remains enlarged during active regeneration and returns to normal size

as the nerve matures. During this time, there is an increase in both RNA and DNA activity within the cell. The increased enzymatic activity and incorporation of amino acids within the cell body reflect the increased metabolic activity. A cell may replace 50 to 100 times the protein and organic material contained in the normal central cell body. The nearer the severance is to the cell body, the more pronounced are these changes.[9, 10, 15–17, 24, 28, 42] In addition, the glial cells that surround the neuron also undergo alterations that aid in supporting the increased metabolic activity in the cell body.[1, 16, 17] The enlargement of the nerve cell body may peak early in the regeneration process and again as myoneural junctions are formed.[16, 17] Injury too close to the cell body may result in its death or, if it survives, the amount of axon that must be regenerated may exceed the metabolic capacity of the cell and axonal regeneration will not occur.[10, 24] Of interest is the discovery that rat peripheral nervous tissue releases two or more soluble substances ("nerve growth factor") that stimulate neuritic growth.[47]

After new protoplasm is synthesized by the cell body, it migrates by axoplasmic flow from the cell body down the axon.[16, 17, 74] Flow of the newly synthesized axoplasm has a slow and a fast component. The slow component (1 mm/day) occurs by microperistalsis within the

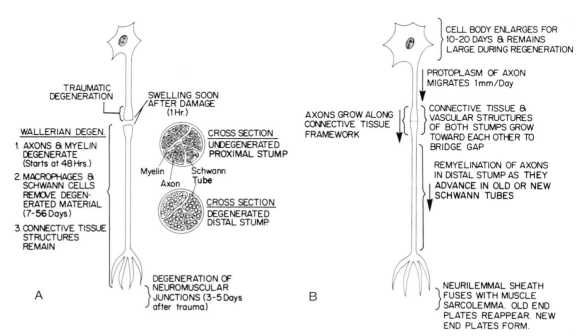

Figure 19–2. A, General schematic summary of nerve degeneration process. B, General schematic summary of nerve regeneration process.

nerve trunk membrane, and the fast component (100 times faster) involves the microtubules.[16, 17] The axon flow has been compared to molten lava or toothpaste.[74] The slowly transported proteins are partially consumed during this passage down the axon and are used to replace catabolized enzymes in the membrane. However, a significant fraction reaches the terminal segments of the axon. At the synaptic regions there are increased nutrient requirements and increased metabolic activity. To supply these needs, the microtubules play a significant role by providing the fast transport of axoplasm.[16, 17]

Following severance of a nerve, the changes that occur at and between the proximal and distal nerve stumps strongly influence nerve regeneration. The regeneration of axons between nerve stumps is dependent on proliferation of epineurial and endoneurial connective tissue, Schwann cells, and capillaries. Within 1 to 3 days following injury, fibroblasts of epineurial origin, the endoneurial connective tissue within the nerve, and capillaries begin proliferation at the proximal and distal nerve stumps. (A greater degree of connective tissue proliferation occurs from the proximal nerve stump.) These tissues migrate toward each other, forming a bridge and capillary bed between the nerve stumps, along which regenerating axons may grow to reach the distal nerve stump. Axons sprout from the proximal nerve stump from 4 to 20 days after injury, in conjunction with the increased metabolic activity of the nerve cell body. In instances of diffuse traumatic severance, axonal budding begins 1 to 3 cm proximal to the point of severance; however, with sharply localized injury, this budding begins a few millimeters retrograde to the last node of Ranvier. The bridge along which regenerating axons will grow is subject to distortion owing to the random growth of intraneural connective tissue elements and to the extraneural connective tissue[1, 10, 17, 24] (See Neuroma Formation below). Connective tissue proliferation at the injury site is marked during the first 3 weeks after severance. Immediate nerve anastomosis may result in the inability of axon sprouts to penetrate this dense connective tissue. However, if nerve repair is delayed for 3 weeks, the new axon sprouts are active and ready to cross the anastomotic site almost immediately.[16, 17] This would apply primarily to nerve severance associated with severe soft tissue trauma rather than to sharp nerve severance.

Schwann cells of the two nerve stumps probably play the most important role in axonal regeneration between stumps. Electron microscopy has revealed a proliferation of Schwann cells that greatly outnumber the connective tissue cells of endoneurial and perineurial origin.[13] As Schwann cells proliferate, they tend to line up longitudinally to form bands of Büngner, which are continuous with the persisting Schwann tubes in each nerve stump.[1] The Schwann cells of each stump grow toward each other and join. According to some, the Schwann cells of the proximal stump slightly precede those of the distal stump. As a result, advancing Schwann cells serve as a guiding mechanism for regenerating axons to follow.[1, 16, 17, 24] There is a theory that Schwann cells totally disintegrate during wallerian degeneration, leaving endoneurial pathways that are maintained by a nondegenerating basement membrane. Monocytes and vascular pericytes migrate into the endoneurial basement membrane sheath, dedifferentiate to form Schwann cells, produce bands of Büngner, and prepare for new axon sprouts.[73]

As axons regenerate, they form numerous sprouts or branches.[10, 30, 73] These have a natural affinity for Schwann cells called homotropism.[30] A regenerating axon sprout can follow a Schwann cell band into an endoneurial tube in the distal stump, where the Schwann cells envelope the axon by multiple concentric enfoldings, and the axon is remyelinated. Schwann cells also envelope and remyelinate the regenerating axons at the injury site.[10] As axon branches enter preexisting tubules in the distal stump they push the Schwann cell of the tubule to one side as many small branches enter the tubule.[30] Although many axon branches may enter a tubule and grow peripherally, only one branch will be myelinated and mature once contact is made with a peripheral end plate.[10, 72] Axon sprouts can penetrate endoneurial tubes in the distal stump and be remyelinated before these tubes have been cleared of degenerated axon and myelin material.[12, 73] Electron microscopic studies of nerve regeneration have demonstrated that Schwann cells form new endoneurial tubes during nerve regeneration and that regenerating axons may utilize either these or old, but different, endoneurial tubes in the distal stump.[12, 43] One study in monkeys showed that some old endoneurial tubes persist in the distal stump at degeneration, and they are less often used as conduits or scaffolds for the regenerating axons than had previously been stated in the literature. If they do act as conduits for regenerating axons, it is rare. Most regenerating fibers, myelinated and unmyelinated, pass down newly formed tubes.[12]

Axonal regeneration at the marginal zone of realignment progresses at the rate of 0.25 mm/day. Beyond this point regeneration occurs at the rate of 1 to 4 mm/day[14] or approximately 2.5 cm/month. Although axon tips may regenerate 3 to 4 mm/day, the rate of functional return is approximately 1 to 2 mm/day.[68] Studies on monkeys have shown axon tips to be across the neurorrhaphy site at 1 week following primary repair and clearly evident 40 mm distal to the repair site by 3 weeks.[12] Actually, the rate of axonal growth peripherally appears to change during the course of regeneration in a single nerve, with lag periods at the beginning and end of regeneration.[44] Growth is more rapid in the proximal areas and slower in the more distal areas. The state of the motor end plate and the health of the muscle fibers control success of peripheral nerve regeneration (Fig. 19–2B). Therefore, physical therapy and care of muscles and skin are important after peripheral nerve repair. These structures must be properly handled or the muscles will lose their neurotrophic and regenerative capacities. In the dog, if it is assumed that regeneration takes place at the rate of 2.5 cm/month, it follows that most nerves could regenerate quickly enough, because few of them would exceed 50 cm in length. However, some dogs' unwillingness to cooperate following surgery and difficulties in preventing crippling muscle atrophy, tendon contracture, and self mutilation during the period of regeneration must be considered. These problems and the longer lengths of peripheral nerves in large animals prompt a more cautious prognosis following neurorrhaphy in these species.

Neuroma Formation

One of the major deterrent factors in nerve regeneration is the formation of a neuroma at the end of the proximal stump and a smaller glioma or schwannoma at the end of the distal stump. They may also occur as neuromas in continuity when axonal damage occurs without nerve severance. Neuromas occur most often when there is a gap between nerve ends that have not been approximated surgically. They start to form soon after a nerve has been severed. A blood clot forms at the end of the proximal nerve stump and organizes into a mass of randomly oriented fibrin strands. The Schwann cells proliferating at the end of the nerve stump encounter the tangled scaffolding of fibrin and follow it. The regenerating axons follow the Schwann cells in the preestablished random pattern. The distortion and blockage of axonal regeneration are further complicated by invasion of extraneural connective tissue into the area between the nerve stumps. A third factor contributing to axonal blockage and disarray is the proliferation of connective tissue elements (endoneurium, perineurium, and epineurium) within the nerve. As regenerating axons migrate distally, they undergo considerable branching. The more extensive the neuroma, the more pronounced is the branching. This branching may be compensatory and a means of producing enough axons so that some will be able to find their way through the neuroma and penetrate the distal nerve stump. The tangled mass of axons soon becomes enveloped by Schwann cells and becomes myelinated[16, 17, 42, 69] (Fig. 19–3).

The schwannoma or peripheral glioma is formed in the same way as a neuroma. However, no axons are in the schwannoma.[16, 17, 42, 69]

In amputations or neurectomies, neuromas on severed nerves have been a source of severe pain. Evans et al[18] reported that neuromas occurred in 25% of the horses in which neurectomies were performed. Painful neuromas do not seem to be as problematic in dogs and cats as in horses, perhaps because the neuromas are small and do not cause distressing pain.

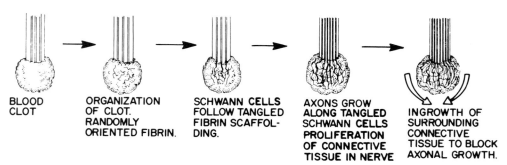

| BLOOD CLOT | ORGANIZATION OF CLOT. RANDOMLY ORIENTED FIBRIN. | SCHWANN CELLS FOLLOW TANGLED FIBRIN SCAFFOLDING. | AXONS GROW ALONG TANGLED SCHWANN CELLS PROLIFERATION OF CONNECTIVE TISSUE IN NERVE | INGROWTH OF SURROUNDING CONNECTIVE TISSUE TO BLOCK AXONAL GROWTH. |

Figure 19–3. Pathogenesis of a neuroma.

Avoidance of painful neuroma formation following neurectomy is a concern of large animal surgeons, and many preventive techniques have been advocated. Silicone rubber caps* have been described for capping cut nerves in horses with a 97% success rate in 178 neurectomies in 52 horses.[18] Cauterization followed by ligation and folding the nerve end back on itself have been described for preventing neuroma formation following posterior digital neurectomy in horses.[19] Another technique for preventing neuroma formation is use of epineurium as a cap for the nerve[71] (see Palmar Digital Neurectomy below).

In summary, a period of dynamic degeneration and phagocytosis occurs in peripheral nerves following certain types of trauma. These two processes occur in the entire distal nerve stump, and in the proximal nerve stump up to the most distal nodes of Ranvier or further in some types of trauma. Nerve regeneration follows these processes and is influenced by several factors: The younger the individual, the better regeneration will be. Nerve regeneration is poorer in patients whose nerve damage has been related to massive trauma and its resultant scar tissue. Because of the dog's position on the phylogenetic scale, nerve regeneration in this animal is generally better than in humans. Neuroma formation is the major problem in nerve regeneration when the trauma results in severance.[69]

SURGICAL TECHNIQUE

Primary Versus Secondary Repair

When peripheral nerve repair is performed depends on the type of injury. In primary (immediate or emergency) repair the severed ends are sutured together within hours of the time of injury. It is generally indicated if nerve severance is partial, if there has been little soft tissue trauma, if there is no contamination, if there are no skin defects, and if there is no problem identifying the nerve ends.[24, 32, 40, 42, 44] Such repair has the advantages that the stumps are easily located and not retracted or encased in connective tissue, and the nerve is repaired at the time of original wound management.[42, 44] With primary repair, it has been found that axons are able to regenerate quickly. Remyelination begins early and occurs within 3 weeks

far distal to the site of injury,[12] thus favoring primary repair. If the primary repair is partially or totally unsuccessful, time may be lost and a second surgery may be necessary.[40, 44]

Secondary nerve repair should be considered when there has been soft tissue and bone trauma and/or contamination or infection associated with nerve severance.[32, 42, 44, 49, 59] At the time of initial examination the severed nerve ends should be tacked together with a suture; a monofilament, brightly colored suture can be placed through the epineurium of each stump and tied to loosely approximate them. This aids in finding the nerve at a later date and helps prevent retraction.[49] After 2 to 3 weeks the wound can be reexplored and the nerve observed for fibrotic changes on either side of the severance site. The nerve is then trimmed of this fibrotic tissue and sutured or a graft is placed in the nerve gap. This type of repair has the advantages that the epineurium is thicker and better able to hold sutures, associated injuries and infections have had time to heal, the surgery is elective, inflammatory reaction associated with degeneration in the distal stump has cleared, and the axonal regeneration activity is optimal at this time. The main disadvantage of secondary repair is that there has been time for connective tissue proliferation to shorten and constrict the nerve, and the end organs may have undergone irreversible atrophy and fibrosis.[15, 24, 29, 40, 42, 44, 49, 51, 59]

Instruments

Instruments needed for peripheral nerve surgery are not elaborate. Optical loupes that provide two- to sixfold magnification are helpful.[49] Instruments should include small ophthalmic needle holders; jeweler's forceps; 1 vs 2 toothed Adson forceps; small, curved, blunt pointed scissors; sharp scalpel blades or razor blades; wooden tongue depressors; lint free surgical sponges*; and 5–0 to 7–0 suture material with a swaged needle. Although numerous suture materials have been advocated for neurorrhaphy, a monofilament, low friction suture such as polypropylene or nylon is preferred.[46]

The instruments are thoroughly cleaned and placed in a sterilization tray that has no linen in it. A piece of foam rubber is placed on the bottom of the tray for instrument padding. With

---

*Nerve caps, Dow Corning International Co, Medical Products Division, Midland, MI.

*Weck-cel, Edward Weck & Co, Inc, Long Island City, NY.

no linen in the tray, the potential problem of transferring lint from the cloth to the anastomotic site is circumvented. Such lint interposed between the nerve ends could cause enough tissue reaction to block axonal regeneration.[72, 73]

Preparation, Positioning, and Approach to Nerves

When preparing for peripheral nerve surgery, the entire limb should be prepared for aseptic surgery because it may be necessary to expose the nerve maximally for effective neurorrhaphy. The surgeon may need to flex or position the limb during surgery to allow nerve repair without tension.[46, 49, 51, 66] Skin drapes should be applied, including a stockinette to cover the entire limb. After incising the stockinette and skin, the edges of the stockinette are affixed to the subcutis with sutures or wound clips.[46]

A nerve should be approached through fascial planes; however, if a muscle must be penetrated it should be done parallel to its fibers. If a muscle must be divided, it should be severed at a point of attachment so that it can be sutured.[49, 54] The goal is minimal tissue damage and good hemostasis because tissue debris and hemorrhage promote scarring, which can attenuate the results of the surgical procedure.[46] Tourniquets should not be used, as they may mask significant bleeding points in both the nerve and the surrounding soft tissues.[42]

Exploratory Surgery and Neuroma Evaluation

When an animal is showing signs of peripheral nerve damage and other diagnostic methods have failed to yield definitive information about the nerve's function or when these methods have indicated a certain area of nerve damage and there has been an 8 to 10 week lapse without neurologic improvement, exploratory surgery is indicated. Three reasons for performing an exploratory operation are to establish an accurate diagnosis and, in particular, to determine how much of a nerve has been divided; to establish a reasonable and accurate prognosis; and to improve nerve function.[75]

When exploratory surgery is being performed, the nerve in question must be freely isolated in all areas of possible injury and positively identified. All points of possible compression and abnormal adhesion should be relieved.

Dissection should begin along normal nerve proximal and distal to the neuroma. Longitudinal, subepineurial blood vessels should be spared, but collateral vessels in the mesoneurium can be sacrificed.[32, 42] The nerves should be examined by inspection, determining the size of the neuroma; by palpation, ascertaining the neuroma's consistency; and by electric stimulation, noting the reaction that occurs. If the nerve sheath is thickened, it may be split along the longitudinal axis of the nerve; this will expose the nerve bundles adequately to assess their condition.[2, 7, 69, 75]

The neuroma is of particular interest during exploratory nerve surgery. Usually a normal or almost normal appearing nerve indicates axonotmesis or intact fibers. A fusiform neuroma is a sign of a combination of axonotmesis and neurotmesis or axonotmesis mainly with intact fibers. It may also indicate intraneural bleeding. If a fusiform neuroma is soft, there is relatively good axonal regeneration across the lesion, and the prognosis for spontaneous recovery is better. However, a fusiform neuroma with a palpable induration may be evidence of intraneural scarring. Intraneural fibrosis with a large, firm, bulbous neuroma usually indicates widespread neurotmesis with poor regeneration of axons across the lesion.[3, 29, 32, 48, 53, 58, 59, 75] Blood vessels within a neuroma are associated with a better prognosis for nerve regeneration.[3] A lateral neuroma indicates partial division of a nerve or partial neurotmesis with the remainder of the nerve containing normal fibers or fibers that have undergone axonotmesis.[32, 48, 75] Lateral neuromas may recover spontaneously, and it is probably best not to excise them.[48, 53] However, nerves that have been cut one half to three fourths of the way through often require resection and repair. A neuroma with a dumbbell configuration suggests that the nerve has been completely transected and the ends are being held in approximation only by scar tissue[58, 59] (Fig. 19–4).

Palpation of thickened enlarged neuromas can be misleading, and direct evoking of distal action potentials by electric stimulation of proximal axons should be used in combination with palpation for complete evaluation. If no potential can be evoked 8 weeks after injury, nerve resection is indicated. Muscle contraction when a nerve is stimulated proximal to a neuroma is a favorable sign and may precede the return of clinical function by as long as a month.[24, 34, 42, 69, 73] When stimulating the nerve proximal to the neuroma, care must be taken because the stimulus may travel in a retrograde direction,

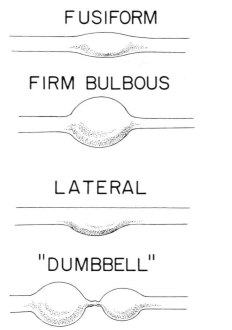

FUSIFORM

FIRM BULBOUS

LATERAL

"DUMBBELL"

Figure 19–4. Neuromas of various shapes that may be formed on traumatized peripheral nerves. (Adapted from Smith JW: Microsurgery of peripheral nerves. *In* Rand RW (ed): Microneurosurgery. St Louis, CV Mosby Co, 1969.)

causing muscles with innervation proximal to the lesion to contract. This apparent function may be misleading unless one palpates and, if possible, inspects the contracting muscles.[32] In

the case of a lateral neuroma, intact fascicles may be dissected free from the neuroma and spared if nerve action potentials can be recorded from them. If no nerve action potentials can be stimulated across the lateral neuroma, repair may be performed with autogenous grafts.[32]

A surgeon may elect to perform external or internal neurolysis of a damaged nerve in an attempt to improve its function. This is generally done when the surgeon decides the lesion in continuity will provide better regeneration if left undisturbed than if it is resected and sutured. External neurolysis is accomplished by freeing the nerve from surrounding scar tissue and laying it in a bed free of scar tissue (Fig. 19–5A). Internal neurolysis involves incising the epineurium longitudinally in the involved area and separating the nerve fascicles with either a sharp blade or scissor points[2, 7, 9, 24, 42, 48, 75] (Fig. 19–5B). The epineurium may be opened either proximal or distal to the neuroma, and dissection is carried out until fascicles are identified. Fascicles are then followed into and through the neuroma.[7]

When a traumatic fibrous neuroma is in a nerve, internal neurolysis is of questionable value, and resection and anastomosis should be considered.[2] Electrodiagnostic testing may be beneficial in deciding whether to perform neurolysis or resect and suture the nerve. If direct stimulation of the nerve just proximal to the neuroma produces some degree of distal motor

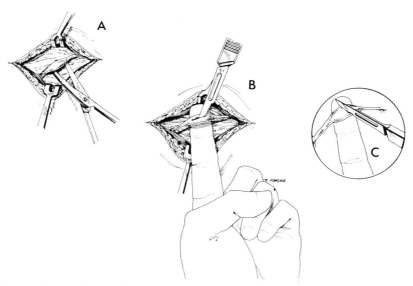

Figure 19–5. Technique for neurolysis and trial section. A, External neurolysis—freeing the nerve from the surrounding connective tissue. B, Internal neurolysis—longitudinal separation of nerve bundles in the area of the lesion. C, Trial section—gradual transverse sectioning of a nerve to ascertain the presence of viable nerve bundles.

function, neurolysis should be performed. Resection and anastomosis are indicated when there is a lack of muscle contraction. Neurolysis rather than resection is also indicated if nerve action potentials can be recorded distal to the neuroma after stimulating the nerve proximally.[29, 34, 42, 69]

Another diagnostic procedure that can be performed at the time of surgery is trial section of the damaged area of the nerve. A transverse incision is made at the point of greatest induration and deepened not more than 0.5 mm at a time until normal nerve bundles are encountered. The fibrous tissue springs apart so that the nerve bundles are seen before they are cut. In general, if the trial section is carried across more than one half to three fourths of the diameter of the nerve, complete resection with anastomosis is indicated[29, 53, 58, 69, 75] (Fig. 19–5C).

The extent of intraneural fibrosis in a neuroma may also be evaluated by *carefully* injecting saline or saline tinted with a harmless dye through a fine gauge needle into the nerve near the neuroma. Diffusion of the saline will be arrested if scar tissue is present; otherwise, the liquid will spread freely between the fascicles and beneath the sheath.[7, 53] This procedure does not constitute a form of neurolysis, but is merely an adjunct to locate the intraneural scar and to facilitate opening the nerve sheath to begin internal neurolysis.[7]

Neuroma Removal and Hemostasis

In instances of clear, sharp nerve laceration when primary repair is to be performed, minimal trimming of the nerve is necessary. However, uneven tags of nerve tissue should be eliminated so that the two nerve ends have flush contact.[49]

When the surgeon has determined through history, clinical neurologic signs, electrodiagnostic testing, and neuroma inspection, that neurorrhaphy is indicated, any neuroma on the nerve must be removed. Prior to removing the neuroma, a marking suture should be placed in the epineurium of normal nerve on each side of the neuroma. These are placed in line with each other and are used to orient the nerve for anastomosis after neuroma removal. After laying the neuroma across a wooden tongue depressor, a single bold cut is made in its center, perpendicular to the long axis of the nerve. A sharp scalpel blade or razor blade should be used. The proximal nerve stump is placed on the tongue depressor. With no tension on the

nerve, 1 to 2 mm thick serial sections are cut from the neuroma (Fig. 19–6). When viable nerve tissue (normal fascicles without excessive connective tissue between them) is exposed, the neuromatous tissue is excised and discarded. When the proper level is reached, the epineurium should retract and the fascicles should appear as multiple small bulges from the cut surface. Ideally, the epineurium will slip back and forth over the fascicular bundles ("prepuce test").[31, 42, 44, 46, 60, 66, 67]

Another technique to trim nerve ends involves wrapping the nerve in a collar of umbilical tape, Penrose drain, polyethylene, paper, or Vi-drape and snugging this collar around the nerve with a pair of right angle forceps. A razor blade or dermatome blade is used to make transverse cuts back along the nerve at 1 mm intervals until a healthy interface is seen[6, 31, 49, 59, 60] (Fig. 19–7).

The distal stump is treated in like manner. This stump is usually between 30 and 40% smaller in diameter than the proximal stump and the funicular pattern is not as easily recognized. Because evaluation of the internal con-

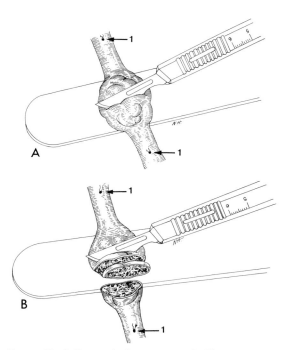

Figure 19–6. Removal of a neuroma. A, The neuroma is laid on a sterile tongue blade and cut in its center perpendicular to its long axis. B, Serial sections are sliced from the neuroma to expose viable nerve tissue. Epineurial marking sutures for nerve alignment (1). (From Swaim SF: Isolated peripheral nerves. *In* Bojrab MJ (ed): Current Techniques in Small Animal Surgery I. Philadelphia, Lea & Febiger, 1975.)

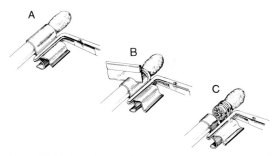

Figure 19–7. A technique for trimming nerve ends. A, A collar of sterile paper or other materials (see text) is held snugly around a nerve end with right angle forceps. B and C, A sharp blade is used to make cuts back along the nerve at 1 mm intervals until viable nerve bundles appear on cross section. (Adapted from Smith JW: Newer techniques in peripheral nerve repair. In Clinical Neurosurgery. Baltimore, Williams & Wilkins Co, 1977.)

dition of the distal stump is less accurate than assessment of the condition of the proximal stump, most surgeons prepare the proximal end first and then excise as much of the distal stump as possible without placing the anastomosis under significant tension.[44]

Any hemorrhage that occurs at the ends of the nerve stump after trimming can be controlled by tamponading a piece of muscle or gelatin foam (Gelfoam) against the nerve stump and then irrigating it free after a few minutes.[31, 42] Removal of any clots or hemorrhage from the area of nerve repair should be done with a lint free sponge material.[66, 67] These sponges can be dipped in 1:100,000 epinephrine solution to help attain hemostasis.[46]

Following neuroma removal or when primary nerve repair is undertaken, the surgeon should consider the use of end-to-end anastomosis of the nerve stumps. It is generally accepted that this form of repair provides the best nerve regeneration. If nerve tissue has been lost at the time of initial injury or if considerable neuroma has been removed from the nerve during secondary repair, a gap may exist between nerve ends. If possible, this gap should be overcome to allow for nerve anastomosis. Anastomotic sites in rats that have 25 g of tension on them have impaired blood flow at the suture site, and return of neurologic function was inferior to that in nerves that had been anastomosed with no tension and nerves that had tension relieved at the neurorrhaphy site by use of a graft.[41]

Freeing a nerve from surrounding tissues and positioning the limb are the two basic techniques for avoiding tension on a nerve anastomotic site.[49] A nerve can be rather extensively freed from surrounding tissues without damaging its blood supply. Neurophysiologic studies have shown that extensive mobilization does not affect subsequent function of normal nerves. With proper dissection, the ends of nerve stumps should be able to move 3 to 4 cm toward the proposed suture site with joint movement. In some instances the proximal segment can be moved distally by meticulously splitting muscle branches from the main nerve without disrupting their continuity.[42] Mobilization of acutely injured nerves should be minimal; however, studies in monkeys indicated that mobilization of nerves is a safe procedure because functional regeneration does not depend on the initial preservation of collateral blood supply.[33] In humans more than 14 cm of nerve has to be freed from surrounding tissue before nutrition and oxygenation are impaired sufficiently to reduce function.[44] Also, tissue surrounding nerves is not significantly restrictive and dissecting the nerve from its areolar tissue bed does not provide the additional length that theory might indicate.[44]

Mobilizing nerve stumps to overcome length deficits is best accomplished by positioning the limb.[44] However, this is not without potential danger. As a flexed limb is slowly extended a few weeks after anastomosis, traction may be placed on the nerve and anastomotic site, which could result in nerve damage.[47] Studies on rats have shown that nerves gain significant strength at the anastomotic site during the first 2 weeks, with a slower gain in strength thereafter. In monkeys anastomotic sites have been found to regain 77% of the bursting strength of a normal nerve 4 weeks after anastomosis.[26] Some of the strength gained at an anastomotic site can be attributed to the adhesions that form around the nerve. These may be sufficient to immobilize the nerve stumps so that tension will not disrupt the anastomosis. It has been stated that 3 weeks is the necessary time for collagen to form around a nerve and splint it internally.[44] Excessive tension favors fibrosis, separation of nerve ends, large neuroma formation, and ultimately poor regeneration.

Thus the surgeon must use some judgment and possibly some compromise of the two techniques to overcome a nerve gap to allow nerve anastomosis. However, a large gap may require a nerve graft.

Nerve Anastomosis

Nerve anastomosis should be used when there has been little or no loss of nerve tissue, either during original injury or when degenerated nerve tissue is trimmed at secondary repair. There are two techniques for performing peripheral nerve anastomosis: epineurial suture technique and fascicular suture technique. The epineurial technique requires the placement of sutures in the epineurium. A large percentage of nerve injuries can be repaired by this technique. It is the least difficult and most rapid method for repairing peripheral nerves.[49] It does not require expensive operating microscopes or expensive small-sized suture material. The fascicular suture technique entails suturing individual nerve fascicles by placing sutures in their perineurium. It necessitates more magnification (ie, with operating microscope) and is more tedious to perform than epineurial repair.[49] Additional training in the use of operating microscopes and the use of small-sized suture materials would be indicated. There is some controversy concerning the quality of nerve regeneration following the use of these two techniques. Some believe that there is no significant difference in the quality of regeneration between the two techniques[6, 11, 36, 72] or that better results are obtained with epineurial sutures.[5] However, others think that the fascicular suture technique gives a better quality of nerve regeneration.[23, 24, 60, 61] When the veterinary practitioner considers the above factors about each technique, along with the facts that relatively few nerve repairs are performed and animals do not require the discrete motor and sensory function in their digits that humans need, it can be concluded that the epineurial suture repair is the most practical. Consequently, emphasis will be placed on this technique.

A light colored, soft material, such as a piece of latex rubber balloon, is placed in the surgical field to serve as a background against which the surgeon can distinguish anatomic detail. This light background also facilitates finding and handling fine suture material when looking through magnification loupes.[49]

Suture material for nerve anastomosis can range from 5–0 to 8–0 in size. Silicone coated silk and monofilament nylon have been described for neurorrhaphy in veterinary surgery.[49, 66, 67] It should be remembered that with large animals and larger nerves, larger diameter suture material will be needed.[63]

The surgeon should avoid placing too many sutures when anastomosing a nerve because the connective tissue reaction within the nerve increases with the number of sutures. In general, four sutures placed equidistant around the nerve will give a stable anastomosis.[66, 67] However, with larger nerves, more sutures may be required to assure adequate alignment.[46]

The nerve stumps should be examined in detail so that the fascicles of the two segments can be matched as closely as possible. Longitudinal blood vessels in the epineurium of each stump should be aligned to help assure that no rotational misalignment has occurred.[49] If marking sutures were placed on each side of the neuroma before it was removed, these can be aligned to assure that no rotation has occurred.

When proper alignment has been established, the first sutures are placed. The nerve is handled only by the epineurium using jeweler's forceps. Using a swaged needle, the first suture is placed 0.5 to 1.0 mm from the end of one nerve stump, placing the suture from the surface of the nerve so it emerges just subepineurially. The process is repeated on the other nerve stump, passing the suture from the free edge of the epineurium up through the surface of the epineurium. This suture is tied with a square knot. The second suture is placed in like manner 180° around the nerve from the first suture. Long ends are left on these sutures to facilitate placement of the remaining sutures. The surgeon then places a suture halfway between the first two sutures on the uppermost surface of the nerve (Fig. 19–8A and B). With the long ends on these three sutures, the nerve is rotated to allow placement of the fourth suture on the lowermost surface of the nerve (Fig. 19–8C). All sutures are tied with equal tension to assure that the nerve ends just appose each other. The neurorrhaphy is examined carefully for alignment and distraction or impaction. Additional sutures may be required, but this decision is based on the appearance of the repair. All suture ends should be cut short, hemostasis should be attained, and clots should be removed from the surgical site.[46, 49] If there is scar tissue in the area of neurorrhaphy, an attempt should be made to remove it or place the anastomosis in an area clear of such tissue. To help prevent tension on the neurorrhaphy site, two epineurial tacking sutures can be placed 180° apart to tack the nerve to underlying tissues. Two sutures are placed on each side of the anastomotic site, about 2 cm from the neurorrhaphy site[6] (Fig. 19–8D).

An alternate suture technique requires placement of a single suture aligned with the longitudinal axis of the nerve trunk. A swaged needle with small diameter monofilament nylon is inserted into the center of the nerve stump 7 to 8 mm proximal to the transection site and is

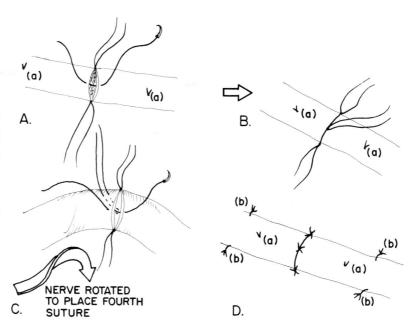

Figure 19-8. Nerve anastomosis. A, First two sutures are placed 180° apart and third suture is halfway between these two on uppermost aspect of the nerve. B, Third suture is tied. C, Nerve is rotated with long ends on the first three sutures and the fourth suture is placed on the underside of the nerve. D, Epineurial tacking sutures (b) tacking the nerve to underlying structures to help keep tension off of the anastomotic site. Epineurial marking sutures for nerve alignment (a).

directed along the nerve parallel to its long axis until it emerges at the end of the stump. The needle is reinserted between the corresponding fibers of the distal stump and is retrieved through the epineurium 7 to 8 mm from the transection site. It emerges on the opposite side of the nerve from where the suture was inserted. Two 3 mm square patches of silicone rubber are used as anchor plates over which

the ends of the suture are tied. These patches serve to stabilize the suture within the nerve and hold the stumps in apposition. The suture is passed through the patch, and one end is secured tying a square knot. After the suture has been placed, the second end is secured by placing a slip knot over the patch, which acts to apply tension for alignment and apposition of the nerve trunks[46, 62, 66, 67] (Fig. 19-9).

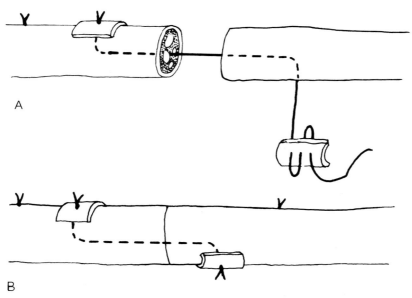

Figure 19-9. Technique for intraneural nerve anastomosis. A, Placement of the suture. B, Completed suture. (Adapted from Raffe MR: Peripheral nerve injuries in the dog (Part II). Comp Contin Educ 1:269, 1979.)

The monosuture technique results in less postsurgical neuroma formation and less ingrowth of extraneural scar tissue. However, the technique has the disadvantages of being difficult to perform and the potential for rotation of the nerve stumps on the single suture, which could interfere with axonal regeneration.[46, 66]

In the past, attempts have been made to protect nerve anastomotic sites to prevent the ingrowth of extraneural connective tissue. One technique involved placing a silicone rubber cuff around the anastomotic site. The cuff's function was to prevent axonal escape into surrounding tissues, stimulate longitudinal axonal growth, and prevent the growth of extraneural connective tissue into the anastomotic site.[66, 67] In spite of the good external appearance of anastomotic sites that have been encased in these cuffing devices, invasion of the suture site by connective tissue cannot be avoided. One of the main sources for proliferating connective tissue is the epineurium, and this remains inside the cuff.[40] These cuffs are apparently not in popular use, because their manufacture has been discontinued. This may be a reflection of the increased popularity of fascicular suturing in the field of human peripheral nerve surgery. However, silicone rubber nerve caps and semirigid silicone tubing* in various diameters are available. Lengths of such tubing can be split along one side and used to surround and protect intact nerves from entrapment by extraneural scar tissue when there has been significant soft tissue trauma to a limb without nerve severance.[20]

---

*Dow Corning International Co, Medical Products Division, Midland, MI.

Nerve Grafts

Nerve grafts are indicated to span large gaps in peripheral nerves. These gaps result from loss of nerve tissue at the time of original trauma or when neuromas and gliomas are removed.[49] As with nerve anastomosis, a graft may be a segment of nerve secured by epineurial sutures (Fig. 19–10), or it may be composed of several individual fascicles anastomosed at either end to fascicles in the nerve stumps. In light of the previously mentioned factors associated with epineurial and fascicular suturing in veterinary surgery, it would follow that grafting a segment of nerve trunk into a nerve gap would be the most feasible for the veterinary practitioner. However, taking an autograft from a nerve of nearly the same diameter as the nerve to be grafted results in motor and/or sensory paralysis at another area of the body. In addition, a whole nerve segment used as a free graft may undergo central fibrotic changes owing to delayed revascularization.[44, 49]

The use of allograft nerve segments in the dog has been described. In early experimental work, allografts were frozen and electron irradiated to reduce their antigenicity. Such grafts were reportedly effective in supplying reinnervation to denervated areas.[39] However, despite promising results in early experiments, disappointing clinical results were obtained with deep frozen irradiated allografts.[52] Short lengths (2 cm) of fresh, nonirradiated nerve allografts have been effective in dogs.[65–67] A study of major canine histocompatibility complex (MHC) and its effect on nerve allografts in dogs has shown that nerves transferred between dogs with identical major histocompatibility complexes had

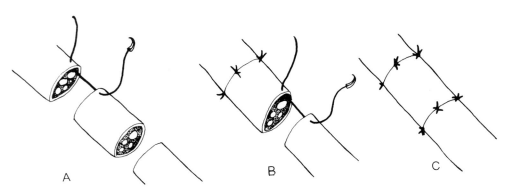

Figure 19–10. A segment of nerve sutured into a nerve gap using epineurial sutures. A, Beginning the first anastomosis. B, First anastomosis complete, beginning second anastomosis. C, Second anastomosis complete.

good nerve regeneration based on electromyographic and histologic findings. Dogs with partially mismatched histocompatibility complexes had better results than dogs that were totally mismatched, and nerve graft survival was not improved by irradiation of grafts in either matched or mismatched groups. It was concluded that a good histocompatibility match was essential for prolonged good functional graft survival and for the survival of longer nerve grafts.[57] Nerve homografts and heterografts evoke an immune response in the host. This eventually leads to graft rejection. Regenerating axons will advance through a graft as long as viable Schwann cells remain present. For a successful graft, the axons must traverse the graft and encounter viable Schwann cells of the distal stump before the graft is destroyed by the inflammatory immune response. Thus, an increase in length of the graft may decrease the chance that regenerating axons will reach the distal nerve stump before the graft has been rejected by the host's immune reaction.[39] Because no histocompatibility studies were performed on the previously mentioned successful allografts,[65] it could be that the success of these grafts may have been related to their short length (2 cm), with axonal regeneration occurring across the graft before graft rejection occurred.

If there still exists a small gap between the nerve stumps after freeing the nerve stumps and flexing the limb to get nerve stumps apposed, the surgeon might consider the use of a fresh allograft. This graft should be approximately the same diameter as the nerve being repaired.

If a long gap exists between nerve stumps, the surgeon could consider using autogenous fascicular nerve grafts or a modification of the fascicular graft technique. As described in the veterinary literature,[49] several segments of the caudal cutaneous sural nerve, which are 10% longer than the gap, can be taken without leaving the patient with a severe nerve deficit. One end of each of these segments is anastomosed to the end of a fascicle in the proximal stump. Using an operating microscope, two sutures of 10–0 nylon are placed through the epineurium of the sural nerve and the perineurium of the fascicle. After all proximal anastomoses have been accomplished, all of the distal anastomoses are performed. Because of the special equipment and time necessary to perform this rather tedious procedure, its practicality is questionable. A modification of this technique entails basically the same procedure;

however, the fascicles of the stumps are not dissected out. Sutures are placed through the epineurium of both the graft segments and the stumps. This would not give the accurate approximation of fascicles that the fascicular suture technique does. However, the grafts could serve to guide regenerating axons from the proximal to the distal stump. The axons might regenerate through the grafts themselves or they might grow along the outside of the individual grafts, as has been reported,[12, 50] to reach the distal nerve stump.

If silicone rubber tubing is used to protect a graft site, it should not completely surround the graft. This would prevent blood vessels from growing into the graft and thus lead to necrosis. Revascularization of grafts occurs from the surrounding tissue as well as from the stumps. Thus, the bed for the graft should be a well-vascularized area that is free of scar tissue.[65, 66]

Nerve Gaps

In two separate studies,[39, 65] nerve gaps 2 cm long have been created in peripheral nerves and the stumps sutured to adjacent musculature. In one of these studies,[39] gaps were created in the peroneal nerves of three dogs. Two of the three dogs showed partial return of function in 7 months; however, the bridged nerve fibers were difficult to identify in the surrounding scar tissue. Electric stimulation showed some proximal fibers had reached the distal stump. Similar histopathologic results were obtained in the second study in which 2 cm gaps were made in radial nerves of three dogs[65] (Fig. 19–11). In this study all three dogs showed evidence of functional recovery at an average of 10.3 weeks following surgery based on neurologic examination. Six months postoperatively, electric stimulation of the affected radial nerves proximal to the gap revealed evidence of fiber regeneration across the gap.

Nerve Biopsy

Peripheral nerve biopsy can be used for diagnostic purposes on the small number of animals with peripheral nerve disease. It is advisable for the technique to be performed by a veterinarian who has some training in fascicular nerve biopsy techniques. The biopsy should be examined at a laboratory equipped for peripheral nerve histologic studies and research.[55]

Peripheral nerve biopsy is indicated when

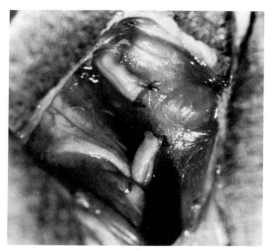

Figure 19–11. Two nerve ends have been sutured in line with each other on a smooth muscle surface. Gap between nerve ends is about 2 cm. (From Swaim SF: Peripheral nerves. In Archibald J (ed): Canine Surgery, 2nd Archibald ed. Santa Barbara, CA, American Veterinary Publications, Inc, 1974.)

peripheral nerve or neuromuscular diseases other than those associated with trauma are suspected. The nerve to be biopsied and the level (proximal or distal) at which it will be biopsied are carefully considered. Degenerative changes in the biopsy specimen unrelated to the disease process can be avoided by selecting a nerve segment that is not subject to recurrent trauma. For example, the segment of the peroneal nerve that is lateral to the stifle joint is prone to recurrent trauma. Sensory nerves are biopsied for disorders affecting sensory function, and mixed nerves (sensory and motor) are biopsied for diseases affecting motor function (Table 19–1). Whenever possible, the biopsied nerve should be one that has been evaluated electrodiagnostically along with the muscle it innervates.[55]

Using aseptic technique, the nerve to be biopsied is approached, avoiding highly vascular areas and using minimal dissection to expose the nerve. The nerve is isolated from surrounding tissues for about 3 to 4 cm to obtain a 2.5 to 3 cm long biopsy. The epineurium is incised

Table 19–1. PERIPHERAL NERVE BIOPSY SITES

Sensory Nerves	Mixed Nerve Trunks
Lateral cutaneous radial	Ulnar
Medial cutaneous radial	Tibial
Saphenous	Peroneal
Superficial peroneal	

longitudinally for the entire length of the exposed segment using a number 11 scalpel blade. This allows identification of the fascicles to be biopsied. After carefully separating fascicles from the nerve, a 4–0 silk or polypropylene suture is placed around the fascicles at the proximal end (Fig. 19–12A). The suture ends are tied and left long, and a transverse cut is made through the fascicles proximal to the tie (Fig. 19–12B). The biopsy sample should be approximately one third of the nerve's diameter. A longitudinal incision is made from proximal to distal along the fascicles to separate them from the rest of the nerve. A transverse incision is made 2.5 to 3 cm distal to the proximal incision, freeing the biopsy sample from its remaining attachment[55] (Fig. 19–12C).

A curved needle that is swaged on a piece of 3–0 stainless steel is passed through and left in the distal end of the biopsy. On the other end of the steel suture is a small weight (Fig. 19–12D). The long ends of the proximal suture are used to suspend the biopsy in a solution of 3% glutaraldehyde for fixation. The weight on the distal end of the specimen keeps it submerged in the fixation solution and maintains its length[55] (Fig. 19–12E).

Palmar Digital Neurectomy

Palmar, or posterior, digital neurectomy is used to relieve pain associated with navicular disease, fracture of the navicular bone, and selected lateral wing fractures of the third phalanx in the horse.[11] The surgery may be performed under local anesthesia with the animal standing or under general anesthesia. If local anesthesia is used, it is injected over the nerves at the level of the abaxial surface of the seasmoid bones. If neurectomy is to be performed immediately following use of a diagnostic block of the palmar digital nerve, the surgery utilizes the same block. General anesthesia should be considered for epineurial capping.[71]

After preparing for aseptic surgery, the guillotine technique of neurectomy can be performed. A 2 cm long incision is made over the dorsal border of the flexor tendons and continued through the subcutaneous tissues (Fig. 19–13A). If epineurial capping is to be used, the incision is made 3 to 4 cm long. Although there may be some variation, the relationships of vein, artery, nerve, and ligament of the ergot aid the surgeon in orientation (Fig. 19–13B). The palmar digital nerve is identified just palmar to the digital artery approximately 1 cm

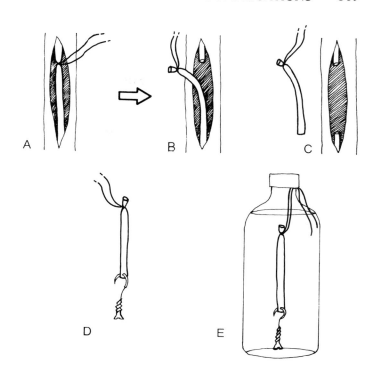

Figure 19–12. Nerve biopsy technique. A, Epineurium has been incised longitudinally and a fascicle separated for biopsy. A 4–0 ligature is placed around the proximal part of fascicle. B, Fascicle is cut proximal to ligature. C, A 2.5 to 3 cm section of fascicle is removed. D, A curved needle on a piece of 3–0 steel is placed and left in the distal aspect of the biopsy and a weight (stainless steel bone screw) is affixed to the end of the wire. E, Specimen is suspended in 3 per cent glutaraldehyde. (Adapted from Shores A, Braund KG, Stockham SL, and Simpson S: Diagnostic methods. *In* Slatter DH (ed): Textbook of Small Animal Surgery. Philadelphia, WB Saunders Co, 1985.)

below the skin surface and deep to the ligament of the ergot. The surgeon should look for accessory branches of the palmar digital nerve commonly located near the ligament of the ergot. If an accessory branch is found, a 2 cm portion is removed using a scalpel.[71]

The main portion of the nerve is dissected free from the subcutaneus fascia. If the structure puckers when it is stretched it is nerve. Scraping its surface should reveal the longitudinal fascicles, and a small incision in the nerve should reveal transversely separated nerve fascicles. After it has been identified, the nerve is severed at the distalmost end of the incision. A hemostat is placed on the nerve just above the point of severance. This is used to stretch the nerve while it is being cut at the proximal end of the incision (Fig. 19–13C). The cut end of the nerve should retract back into the tissues and out of sight. This is believed to be helpful in preventing painful neuromas.[70]

Another technique for neurectomy involves epineurial capping of the nerve to prevent neuromas. The approach to the nerve is the same as for the guillotine technique, except the incision is longer. After a 3 to 4 cm length of nerve is exposed, the nerve is severed as distally as possible and raised from the incision. The end of the nerve is held in forceps, while the epineurium is carefully reflected (Fig. 19–13D). The epineurium is reflected for 2 to 3 cm, and

two incisions are made halfway through the nerve on each side (Fig. 19–13E). The nerve is severed distal to these cuts, and the epineurium is pulled back over the nerve's end and ligated with 2–0 silk[71] (Fig. 19–13F).

POSTOPERATIVE CARE AND COMPLICATIONS

The extent of postoperative limb protection and immobilization required following nerve repair varies with the severity of injury and the type of neurorrhaphy performed.[49] A padded bandage for 7 to 10 days should be sufficient after epineurial or perineurial neurorrhaphy if there was no tension on the repair site. However, if moderate tension was present on the neurorrhaphy site, the limb should be immobilized for 3 weeks.[64] If joints have been positioned to avoid tension on the repaired nerve, the limb should be rigidly fixed in its operative position for 3 weeks. Then at weekly intervals for the next 2 to 4 weeks, the limb should be returned gradually to a neutral position.[49] Three weeks of strict immobilization is suggested because this is the length of time necessary for adequate collagen synthesis and deposition to splint the nerve internally, but it is not long enough for collagen remodeling around the collateral ligaments and capsule of joints in

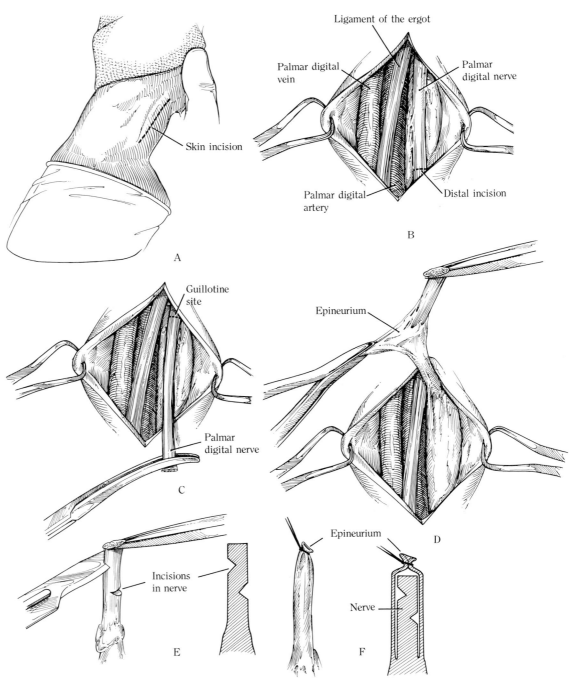

Figure 19–13. Palmar digital neurectomy. A, Site of skin incision. B, Location of the nerve. C, Distal aspect of the nerve has been severed; proximal aspect will be severed for the guillotine technique. D, Epineurial capping technique, stripping epineurium from the nerve after it was cut distally. E, Incising halfway through the nerve at two locations. F, Epineurium pulled back over nerve end and ligated with 2–0 silk. (From Turner AS and McIlwraith CW: Techniques in Large Animal Surgery. Philadelphia, Lea & Febiger, 1982.)

extreme flexion or extension to produce permanent joint fixation. After all external immobilization has been removed, there is still an additional 7 days or more of partial immobility caused by pain and inflexibility of the limb. These prevent sudden forced extension of a joint that was acutely flexed.[44] After nerve grafting, the limb should be protected in semirigid fixation for 7 to 10 days before full mobilization is permitted.[49]

The insensitive portions of a limb must be protected during the reinnervation process to prevent mutilation and self mutilation. Padded bandages, splints, and moldable casts may be used for this purpose.[46, 49] These devices also help prevent tendon contracture in the limbs.

Mutilation of a limb, usually the distal portions of a limb, is not an uncommon problem with denervation. This has generally been attributed to the animal unknowingly and continually traumatizing the digits because of their lack of sensation. However, other factors may be involved in the tissue breakdown. An increased collagenase production has been noted in denervated dermis, along with high levels of collagenase in the necrotic ulcers in denervated skin of paraplegics.[44] It is possible that denervated tissues are more susceptible to trauma, and minor trauma may result in wounds.

The author has encountered instances when animals become incessant in attempts to self mutilate a denervated limb regardless of the covering placed on the limb. In such instances, wire basket-type muzzles have been beneficial in addition to covering the limb. This self mutilation has been hypothesized to be correlated with the early stages of axonal regeneration to sensory deprived areas.[46] There may be paresthesias related to reinnervation that stimulate self mutilation.

Good general nursing and wound care principles should be followed to enhance functional recovery of the limb. Physical therapy, to include active and passive exercise, should be started as soon as possible to help maintain joint motion and muscle tone.[49]

Following a palmar digital neurectomy a sterile dressing and pressure bandage are maintained over the sutured skin wound for at least 10 days. To reduce postoperative inflammation, 2 g of phenylbutazone are given following surgery. Sutures are removed 10 days after surgery, and the horse is rested for 4 to 6 weeks. Complications of neurectomy include painful neuroma formation, rupture of the deep digital flexor tendon, reinnervation, persistence of sensation because of failure to identify and sever

accessory branches of the nerve, and loss of the hoof wall.[71]

REFERENCES

1. Asbury AK and Johnson PC: Pathology of Peripheral Nerves. Philadelphia, WB Saunders Co, 1978.
2. Babcock WW: A standard technique for operations on peripheral nerves. With special reference to the closure of large gaps. Surg Gynecol Obstet 45:364, 1927.
3. Bateman JE: Trauma to the Nerves in Limbs. Philadelphia, WB Saunders Co, 1962.
4. Blumke, S, Niedorf HR, and Rode J: Axoplasmic alterations in the proximal and distal stumps of transected nerves. Acta Neuropathol 7:44, 1966.
5. Bora FW: A comparison of epineurial, perineurial, and epiperineurial methods of nerve suture. Clin Orthop 133:91, 1978.
6. Braun, RM: Epineurial nerve suture. Clin Orthop 163:50, 1982.
7. Brown BA: Internal neurolysis in traumatic peripheral nerve lesions in continuity. Surg Clin North Am 52:1167, 1972.
8. Brown DD and Doherty MM: Effects of transient stretching of peripheral nerve. Arch Neurol Psychiat 54:116, 1945.
9. Brown HA and Brown BA: Treatment of peripheral nerve injuries. Rev Surg 24:1, 1967.
10. Bryant WM: Wound healing. Clin Symp 29:23, 1977.
11. Cabaud HE, Rodkey WG, McCarroll HR, et al: Epineurial and perineurial fascicular nerve repairs: A critical comparison. J Hand Surg 1:131, 1976.
12. Cabaud HE, Rodkey WG, and Nemeth TJ: Progressive ultrastructural changes after peripheral nerve transection and repair. J Hand Surg 7:353, 1982.
13. Causey G: The Cell of Schwann. London, E and S Livingstone, 1960.
14. deLahunta A: Veterinary Neuroanatomy and Clinical Neurology, 2nd ed. Philadelphia, WB Saunders Co, 1983.
15. Ducker TB, Kempe LG, and Hayes GJ: The metabolic background for peripheral nerve surgery. J Neurosurg 30:270, 1969.
16. Ducker TB: Metabolic factors in surgery of peripheral nerves. Surg Clin North Am 52:1109, 1972.
17. Ducker, TB and Kauffman FC: Metabolic factors in surgery of peripheral nerves. Clin Neurosurg 24:406, 1977.
18. Evans LH, Campbell JB, Pinner-Poole B, and Jenny J: Prevention of painful neuromas in the horse. JAVMA 153:313, 1968.
19. Fackelman GE and Clodius L: New techniques for posterior digital neurectomy in the horse. Vet Med Small Anim Clin 67:1339, 1972.
20. Finsterbush A, Porat S, Rousso M, and Ashur H: Prevention of peripheral nerve entrapment following extensive soft tissue injury, using silicone cuffing. Clin Orthop 162:276, 1982.
21. Fisher ER and Turano A: Schwann cells in wallerian degeneration. Arch Pathol 75:517, 1963.
22. Grabb WC: The healing nerve. In Kernahan DA and Vistnes LM (ed): Biological Aspects of Reconstructive Surgery. Boston, Little, Brown, and Co, 1977.
23. Grabb WC, Bement SL, Koepke GH, and Greene RA: Comparison of methods of peripheral nerve suturing in monkeys. Plast Reconst Surg 46:31, 1970.
24. Grabb WC and Smith JW: Repair of peripheral nerves.

In Converse JM (ed): Reconstructive Plastic Surgery, vol 6, 2nd ed. Philadelphia, WB Saunders Co, 1977.

25. Haftek J: Stretch injury of peripheral nerve. Acute effects of stretching on rabbit nerve. J Bone Joint Surg (Br) 52:354, 1970.

26. Higgs PE and Weeks PM: The rate of bursting strength gain in repaired nerves. Ann Plast 3:338, 1979.

27. Horch K: Guidance of regrowing sensory axons after cutaneous nerve lesions in the cat. J Neurophysiol 42:1437, 1979.

28. Hubbard JH: The quality of nerve regeneration: Factors independent of the most skillful repair. Surg Clin North Am 52:1099, 1972.

29. Hudson AR and Hunter RT: Timing of peripheral nerve repair: Important local neuropathological factors. Clin Neurosurg 24:391, 1976.

30. Ketchum LD: Peripheral nerve repair. *In* Fundamentals of Wound Management in Surgery. Smith, Kline, and French Labs, 1978.

31. Kline DG: Macroscopic and microscopic concomitants of nerve repair. Clin Neurosurg 26:582, 1979.

32. Kline DG: Timing for exploration of nerve lesions and evaluation of the neuroma-in-continuity. Clin Orthop 163:42, 1982.

33. Kline DG, Hackett ER, Davis GD, and Myers MB: Effect of mobilization on the blood supply and regeneration of injured nerves. J Surg Res 12:254, 1972.

34. Kline DG and Nulsen FE: The neuroma in continuity: Its preoperative and operative management. Surg Clin North Am 52:1189, 1972.

35. Lehman RAW and Hayes GJ: Degeneration and regeneration in peripheral nerves. Brain 90:285, 1977.

36. Levinthal R, Brown J, and Rand RW: Comparison of fascicular, interfascicular, and epineurial suture techniques in the repair of simple nerve lacerations. J Neurosurg 47:744, 1977.

37. Lundborg G: Ischemic nerve injury. Scand J Plast Surg (Suppl) 6, 1970.

38. Mackinnon SE, Hudson AR, Gentili F, et al: Peripheral nerve injection injury with steroid agents. Plast Reconstr Surg 69:482, 1982.

39. Marmor L: Peripheral Nerve Regeneration Using Nerve Grafts. Springfield, IL, Charles C Thomas, 1967.

40. Millesi H: Microsurgical repair of peripheral nerves. *In* Grabb WC and Smith JW (ed): Plastic Surgery, 3rd ed. Boston, Little, Brown and Co, 1979.

41. Miyamoto Y: Experimental study of results of nerve suture under tension vs. nerve grafting. Plast Reconstr Surg 64:540, 1979.

42. Nulsen FE and Kline DG: Acute injuries of peripheral nerves. *In* Youmans JR (ed): Neurological Surgery, vol 2. Philadelphia, WB Saunders Co, 1973.

43. O'Daly JA and Imaeda T: Electron microscopic study of wallerian degeneration in cutaneous nerves caused by mechanical injury. Lab Invest 17:744, 1967.

44. Peacock EE: Wound Repair, 3rd ed. Philadelphia, WB Saunders Co, 1984.

45. Raffe MR: Peripheral nerve injuries in the dog. Part I. Comp Cont Ed Prac Vet 1:207, 1979.

46. Raffe MR: Peripheral nerve injuries in the dog. Part II. Comp Cont Ed Pract Vet 1:269, 1979.

47. Richardson PM and Ebendal T: Nerve growth activities in rat peripheral nerve. Brain Res 246:57, 1982.

48. Rizzoli HV: Treatment of peripheral nerve injuries. *In* Neurological Surgery of Trauma. Washington, DC, US Government Printing Office, 1965.

49. Rodkey WG and Cabaud HE: Peripheral nerve injury and repair. *In* Bojrab MJ (ed): Current Techniques in Small Animal Surgery, 2nd ed. Philadelphia, Lea & Febiger, 1983.

50. Rodkey WG, Cabaud HE, and McCarroll HR: Neurorrhaphy after loss of a nerve segment: Comparison of epineurial suture under tension versus multiple nerve grafts. J Hand Surg 5:366, 1980.

51. Rowe SN: The surgical treatment of nerve lesions. *In* Vinken PJ and Bruyn GW (ed): Handbook of Clinical Neurology. New York, American Elsevier Publishing Co, Inc, 1970.

52. Seddon HJ: Three types of nerve injury. Brain 66:238, 1943.

53. Seddon HJ: Surgical Disorders of the Peripheral Nerves. Baltimore, Williams & Wilkins Co, 1972.

54. Seletz E: Surgery of Peripheral Nerves. Springfield, IL, Charles C Thomas, 1951.

55. Shores A, Braund KG, Stockham SL, and Simpson ST: Diagnostic methods. *In* Slatter DH (ed): Textbook of Small Animal Surgery. Philadelphia, WB Saunders Co, 1985.

56. Sims MH and Redding RW: Failure of neuromuscular transmission after complete nerve section in the dog. Am J Vet Res 40:931, 1979.

57. Singh R, Vriesendorp HM, Mechelse K, and Stefanko S: Nerve allografts and histocompatibility in dogs. J Neurosurg 47:737, 1977.

58. Smith JW: Microsurgery of peripheral nerves. *In* Rand RW (ed): Microneurosurgery. St Louis, CV Mosby Co, 1969.

59. Smith JW: Injuries of the nerves. *In* Grabb WC and Smith JW (ed): Plastic Surgery: A Concise Guide to Clinical Practice, 2nd ed. Boston, Little Brown and Co, 1973.

60. Smith JW: Newer techniques in peripheral nerve repair. Clin Neurosurg 24:456, 1977.

61. Smith JW and Gillen FJ: Current techniques in peripheral nerve repair. *In* Rand RW (ed): Microneurosurgery, 2nd ed. St Louis, CV Mosby Co, 1978.

62. Synder CC, Webster HD, Pickens JE, et al: Intraneural neurorrhaphy: A preliminary clinical and histological evaluation. Ann Surg 167:691, 1968.

63. Stashak TS and Mayhew IG: The nervous system. *In* Jennings PB (ed): The Practice of Large Animal Surgery. Philadelphia, WB Saunders Co, 1984.

64. Sunderland S: Nerves and Nerve Injuries. Edinburgh, Churchill-Livingstone, 1978.

65. Swaim SF: Peripheral Nerve Surgery in the Dog. Thesis (MS), Auburn University, Auburn, AL, 1971.

66. Swaim SF: Peripheral nerve surgery in the dog. JAVMA 161:905, 1972.

67. Swaim SF: Isolated peripheral nerves. *In* Bojrab MJ (ed): Current Techniques in Small Animal Surgery I. Philadelphia, Lea & Febiger, 1975.

68. Swaim SF: Peripheral nerve surgery. *In* Hoerlein BF (ed): Canine Neurology, 3rd ed. Philadelphia, WB Saunders Co, 1978.

69. Swaim SF: Peripheral neuropathies. *In* Bojrab MJ (ed): Pathophysiology of Small Animal Surgery. Philadelphia, Lea & Febiger, 1981.

70. Tomson FN and Gattuso JL: Peripheral nerve tumors in the dog. Canine Pract 4:23, 1977.

71. Turner AS and McIlwraith CW: Techniques in Large Animal Surgery. Philadelphia, Lea & Febiger, 1982.

72. Urbaniak JR: Fascicular nerve suture. Clin Orthop 163:57, 1982.

73. Van Beek A and Kleinert HE: Peripheral nerve injuries and repair. *In* Rand RW (ed): Microneurosurgery, 2nd ed. St Louis, CV Mosby Co, 1978.

74. Weiss P: "Panta Rhei"—And so flow our nerves. Am Sci 57:287, 1969.

75. Zachary RB and Roaf F: Lesions in continuity. Med Res Coun, Special Report Series, 282:57, 1954.

Problems Caused by Disorders of the Nervous System

This appendix is designed to assist the reader in identifying the diseases that are most likely to cause a particular clinical problem. Major problems, such as monoparesis, pelvic limb paresis, and seizures, are listed in separate tables. Each table cites the most common causes of the syndrome for each species. Separate tables are provided for (1) dogs and cats and (2) horses and food animals. The diseases are arranged according to whether they are acute or chronic and progressive or nonprogressive. If age predilection is a factor it is indicated (y, young; o, old). All species may be affected unless indicated otherwise. For each disease or group of diseases there is a cross reference to the chapter in which it is discussed.

PROBLEM: MONOPARESIS–DOG AND CAT

Thoracic Limb

    Acute nonprogressive
        Allergic
            Brachial plexus neuritis   Ch 14
        Traumatic
            Brachial plexus avulsion   Ch 14
            Individual nerves   Ch 14

    Chronic progressive
        Neoplastic (o)
            Neurofibroma   Ch 9
            Other   Ch 9

Pelvic Limb

    Acute nonprogressive
        Traumatic
            Individual nerves   Ch 14
    Chronic progressive
        Neoplastic (o)
            Neurofibroma   Ch 9
            Other   Ch 9
    Acute or chronic progressive
        Inflammatory   Ch 7
        Rabies
        Postvaccinal rabies

o, Older animals usually affected; y, younger animals usually affected.

PROBLEM: MONOPARESIS—HORSE AND FOOD ANIMAL

Thoracic Limb
  Acute nonprogressive
    Physical   Ch 14
      Sweeny—suprascapular
        nerve
      Brachial compression, avul-
        sion
      Radial fractures
      Postanesthetic myoneurop-
        athy
  Chronic progressive
    Neoplastic   Ch 9
      Neurofibroma (E,B)
      Lymphosarcoma (E,B)
  Acute or chronic progressive
    Inflammatory   Ch 7
      Equine protozoal myeloen-
        cephalitis (E)
      Rabies
      Caprine arthritis encephalitis
        (C)
      Cervical vertebral osteoar-
        thropathy (E)

Pelvic Limb
  Acute nonprogressive
    Physical   Ch 14
      Sciatic—perineurial injection
      Femoral—calving paralysis
        (calf) (B)
      L$_5$-L$_6$—calving paralysis (B)
      Postanesthetic myoneurop-
        athy (E,B)
  Acute or chronic progressive
    Neoplastic   Ch 9
      Neurofibroma (E,B)
      Lymphosarcoma (E,B)
    Inflammatory   Ch 7
      Equine protozoal myeloen-
        cephalitis (E)
      Injection abscess
      Rabies
      Caprine arthritis encephalitis
        (C)
    Idiopathic   Ch 14
      Stringhalt (E)
      Fibrotic myopathy (E)

B, Bovine; C, caprine; E, Equine; O, ovine; P, porcine.

PROBLEM: PELVIC LIMB PARESIS—DOG AND CAT

Spinal Cord T$_3$–L$_3$
  Acute nonprogressive
    Traumatic   Ch 11
    Vascular
      Fibrocartilaginous emboli   Ch 7
  Acute progressive
    Degenerative
      Intervertebral disk disease   Ch 12
    Neoplastic (o)   Ch 9
    Inflammatory   Ch 7
      Canine distemper (y)
      Bacterial myelitis
      Bacterial osteomyelitis, dis-
        kospondylitis
      Toxoplasmosis
      Systemic mycoses
      Feline polioencephalomyeli-
        tis
    Traumatic   Ch 11
    Idiopathic
      Scotty cramp (y)   Ch 6
  Chronic progressive
    Degenerative
      Intervertebral disk disease   Ch 12
      Degenerative myelopathy (o)   Ch 6

Hereditary myelopathy (Af-   Ch 6
  ghan) (y)
Demyelinating diseases, glo-   Ch 6
  boid cell leukodystrophy
  (y)
Demyelinating myelopathy   Ch 6
  (poodle) (y)
Neuronal and axonal degen-   Ch 6
  erations
Axonopathy (boxer) (y)   Ch 6
Spinocerebellar tract degen-   Ch 6
  eration (y)
Anomalous
  Vertebral malformations (y)   Ch 6
  Spinal dysraphism (y)   Ch 6
  Multiple cartilaginous exos-   Ch 6
    toses (y)
Neoplastic (o)   Ch 9
Nutritional
  Hypervitaminosis A   Ch 8
Inflammatory   Ch 7
  Feline infectious peritonitis
  Canine distemper myelitis
  Toxoplasmosis
  Systemic mycoses

PROBLEM: PELVIC LIMB PARESIS—DOG AND CAT *Continued*

Granulomatous meningoen-
  cephalomyelitis

Spinal Cord L_4–S_3
  Acute nonprogressive
    Anomalous   Ch 6
      Vertebral malformation (y)
      Meningomyelocele (y)
      Myelodysplasia (y)
    Traumatic   Ch 18
    Vascular
      Fibrocartilaginous emboli   Ch 7
      Aortic thromboembolism (is-   Ch 14
        chemic neuropathy in the
        cat)
  Acute progressive
    Degenerative
      Intervertebral disk disease   Ch 12
    Neoplastic   Ch 9
    Inflammatory   Ch 7
      Canine distemper (y)
      Bacterial myelitis
      Bacterial osteomyelitis, dis-
        kospondylitis
      Toxoplasmosis

Systemic mycoses
  Postvaccinal rabies   Ch 11
  Traumatic   Ch 11
Chronic progressive
  Degenerative
    Intervertebral disk disease   Ch 12
    Stockard's paralysis (y)   Ch 6
  Anomalous   Ch 6
    Myelodysplasia (y)
    Vertebral anomalies
    Lumbosacral malformation-
      malarticulation (o)
  Neoplastic (o)   Ch 9
  Inflammatory   Ch 7
    Bacterial osteomyelitis,
      diskospondylitis
    Systemic mycoses
    Feline infectious peritonitis
    Postvaccinal rabies
    Canine distemper
    Toxoplasmosis
  Traumatic   Ch 11
  Toxic
    Chronic organophosphate   Ch 8

---

o, Older animals usually affected; y, younger animals usually affected.

PROBLEM: PELVIC LIMB PARESIS—HORSE AND FOOD ANIMAL

Spinal Cord T_3–L_3

  Acute nonprogressive
    Traumatic   Ch 11
    Vascular   Ch 7
      Fibrocartilaginous emboli
        (E,P,O)

  Acute progressive
    Neoplastic   Ch 9
      Lymphosarcoma (E,B)
    Inflammatory   Ch 7
      Equine herpesvirus I myeli-
        tis (E)
      Equine protozoal myeloen-
        cephalitis (E)
      Caprine arthritis encephalitis
        (C)
      Enteroviral encephalomyeli-
        tis (P)
      Rabies
      Bacterial infection
      Systemic fungal infection
      Parasitic larval migration
    Toxic   Ch 8

Chronic progressive
  Degenerative   Ch 6
    Degenerative myelopathy (E)
    Myelin disorder of Charolais
      (B)
    Bovine progressive degener-
      ative myeloencephalopathy
      (B)
  Neoplastic   Ch 9
    Lymphosarcoma (B)
    Other
  Nutritional   Ch 8
    Poliomyelomalacia (P)
    Pantothenic acid deficiency
      (P)
  Inflammatory   Ch 7
    Bacterial infections, abscess
    Systemic fungal infections
  Toxic   Ch 8
    Sorghum sp (E,B)
    Organophosphates
    Arsanilic acid (P)
    Selenium (P)
    Braken fern (E)

PROBLEM: PELVIC LIMB PARESIS—HORSE AND FOOD ANIMAL *Continued*

Spinal Cord L$_4$–S$_2$, Peripheral
Nerves and Muscle
  Acute nonprogressive
    Anomalous   Ch 6
      Myelodysplasia
      Meningomyelocele
    Traumatic   Ch 11
    Vascular   Ch 7
      Fibrocartilaginous emboli
        (P,E,O)
      Aortoiliac thromboembolism,
        ischemic neuromyopathy
        (E)
      Postanesthetic hemorrhagic
        myelopathy (E)
  Acute progressive
    Inflammatory   Ch 7
      Protozoal myelitis (E)
      Herpes virus I myelitis
      Rabies
      Bacterial infections
      Parasitic larval migration

      Neuritis of cauda equina,   Ch 14
        polyneuritis (E)
    Toxic   Ch 8
      Sorghum ingestion (E,B)
      Selenium ingestion (P)
      Nutritional myodegeneration   Ch 14
        (B,O,E)
    Physical
      Exertional rhabdomyolysis   Ch 14
        (E)
  Chronic progressive
    Neoplastic   Ch 9
    Inflammatory
      Neuritis of cauda equina (E)   Ch 14
      Equine infectious anemia (E)   Ch 7
    Toxic   Ch 8
      Sorghum ingestion (E,B)
      Swayback (O,C)
    Vascular   Ch 7
      Aortoiliac thromboembolism,
        ischemic neuropathy (E)

B, Bovine; C, caprine; E, equine; O, ovine; P, porcine.

PROBLEM: TETRAPARESIS—DOG AND CAT

Spinal Cord C$_1$–T$_2$
  Acute nonprogressive
    Traumatic   Ch 10
    Vascular   Ch 7
      Fibrocartilaginous emboli
  Acute progressive
    Degenerative   Ch 12
      Intervertebral disk disease
    Neoplastic (o)   Ch 9
    Inflammatory   Ch 7
      Canine distemper
      Bacterial myelitis
      Bacterial osteomyelitis, dis-
        kospondylitis
      Toxoplasmosis
      Systemic mycoses
      Feline polioencephalomyeli-
        tis
      Angiostrongylus cantonensis
        (dog)
    Traumatic   Ch 10
    Vascular   Ch 7
      Fibrocartilaginous emboli
  Chronic progressive
    Degenerative   Ch 6
      Storage diseases (y)
      Demyelinating diseases (y)

      Spinal tract degeneration (y)
    Anomalous   Ch 6
      Vertebral malformations: at-
        lantoaxial malformation (y);
        cervical malformation (y);
        myelodysplasia (y)
    Neoplastic (o)   Ch 9
    Nutritional   Ch 8
      Hypervitaminosis A
    Inflammatory   Ch 7
      Feline infectious peritonitis
      Canine distemper myelitis
      Toxoplasmosis
      Systemic mycoses
      Granulomatous meningoen-
        cephalomyelitis
    Traumatic   Ch 11

Generalized LMN
  Acute progressive
    Inflammatory (immune)   Ch 14
      Polyradiculoneuritis (coon-
        hound paralysis)
      Idiopathic polyneuropathy
    Toxic
      Tick paralysis   Ch 14
      Botulism   Ch 7

PROBLEM: TETRAPARESIS—DOG AND CAT *Continued*

Chronic progressive
  Degenerative
    Motor neuronopathies   Ch 6
  Axonopathies   Ch 14
  Demyelinating (axons some-   Ch 14
    times involved)
  Metabolic   Ch 14
    Diabetic neuropathy
  Neoplastic   Ch 14
    Paraneoplastic neuromyopa-
      thy (o)
  Inflammatory (immune)   Ch 14
    Chronic relapsing polyradi-
      culoneuritis
Episodic progressive
  Immune   Ch 14
    Myasthenic syndromes
  Metabolic   Ch 8
    Hypoglycemia
    Electrolyte abnormalities

Muscle
  Acute progressive
    Degenerative   Ch 14
      Myotonic myopathy (chow-
        chow and others) (y)
      X-linked myopathy (Irish ter-
        rier) (y)
    Metabolic   Ch 8,
      Exertional myopathy   14
      Malignant hyperthermia

Idiopathic   Ch 14
  Idiopathic feline polymyopa-
    thy
Inflammatory (immune)   Ch 14
  Polymyositis
Chronic progressive
  Degenerative   Ch 14
    Muscular dystrophy (Labra-
      dor retriever) (y)
    Canine hypotrophic myopa-
      thy
  Metabolic   Ch 14
    Hyperadrenocortical myopa-
      thy
    Steroid myopathy
    Hypothyroid myopathy
  Neoplastic   Ch 14
    Paraneoplastic neuromyopa-
      thy (o)
  Nutritional   Ch 14
    Vitamin E-Selenium defi-
      ciency
  Idiopathic   Ch 14
    Immobilization myopathy
      (dogs)
  Inflammatory   Ch 14
    Toxoplasma myositis
  Traumatic   Ch 14
    Myositis ossificans
    Fibrotic myopathy

o, Older animals usually affected; y, younger animals usually affected.

PROBLEM: TETRAPARESIS—HORSE AND FOOD ANIMAL

Spinal Cord C_1–T_2
  Acute nonprogressive
    Degenerative   Ch 6
      Hereditary neuraxial edema
        (B)
      Congenital brain edema (B)
      Inherited paralysis (B)
    Traumatic   Ch 10
    Vascular   Ch 7
      Fibrocartilaginous emboli
        (E,P,O)
  Acute progressive
    Anomalous   Ch 6
      Cervical vertebral malforma-
        tion-malarticulation (E)
      Occipitoatlantoaxial malfor-
        mation (E,B)
    Neoplastic   Ch 9

    Lymphosarcoma (B,E)
  Nutritional   Ch 8
    Nicotinic acid deficiency (P)
  Inflammatory   Ch 7
    Rabies
    Equine herpesvirus I myeli-
      tis (E)
    Equine protozoal myeloen-
      cephalitis (E)
    Caprine arthritis encephalitis
      (C)
    Polioencephalomyelitis (P)
    Bacterial infection
    Vertebral osteomyelitis
    Systemic fungal infection
    Parasitic larval migration
  Toxic   Ch 8

PROBLEM: TETRAPARESIS—HORSE AND FOOD ANIMAL *Continued*

Chronic progressive
  Degenerative — Ch 6
    Degenerative myeloen-
      cephalopathy (E,B)
    Myelin disorder of Charolais
      (B)
    Storage diseases
  Anomalous — Ch 6
    Cervical vertebral malforma-
      tion-malarticulation (E)
    Occipitoatlantoaxial malfor-
      mation (E,B)
    Vascular anomalies (E)
  Neoplastic — Ch 9
  Nutritional — Ch 8
    Copper deficiency (O,P,C)
  Inflammatory — Ch 7
    Caprine arthritis encephalitis
      (C)
    Equine protozoal myeloen-
      cephalitis (E)
    Systemic fungal infection
    Parasitic larval migration
    Equine infectious anemia (E)
  Toxic — Ch 8
    Heavy metals
    Organophosphates
    Poisonous plants
    Selenium (P)
    Tetanus — Ch 7

Generalized LMN
  Acute progressive
    Inflammatory — Ch 7
      Polyneuritis

Toxic — Ch 8
  Botulism
  Tick paralysis
  Postanesthetic myasthenia
Acute nonprogressive
  Arthrogryposis — Ch 6
Episodic progressive — Ch 8
  Metabolic derangements

Muscle — Ch 14
  Acute progressive
    Degenerative — Ch 14
      Myotonia (C,E)
    Metabolic — Ch 8, 14
      Exertional rhabdomyolysis
        (E)
      Malignant hyperthermia
        (E,P)
    Nutritional — Ch 8, 14
      Vitamin E-Selenium defi-
        ciencies (B,C,E,O)
    Inflammatory
      Polymyositis (*Clostridium* sp) — Ch 14
    Physical
      Downer cow syndrome (B) — Ch 14
      Postanesthetic myoneuropa- — Ch 14
        thy (E,B)
  Chronic progressive
    Degenerative — Ch 14
      Myotonia (C,E)
    Nutritional — Ch 8, 14
      Vitamin E-Selenium defi-
        ciency (B,C,E,O)
    Idiopathic fibrotic myopathy — Ch 14
      (E)

B, Bovine; C, caprine; E, equine; O, ovine; P, porcine.

PROBLEM: VESTIBULAR AND CEREBELLAR ATAXIA*—DOG AND CAT

Peripheral Vestibular Diseases
  Acute nonprogressive
    Anomalous
      Congenital vestibular syn- — Ch 6
        drome
    Idiopathic
      Vestibular syndrome — Ch 7
    Traumatic — Ch 11
  Acute progressive
    Inflammatory — Ch 7
      Otitis media interna
  Chronic progressive
    Neoplasia — Ch 9
    Toxic — Ch 8

Central Vestibular Disease
  Acute nonprogressive
    Traumatic — Ch 11
    Vascular — Ch 7
      Hemorrhage or infarct
  Acute progressive
    Inflammatory — Ch 6
      Canine distemper
      Feline infectious peritonitis
      Bacterial infections
      Fungal infections
      Granulomatous meningoen-
        cephalitis (dog)
    Nutritional — Ch 8

PROBLEM: VESTIBULAR AND CEREBELLAR ATAXIA*—DOG AND CAT Continued

Thiamine deficiency
Chronic progressive
  Inflammatory — Ch 7
    Granulomatous meningoen-
      cephalitis
    Feline infectious peritonitis
    Fungal infections
  Neoplasia (o) — Ch 9

Cerebellar Ataxia
  Acute nonprogressive
    Anomalous
      Malformations (y) — Ch 6
    Inflammatory — Ch 7
      In utero panleukopenia viral
        infection (cats) (y)
    Traumatic — Ch 11
  Acute progressive

    Inflammatory — Ch 7
      Canine distemper
      Feline infectious peritonitis
      Toxoplasmosis
      Fungal infections
      Bacterial infections
  Chronic progressive
    Degenerative — Ch 6
      Storage diseases (y)
      Abiotrophies (y)
    Inflammatory — Ch 7
      Granulomatous meningoen-
        cephalitis
      Fungal infections
    Neoplastic (o) — Ch 9
    Toxic — Ch 8
      Lead
      Hexachlorophene (y)

*Ataxia without head signs—spinal cord, see Tetraparesis and Pelvic Limb Paresis.
o, Older animals usually affected; y, younger animals usually affected.

PROBLEM: VESTIBULAR AND CEREBELLAR ATAXIA*—HORSE AND FOOD ANIMAL

Peripheral Vestibular Diseases
  Acute nonprogressive
    Traumatic — Ch 11
  Acute progressive
    Inflammatory — Ch 7
      Otitis media interna
      Ear mites (C)
      Guttural pouch mycosis (E)
      Polyneuritis-neuritis of cauda
        equina (E)
    Physical — Ch 11
      Osteoarthrosis and fractures
        of temperohyoid region (E)
    Idiopathic
      Vestibular syndrome — Ch 7

Central Vestibular Disease
  Acute nonprogressive
    Traumatic — Ch 11
    Vascular — Ch 7
  Acute progressive
    Inflammatory — Ch 7
      Equine protozoal encepha-
        litis (E)
      Caprine arthritis encephalitis
        (C)
      Equine herpesvirus I en-
        cephalitis (E)
      Bacterial infections, Listeria
        (B,O,C)

      Systemic fungal infections
      Parasitic larval migration
      Basilar empyema (P,B)
  Chronic progressive
    Inflammatory — Ch 7
      Equine protozoal encepha-
        litis (E)
    Neoplastic — Ch 9

Cerebellar Ataxia
  Acute nonprogressive
    Anomalous — Ch 6
      Congenital malformations (B)
    Inflammatory — Ch 7
      In utero degenerations
        (B,O,P)
    Traumatic — Ch 11
  Acute progressive
    Inflammatory — Ch 7
      Bacterial infection
      Equine protozoal encepha-
        litis (E)
      Parasitic larval migration
  Chronic progressive
    Degenerative — Ch 6
      Storage diseases
      Abiotrophies (B,E,O,P)
      Ataxia and convulsions of
        Angus calves (B)

PROBLEM: VESTIBULAR AND CEREBELLAR ATAXIA*—HORSE AND FOOD ANIMAL *Continued*

Inflammatory
  Equine protozoal myeloen-
    cephalitis (E)
  Parasitic larval migration
Neoplastic   Ch 9
  Lymphosarcoma, medulo-
    blastoma (B)

Toxic   Ch 8
  Heavy metals
  Plants
  Mycotoxins

*Ataxia without head signs—spinal cord, see Tetraparesis and Pelvic Limb Paresis.
B, Bovine; C, caprine; E, equine; O, ovine; P, porcine.

PROBLEM: SEIZURES*

*See Ch 10, Tables 10–2 and 10–3.

PROBLEM: STUPOR OR COMA—DOG AND CAT

Brain Stem or Cerebrum
  Acute nonprogressive
    Anomalous
      Brain malformations (y)   Ch 6
    Traumatic   Ch 11
    Vascular   Ch 7
  Acute progressive
    Metabolic   Ch 8
      Hypoglycemia
      Hepatic Encephalopathy
      Uremic encephalopathy
      Diabetic coma
      Heat stroke
      Hypoxia
    Neoplastic (o)   Ch 9
      Metastatic
      Neoplasm with hemorrhage
    Nutritional   Ch 8
      Thiamine deficiency
    Idiopathic   Ch 10
      Epilepsy
      Narcolepsy-cataplexy
    Inflammatory   Ch 7
      Canine distemper
      Rabies
      Feline infectious peritonitis
      Infectious canine hepatitis
      Aujeszky's disease (pseudora-
        bies)
      Herpesvirus

      Toxoplasmosis
      Systemic fungal diseases
      Bacterial encephalitis
      Granulomatous meningoen-
        cephalitis
      Feline polioencephalomyeli-
        tis
      Chronic encephalitis of pug
        dogs
      Babesiosis
      Encephalitozoonosis
      Rickettsial diseases
      Trypanosomiasis
      Parasitic larval migration
    Toxic   Ch 8
      Lead
      Many other toxins
    Trauma   Ch 11
  Chronic progressive
    Degenerative   Ch 6
      Storage diseases (y)
    Anomalous   Ch 6
      Hydrocephalus (y)
    Metabolic (see Acute progres-   Ch 8
      sive)
    Neoplastic (o)   Ch 9
    Inflammatory (see Acute pro-   Ch 7
      gressive)
    Toxic   Ch 8
      Heavy metals

y, Younger animals usually affected; o, older animals usually affected.

PROBLEM: STUPOR OR COMA—HORSE AND FOOD ANIMAL

Brain Stem or Cerebrum
  Acute nonprogressive
    Anomalous   Ch 6
      Brain malformations
    Traumatic   Ch 11
    Vascular   Ch 7
      Parasitic thromboembolism
        (E)
      Intracarotid injections
  Acute progressive
    Metabolic   Ch 8
      Hypoglycemia
      Hypocalcemia
      Hepatic encephalopathy
      Hypoxia
      Heat stroke
    Neoplastic   Ch 9
    Nutritional   Ch 8
      Thiamine deficiency (B,C,O)
    Idiopathic *or* Vascular
      Neonatal maladjustment syn- Ch 7
        drome (E)
    Idiopathic
      Narcoplepsy-cataplexy (E,B) Ch 10
    Inflammatory   Ch 7
      Equine viral encephalomyeli-
        tides (E)
      Rabies
      Thrombotic meningoen-
        cephalitis (B)
      Sporadic bovine encephalo-
        myelitis (B)
      Malignant catarrhal fever (B)
      Porcine polioencephalomyeli-
        tis (P)

      Pseudorabies
      Hemagglutinating encepha-
        lomyocarditis (P)
      Infectious bovine rhinotra-
        cheitis (B)
      Borna (O,C,B)
      Louping ill (O,E,P)
      Glasser's disease (P)
      Equine protozoal myeloen-
        cephalitis (E)
      Bacterial infections
      Systemic fungal infections
      Parasitic larval migration
    Toxic   Ch 8
      Heavy metals (B)
      Organophosphates
      Moldy corn (leukoencepha-
        lomalacia) (E)
      Water intoxication or salt
        poisoning (B,P)
      Urea (B,E)
      Clostridium and coliform en-
        terotoxemia (C,O,P)
      Various plants
  Chronic progressive
    Degenerative   Ch 6
      Storage diseases (B,C,O,P)
    Anomalous   Ch 6
      Hydrocephalus
    Metabolic (see Acute progres- Ch 8
      sive)
    Neoplastic   Ch 9
    Inflammatory (see Acute pro- Ch 7
      gressive)
    Toxic (see Acute progressive) Ch 8

B, Bovine; C, caprine; E, equine; O, ovine; P, porcine.

PROBLEM: DIFFUSE OR MULTIFOCAL SIGNS—DOG AND CAT

Acute progressive
  Metabolic   Ch 8
    Hypoglycemia
    Hepatic encephalopathy
    Uremic encephalopathy
    Endocrine disorders
  Neoplastic   Ch 9
    Metastatic (o)
  Nutritional   Ch 8
    Thiamine deficiency
  Inflammatory   Ch 7
    Canine distemper
    Rabies
    Feline infectious peritonitis

    Infectious canine hepatitis
    Aujeszky's disease (pseudora-
      bies)
    Canine herpesvirus (y)
    Toxoplasmosis
    Systemic fungal diseases
    Bacterial infections
    Granulomatous meningoen-
      cephalitis
    Chronic encephalitis of pug
      dogs
    Babesiosis
    Encephalozoonosis (y)
    Rickettsial diseases

PROBLEM: DIFFUSE OR MULTIFOCAL SIGNS—DOG AND CAT *Continued*

Trypanosomiasis
Parasitic larval migrations
Toxic   Ch 8
  Most toxins
Chronic progressive
  Degenerative   Ch 6
    Storage diseases (y)
    Abiotrophies (y)
    Motor neuronopathies (y)
    Axonal degenerations (y)
    Demyelinating diseases (y)
  Metabolic   Ch 8
    Hepatic encephalopathy
    Endocrine disorders
  Neoplastic   Ch 9
  Inflammatory   Ch 7
    Canine distemper, old dog
      encephalitis

Feline infectious peritonitis
Toxoplasmosis
Systemic fungal diseases
Bacterial meningitis
Granulomatous meningoen-
  cephalitis
Chronic encephalitis of pug
  dogs
Babesiosis
Rickettsial diseases
Trypanosomiasis
Parasitic larval migration
Prototheocosis
Toxic
  Heavy metals

o, Older animals usually affected; y, younger animals usually affected.

PROBLEM: DIFFUSE OR MULTIFOCAL SIGNS—HORSE AND FOOD ANIMAL

Acute progressive
  Metabolic   Ch 8
    Hypoglycemia
    Hypocalcemia and other
      electrolyte imbalances
    Hepatic encephalopathy
  Neoplastic   Ch 9
    Lymphosarcoma
  Nutritional   Ch 8
    Thiamine deficiency
  Inflammatory   Ch 7
    Rabies
    Viral encephalomyelitis (E)
    Aujeszky's disease (pseudora-
      bies)
    Polioencephalomyelitis (P)
    Equine herpesvirus I en-
      cephalomyelitis (E)
    Scrapie (o)
    Visna, maedi (o)
    Malignant catarrhal fever (B)
    Caprine arthritis encephalitis
      (C)
    Sporadic bovine encephalo-
      myelitis (B)
    Thrombotic meninogen-
      cephalitis (B)
    Hemagglutinating encepha-
      lomyocarditis (P)
    Neuritis of the cauda equina,
      polyneuritis equi (E)

Listeriosis (B,C,O)
Bacterial infections
Systemic fungal infections
Toxoplasmosis
Equine protozoal encephalo-
  myelitis (E)
Parasitic larval migration
Toxic   Ch 8
  Most toxins
Vascular   Ch 7
  Neonatal maladjustment syn-
    drome (E)
Chronic progressive
  Degenerative   Ch 6
    Storage diseases
    Abiotrophies
    Demyelinating diseases
  Metabolic   Ch 8
    Hepatic encephalopathy
    Endocrine disorders
  Neoplasia   Ch 9
  Nutritional   Ch 8
    Hypo- or Hypervitaminoses
  Inflammatory   Ch 7
    Viral encephalomyelitis (E)
    Herpesvirus I encephalo-
      myelitis (E)
    Scrapie (o)
    Visna, maedi (o)
    Caprine arthritis encephalitis
      (C)

PROBLEM: DIFFUSE OR MULTIFOCAL SIGNS—HORSE AND FOOD ANIMAL *Continued*

Malignant catarrhal fever (B)
Neuritis of the cauda equina, polyneuritis equi (E)
Equine infectious anemia (E)
Sporadic bovine encephalomyelitis (B)
Hemagglutinating encephalomyocarditis (P)

Listeriosis
Systemic fungal infections
Guttural pouch mycosis (E)
Toxoplasmosis
Parasitic larval migration
Toxic   Ch 8
Heavy metals

B, Bovine; C, caprine; E, equine; O, ovine; P, porcine.

PROBLEM: MOVEMENT DISORDERS (TETANY, TETANUS, TREMOR, MYOCLONUS, SPASTICITY, MUSCLE SPASMS, AND OPISTHOTONOS)—DOG AND CAT

Acute nonprogressive
  Anomalous   Ch 6
    Cerebellar malformations (y)
    Hypomyelination (y)
  Idiopathic
    Myotonia (y)   Ch 14
    Scotty cramp (y)   Ch 6
    Tremor of adult dogs   Ch 7
Acute progressive
  Metabolic   Ch 8
    Hyperadrenocorticism   Ch 14
    Hypocalcemia
    Hypoglycemia
    Liver failure
    Uremia
  Inflammatory   Ch 7
    Canine distemper
  Toxic   Ch 8
    Chlorinated hydrocarbons
    Hexachlorophene

    Metaldehyde
    Neurotoxin, *Clostridium tetani*
    Organophosphate
    Strychnine
    Many other toxic plants and chemicals
  Trauma
    Severe brain trauma   Ch 11
Chronic progressive
  Degenerative   Ch 6
    Cerebellar neuronal degeneration (y)
    Demyelinating diseases (y)
    Storage diseases
  Inflammatory   Ch 7
    Canine distemper (myoclonus)
  Toxic   Ch 8
    Heavy metals (lead)

---

y, Younger animals usually affected.

PROBLEM: MOVEMENT DISORDERS (TETANY, TETANUS, TREMOR, MYOCLONUS, SPASTICITY, MUSCLE SPASMS, AND OPISTHOTONOS)—HORSE AND FOOD ANIMAL

Acute nonprogressive
  Anomalous   Ch 6
    Cerebellar malformation (B,O,E,P)
    Hypomyelination (B,O,P)
  Idiopathic
    Myotonia (C,E)   Ch 14
    Spastic paresis (B)   Ch 6
    Tremor of horses (E)   Ch 6
Acute progressive
  Degenerative   Ch 6
    Neuraxial edema (B)

    β-Mannosidosis (C)
  Idiopathic
    Spastic syndrome (B)   Ch 6
    Stringhalt, "shivering" (E)   Ch 14
  Metabolic   Ch 8
    Hypocalcemia (B,E,O)
    Hypomagnesemia (B,O)
    Uremia
  Toxic   Ch 8
    Australian Stringhalt (buttercup) (E)   Ch 14
    Chlorinated hydrocarbons

PROBLEM: MOVEMENT DISORDERS (TETANY, TETANUS, TREMOR, MYOCLONUS, SPASTICITY, MUSCLE SPASMS, AND OPISTHOTONOS)— HORSE AND FOOD ANIMAL *Continued*

Lathyrism (E)
Metaldehyde
Mycotoxicoses
Neurotoxin, *Clostridium*
  tetani
Organophosphate

Other toxic plants and chemicals
Chronic progressive
  Degenerative   Ch 6
    Cerebellar degenerations
    Demyelinating diseases
    Storage diseases

B, Bovine; C, caprine; E, equine; O, ovine; P, porcine.

Species and Breed Predisposition for Noninfectious Diseases

BOVINE DISEASES

Breed	Classification of Disease	Name of Disease	Eponym	Inherited	References
Aberdeen Angus	Anomalous	Cerebellar hypoplasia		Unknown	81
	Degenerative	α-Mannosidosis		Yes	119
	Idiopathic	Cerebellar ataxia with seizures		Yes	14
		Spastic paresis		Unknown	67, 145
Angus-shorthorn	Anomalous	Hypomyelination		Yes	255
Ayrshire	Degenerative	Cerebellar abiotrophy		Yes	135
	Idiopathic	Spastic paresis		Unknown	67, 145
Beefmaster	Degenerative	Neuronal lipodystrophy		Yes	207
Brahman	Degenerative	Glycogenosis	Pompe's disease	Yes	176, 190
Brown Swiss	Degenerative	Degenerative myeloencephalopathy		Unknown	226
	Idiopathic	Epilepsy		Yes	3
		Spastic paresis		Unknown	67, 145
Charolais	Anomalous	Myelodysplasia, arthrogryposis		Yes	69, 157
	Degenerative	Myelin disorder		Unknown	23, 192
	Idiopathic	Spastic paresis		Unknown	67, 145
Guernsey	Idiopathic	Spastic syndrome		Unknown	27
Hereford	Anomalous	Brain edema		Yes	139
		Cerebellar hypoplasia		Yes	63, 132
		Hydrocephalus		Yes	100
		Retinal dysplasia		Yes	220
	Degenerative	Cerebellar abiotrophy		Yes	130
		Neuronal degeneration		Yes	211
	Idiopathic	Spastic paresis		Unknown	67, 145
Holstein Friesian	Anomalous	Atlantoaxial luxation		Unknown	247
	Degenerative	Cerebellar neuronal abiotrophy		Yes	62, 248
		Gangliosidosis GM1		Yes	71, 72
	Idiopathic	Spastic paresis		Unknown	67, 145
		Spastic syndrome		Unknown	27
Jersey	Anomalous	Hypomyelination		Yes	216
	Idiopathic	Spastic paresis		Unknown	67, 145
Murray grey	Degenerative	α-Mannosidosis		Yes	119
Norwegian red poll	Idiopathic	Pelvic limb paralysis		Yes	132
Polled Hereford	Degenerative	Hereditary neuraxial edema		Yes	24, 44, 139
Red Danish	Degenerative	Paralysis		Yes	132
Shorthorn	Anomalous	Cerebellar hypoplasia		Yes	62
		Hydrocephalus		Yes	101
		Hypomyelination		Yes	130
	Degenerative	Glycogenosis	Pompe's disease	Yes	209
	Idiopathic	Spastic paresis		Unknown	67, 145
Simmental	Idiopathic	Spastic paresis		Unknown	67, 145

CANINE DISEASES

Breed	Classification of Disease	Name of Disease	Eponym	Inherited	References
Afghan hound	Degenerative	Myelopathy		Yes	5, 40, 56
		Retinal degeneration		Yes	220
Airedale terrier	Degenerative	Cerebellar neuronal abiotrophy		Yes	45, 62, 74
Akita	Idiopathic	Congenital vestibular disease		Unknown	63
Alaskan malamute	Degenerative	Retinal degeneration		Yes	220
Australian heeler	Anomalous	Deafness		Yes	63, 117
Australian shepherd	Anomalous	Deafness		Yes	63, 117
Basset hound	Anomalous	Cervical malformation		Unknown	191
	Degenerative	Globoid leukodystrophy	Krabbe's disease	Unknown	166
		Glycoproteinosis	Lafora's disease	Unknown	127
Beagle	Anomalous	Retinal dysplasia		Yes	220
	Degenerative	Cerebellar neuronal abiotrophy		Yes	63
		Gangliosidosis GM1		Yes	9, 10, 205
		Globoid leukodystrophy	Krabbe's disease	Unknown	136
		Glycoproteinosis	Lafora's disease	Unknown	122, 127, 230
	Idiopathic	Epilepsy		Yes	16, 80
Bedlington terriers	Anomalous	Retinal dysplasia		Yes	220
Bern running dog	Degenerative	Cerebellar neuronal abiotrophy		Yes	62
Bernese mountain dog	Degenerative	Cerebellar abiotrophy		Yes	63
Blue tick hound	Degenerative	Globoid leukodystrophy	Krabbe's disease	Yes	26
Border collie	Degenerative	Cerebellar degeneration		Yes	96
		Ceroid lipofuscinosis		Yes	63
		Retinal degeneration		Yes	220
Boston terrier	Anomalous	Deafness		Yes	63, 117
		Hemivertebrae		Yes	6, 70, 181
		Hydrocephalus		Unknown	217
		Myelodysplasia		Yes	6
	Neoplastic	Gliomas		Unknown	88, 116, 163
		Pituitary tumors		Unknown	88, 116, 163
Bouvier des Flandres	Degenerative	Laryngeal paralysis		Yes	239, 240
Boxer	Degenerative	Central-peripheral neuropathy		Yes	105
	Neoplastic	Glioma		Unknown	116, 118, 164
		Pituitary tumors		Unknown	88, 116, 164
Brittany spaniel	Degenerative	Spinal muscular atrophy		Yes	46, 47, 160
Bull mastiff	Degenerative	Cerebellar neuronal abiotrophy		Yes	35
Bull terrier	Anomalous	Deafness		Yes	132
Cairn terrier	Degenerative	Globoid leukodystrophy	Krabbe's disease	Yes	91, 175, 227
Cardigan corgi	Degenerative	Retinal degeneration		Yes	220
Chihuahua	Anomalous	Hydrocephalus		Unknown	217
	Degenerative	Ceroid lipofuscinosis		Yes	204
Chondrodystrophic breeds	Degenerative	Intervertebral disk disease		Unknown	29, 108, 126
Chow chow	Anomalous	Cerebellar hypoplasia		Unknown	148
	Degenerative	Hypomyelination		Yes	234
		Myotonia		Yes	89, 141, 245
Cocker spaniel	Anomalous	Deafness		Unknown	117
		Retinal dysplasia		Yes	220
	Degenerative	Ceroid lipofuscinosis		Yes	184
		Retinal degeneration		Yes	220
	Idiopathic	Congenital vestibular disease		Unknown	63
		Facial paralysis		Unknown	28
Collie	Anomalous	Collie eye syndrome		Yes	254
		Deafness		Yes	165
	Degenerative	Cerebellar neuronal abiotrophy		Yes	111
		Neuroaxonal dystrophy		Yes	37, 66
		Retinal degeneration		Yes	220
	Immune	Dermatomyositis		Yes	110
Dachshund	Degenerative	Ceroid lipofuscinosis		Yes	55
		Retinal degeneration		Yes	220
	Idiopathic	Epilepsy		Yes	128
Dachshund, long haired	Degenerative	Ceroid lipofuscinosis		Yes	236
		Sensory neuropathy		Yes	78
Dalmatian	Anomalous	Deafness		Yes	117, 129, 165
		Hypomyelination		Yes	99
		Spinal dysraphism		Unknown	183
	Degenerative	Leukodystrophy		Yes	17
	Idiopathic	Hyperkinesis		Unknown	252
Doberman pinscher	Anomalous	Cervical vertebral malformation		Unknown	170, 198, 253
	Idiopathic	Congenital vestibular disease		Unknown	63
		Narcolepsy-cataplexy		Yes	9
English bulldog	Anomalous	Deafness		Unknown	117
		Hemivertebrae		Yes	6, 75, 181
		Myelodysplasia		Yes	6, 196, 249
	Neoplastic	Pituitary tumors		Unknown	88, 116, 164
English pointer	Degenerative	Sensory neuropathy		Yes	57–59

CANINE DISEASES *Continued*

Breed	Classification of Disease	Name of Disease	Eponym	Inherited	References
English setter	Anomalous	Deafness		Yes	117
	Degenerative	Ceroid lipofuscinosis		Yes	149, 150, 199
Finnish harrier	Degenerative	Cerebellar neuronal abiotrophy		Yes	231
Fox hound	Anomalous	Deafness		Yes	1
Fox terrier	Anomalous	Congenital myasthenia gravis		Yes	133, 180
	Degenerative	Spinocerebellar degeneration		Unknown	18, 20
German shepherd	Anomalous	Esophageal hypomotility		Unknown	225
	Degenerative	Degenerative myelopathy		Unknown	4, 30, 103
		Giant axonal neuropathy		Yes	76, 104, 106
		Lumbosacral malformation		Unknown	188, 229
	Idiopathic	Congenital vestibular disease		Unknown	63
		Epilepsy		Yes	85
German shorthair pointer	Degenerative	Gangliosidosis GM2	Tay-Sachs disease	Yes	142, 143
Golden retriever	Degenerative	Retinal degeneration		Yes	220
	Idiopathic	Myotonia		Unknown	63
Gordon setter	Degenerative	Cerebellar neuronal abiotrophy		Yes	50, 65
		Retinal degeneration		Yes	220
Great Dane	Anomalous	Cervical vertebral malformation		Unknown	121, 218, 253
		Esophageal hypomotility		Unknown	225
Great Dane cross-breeds	Degenerative	Neuronal abiotrophy	Stockard's paralysis	Yes	224
Irish setter	Anomalous	Cerebellar hypoplasia		Unknown	61–63
		Esophageal hypomotility		Unknown	225
		Lissencephaly		Unknown	63
	Degenerative	Cerebellar abiotrophy		Yes	61–63
		Quadriplegia and amblyopia		Yes	195
		Retinal degeneration		Yes	220
Irish terrier	Degenerative	X-linked myopathy		Yes	246
Jack Russell terrier	Anomalous	Congenital myasthenia gravis		Yes	194
	Degenerative	Spinocerebellar degeneration		Yes	114
Keeshond	Idiopathic	Epilepsy		Yes	242
Kerry blue terrier	Degenerative	Cerebellar neuronal abiotrophy		Yes	64
Labrador retriever	Anomalous	Retinal dysplasia		Yes	220
	Degenerative	Retinal degeneration		Yes	220
		Muscular dystrophy		Yes	151, 152
	Idiopathic	Narcolepsy-cataplexy		Yes	12
		Reflex myoclonus		Unknown	92
Lapland dog	Degenerative	Glycogenosis	Pompe's disease	Yes	243
		Neuronal abiotrophy		Yes	213, 214
Lhasa apso	Anomalous	Lissencephaly		Unknown	98, 256
Lurcher	Anomalous	Hypomyelination		Unknown	171
Miniature pinscher	Degenerative	Retinal degeneration		Yes	220
Miniature schnauzer	Anomalous	Esophageal hypomotility		Yes	39, 53
Norwegian dunkerhound	Anomalous	Deafness		Yes	63
Norwegian elkhound	Degenerative	Retinal degeneration		Yes	220
Old English sheepdog	Anomalous	Deafness		Yes	132
Pointer	Degenerative	Neurogenic amyotrophy		Yes	133
Poodle	Anomalous	Agenesis vermis cerebellum	Dandy-Walker disease	Unknown	144, 185
		Cerebellar hypoplasia		Unknown	63
	Degenerative	Demyelination		Unknown	73, 222
		Globoid leukodystrophy	Krabbe's disease	Yes	257
		Glycoproteinosis	Lafora's disease	Unknown	127
		Retinal degeneration		Yes	220
		Sphingomyelin lipidosis	Niemann-Pick disease	Yes	33
Red bone coonhound	Degenerative	Retinal degeneration		Yes	220
Rottweiler	Degenerative	Leukoencephalomyelopathy		Yes	94
		Neuroaxonal dystrophy		Yes	51
Saluki	Degenerative	Ceroid lipofuscinosis		Yes	2
		Retinal degeneration		Yes	220
Samoyed	Degenerative	Cerebellar neuronal abiotrophy		Yes	63
		Retinal degeneration		Yes	220
		Spongiform degeneration		Unknown	169
Scottish terrier	Idiopathic	Scotty cramp		Yes	177–179
Sealyham terrier	Anomalous	Retinal dysplasia		Yes	220
Shetland sheepdog	Degenerative	Retinal degeneration		Yes	220
Siberian husky	Degenerative	Laryngeal paralysis		Yes	208
Silky terrier	Degenerative	Glucocerebrosidosis	Gaucher's disease	Yes	112, 238
		Spongiform degeneration		Unknown	210

Table continued on following page

CANINE DISEASES *Continued*

Breed	Classification of Disease	Name of Disease	Eponym	Inherited	References
Springer spaniel	Anomalous	Congenital myasthenia gravis		Yes	138
		Retinal dysplasia		Yes	220
	Degenerative	α-L-Fucosidosis		Yes	113, 147, 159
		Hypomyelination		Yes	107
		Retinal degeneration		Yes	220
	Idiopathic	Rage syndrome		Unknown	63
Tervuren shepherd	Idiopathic	Epilepsy		Yes	233
Tibetan mastiff	Degenerative	Hypertrophic neuropathy		Yes	54
Tibetan terrier	Degenerative	Retinal degeneration		Yes	220
Toy breeds	Anomalous	Atlantoaxial luxation		Unknown	95, 153, 186
		Hydrocephalus		Unknown	86, 97, 217
		Occipital dysplasia		Unknown	13, 197
Weimaraner	Anomalous	Spinal dysraphism		Yes	83, 84, 174
West Highland white terrier	Degenerative	Globoid leukodystrophy	Krabbe's disease	Yes	87, 91, 175
Wire haired fox terrier	Anomalous	Lissencephaly		Unknown	62
		Cerebellar hypoplasia		Unknown	62, 63
		Esophageal hypomotility		Yes	189

CAPRINE DISEASES

Breed	Classification of Disease	Name of Disease	Inherited	References
Goats	Degenerative	Myotonia	Yes	31, 32
Nubian	Degenerative	β-Mannosidosis	Yes	120

EQUINE DISEASES

Breed	Classification of Disease	Name of Disease	Inherited	References
Appaloosa	Anomalous	Night blindness	Unknown	220
Arabian	Anomalous	Atlantooccipital malformation	Yes	156, 172, 173
	Degenerative	Cerebellar neuronal abiotrophy	Yes	79, 193
Arabian Foals	Idiopathic	Epilepsy	Unknown	63
Gotland pony	Degenerative	Cerebellar neuronal abiotrophy	Yes	19
Horses	Anomalous	Cervical vertebral malformation	Unknown	172
	Degenerative	Degenerative myeloencephalopathy	Unknown	172
		Myotonia	Unknown	223
Shetland ponies	Idiopathic	Narcolepsy-cataplexy	Unknown	63
Suffolk draft horses	Idiopathic	Narcolepsy-cataplexy	Unknown	63
Thoroughbred	Anomalous	Cervical vertebral malformation	Unknown	68, 93, 172
Thoroughbred (and others)	Degenerative	Laryngeal paralysis	Unknown	41, 42, 77
Zebra	Degenerative	Degenerative myeloencephalopathy	Unknown	125

FELINE DISEASES

Breed	Classification of Disease	Name of Disease	Eponym	Inherited	References
Abyssinian	Degenerative	Glucocerebrosidosis	Gaucher's disease	Yes	154, 232
Burmese	Anomalous	Encephalocele		Yes	258
	Idiopathic	Congenital vestibular disease		Unknown	63
Cats (white, blue eyes)	Anomalous	Deafness		Yes	15, 25, 250
Domestic	Degenerative	Gangliosidosis GM1		Yes	7, 10, 22
		Gangliosidosis GM2	Sandhoff's disease	Yes	10, 48, 49
		Globoid leukodystrophy	Krabbe's disease	Yes	90, 137
		Glycogenosis	Pompe's disease	Yes	215
		Metachromatic leukodystrophy		Yes	123
		Mucopolysaccharidosis		Yes	115
		Neuroaxonal dystrophy		Yes	251
		Neurofilament accumulation		Yes	237
		Sphingomyelin lipidosis	Niemann-Pick disease	Yes	36, 201
		α-Mannosidosis		Yes	34, 241
	Neoplastic	Meningioma		Unknown	162
Egyptian Mau	Degenerative	Spongiform degeneration		Yes	146
Korat	Degenerative	Gangliosidosis GM1		Yes	9–11
Manx	Anomalous	Myelodysplasia		Yes	60, 158, 168
Persian	Degenerative	α-Mannosidosis		Yes	235
Siamese	Anomalous	Hydrocephalus		Yes	219
		Optic pathway anomaly		Yes	21, 186
	Degenerative	Ceroid lipofuscinosis		Yes	102
		Esophageal hypomotility		Unknown	38
		Gangliosidosis GM1		Yes	7–9
		Mucopolysaccharidosis		Yes	52, 115, 155
		Sphingomyelin lipidosis	Niemann-Pick disease	Yes	221, 244
	Idiopathic	Congenital vestibular disease		Unknown	63

OVINE DISEASES

Breed	Classification of Disease	Name of Disease	Eponym	Inherited	References
Corriedale	Degenerative	Cerebellar atrophy		Yes	62, 63
		Glycogenosis	Pompe's disease	Yes	167
Polled Dorset	Degenerative	Globoid leukodystrophy	Krabbe's disease	Yes	203
Sheep	Degenerative	Glucocerebrosidosis	Gaucher's disease	Yes	69
South Hampshire	Degenerative	Ceroid lipofuscinosis	Batten's disease	Yes	140
Suffolk	Degenerative	Congenital myopathy		Unknown	182
		Neuroaxonal dystrophy		Yes	43
Welsh mountain	Degenerative	Cerebellar atrophy		Yes	131

PORCINE DISEASES

Breed	Classification of Disease	Name of Disease	Eponym	Inherited	References
British saddleback	Anomalous	Hypomyelination		Yes	69, 200
Landrace	Anomalous	Hypomyelination		Yes	69, 109
	Metabolic	Malignant hyperthermia		Yes	82, 161, 228
Pietrain	Metabolic	Malignant hyperthermia		Yes	82, 161, 228
Poland China	Metabolic	Malignant hyperthermia		Yes	82, 161, 228
Swine	Degenerative	Glucocerebrosidosis	Gaucher's disease	Unknown	69
Yorkshire	Degenerative	Cerebellar neuronal abiotrophy		Yes	62
		Gangliosidosis GM2	Tay-Sachs disease	Yes	202, 206
		Neuronal degeneration		Unknown	124

REFERENCES

1. Adams EW: Hereditary deafness in a family of foxhounds. JAVMA 128:302, 1956.
2. Appleby EC, Longstaffe JA, and Bell FR: Ceroid-lipofuscinosis in two saluki dogs. J Comp Pathol 92:375, 1982.
3. Atkeson FW, Ibsen HL, and Eldridge E: Inheritance of an epileptic type character in Brown Swiss cattle. J Hered 34:45, 1944.
4. Averill DR: Degenerative myelopathy in the aging German shepherd dog. JAVMA 162:1045, 1973.
5. Averill DR and Bronson RT: Inherited necrotizing myelopathy of Afghan hounds. J Neuropathol Exp Neurol 36:734, 1977.
6. Bailey CS: An embryological approach to the clinical significance of congenital vertebral and spinal cord abnormalities. J Am Anim Hosp Assoc 11:426, 1975.
7. Baker HJ and Lindsey JR: Animal model of human disease: Human GM1 gangliosidosis. Animal model: Feline GM1 gangliosidosis. Am J Pathol 74:649, 1974.
8. Baker HJ, Lindsey JR, McKann GM, and Farrell DF: Neuronal GM1 gangliosidosis in a Siamese cat with β-galactosidase deficiency. Science 174:838, 1971.
9. Baker HJ, Mole JA, Lindsey JR, and Creel RM: Animal models of human ganglioside storage diseases. Fed Proc 35:1193, 1976.
10. Baker HJ, Reynolds GD, Walkley SU, et al: The gangliosidosis: Comparative features and research applications. Vet Pathol 16:635, 1979.
11. Baker HJ, Walkley SU, Rattazi MC, et al.: Feline gangliosidoses as models of human lysosomal storage diseases. In Animal Models of Inherited Metabolic Diseases. New York, Alan R Liss, Inc, 1982.
12. Baker TL, Mitler MM, Foutz AS, and Dement WC: Diagnosis and treatment of narcolepsy in animals. In Kirk RW (ed): Current Veterinary Therapy VIII. Philadelphia, WB Saunders Co, 1983.
13. Bardens JW: Congenital malformations of the foramen magnum in dogs. Southwest Vet 18:295, 1965.
14. Barlow RM, Linklater KA, and Young GB: Familial convulsions and ataxia in Angus calves. Vet Rec 83:60, 1968.
15. Bergsma DR and Brown KS: White fur, blue eyes, and deafness in the domestic cat. J Hered 62:171, 1971.
16. Biefelt SW, Redman HC, and Broadhurst JJ: Sire and sex-related differences in rates of epileptiform seizures in a purebred beagle dog colony. Am J Vet Res 32:2039, 1971.
17. Bjerkas I: Hereditary "cavitating" leukodystrophy in Dalmatian dogs. Acta Neuropathol 40:163, 1977.
18. Bjorck G, Dyrendahl S, and Olsson SE: Hereditary ataxia in smooth-haired fox terriers. Vet Rec 69:87, 1957.
19. Bjorck G, Everz KE, Hansen HJ, and Henrickson B: Congenital cerebellar ataxia in the Gotland pony breed. Zentralbl Veterinarmed 20:341, 1973.
20. Bjorck G, Mair W, Olsson SE, and Sourander P: Hereditary ataxia in fox terriers. Acta Neuropathol (Suppl) 1:45, 1962.
21. Blake R and Crawford MLJ: Development of strabismus in Siamese cats. Brain Res 77:492, 1974.
22. Blakemore WF: GM1 gangliosidosis in a cat. J Comp Pathol 82:179, 1972.
23. Blakemore WF, Palmer AC, and Barlow RM: Progressive ataxia of Charolais cattle associated with disordered myelin. Acta Neuropathol 29:127, 1974.
24. Blood DC and Gay CC: Hereditary neuroaxial edema of calves. Aust Vet J 47:520, 1971.
25. Bosher SK and Hallpike CS: Observations on the histologic features, development, and pathogenesis of the inner ear degeneration of the deaf white cat. Proc R Soc Lond (Biol) 162:147, 1965.
26. Boysen BG, Tryphonas L, and Harries NW: Globoid cell leukodystrophy in the bluetick hound dog. 1. Clinical manifestations. Can Vet J 15:303, 1974.
27. Bradley R and Wijeratne WVS: A locomotor disorder clinically similar to spastic paresis in an adult Friesian bull. Vet Pathol 17:305, 1980.
28. Braund KG, Luttgen PJ, Sorjonen DC, and Redding RW: Idiopathic facial paralysis in the dog. Vet Rec 105:297, 1979.
29. Braund KG, Taylor TKF, Ghosh P, and Sharwood AA: Spinal mobility in the dog. A study in chondrodystrophoid and non-chondrodystrophoid animals. Res Vet Sci 22:78, 1977.
30. Braund KG and Vandevelde M: German shepherd dog myelopathy. A morphologic and morphometric study. Am J Vet Res 39:1309, 1978.
31. Bryant SH: Altered membrane potentials in myotonia. In Bolis L, Hoffman JF, and Leaf A (ed): Membranes and Diseases. New York, Raven Press, 1976, p 197.
32. Bryant SH: Myotonia in the goat. Ann NY Acad Sci 317:314, 1979.
33. Bundza A, Lowden JA, and Charlton KM: Niemann-Pick disease in a poodle dog. Vet Pathol 16:530, 1979.
34. Burditt LJ, Chotai K, Hirani S, et al: Biochemical studies on a case of feline mannosidosis. Biochem J 189:467, 1980.
35. Carmichael S, Griffiths IR, and Harvey MJA: Familial cerebellar ataxia with hydrocephalus in bull mastiffs. Vet Rec 112:354, 1983.
36. Chrisp CE, Ringle DH, Abrams GD, et al: Lipid storage disease in a Siamese cat. JAVMA 156:616, 1970.
37. Clark RG, Hartley WJ, Burgess GS, et al: Suspected neuroaxonal dystrophy in collie sheep dogs. NZ Vet J 30:102, 1982.
38. Clifford DH, Soifer FK, Wilson MD, and Guillord GL: Congenital achalasia of the esophagus in 4 cats of common ancestry. JAVMA 158:1554, 1971.
39. Clifford DH, Waddell ED, Patterson DR, et al: Management of esophageal achalasia in miniature schnauzers. JAVMA 161:1012, 1972.
40. Cockrell BY, Herigsted RR, Flo GJ, and Lengendre AB: Myelomalacia in Afghan hounds. JAVMA 162:362, 1973.
41. Cole CR: Changes in the equine larynx associated with laryngeal hemiplegia. Am J Vet Res 7:69, 1946.
42. Cook WR: The diagnosis of respiratory unsoundness in the horse. Vet Rec 77:516, 1965.
43. Cordy DR, Richards WPC, and Bradford GE: Systemic neuroaxonal dystrophy in Suffolk sheep. Acta Neuropathol 8:133, 1967.
44. Cordy DR, Richards WPD, and Stormont C: Hereditary neuraxial edema in Hereford calves. Pathol Vet 6:487, 1969.
45. Cordy DR and Snelbaker HA: Cerebellar hypoplasia and degeneration in a family of Airedale dogs. J Neuropathol Exp Neurol 11:324, 1952.
46. Cork LC, Griffin JW, Adams RJ, and Price DL: Hereditary canine spinal muscular atrophy. Am J Pathol 100:599, 1980.
47. Cork LC, Griffin JW, Choy C, et al.: Pathology of motor neurons in accelerated hereditary canine spinal muscular atrophy. Lab Invest 46:89, 1982.

48. Cork LC, Munnell JF, and Lorenz MD: The pathology of feline GM2 gangliosidosis. Am J Pathol 90:723, 1978.

49. Cork LC, Munnell JF, Lorenz MD, et al: GM2 ganglioside lysosomal storage disease in cats with β-hexosaminidase deficiency. Science 196:1014, 1977.

50. Cork LC, Troncoso JC, and Price DL: Canine inherited ataxia. Ann Neurol 9:492, 1981.

51. Cork LC, Troncoso JC, Price DL, et al: Canine neuroaxonal dystrophy. J Neuropathol Exp Neurol 42:286, 1983.

52. Cowell KR, Jezyk PF, Haskins ME, and Patterson DF: Mucopolysaccharidosis in a cat. JAVMA 169:334, 1976.

53. Cox VS, Wallace LJ, Anderson VE, and Rushmer RA: Hereditary esophageal dysfunction in the miniature schnauzer dog. Am J Vet Res 41:326, 1980.

54. Cummings JF, Cooper BJ, deLahunta A, and Van Winkle TJ: Canine inherited hypertrophic neuropathy. Acta Neuropathol 53:137, 1981.

55. Cummings JF and deLahunta A: An adult case of canine neuronal ceroid-lipofuscinosis. Acta Neuropathol 39:43, 1977.

56. Cummings JF and deLahunta A: Hereditary myelopathy of Afghan hounds, a myelinolytic disease. Acta Neuropathol 42:173, 1978.

57. Cummings JF, deLahunta A, Braund KG, and Mitchell WJ: Animal model of human disease: Hereditary sensory neuropathy: Nociceptive loss and acral mutilation in pointer dogs: Canine hereditary sensory neuropathy. Am J Pathol 112:136, 1983.

58. Cummings JF, deLahunta A, Simpson ST, and McDonald JM: Reduced substance P-like immunoreactivity in hereditary sensory neuropathy of pointer dogs. Acta Neuropathol 63:33, 1984.

59. Cummings JF, deLahunta A, and Winn SS: Acral mutilation and nociceptive loss in English pointer dogs. Acta Neuropathol 53:119, 1981.

60. Deforest ME, and Basrur PK: Malformations and the Manx syndrome in cats. Can Vet J 20:304, 1979.

61. deLahunta A: Diseases of the cerebellum. Vet Clin North Am 10:91, 1980.

62. deLahunta A: Comparative cerebellar disease in domestic animals. Comp Cont Ed Pract Vet 2:8, 1980.

63. deLahunta A: Veterinary Neuroanatomy and Clinical Neurology, 2nd ed. Philadelphia, WB Saunders Co, 1983.

64. deLahunta A and Averill DR: Hereditary cerebellar cortical and extrapyramidal nuclear abiotrophy in Kerry blue terriers. JAVMA 168:1119, 1976.

65. deLahunta A, Fenner WR, Indrieri RJ, et al: Hereditary cerebellar cortical abiotrophy in the Gordon setter. JAVMA 177:538, 1980.

66. deLahunta A and Shively GN: Neurofibrillary accumulation in a puppy. Cornell Vet 65:240, 1975.

67. Denniston JC, Shive RJ, Friedli U, and Boucher WB: Spastic paresis syndrome in calves. JAVMA 152:1138, 1968.

68. Dimock WW and Errington BJ: Incoordination of equidae: Wobblers. JAVMA 95:261, 1939.

69. Done JT: Developmental disorders on the nervous system in animals. Adv Vet Sci Comp Med 21:69, 1977.

70. Done SH, Drew RA, Robins GM, and Lane JG: Hemivertebra in the dog: Clinical and pathological observations. Vet Rec 96:313, 1975.

71. Donnelly WJC, Hannon J, Sheahan BJ, and O'Connor PJ: Cerebrospinal lipidosis in Friesian calves. Vet Rec 91:225, 1972.

72. Donnelly WJC, Sheahan BJ, and Rogers TA: GM1 gangliosidosis in Friesian calves. J Pathol 111:173, 1973.

73. Douglas SW and Palmer AC: Idiopathic demyelination of brain-stem and cord in a miniature poodle puppy. J Pathol Bact 82:67, 1961.

74. Dow RW: Partial agenesis of the cerebellum in dogs. J Comp Neurol 72:569, 1940.

75. Drew RA: Possible association between abnormal vertebral development and neonatal mortality in bulldogs. Vet Rec 94:480, 1974.

76. Duncan ID and Griffiths IR: Canine giant axonal neuropathy: Some aspects of its clinical, pathological and comparative features. J Small Anim Pract 22:491, 1981.

77. Duncan ID, Griffiths IR, McQueen A, and Baker GO: The pathology of equine laryngeal hemiplegia. Acta Neuropathol 27:337, 1974.

78. Duncan ID, Griffiths IR, and Munz M: The pathology of a sensory neuropathy affecting long haired dachshund dogs. Acta Neuropathol 58:141, 1982.

79. Dungworth DL and Fowler ME: Cerebellar hypoplasia and degeneration in a foal. Cornell Vet 56:17, 1966.

80. Edmonds HL, Hegreberg GA, Van Gelder NM, et al: Spontaneous convulsions in beagle dogs. Fed Proc 39:2424, 1979.

81. Edmonds L, Crenshaw D, and Selby LA: Micrognathia and cerebellar hypoplasia in an Aberdeen Angus herd. J Hered 64:62, 1973.

82. Eikelenboom G and Minkema D: Prediction of pale soft and exudative muscle with a non-lethal test for the halothane-induced porcine malignant hyperthermia syndrome. Neth J Vet Sci 99:421, 1974.

83. Engel HN and Draper DD: Comparative prenatal development of the spinal cord in normal and dysraphic dogs: Embryonic stage. Am J Vet Res 43:1729, 1982.

84. Engel HN and Draper DD: Comparative prenatal development of the spinal cord in normal and dysraphic dogs: Fetal stage. Am J Vet Res 43:1735, 1982.

85. Falco MJ, Barker J, and Wallace ME: The genetics of epilepsy in the British Alsatian. J Small Anim Pract 15:685, 1974.

86. Fankhauser R: Hydrocephalus studien. Schweiz Arch Tierheilkd 101:407, 1959.

87. Fankhauser R, Luginbuhl H, and Hartley WJ: Leukodystrophie von Typus Krabbe beim Hund. Schweiz Arch Tierheilkd 105:198, 1965.

88. Fankhauser R, Luginbuhl H, and McGrath JT: Tumors of the nervous system. Bull WHO 50:53, 1974.

89. Farrow BRH and Malik R: Hereditary myotonia in the chow chow. J Small Anim Pract 22:451, 1981.

90. Fatzer R: Leukodystrophische Eskrankungen im Gehirn junger Katzen. Schweiz Arch Tierheilkd 117:641, 1975.

91. Fletcher TF, Kurtz HJ, and Low DG: Globoid cell leukodystrophy (Krabbe type) in the dog. JAVMA 149:165, 1966.

92. Fox JG, Averill DR, Hallett M, and Schunk K: Familial reflex myoclonus in Labrador retrievers. Am J Vet Res 45:2367, 1985.

93. Fraser H and Palmer AC: Equine incoordination and wobbler disease of young horses. Vet Rec 80:338, 1967.

94. Gamble DA and Chrisman CL: A leukoencephalomyelopathy of Rottweiler dogs. Vet Pathol 21:274, 1984.

95. Geary JC, Oliver JE Jr, and Hoerlein BF: Atlanto-

axial subluxation in the canine. J Small Anim Pract 8:577, 1967.

96. Gill JM and Hewland ML: Cerebellar degeneration in the border collie. NZ Vet J 8:170, 1980.

97. Gilmore JPW: Congenital hydrocephalus in domestic animals. Cornell Vet 46:487, 1956.

98. Greene CE, Vandevelde M, and Braund KG: Lissencephaly in two Lhasa apso dogs. JAVMA 169:405, 1978.

99. Greene CE, Vandevelde M, and Hoff EJ: Congenital cerebrospinal hypomyelinogenesis in a pup. JAVMA 171:534, 1977.

100. Greene HJ, Leipold HW, and Hibbs CM: Bovine congenital defects: Variations of internal hydrocephalus. Cornell Vet 64:596, 1974.

101. Greene HJ, Saperstein G, Schalles R, and Leipold HW: Internal hydrocephalus and retinal dysplasia in shorthorn cattle. Ir Vet 32:65, 1978.

102. Greene PD and Little PB: Neuronal ceroid-lipofuscin storage in Siamese cats. Can J Comp Med 38:207, 1974.

103. Griffiths IR and Duncan ID: Chronic degenerative radiculomyelopathy in the dog. J Small Anim Pract 16:461, 1975.

104. Griffiths IR and Duncan ID: The central nervous system in canine giant axonal neuropathy. Acta Neuropathol 46:169, 1979.

105. Griffiths IR, Duncan ID, and Barker J: A progressive axonopathy of boxer dogs affecting the central and peripheral nervous systems. J Small Anim Pract 21:29, 1980.

106. Griffiths IR, Duncan ID, McCulloch M, and Carmichael S: Further studies of the central nervous system in canine giant axonal neuropathy. Neuropathol Appl Neurobiol 6:421, 1980.

107. Griffiths IR, Duncan ID, McCulloch M, and Harvey MJA: Shaking pups: A disorder of central myelination in the spaniel dog. Part 1. Clinical, genetic, and light microscopical observations. J Neurol Sci 50:423, 1981.

108. Hansen HJ: A pathologic-anatomical study on disk degeneration in the dog. Acta Orthop Scand (Suppl) 11, 1952.

109. Harding JDJ, Done JT, Harbourne JF, and Gilbert FR: Congenital tremor type A III in pigs: An hereditary sex-linked cerebrospinal hypomyelinogenesis. Vet Rec 92:527, 1973.

110. Hargis AM, Haupt KH, Hegreberg GA, et al: Familial canine dermatomyositis. Am J Pathol 116:234, 1984.

111. Hartley WJ, Barker JSF, Wanner RA, and Farrow BRH: Inherited cerebellar degeneration in the rough coated collie. Aust Vet Pract June:1, 1978.

112. Hartley WJ and Blakemore WF: Neurovisceral glucocerebroside storage (Gaucher's disease) in a dog. Vet Pathol 10:191, 1973.

113. Hartley WJ, Canfield PJ, and Donnelly TM: A suspected new canine storage disease. Acta Neuropathol 56:225, 1982.

114. Hartley WJ and Palmer AC: Ataxia in Jack Russell terriers. Acta Neuropathol 26:71, 1973.

115. Haskins ME, Jezyk PF, Desnick RJ, et al: Mucopolysaccharidosis in a domestic short-haired cat—a disease distinct from that seen in the Siamese cat. JAVMA 175:384, 1979.

116. Hayes HM, Priester WA, and Pendergrass TW: Occurrence of nervous-tissue tumors in cattle, horses, cats and dogs. Int J Cancer 15:39, 1975.

117. Hayes HM, Wilson GP, Fenner WR, and Wyman M: Canine congenital deafness: Epidemiologic study of 272 cases. J Am Anim Hosp Assoc 17:473, 1981.

118. Hayes KC and Schiefer B: Primary tumors in the CNS of carnivores. Pathol Vet 6:94, 1969.

119. Healy PJ and Cole AE: Heterozygotes for mannosidosis in Angus and Murray grey cattle. Aust Vet J 52:385, 1976.

120. Healy PJ, Seaman JT, Gardner IA, and Sewell CA: β-Mannosidase deficiency in Anglo Nubian goats. Aust Vet J 57:504, 1981.

121. Hedhammar A, Wu FM, Krook L, et al: Overnutrition and skeletal diseases: An experimental study in growing Great Dane dogs. Cornell Vet (Suppl 5) 64:1, 1974.

122. Hegreberg GA and Padget GA: Inherited progressive epilepsy of the dog with comparisons to Lafora's disease of man. Fed Proc 35:1202, 1976.

123. Hegreberg GA, Thuline HC, and Francis BH: Morphologic changes in feline leukodystrophy. Fed Proc 30:341, 1971.

124. Higgins RJ, Rings DM, Fenner WR, and Stevenson S: Spontaneous lower motor neuron disease with neurofibrillary accumulation in young pigs. Acta Neuropathol 59:288, 1983.

125. Higgins RJ, Vandevelde M, Hoff EJ, et al: Neurofibrillary accumulation in the zebra (Equus burchelli). Acta Neuropathol 37:1, 1977.

126. Hoerlein BF: Canine Neurology, 3rd ed. Philadelphia, WB Saunders Co, 1978.

127. Holland JM, Davis WC, Prieur DJ, and Collins GH: Lafora's disease in the dog. Am J Pathol 58:509, 1970.

128. Holliday TA, Cunningham JG, and Gutnick MJ: Comparative clinical and electroencephalographic studies of canine epilepsy. Epilepsia 11:281, 1971.

129. Hudson WR and Ruben RJ: Hereditary deafness in the Dalmatian dog. Arch Otolaryngol 75:213, 1962.

130. Hulland TJ: Cerebellar ataxia in calves. Can J Comp Med 21:72, 1957.

131. Innes JRM, Rowlands WT, and Parry HB: An inherited form of cortical cerebellar atrophy in ("daft") lambs in Great Britain. Vet Rec 61:225, 1949.

132. Innes JRM and Saunders LA: Comparative Neuropathology. New York, Academic Press, 1962.

133. Izumo S, Ikuta F, Igata A, et al: Morphological study on the hereditary neurogenic amyotrophic dogs: Accumulation of lipid compound-like structures in the lower motor neuron. Acta Neuropathol (Berl) 61:270, 1983.

134. Jenkins WL, Van Dyk E, and McDonald CB: Myasthenia gravis in a fox terrier litter. J South Afr Vet Assoc 47:59, 1976.

135. Jennings A and Summer G: Cortical cerebellar disease in an Ayrshire. Vet Rec 63:60, 1951.

136. Johnson GR, Oliver JE Jr, and Selcer R: Globoid cell leukodystrophy in a beagle. JAVMA 167:380, 1975.

137. Johnson KH: Globoid leukodystrophy in the cat. JAVMA 157:2057, 1970.

138. Johnson RP, Watson ADJ, Smith J, and Cooper BJ: Myasthenia in springer spaniel littermates. J Small Anim Pract 16:641, 1975.

139. Jolly RD: Congenital brain oedema of Hereford calves. J Pathol 114:199, 1974.

140. Jolly RD, Janmaat A, West DM, and Morrison I: Ovine ceroid lipofuscinosis: A model of Batten's disease. Neuropathol Appl Neurobiol 6:195, 1980.

141. Jones BR, Anderson LJ, Barnes GRG, et al: Myotonia in related chow chow dogs. NZ Vet J 25:217, 1977.

142. Karbe E: Animal model of human disease: GM2-gangliosidosis (amaurotic idiocies) types I, II, and III. Animal model: Canine GM2-gangliosidosis. Am J Pathol 71:151, 1973.

143. Karbe E and Schiefer B: Familial amaurotic idiocy in male German shorthair pointers. Pathol Vet 4:223, 1967.

144. Kay WJ and Budelovich GN: Cerebellar hypoplasia and agenesis in the dog. J Neuropathol Exp Neurol 29:156, 1970.

145. Keith JR: Spastic paresis in beef and dairy cattle. Vet Med Small Anim Clin 76:1043, 1981.

146. Kelly DF and Gaskell CJ: Spongy degeneration of the central nervous system in kittens. Acta Neuropathol 35:151, 1976.

147. Kelly WR., Clague AE, Barns RJ, Bate MJ, MacKay BM: Canine α-L-fucosidosis: A storage disease of springer spaniels. Acta Neuropathol 60:9, 1983.

148. Knecht CD, Lamar CH, Schaible R, and Pflum K: Cerebellar hypoplasia in chow chows. J Am Anim Hosp Assoc 15:51, 1979.

149. Koppang N: Canine ceroid-lipofuscinosis in English setters. J Small Anim Pract 10:639, 1970.

150. Koppang N: Canine cereoid-lipofuscinosis. A model for human neuronal ceroid-lipofuscinosis and aging. Mech Ageing Dev 2:421, 1973/1974.

151. Kramer JW, Hegreberg GA, Bryan GM, et al: A muscle disorder of Labrador retrievers characterized by deficiency of type II muscle fibers. JAVMA 169:817, 1976.

152. Kramer JW, Hegreberg GA, and Hamilton MJ: Inheritance of a neuromuscular disorder of Labrador retriever dogs. JAVMA 179:380, 1981.

153. Ladds F, Guffy M, Blauch B, and Splitter G: Congenital odontoid process separation in two dogs. J Small Anim Pract 12:463, 1970.

154. Lange AL, Van Den Berg PB, and Baker MK: A suspected lysosomal storage disease in Abyssinian cats. Part II. Histopathological and ultrastructural aspects. J South Afr Vet Assoc 48:201, 1977.

155. Langweiler M, Haskins ME, and Jezyk PF: Mucopolysaccharidosis in a litter of cats. J Am Anim Hosp Assoc 14:748, 1978.

156. Leipold HW, Brandt GW, Guffy M, and Blauch B: Congenital atlanto-occipital fusion in a foal. Vet Med Small Anim Clin 69:1312, 1974.

157. Leipold HW, Cates WF, Radostits OM, and Howell WE: Spinal dysraphism, arthrogryposis and cleft palate in newborn Charolais calves. Can Vet J 10:268, 1969.

158. Leipold HW, Huston K, Blauch B, and Guffy MM: Congenital defects of the caudal vertebral column and spinal cord in Manx cats. JAVMA 164:520, 1974.

159. Littlewood JD, Herrtage ME, and Palmer AC: Neuronal storage disease in English springer spaniels. Vet Rec 112:86, 1983.

160. Lorenz MD, Cork LC, Griffin JW, et al: Hereditary muscular atrophy in Brittany spaniels: Clinical manifestations. JAVMA 175:833, 1979.

161. Lucke JN, Hall GM, and Lister D: Malignant hyperthermia in the pig and the role of stress. Ann NY Acad Sci 317:326, 1979.

162. Luginbuhl H: Studies on meningiomas in cats. Am J Vet Res 22:1030, 1961.

163. Luginbuhl H: A comparative study of neoplasms of the central nervous system in animals. Acta Neurochir (Suppl) 10:30, 1964.

164. Luginbuhl H, Fankhauser R, and McGrath JT: Spontaneous neoplasms of the nervous system in animals. Prog Neurol Surg 2:85, 1968.

165. Lurie MH: The membranous labyrinth in the congenitally deaf collie and Dalmatian dog. Laryngoscope 58:279, 1948.

166. Luttgen PJ, Braund KG, and Storts RW: Globoid cell leukodystrophy in a basset hound. J Small Anim Pract 24:153, 1983.

167. Manktelow CD and Hartley WJ: Generalized glycogen storage disease in sheep. J Comp Pathol 85:139, 1975.

168. Martin A: A congenital defect in the spinal cord of the Manx cat. Vet Pathol 8:232, 1971.

169. Mason RW, Hartley WJ, and Randall M: Spongiform degeneration of the white matter in a Samoyed pup. Aust Vet Pract 9:11, 1979.

170. Mason TA: Cervical vertebral instability (wobbler syndrome) in the Doberman. Aust Vet J 53:440, 1977.

171. Mayhew IG, Blakemore WF, Palmer AC, and Clarke CJ: Tremor syndrome and hypomyelination in Lurcher pups. J Small Anim Pract 25:551, 1984.

172. Mayhew IG, deLahunta A, Whitlock RH, et al: Spinal cord disease in the horse. Cornell Vet (Suppl 6) 68:1, 1978.

173. Mayhew IG, Watson AG, and Heissan JA: Congenital occipitoatlantoaxial malformation in the horse. Equine Vet J 10:103, 1978.

174. McGrath JT: Spinal dysraphism in the dog. Pathol Vet (Suppl) 2:1, 1965.

175. McGrath JT, Schutta H, Yaseen A, and Steinberg S: A morphologic and biochemical study of canine globoid cell leukodystrophy. J Neuropathol Exp Neurol 28:171, 1969.

176. McHowell J, Dorling PR, Cook RD, et al: Infantile and late onset form of generalised glycogenosis type II in cattle. J Pathol 134:266, 1981.

177. Meyers KM, Dickson WM, Lund JE, and Padgett GA: Muscular hypertonicity. Arch Neurol 25:61, 1971.

178. Meyers KM, Lund JE, Padgett G, and Dickerson WM: Hyperkinetic episodes in Scottish terrier dogs. JAVMA 155:129, 1969.

179. Meyers KM and Schaub RG: The relationship of serotonin to a motor disorder of Scottish terrier dogs. Life Sci 14:1895, 1974.

180. Miller LM, Lennon VA, Lambert EH, et al: Congenital myasthenia gravis in 13 smooth fox terriers. JAVMA 182:694, 1983.

181. Morgan JP: Congenital anomalies of the vertebral column of the dog: A study of the incidence and significance based on a radiographic and morphometric study. J Am Vet Radiol Soc 9:21, 1968.

182. Nisbet DI and Renwick CC: Congenital myopathy in lambs. J Comp Pathol 71:177, 1961.

183. Neufeld JL and Little PB: Spinal dysraphism in a Dalmatian dog. Can Vet J 15:335, 1974.

184. Nimmo Wilkie JS and Hudson EB: Neuronal and generalized ceroid-lipofuscinosis in a cocker spaniel. Vet Pathol 19:623, 1982.

185. Oliver JE Jr and Geary JC: Cerebellar anomalies—two cases. Vet Med Small Anim Clin 60:697, 1965.

186. Oliver JE Jr and Lewis RE: Lesions of the atlas and axis in dogs. J Am Anim Hosp Assoc 9:304, 1973.

187. Oliver JE Jr and Lorenz MD: Handbook of Veterinary Neurologic Diagnosis. Philadelphia, WB Saunders Co, 1983.

188. Oliver JE Jr, Selcer RR, and Simpson S: Cauda equina compression from lumbosacral malarticulation and malformation in the dog. JAVMA 173:207, 1978.

189. Osborne CA, Clifford DH, and Jessen C: Hereditary esophageal achalasia in dogs. JAVMA 151:572, 1967.

190. O'Sullivan BM, Healy PJ, Fraser IR, et al: Generalised glycogenosis in Brahman cattle. Aust Vet J 57:227, 1981.

191. Palmer, AC: Deformation of cervical vertebrae in basset hounds. Vet Rec 80:430, 1967.

192. Palmer AC, Blakemore WF, Barlow RM, et al: Progressive ataxia of Charolais cattle associated with a myelin disorder. Vet Rec 91:592, 1972.

193. Palmer AC, Blakemore WF, Cook WR, et al: Cerebellar hypoplasia and degeneration in the young Arab horse. Clinical and neuropathological features. Vet Rec 93:62, 1973.

194. Palmer AC and Goodyear JV: Congenital myasthenia in the Jack Russell terrier. Vet Rec 103:433, 1978.

195. Palmer AC, Payne JE, and Wallace ME: Hereditary quadriplegia and amblyopia in the Irish setter. J Small Anim Pract 14:343, 1973.

196. Parker AJ and Byerly CS: Meningomyelocele in a dog. Vet Pathol 10:266, 1973.

197. Parker AJ and Park RD: Occipital dysplasia in the dog. J Am Anim Hosp Assoc 10:520, 1974.

198. Parker AJ, Park RD, Cusick PK, and Jeffers CB: Cervical vertebral instability in the dog. JAVMA 163:71, 1983.

199. Patel V, Koppang N, Patel B, and Zeman W: p-Phenylene diamine-mediated peroxidase deficiency in English setters with neuronal ceroid-lipofuscinosis. Lab Invest 30:366, 1974.

200. Patterson DSP, Sweasey D, Brush PJ, and Harding JDJ: Neurochemistry of the spinal cord in British saddleback piglets affected with congenital tremor type A-IV, a second form of hereditary cerebrospinal hypomyelinogenesis. J Neurochem 21:397, 1973.

201. Percy DH and Jortner BS: Feline lipidosis. Arch Pathol 92:136, 1971.

202. Pierce KR, Kosanke SD, Bay WW, and Bridges CH: Animal model of human disease: GM2 gangliosidosis. Animal model: Porcine cerebrospinal lipodystrophy (GM2 gangliosidosis). Am J Pathol 83:419, 1976.

203. Pritchard DH, Napthine DV, and Sinclair AJ: Globoid cell leukodystrophy in polled Dorset sheep. Vet Pathol 17:399, 1980.

204. Rac R and Giesecke PR: Lysosomal storage disease in Chihuahuas. Aust Vet J 51:403, 1975.

205. Read DH, Harrington DD, Keenan TW, and Hinsman EJ: Neuronal-visceral GM$_1$ gangliosidosis in a dog with β-galactosidase deficiency. Science 194:442, 1976.

206. Read WK and Bridges CH: Cerebrospinal lipodystrophy in swine. Pathol Vet 5:67, 1968.

207. Read WK and Bridges CH: Neuronal lipodystrophy—occurrence in an inbred strain of cattle. Pathol Vet 6:235, 1969.

208. Reinke JD and Suter PF: Laryngeal paralysis in a dog. JAVMA 172:714, 1978.

209. Richards RB, Edwards JR, Cook RD, and White RR: Bovine generalized glycogenosis. Neuropathol Appl Neurobiol 3:45, 1977.

210. Richards RB and Kakulas BA: Spongiform leukencephalopathy associated with congenital myoclonia syndrome in the dog. J Comp Pathol 88:317, 1978.

211. Rousseaux CG, Klavanon GG, Johnson ES, et al: A newly recognized neurodegenerative disorder of horned Hereford calves. Can Vet J 24:296, 1983.

212. Sahar A, Hochwald GM, Kay WJ, and Ransohoff J: Spontaneous canine hydrocephalus: Cerebrospinal fluid dynamics. J Neurol Neurosurg Psychiatr 34:308, 1971.

213. Sandefeldt E, Cummings JF, deLahunta A, et al: Hereditary neuronal abiotrophy in the Swedish Lapland dog. Cornell Vet 63 (Suppl 3):1, 1973.

214. Sandefeldt E, Cummings JF, deLahunta A, et al: Hereditary neuronal abiotrophy in Swedish Lapland dogs. Am J Pathol 82:649, 1976.

215. Sandstrom B, Westman J, and Ockerman PA: Glycogenosis of the central nervous system in the cat. Acta Neuropathol 14:194, 1969.

216. Saunders LZ, Sweet JD, Martin SM, et al: Hereditary congenital ataxia in Jersey calves. Cornell Vet 42:559, 1952.

217. Selby L, Hayes H, and Becker S: Epizootiologic features of canine hydrocephalus. Am J Vet Res 40:411, 1979.

218. Selcer R and Oliver J: Cervical spondylopathy—wobbler syndrome in dogs. J Am Anim Hosp Assoc 11:175, 1975.

219. Silson M and Robinson R: Hereditary hydrocephalus in the cat. Vet Rec 84:477, 1969.

220. Slatter D: Fundamentals of Veterinary Ophthalmology. Philadelphia, WB Saunders Co, 1981.

221. Snyder S, Kingston R, and Wenger D: Animal model of human disease: Niemann-Pick disease. Sphingomyelinosis of Siamese cats. Am J Pathol 108:252, 1982.

222. Steinberg S: Clinico-pathologic conference. JAVMA 143:404, 1963.

223. Steinberg S and Bothelo S: Myotonia in a horse. Science 137:979, 1962.

224. Stockard C: An hereditary lethal factor for localized motor and preganglionic neurons. Am J Anat 59:1, 1936.

225. Strombeck DR: Small Animal Gastroenterology. Davis, CA, Stonegate Publishing, 1979.

226. Stuart LD and Leipold HW: Lesions in bovine progressive degenerative myeloencephalopathy ("Weaver") of Brown Swiss cattle. Vet Pathol 22:13, 1985.

227. Suzuki Y, Austin J, Armstrong D, et al: Studies in globoid leukodystrophy: Enzymatic and lipid findings in the canine form. Exp Neurol 29:65, 1970.

228. Sybesma W and Eikelenboom G: Malignant hyperthermia in pigs. Neth J Vet Sci 2:155, 1969.

229. Tarvin G and Prata R: Lumbosacral stenosis in dogs. JAVMA 177:154, 1980.

230. Tomchick T: Familial Lafora's disease in the beagle dog. Fed Proc 32:8, 1973.

231. Tontitila P and Lindberg LA: ETT fall av cerebellar ataxi hos finsk stovare. Svoman Elainlaakarilehti 77:135, 1971.

232. Van Den Berg P, Baker M, and Lange A: A suspected lysosomal storage disease in Abyssinian cats. Part I: Genetic, clinical and clinical pathological aspects. J South Afr Vet Assoc 48:195, 1977.

233. Van Der Velden A: Fits in Tervuren shepherd dogs: A presumed hereditary trait. J Small Anim Pract 9:63, 1968.

234. Vandevelde M, Braund KG, Walker T, and Kornegay J: Dysmyelinaton of the central nervous system in the chow-chow dog. Acta Neuropathol 42:211, 1978.

235. Vandevelde M, Fankhauser R, Bichsel P, et al: Hereditary neurovisceral mannosidosis associated with α-mannosidase deficiency in a family of Persian cats. Acta Neuropathol 58:64, 1982.

236. Vandevelde M and Fatzer R: Neuronal ceroid-lipofuscinosis in older dachshunds. Vet Pathol 17:686, 1980.

237. Vandevelde M, Greene C, and Hoff E: Lower motor neuron disease with accumulation of neurofilaments in a cat. Vet Pathol 13:428, 1976.

238. Van De Water N, Jolly R, and Farrow B: Canine Gaucher disease—the enzymatic defect. Aust J Exp Biol Med Sci 57:551, 1979.

239. Venker-van Haagen AJ, Bouw J, and Hartman W: Hereditary transmission of laryngeal paralysis in young Bouviers. J Am Anim Hosp Assoc 17:75, 1981.

240. Venker-van Haagen AJ, Hartman W, and Goedoge-buure SA: Spontaneous laryngeal paralysis in young Bouviers. J Am Anim Hosp Assoc 14:714, 1978.

241. Walkley SU, Blakemore WF, and Purpura DP: Alterations in neuron morphology in feline mannosidosis. Acta Neuropathol 53:75, 1981.

242. Wallace ME: Keeshounds: A genetic study of epilepsy and EEG readings. J Small Anim Pract 16:1, 1975.

243. Walvoort HC, VanNes JJ, Stokhof AA, and Wolve-kamp WTC: Canine glycogen storage disease type II: A clinical study of four affected Lapland dogs. J Am Anim Hosp Assoc 20:279, 1984.

244. Wenger DA, Sattler M, Kudoh T, et al: Niemann-Pick disease: A genetic model in Siamese cats. Science 208:1472, 1980.

245. Wentink GH, Hartman W, and Koeman JP: Three cases of myotonia in a family of chows. Tijdschr Diergeneeskd 14:729, 1974.

246. Wentink GH, Van Der Linde-Sipman JS, Meijer, AEF, et al: Myopathy with a possible recessive X-linked inheritance in a litter of Irish terriers. Vet Pathol 9:328, 1972.

247. White ME, Pennock PW, and Seiler RJ: Atlanto-axial subluxation in five young cattle. Can Vet J 19:79, 1978.

248. White ME, Whitlock RH, and deLahunta A: A cerebellar abiotrophy of calves. Cornell Vet 65:476, 1979.

249. Wilson JW, Kurtz HJ, Leipold HW, and Lees GE: Spina bifida in the dog. Vet Pathol 16:165, 1979.

250. Wolff D: Three generations of deaf white cats. J Hered 33:39, 1942.

251. Woodard JC, Collins GH, and Hessler JR: Feline hereditary neuroaxonal dystrophy. Am J Pathol 74:551, 1974.

252. Woods CB: Hyperkinetic episodes in two Dalmatians. J Am Anim Hosp Assoc 13:255, 1977.

253. Wright F, Rest JR, and Palmer AC: Ataxia of the Great Dane caused by stenosis of the cervical vertebral canal: Comparison with similar conditions in the basset hound, Doberman pinscher, and the thoroughbred horse. Vet Rec 92:1, 1973.

254. Yakely WL, Wyman M, Donovan EF, and Fechheimer NS: Genetic transmission of an ocular fundus anomaly in collies. JAVMA 152:457, 1968.

255. Young, S: Hypomyelinogenesis congenita (cerebellar ataxia) in Angus-shorthorn calves. Cornell Vet 52:84, 1962.

256. Zake FA: Lissencephaly in Lhasa apso dogs. JAVMA 169:1165, 1976.

257. Zaki FA and Kay WJ: Globoid cell leukodystrophy in a miniature poodle. JAVMA 163:248, 1973.

258. Zook B, Sostaric BR, Draper DJ, and Graf-Webster E: Encephalocele and other congenital craniofacial anomalies in Burmese cats. Vet Med Small Anim Clin 78:695, 1983.

Index